48

Pediatric Disease

(Fifth Series)

Test and Syllabus

John R. Sty, M.D.
Section Chair

Lane F. Donnelly, M.D.

Donald P. Frush, M.D.

Marta Hernanz-Schulman, M.D.

Marilyn J. Siegel, M.D.

Library of Congress Data

Pediatric Disease (fifth series) test and syllabus / John R. Sty, section chair; Lane F. Donnelly, Donald P. Frush, Marta Hernanz-Schulman, Marilyn J. Siegel [co-authors].

p. cm. — (Professional self-evaluation program; set 48)

"Committee on Professional Self-Evaluation, Commission on Education"—Cover.

Includes bibliographical references and index.

ISBN 1-55903-048-8 — ISBN 1-55903-000-3 (series)

Library of Congress Control Number: 2001092173

Note: While the American College of Radiology and the editors of the publication have attempted to include the most current and accurate information possible, errors may inadvertently appear. Diagnostic and interventional decisions should be based on the individual circumstances of each case.

Volume 48

Pediatric Disease

(Fifth Series)

Test and Syllabus

CONTRIBUTORS

Section Chair

John R. Sty, M.D.
Chief of Radiology, Children's Hospital of Wisconsin; Clinical Professor of Radiology, Medical College of Wisconsin, Milwaukee, Wisconsin and University of Wisconsin, Madison, Wisconsin

Co-Authors

Lane F. Donnelly, M.D.
Associate Director, Department of Radiology, Children's Hospital Medical Center; Associate Professor of Radiology and Pediatrics, University of Cincinnati College of Medicine, Cincinnati, Ohio

Donald P. Frush, M.D.
Associate Professor of Radiology, Chief, Division of Pediatric Radiology, Department of Radiology, Duke University Medical Center, Durham, North Carolina

Marta Hernanz-Schulman, M.D.
Professor of Radiology and Radiological Sciences, Professor of Pediatrics, Vanderbilt University Medical Center, Nashville, Tennessee

Marilyn J. Siegel, M.D.
Professor of Radiology and Pediatrics, Mallinckrodt Institute of Radiology, Washington University School of Medicine, St. Louis, Missouri

EDITORS

Editor in Chief

Barry A. Siegel, M.D.
Professor of Radiology and Medicine and Director, Division of Nuclear Medicine, Mallinckrodt Institute of Radiology, Washington University School of Medicine, St. Louis, Missouri

Associate Editor

Marilyn J. Siegel, M.D.
Professor of Radiology and Pediatrics, Mallinckrodt Institute of Radiology, Washington University School of Medicine, St. Louis, Missouri

American College of Radiology

Professional Self-Evaluation Program
Commission on Education
American College of Radiology

Professional Self-Evaluation Committee

ACR Publishing Coordinator: Cary Boshamer
Administrative Assistant: Beth Meehan
Copy Editor: Paula R. Ellison
Graphic & Design Support: Keith Stanger and Paul Wiegmann
Index: EEI Communications, Alexandria, Va.
Image Scanning: EU Services, Rockville, Md.
Printing: John D. Lucas Printing, Baltimore, Md.

ADDITIONAL CONTRIBUTORS

Michele H. Johnson, M.D.
Associate Professor and Director, Interventional Neuroradiology, Department of Diagnostic Imaging, Yale University School of Medicine, New Haven, Connecticut

Lisa H. Lowe, M.D.
Pediatric Radiologist, Department of Radiology, Children's Mercy Hospital; Associate Professor, University of Missouri-Kansas City, Kansas City, Missouri

Richard B. Towbin, M.D.
Professor and Chairman, Van Alen Chair in Pediatric Radiology, Children's Hospital of Philadelphia, University of Pennsylvania School of Medicine, Philadelphia, Pennsylvania

Section Chair's Preface

Following the seminal 1974 publication of the first pediatric disease syllabus for the Professional Self-Evaluation (PSE) Program of the American College of Radiology (ACR), it has become widely accepted that a combination of a thorough clinical history and high-quality imaging enables the pediatric radiologist and clinician to diagnose or significantly narrow the differential diagnosis of pediatric disease. Both are mandatory for good outcomes. Further advances in diagnostic imaging technology have taken place since the publication of the last volume in this series, the *Pediatric Disease (Fourth Series) Test and Syllabus*, resulting in modifications in the imaging evaluation of a variety of pediatric problems. Despite the value of standard radiography, it is clear that this modality has limitations. Partly because of the recognition of these limitations and partly because of the development of new technology, pediatric radiology underwent a marked transformation in the 1990s, particularly because of the availability and increased diagnostic accuracy of high-resolution CT and spiral CT. The former enables the practitioner to make a better assessment of the morbid anatomy and full extent of disease. MRI has proved to be an important modality in the assessment of the central nervous system, musculoskeletal system, and vascular abnormalities. The contents of this publication reflect the contributions of changing technology in the diagnosis of pediatric disorders. Although the newer innovations are emphasized, the important roles of standard radiography, nuclear medicine, and sonography are included. Rather than present a syllabus based on state-of-the-art information, we decided to present subject matter from the broad base of pediatric conditions, emphasizing the full roles of standard and advanced imaging technologies. This syllabus includes relevant clinical and diagnostic information necessary to understand the etiology, pathogenesis, and diagnosis of the selected pediatric diseases discussed. This work is intended for radiologists in training as well as those in current practice who are seeking a relatively concise view of the imaging assessment of pediatric disease. When appropriate, differential diagnosis is emphasized.

The individuals who assisted me in this task were chosen because of their unbiased, but special interest, in pediatric radiology. The members of this committee, as well as several additional contributors, have worked diligently and spent a great deal of time in the preparation of this syllabus. All are accomplished pediatric radiologists who derive a wealth of information from their daily practices. I wish to thank Drs. Lane F. Donnelly, Donald P. Frush, Marta Hernanz-Schulman, Michele H. Johnson, Lisa H. Lowe, Marilyn J. Siegel, and Richard Towbin for their efforts. Preparation of a syllabus for the College's self-evaluation program is very time-consuming. I thank these individuals for responding to the suggested revisions in their manuscripts. I especially wish to acknowledge Dr. Barry A. Siegel for his literary, scientific, and efficient oversight. He was able to ensure order and concise presentations throughout the text. Finally, I wish to thank the dedicated ACR staff for their patience in the completion of this publication.

John R. Sty, M.D.
Section Chair

Editor's Preface

On behalf of the editors of the American College of Radiology (ACR) Professional Self-Evaluation (PSE) Program, I am proud to introduce this *Pediatric Disease (Fifth Series) Test and Syllabus* to our readers. This volume is the 48th in the series of PSE educational packages published by the College during its sponsorship of this program over the last 30 years. This book, like its predecessors in this series, is intended to challenge program participants with a collection of diagnostic exercises for self-assessment and to provide current information about selected important topics in pediatric radiology. Given the wide scope of pediatric radiology, this volume is not a comprehensive textbook on this subject, and it is not intended to substitute for a textbook; rather, the material selected for inclusion represents topics the authors believe to be of current importance on the basis of their extensive experience and their educational encounters with practicing radiologists and radiologists in training. Selection of material for inclusion also was based on a careful evaluation of new developments since publication of the last pediatric disease syllabus in 1993. Much of the book's content addresses the impact of cross-sectional imaging on pediatric radiology practice. The test illustrations for three-fourths of the case discussions in this book include CT scans, MR images, or sonograms.

The educational goals and format of instruction for the *Pediatric Disease (Fifth Series) Test and Syllabus* are essentially unchanged by comparison with earlier volumes in the PSE series. In each case discussion (chapter), the primary test question is based generally on the findings in one or more images obtained in an infant or child presenting to a radiology department for diagnostic evaluation. The authors and editors strived to design these exercises to simulate, as realistically as possible, the clinical problems radiologists encounter in daily practice. The syllabus discussions of the primary questions are intended to illustrate how experts evaluate the imaging findings and the accompanying clinical information to arrive at a logical differential diagnosis. The satellite questions accompanying each case are designed to test the readers' knowledge about both the clinical and the radiological features of the various disorders introduced by the primary question, as well as about the general principles underlying the imaging approaches for evaluating these disorders. The syllabus discussion of each satellite question is a brief topical review, emphasizing recent developments. The test questions are intentionally of varying levels of difficulty, because this program is intended to provide material of interest to individuals ranging from radiologists in training to practicing subspecialists. The editors and authors believe that program participants who are willing to work through the test will find useful information in the syllabus.

The conception and production of a self-evaluation test and syllabus are part of a now well-established, but arduous, process that involves many individuals with different skills. The goal of this process is the development of a final product of high quality with maximum educational value. The Section Chair and the committee members choose the cases, write and critique the questions, and prepare the syllabus discussions for each case; the efforts of these individuals represent the most important intellectual ingredient needed to accomplish the task. As Section Chair for this volume, John R. Sty, M.D., has performed a substantial service for the ACR and its members by conceiving the overall plan for this syllabus and by guiding the work of the authors during each step of the process. Jack was joined in this work by an outstanding group of experienced pediatric radiologists—Lane F. Donnelly, M.D., Donald P. Frush, M.D., Marta Hernanz-Schulman, M.D., and Marilyn J. Siegel, M.D. Several additional case discussions were contributed by Michele H. Johnson, M.D., and Richard B. Towbin, M.D. Our gratitude is due to all of these physicians for their significant voluntary efforts on behalf of the College and its members.

In addition to her contributions as an author, Dr. Marilyn J. Siegel also served as an Associate Editor for this volume and thus participated in the rigorous peer review that all PSE syllabi routinely undergo. We also thank Dr. Reed Dunnick, chairman of the College's Committee on Professional Self-Evaluation, who provides the overall guidance of the PSE program. The strong support for this program of the College's Commission on Education and its Board of Chancellors is also key to the program's success. Several members of the American College of Radiology staff have worked on the creation of this volume. Thanks for his dedicated efforts are owed most notably to Cary Boshamer, ACR Publishing Coordinator.

The editors and authors recognize the long-standing and unwavering support of the many radiologists who participate in the PSE program; it is ultimately this support that has made the program successful. It is indeed our great privilege to participate in the continuing education of the membership. We trust that our readers will find the *Pediatric Disease (Fifth Series) Test and Syllabus* worthy of their continuing support.

I conclude this Preface with a personal note. With the completion of this volume, I end my tenure as Editor in Chief of the PSE program. PSE has been an important part of nearly my entire professional life. My involvement began (as a resident) in 1971, when I was asked to serve as a committee member and author for the first nuclear radiology syllabus. I subsequently was the Section Chair for the second nuclear radiology volume and have contributed as an author to the third, fourth, and fifth books in the nuclear radiology series. In 1986, I became an Associate Editor of the program, and I assumed the role of Editor in Chief in 1988. I have thus had the privilege of contributing as author, editor, or both to 29 of the 48 volumes published by the College. This participation has involved a lot of work; it seemed as if one or more case discussions awaiting review were permanent features of my "in-box." It also was great fun and gave me substantial reward. I have had a continuing opportunity to maintain my personal education in diagnostic radiology by immersion in the process of PSE syllabus creation and thus have had the "stars" of academic radiology as my "personal trainers" for all these years. I thank all of these radiologists for their willingness to teach (me and the membership). I also thank the members of the ACR leadership who entrusted me with this responsibility and afforded me this unique privilege, as well as the many ACR staff members, who did all the really hard stuff and made my job easy by comparison. This list of colleagues is too extensive to name and thank individually (and the chances I might forget someone important and thus offend too great), so please accept this collective statement of my gratitude. However, I am compelled to mention the special support given to me by two individuals. The late Elias G. Theros, M.D., who "invented" the PSE program and served as Editor in Chief before me, was most directly responsible for teaching me how to do this job. Marilyn J. Siegel, M.D., my spouse, not only cheerfully tolerated the hours of attention I stole from her to work on PSE, but also joined in the work, making my involvement all the more rewarding.

The PSE program will, of course, go on. I am pleased to announce that Dr. Harris Cohen will succeed me as Editor in Chief and that the sixth gastrointestinal disease syllabus will be the next installment. I wish Harris great success and hope that he will find as much enjoyment from this task as have I.

Barry A. Siegel, M.D.
Editor in Chief

Pediatric Disease

(Fifth Series)

Test

NOTE: For you to derive the maximum benefit from this program, you should complete the following test and send your answer sheet to the ACR for scoring before you proceed to the syllabus. If for any reason you refer to the syllabus material or any other references in answering the questions, please be sure to so indicate when answering Question 121, the first demographic question. Your score will then be used in developing the norm tables.

CME Information

Program Objective

After completing this program, the diagnostic radiologist should be able to successfully answer the questions that comprise the program's evaluation component. The intent of the course is to provide the reader with recent scientific information relating to the diagnosis and treatment of pediatric disease, including the presentation of issues relating to the effective use of various imaging methods. This course should also provide the reader with a review of the current state of scientific options relating to specific disease entities.

CME Credit Award: 20 Credit Hours

The American College of Radiology (ACR) is accredited by the Accreditation Council for Continuing Medical Education (ACCME) to sponsor continuing medical education for physicians.

The ACR designates this educational activity for a maximum of 20 hours in Category 1 credit towards the AMA's Physician's Recognition Award. Each physician should claim only those hours of credit that he or she actually spent in the educational activity.

The Pediatric Disease V Test and Syllabus program has been approved for ACR and AMA/PRA Category 1 CME credit for the period from August 2002 through August 2005.*

CME Credit Award Process

To receive the Category 1 credit, participants must complete the accompanying answer sheet and return it to the ACR.

Within 40 days of receipt of the answer sheet, the ACR will provide you with a credit award letter. The letter will indicate your score, the date it was recorded, and a credit award statement.

This CME activity was planned and produced in accordance with the ACCME Essentials. The estimated study time is 20 hours. Category 1 CME credit for this program is not transferable. Only the purchaser may apply for and receive Category 1 credit.

---

* If you receive these materials after August 2005, please consult the enclosed "Information Sheet" for the current designation period. At the conclusion of each period, the program is extensively reviewed by the ACR Committee on Accreditation for Continuing Medical Education to ensure the validity and timeliness of the content.

Case 1: Questions 1 through 4

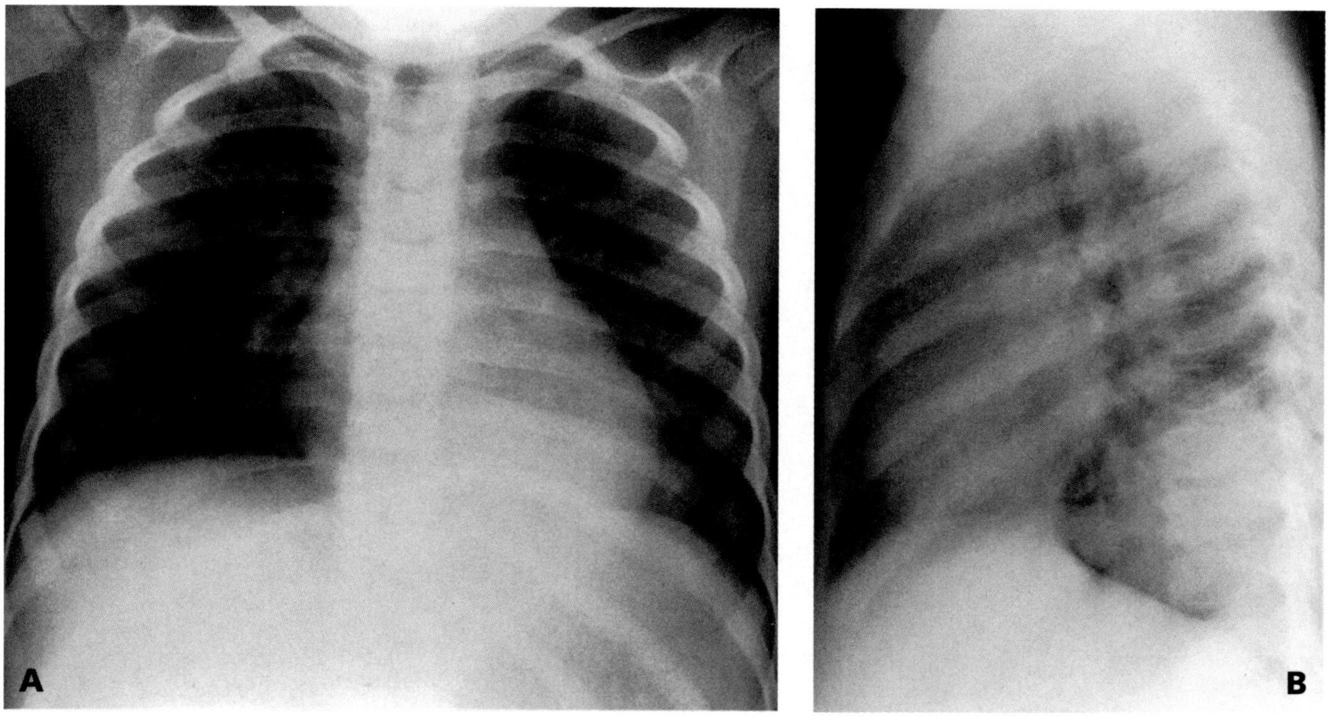

Figure 1-1

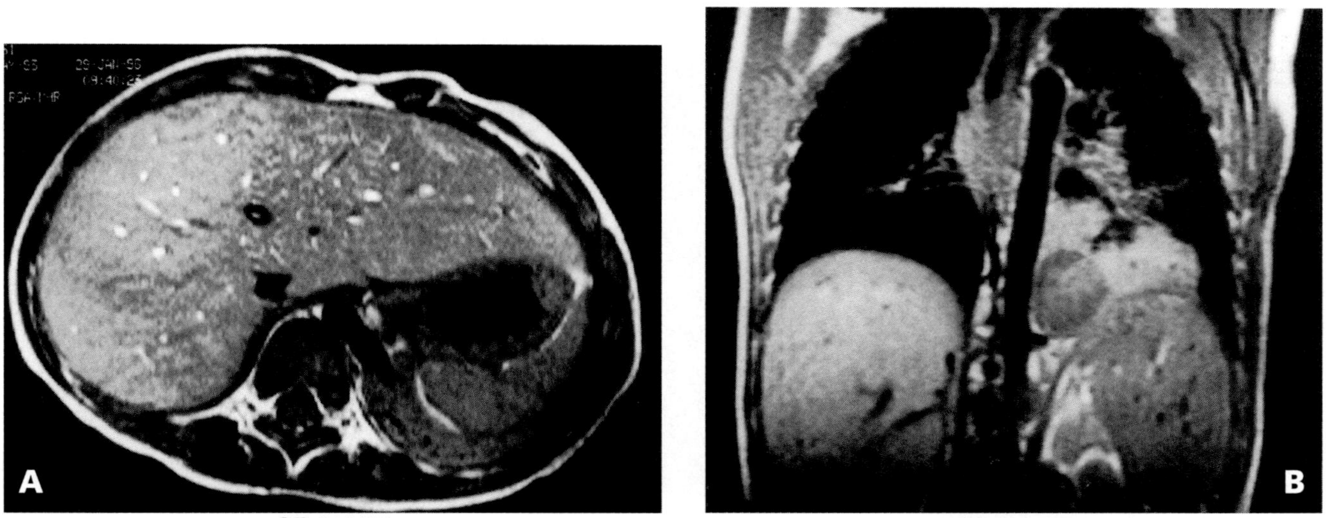

SE 641/15 SE 641/15

Figure 1-2

This 7-year-old girl has been treated for pneumonia for 3 weeks and has not responded to antibiotic therapy. You are shown frontal (A) and lateral (B) chest radiographs (Figure 1-1) and axial (A) and coronal (B) T1-weighted MR images (Figure 1-2).

1. Which *one* of the following is the MOST likely diagnosis?

   (A) Lung abscess
   (B) Pulmonary blastoma
   (C) Infected pulmonary cyst
   (D) Bronchopulmonary sequestration
   (E) Neuroblastoma

QUESTIONS 2 THROUGH 4: MARK YOUR ANSWER SHEET TRUE (T) OR FALSE (F) FOR EACH OF THE RESPONSE CHOICES

2. Concerning lung abscess,

(A) in a neonate, it usually is associated with sepsis
(B) an underlying congenital anomaly is usually present
(C) the diagnosis should be suspected in a patient with pneumonia unresponsive to antibiotic treatment
(D) an air-fluid level is present on CT in virtually all patients
(E) surgical treatment is usually necessary

3. Concerning imaging of bronchopulmonary sequestration,

(A) the feeding vessel usually arises from the subdiaphragmatic aorta
(B) identification of systemic arterial supply is pathognomonic for sequestration
(C) angiographic evaluation is usually necessary to delineate the feeding vessel
(D) sonography is a reliable diagnostic technique in neonates
(E) on CT, the feeding vessel enhances at the same time as the aorta

4. Concerning thoracic neuroblastoma,

(A) it accounts for about 10% to 15% of all neuroblastomas
(B) it is the most common cause of Horner's syndrome in infancy
(C) opsoclonus-myoclonus at presentation is associated with a poor prognosis
(D) it is less often calcified than abdominal neuroblastoma
(E) the prognosis is better than that of abdominal neuroblastoma

Case 2: Questions 5 through 9

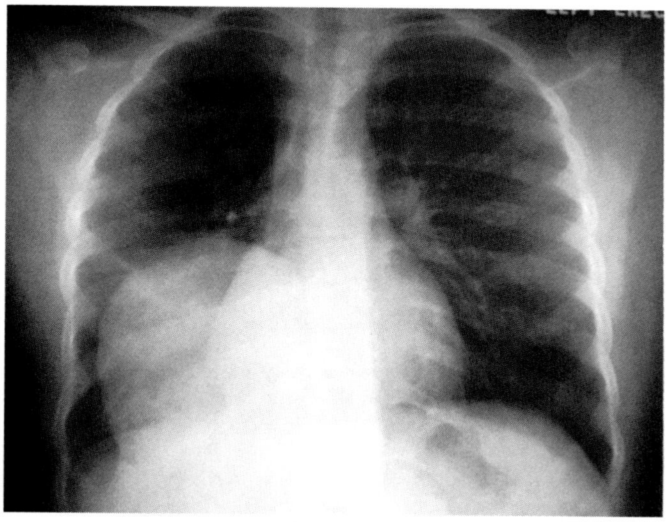

Figure 2-1

This 8-year-old girl has right-sided chest pain. You are shown a posteroanterior chest radiograph (Figure 2-1).

5. Which *one* of the following is the MOST likely diagnosis?

   (A) Thymolipoma
   (B) Pericardial cyst
   (C) Bronchogenic cyst
   (D) Askin tumor
   (E) Ganglioneuroma

6. Which *one* of the following is the MOST appropriate next study for the evaluation of the test patient?

   (A) MRI
   (B) CT
   (C) Biopsy
   (D) Bone scintigraphy
   (E) Barium esophagram

QUESTIONS 7 THROUGH 9: MARK YOUR ANSWER SHEET TRUE (T) OR FALSE (F) FOR EACH OF THE RESPONSE CHOICES

7. Concerning posterior mediastinal masses in children,

   (A) at least 85% are neurogenic in origin
   (B) most patients present with neurologic symptoms
   (C) percutaneous biopsy is the preferred method of histologic diagnosis
   (D) nerve cell tumors are more common than in adults
   (E) they are less common than middle mediastinal masses

8. Concerning thymolipomas,

   (A) they account for approximately 10% of mediastinal masses
   (B) most patients are asymptomatic
   (C) they are often associated with myasthenia gravis
   (D) large ones simulate pericardial masses
   (E) they are typically of homogeneous attenuation on CT

9. Concerning ganglioneuroma in children,

   (A) it arises from the sympathetic chain
   (B) it occurs most often in children younger than 5 years
   (C) it is associated with neurofibromatosis type 1
   (D) it usually contains calcifications visible by CT
   (E) it usually is limited to a single vertebral segment

Case 3: Questions 10 through 16

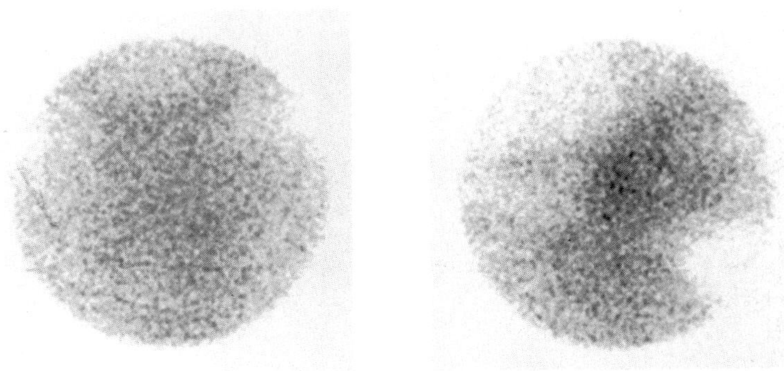

Figure 3-1

This 2-day-old girl has neonatal hypothyroidism diagnosed on the basis of a screening thyroxine measurement. A fetal sonogram had shown multiple ovarian cysts. You are shown anterior and right lateral Tc-99m pertechnetate thyroid scintigrams (Figure 3-1).

10. Which *one* of the following is the BEST explanation for the scintigraphic and clinical findings?

    (A) Peroxidase deficiency
    (B) Thyroid aplasia
    (C) Lingual thyroid
    (D) Turner's syndrome
    (E) Treatment of maternal hyperthyroidism

QUESTION 11: MARK YOUR ANSWER SHEET TRUE (T) OR FALSE (F) FOR EACH OF THE RESPONSE CHOICES

11. Concerning neonatal hypothyroidism,

    (A) it is due to thyroid dysgenesis in approximately 80% of patients
    (B) it is clinically evident at birth in most patients
    (C) elevated serum thyroglobulin levels are typical in infants with aplasia
    (D) dyshormonogenesis is most often inherited as an autosomal recessive trait
    (E) deafness is associated with thyroid dysgenesis

For each of the numbered thyroid abnormalities listed below (Questions 12 through 15), select the *one* lettered pattern of Tc-99m pertechnetate scintigraphic findings and laboratory data (A, B, C, D, or E) that is MOST closely associated with it. Each lettered pattern may be used once, more than once, or not at all.

12. Aplasia
13. Chronic lymphocytic thyroiditis
14. Dyshormonogenesis syndrome
15. Graves' disease

	Scintigraphy	*Serum thyroxine*	*Serum thyrotropin*
(A)	Nonvisualization of the thyroid	Increased	Decreased
(B)	Nonvisualization of the thyroid	Decreased	Increased
(C)	Normal	Normal	Normal
(D)	Enlarged thyroid	Increased	Decreased
(E)	Enlarged thyroid	Decreased	Increased

QUESTION 16: MARK YOUR ANSWER SHEET TRUE (T) OR FALSE (F) FOR EACH OF THE RESPONSE CHOICES

16. Concerning neonatal Graves' disease,

    (A) it results from transplacental transfer of maternal thyroid-stimulating immunoglobulins
    (B) it is associated with premature suture closure
    (C) it is associated with mental retardation
    (D) Tc-99m pertechnetate thyroid images appear similar to those of infants with peroxidase deficiency
    (E) it occurs in 50% of infants of mothers with Graves' disease

Case 4: Questions 17 through 25

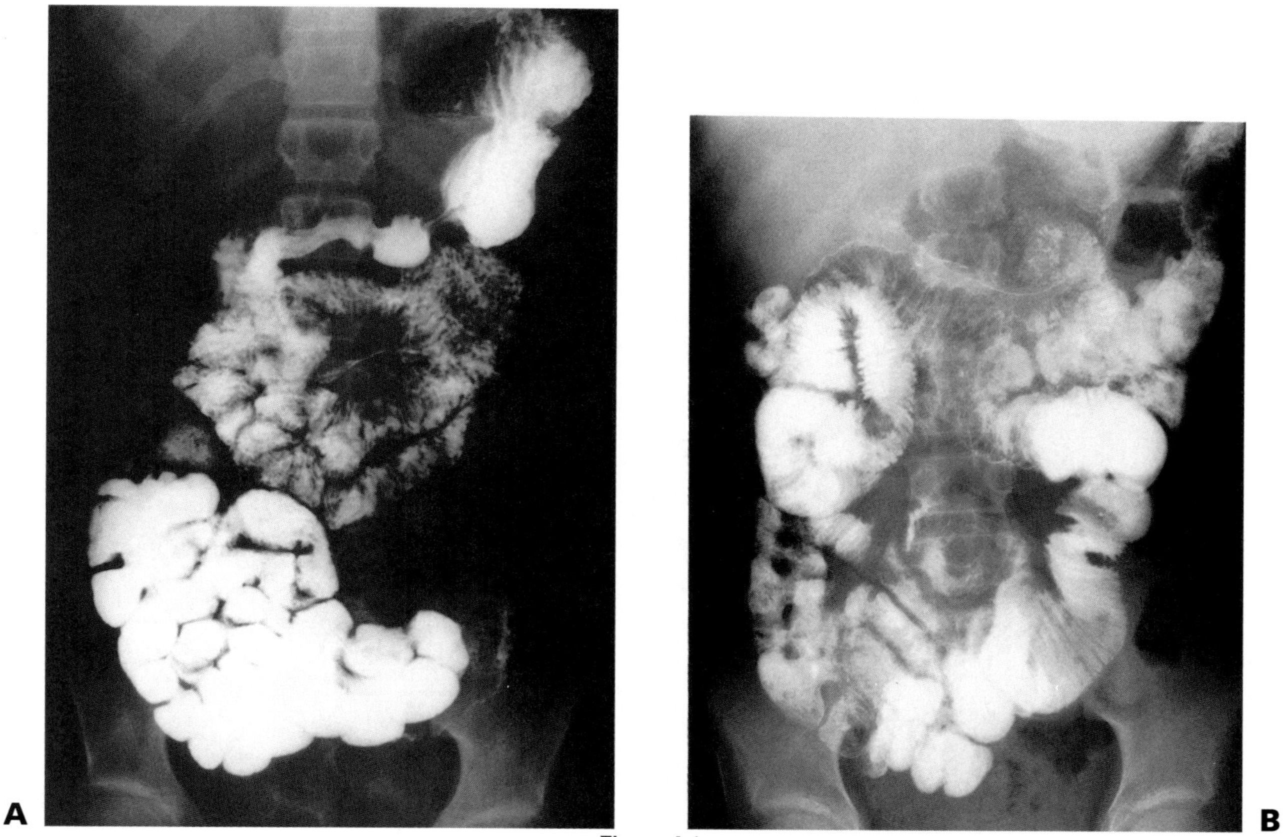

Figure 4-1

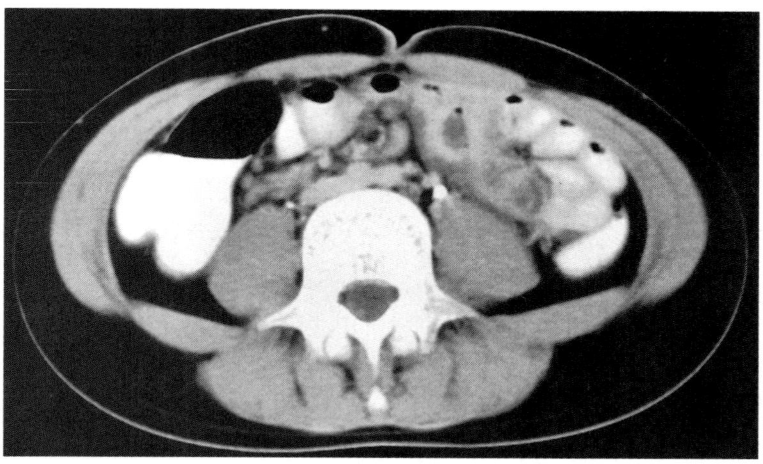

Figure 4-2

This 14-year-old boy has a history of intermittent abdominal pain and guaiac-positive stools. You are shown abdominal radiographs obtained 60 minutes (Figure 4-1A) and 90 minutes (Figure 4-1B) after the ingestion of barium and a postcontrast CT image (Figure 4-2).

QUESTION 17: MARK YOUR ANSWER SHEET TRUE (T) OR FALSE (F) FOR EACH OF THE RESPONSE CHOICES

17. The diagnoses that should be considered include:

    (A) regional enteritis
    (B) intussusception
    (C) B-cell lymphoma
    (D) Henoch-Schönlein purpura
    (E) enteric duplication

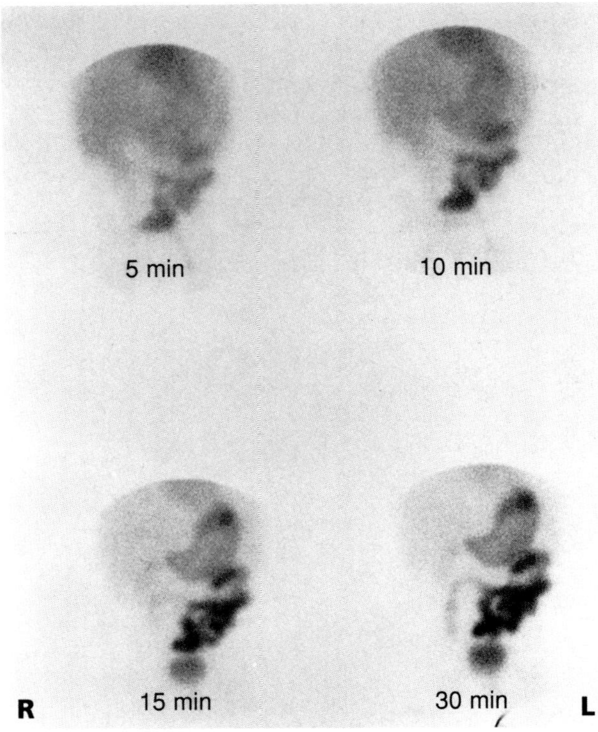

Figure 4-3

The patient then underwent abdominal imaging with Tc-99m pertechnetate. You are shown sequential anterior images (Figure 4-3).

18. Which *one* of the following is the MOST likely diagnosis?

    (A) Regional enteritis
    (B) Intussusception
    (C) B-cell lymphoma
    (D) Henoch-Schönlein purpura
    (E) Enteric duplication

For each of the numbered causes of rectal bleeding listed below (Questions 19 through 23), select the *one* lettered age range (A, B, C, or D) that is MOST closely associated with it. Each lettered age range may be used once, more than once, or not at all.

19. Necrotizing enterocolitis
20. Intussusception
21. Meckel's diverticulum
22. Juvenile polyps
23. Regional enteritis

    (A) birth to 1 month
    (B) 1 month to 3 years
    (C) 3 to 6 years
    (D) 6 to 18 years

QUESTIONS 24 AND 25: MARK YOUR ANSWER SHEET TRUE (T) OR FALSE (F) FOR EACH OF THE RESPONSE CHOICES

24. Extraintestinal manifestations of regional enteritis include:

    (A) gallstones
    (B) sclerosing cholangitis
    (C) urolithiasis
    (D) retroperitoneal fibrosis
    (E) hypertrophic osteoarthropathy

25. Concerning Henoch-Schönlein purpura,

    (A) the renal findings on ultrasonography are similar to those of acute glomerulonephritis
    (B) associated hydronephrosis is usually attributable to an intramural hematoma of the ureter
    (C) testicular involvement occurs in about 50% of patients
    (D) skin manifestations resemble erythema nodosum
    (E) hydrops of the gallbladder is characteristic

Case 5: Questions 26 through 29

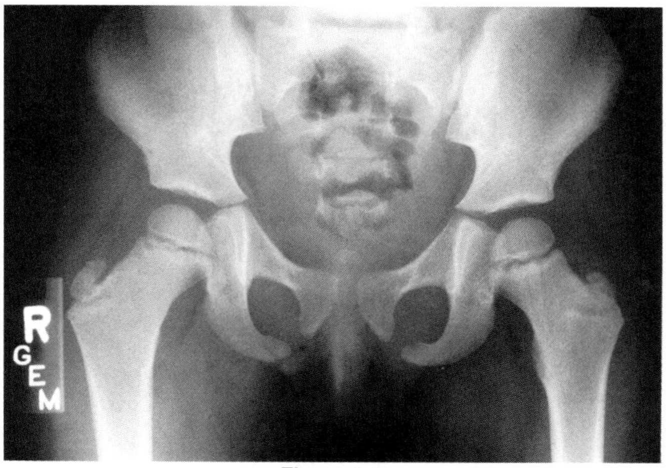

Figure 5-1

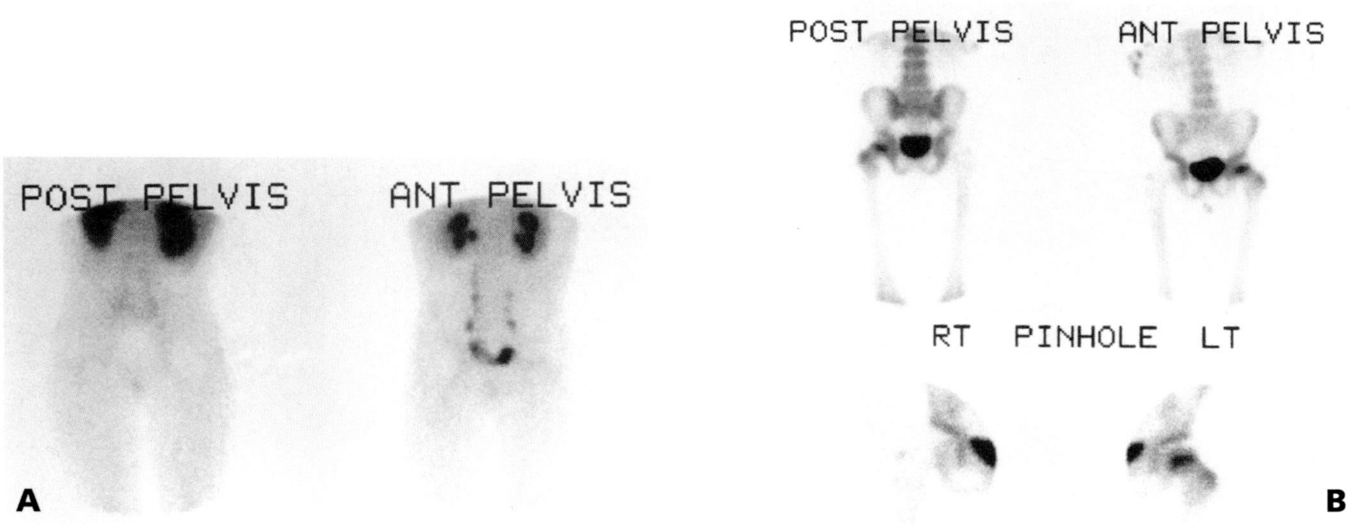

Figure 5-2

This 4-year-old boy has acute limp, thigh swelling, and fever. You are shown an anteroposterior radiograph (Figure 5-1) and immediate (A) and delayed (B) Tc-99m methylene diphosphonate scintigrams (Figure 5-2).

26. Which *one* of the following is the MOST likely diagnosis?

    (A) Leukemia
    (B) Metastatic neuroblastoma
    (C) Legg-Perthes disease
    (D) Osteomyelitis
    (E) Transient synovitis

QUESTIONS 27 THROUGH 29: MARK YOUR ANSWER SHEET TRUE (T) OR FALSE (F) FOR EACH OF THE RESPONSE CHOICES.

27. Concerning skeletal manifestations of childhood leukemia,

    (A) the transverse radiolucent metaphyseal bands represent leukemic infiltration
    (B) the metadiaphyseal lesions mimic those seen in patients with metastatic neuroblastoma
    (C) skeletal radiographs are abnormal in about 40% of patients
    (D) the signal intensity in long bones is slightly higher than normal on T1-weighted MR images
    (E) necrosis is a sequela of treatment

28. Concerning skeletal manifestations of neuroblastoma,

(A) about 30% of children present with bone pain
(B) sutural widening is secondary to cerebral metastases
(C) the diaphyses are the most common site of osseous metastases
(D) cortical metastasis is a unique feature of stage 4S disease
(E) bone scintigraphy is less sensitive than I-131 metaiodobenzylguanidine scintigraphy for diagnosis of bone marrow involvement

29. Concerning Legg-Perthes disease,

(A) most patients have normal radiographs at the time of presentation
(B) bilateral involvement occurs in fewer than 10% of patients
(C) widening of the joint space is related to thickening of the cartilage
(D) bone scintigraphy typically demonstrates a photopenic growth plate
(E) MRI is essential for assessing the response to treatment in most patients

Case 6: Questions 30 through 34

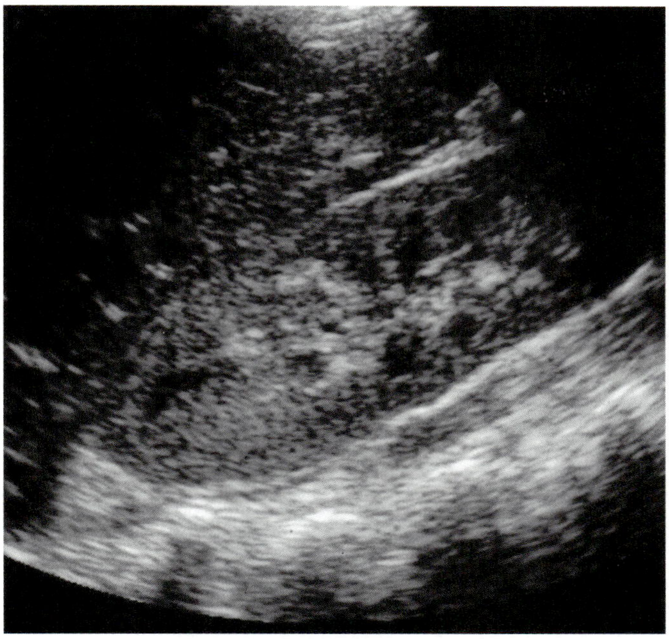

Figure 6-1

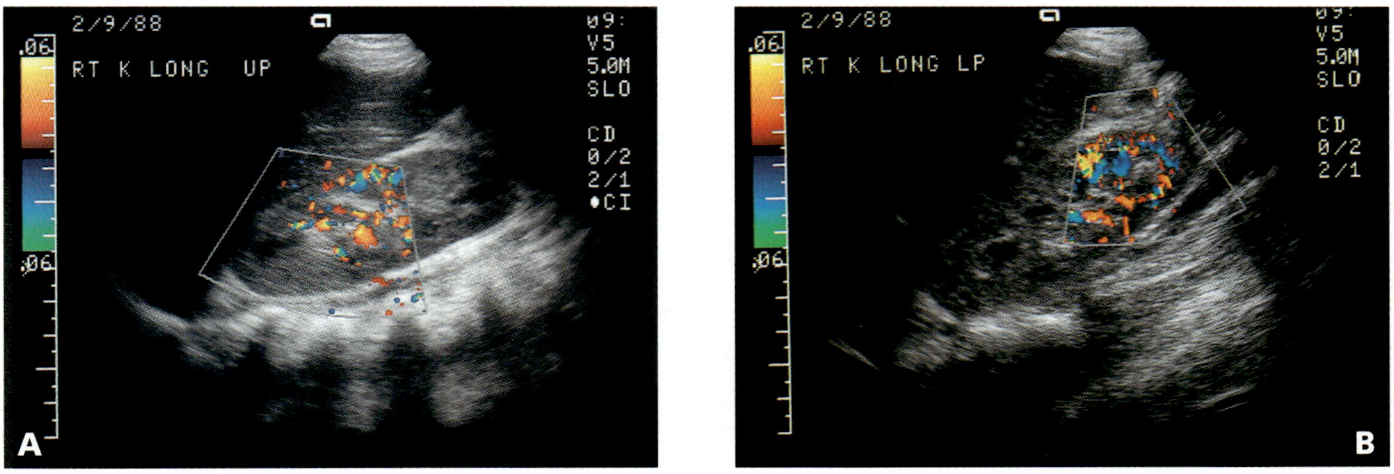

Figure 6-2

This 7-year-old boy has low-grade fever and abdominal pain. You are shown gray-scale (Figure 6-1) and color Doppler (Figure 6-2) images.

30. Which *one* of the following is the MOST likely diagnosis?

    (A) Acute pyelonephritis
    (B) Reflux nephropathy
    (C) Wilms' tumor
    (D) Hemolytic uremic syndrome
    (E) Infected upper pole moiety of a duplex system

QUESTIONS 31 THROUGH 34: MARK YOUR ANSWER SHEET TRUE (T) OR FALSE (F) FOR EACH OF THE RESPONSE CHOICES.

31. Concerning imaging in children with acute pyelonephritis,

    (A) its principal role is to confirm the diagnosis
    (B) cystography is routinely performed in children younger than 5 years
    (C) the sensitivity of gray-scale sonography for diagnosis is about 80%
    (D) the sensitivity of cortical scintigraphy for diagnosis is approximately 90%
    (E) striated parenchymal opacification is a typical pattern on CT

32. Concerning complications of acute renal infection in children,

(A) a frequent CT feature of renal abscess is thickening of Gerota's fascia
(B) most patients with pyonephrosis have obstruction secondary to ureteral calculi
(C) echogenic material in a dilated collecting system is a specific sign of pyonephrosis
(D) fungal balls are characterized sonographically by nonshadowing echogenic masses

33. Concerning vesicoureteral reflux,

(A) there is a familial tendency
(B) it is usually related to a short intramural ureter
(C) intrarenal reflux predisposes to cortical scarring
(D) associated renal injury is usually diffusely distributed
(E) it cannot be graded reliably by radionuclide cystography
(F) a normal renal sonogram excludes high-grade reflux

34. Concerning hemolytic uremic syndrome,

(A) hemorrhagic colitis usually precedes the development of renal failure when the syndrome is associated with *Escherichia coli* infection
(B) patchy echogenicity of the kidneys is noted on sonography
(C) the resistance in intrarenal arteries is elevated
(D) the prognosis is related more closely to extrarenal than to renal complications

Case 7: Questions 35 through 39

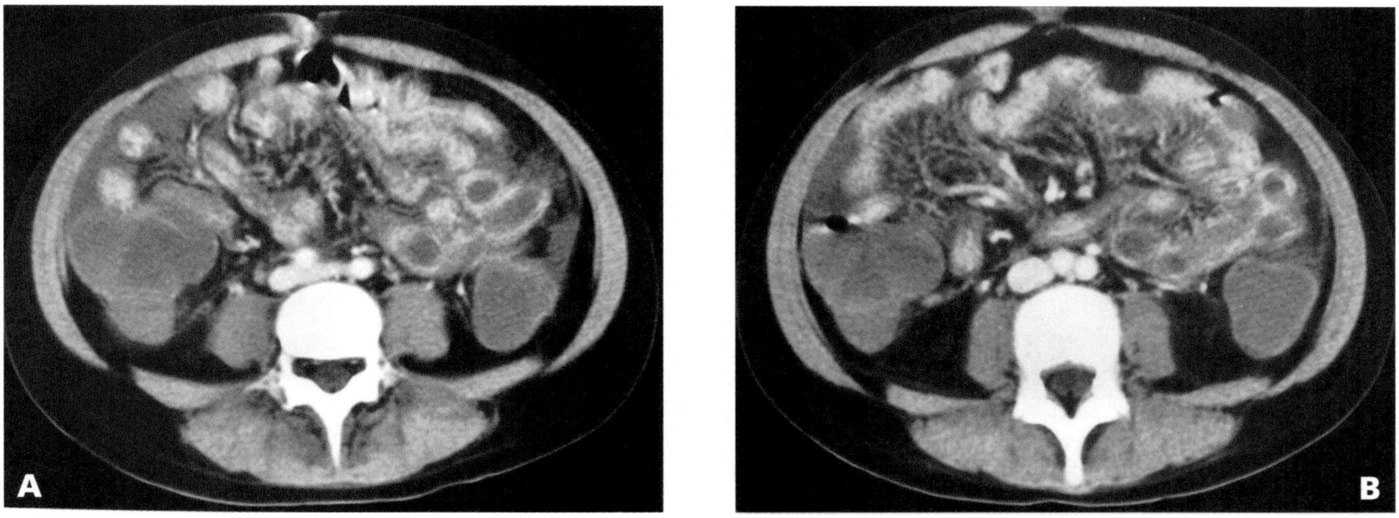

Figure 7-1

This 6-year-old boy underwent bone marrow transplantation for acute myelogenous leukemia 1 month ago and now has abdominal pain, nausea and vomiting, diarrhea, and fever. You are shown two postcontrast CT images (Figure 7-1).

35. Which *one* of the following is the MOST likely diagnosis?

    (A) Typhlitis
    (B) Lymphoproliferative disorder
    (C) Pseudomembranous colitis
    (D) Graft-versus-host disease
    (E) Radiation enterocolitis

QUESTIONS 36 THROUGH 39: MARK YOUR ANSWER SHEET TRUE (T) OR FALSE (F) FOR EACH OF THE RESPONSE CHOICES.

36. Concerning pseudomembranous colitis,

    (A) it is most commonly a pancolitis
    (B) colonic wall thickness is usually greater than 10 mm
    (C) pericolonic inflammatory changes are usually disproportionately greater than the degree of bowel wall thickening
    (D) on CT, the "accordion sign" is seen most often in the transverse colon

37. Concerning graft-versus-host disease,

    (A) it is attributable to epithelial damage of recipient target organs by donor T-cell lymphocytes
    (B) it occurs in fewer than 20% of matched allogeneic bone marrow transplant recipients
    (C) the skin is the most common target organ
    (D) patients rarely present with gastrointestinal symptoms

38. Concerning the appearance of graft-versus-host disease on abdominal CT scans,

    (A) the bowel wall thickness is usually more than 6 mm
    (B) mucosal enhancement is a feature
    (C) infiltration of the mesenteric fat is common
    (D) involvement of both the large and small bowels indicates severe disease

39. Concerning acute abdominal disease in immunocompromised children,

(A) abscess is the most common cause of abdominal symptoms
(B) abscess is more often attributable to fungal infection than to bacterial infection
(C) percutaneous drainage of an intraperitoneal abscess is contraindicated
(D) on CT, cecal thickening with surrounding inflammatory changes reliably indicates typhlitis
(E) severe colonic wall thickening is an indication for colostomy

Case 8: Questions 40 through 47

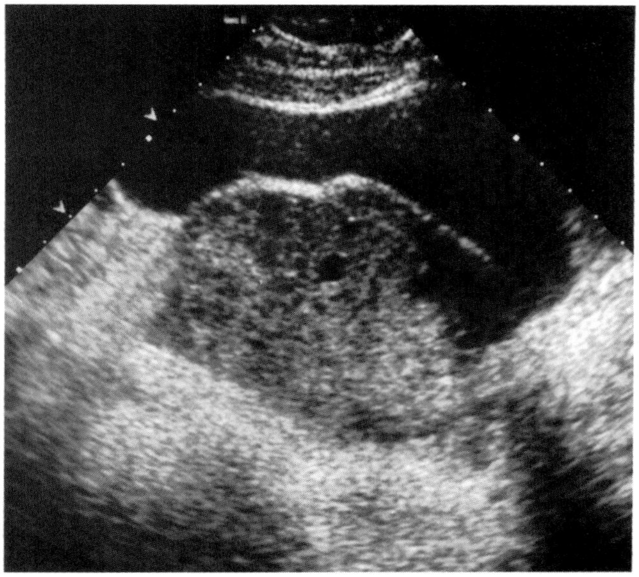

Figure 8-1

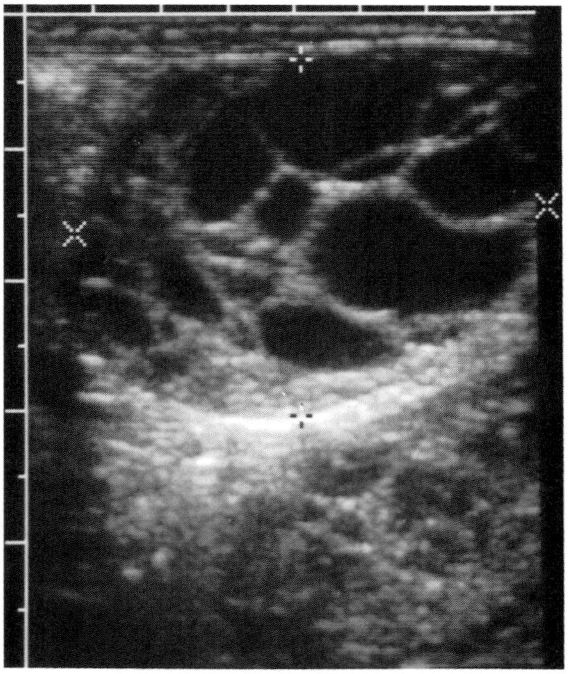

Figure 8-2

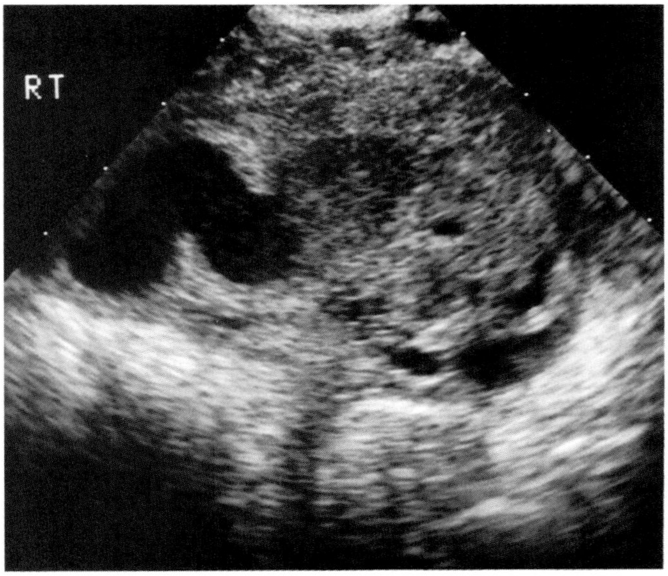

Figure 8-3

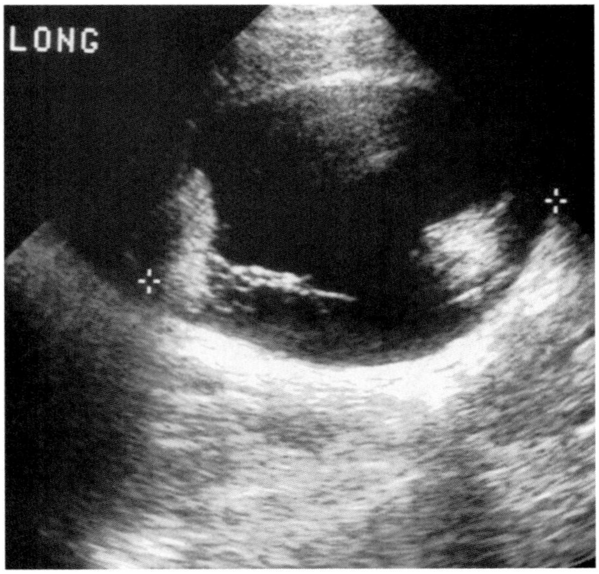

Figure 8-4

You are shown sonograms of four girls with pelvic pain. For each of the numbered images listed below (Figures 8-1 through 8-4), select the *one* lettered diagnosis (A, B, C, D, or E) that is MOST closely associated with it. Each lettered diagnosis may be used once, more than once, or not at all.

40. Figure 8-1
41. Figure 8-2
42. Figure 8-3
43. Figure 8-4

(A) Theca lutein cyst
(B) Pyosalpinx
(C) Torsion
(D) Teratoma
(E) Cystadenoma

QUESTIONS 44 THROUGH 47: MARK YOUR ANSWER SHEET TRUE (T) OR FALSE (F) FOR EACH OF THE RESPONSE CHOICES.

44. Concerning ovarian anatomy and development,

(A) the ovaries in neonates are posterolateral to the uterus
(B) the ovaries are infrequently seen in prepubertal girls
(C) multiple follicles are a normal finding in prepubertal girls
(D) most mature follicles are less than 1.5 cm in diameter
(E) the number of immature follicles is increased in patients with polycystic ovary disease
(F) the ovary is supplied by both uterine and ovarian arteries

45. Concerning pathologic ovarian cysts in childhood,

(A) they are a cause of true isosexual precocious puberty
(B) most are 1 to 2 cm in diameter
(C) the typical sonographic appearance of a hemorrhagic cyst is that of a heterogeneous, echogenic mass
(D) acute hemorrhagic cysts have a high signal intensity on both T1- and T2-weighted MR images
(E) short-tau inversion-recovery images are useful in differentiating between hemorrhagic ovarian cyst and teratoma

46. Concerning ovarian teratomas in children and adolescents,

(A) most are malignant
(B) most benign lesions are hypoechoic
(C) hair or fat lies in a dependent position with aqueous fluid on top
(D) hair causes low signal intensity on T1- and T2-weighted MR images
(E) tumors that contain more than 50% soft tissue elements by volume are usually malignant
(F) Doppler sonography shows peripheral flow in benign lesions

47. Concerning ovarian torsion,

(A) about 50% of patients have a history of recurrent pain
(B) most adolescent girls have a concomitant ovarian mass
(C) in neonates, the typical sonographic appearance is an enlarged ovary with peripheral follicles
(D) an extra-adnexal location in the pelvis is frequent
(E) flow is demonstrated by Doppler sonography in fewer than 5% of patients

Case 9: Questions 48 through 51

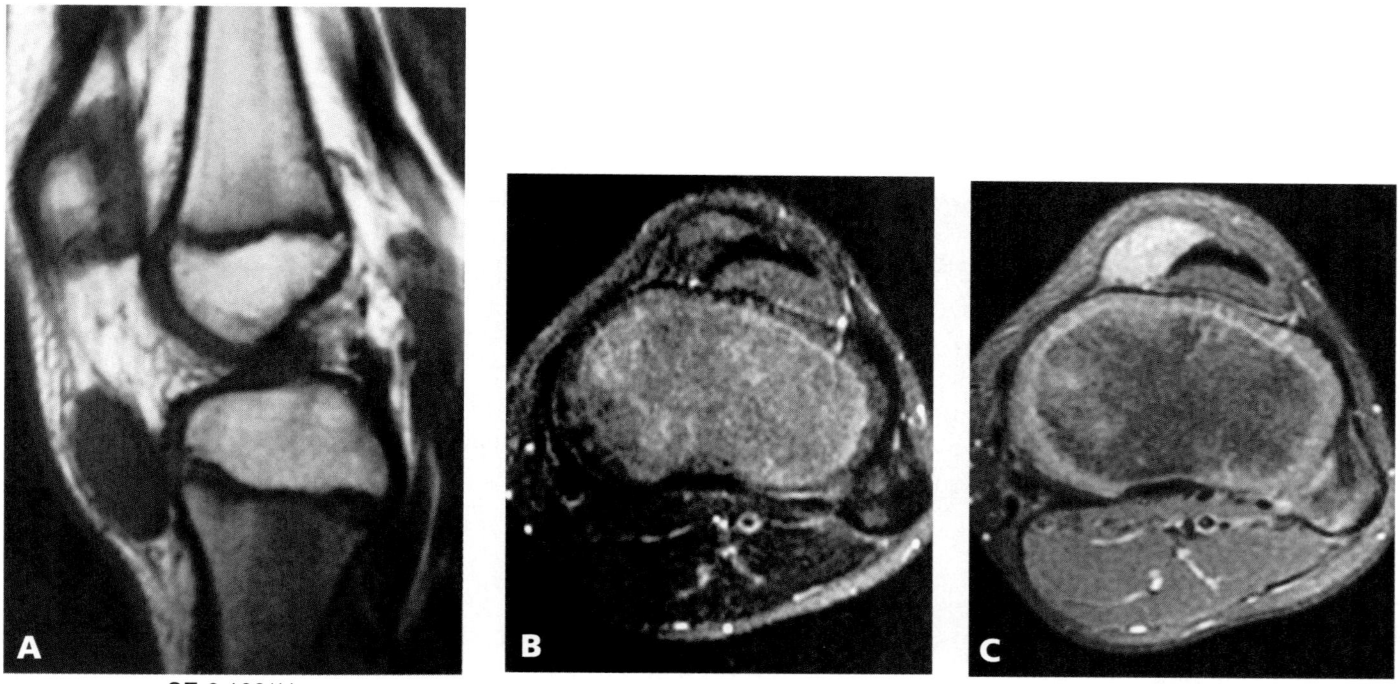

SE 6,100/11 FSE 3,000/81 SE 650/20

Figure 9-1

This 9-year-old boy has a nontender palpable mass in the infrapatellar region. You are shown sagittal T1-weighted (A), fat-saturated axial T2-weighted (B), and postcontrast T1-weighted (C) MR images (Figure 9-1).

48. Which *one* of the following is the MOST likely diagnosis?

    (A) Hematoma
    (B) Pigmented villonodular synovitis
    (C) Giant cell tumor of tendon sheath
    (D) Aggressive fibromatosis
    (E) Synovial sarcoma

QUESTIONS 49 THROUGH 51: MARK YOUR ANSWER SHEET TRUE (T) OR FALSE (F) FOR EACH OF THE RESPONSE CHOICES.

49. Concerning giant cell tumor of tendon sheath,

    (A) it most commonly occurs adjacent to small joints
    (B) the most common radiographic pattern is a soft tissue mass with associated osseous pressure erosions
    (C) it most commonly presents during the second decade of life
    (D) it is histologically identical to giant cell tumor of bone

50. Concerning aggressive fibromatosis,

    (A) the fibrous nature of the lesion results in low signal intensity on all MRI pulse sequences in most patients
    (B) it is a histologically benign lesion
    (C) it arises from fascial or musculoaponeurotic coverings
    (D) there is a high recurrence rate after surgical resection
    (E) there is often a history of previous trauma or surgery

51. Concerning MRI of focal soft tissue masses in children,

(A) well-defined margins reliably indicate a benign lesion
(B) its primary role is to determine the extent of the disease process
(C) postcontrast T1-weighted images reliably distinguish the margin of a tumor from surrounding edema
(D) a chronic hematoma is often indistinguishable from a hemorrhagic tumor
(E) subcutaneous masses are more likely to be malignant than are masses in muscle

Case 10: Questions 52 through 56

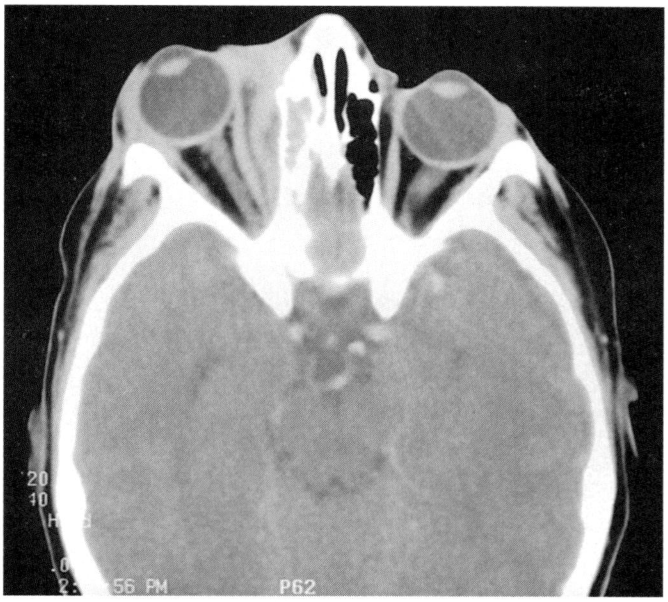

Figure 10-1

This 3-year-old girl has periorbital swelling, redness, and slowly progressive proptosis. You are shown an axial post-contrast CT image (Figure 10-1).

52. Which *one* of the following is the MOST likely diagnosis?

    (A) Pseudotumor
    (B) Orbital cellulitis
    (C) Capillary hemangioma
    (D) Rhabdomyosarcoma
    (E) Metastatic neuroblastoma

QUESTIONS 53 THROUGH 56: MARK YOUR ANSWER SHEET TRUE (T) OR FALSE (F) FOR EACH OF THE RESPONSE CHOICES.

53. Concerning orbital pseudotumor,

    (A) it is more common in children than in adults
    (B) it is rarely bilateral
    (C) the muscle tendons are spared
    (D) CT frequently demonstrates destruction of bone
    (E) it is indistinguishable from Graves' ophthalmopathy

54. Concerning orbital cellulitis,

    (A) preseptal cellulitis usually cannot be distinguished from postseptal cellulitis on physical examination
    (B) preseptal cellulitis is confined to the eyelid
    (C) postseptal cellulitis usually involves the intraconal space
    (D) CT reliably differentiates subperiosteal abscess from phlegmon
    (E) intracranial complications occur in fewer than 5% of children with postseptal cellulitis

55. Concerning capillary hemangioma of the orbit,

    (A) it is usually diagnosed in infancy
    (B) it is associated with cutaneous hemangiomas
    (C) it often presents with proptosis
    (D) it is often associated with spontaneous bleeding
    (E) CT often shows bone destruction
    (F) it is an extraconal lesion

56. Concerning orbital rhabdomyosarcoma,

    (A) it is the most common primary malignant orbital tumor in children
    (B) the embryonal type is the most common histologic form
    (C) CT often shows bone destruction
    (D) it invades the optic nerve

Case 11: Questions 57 through 60

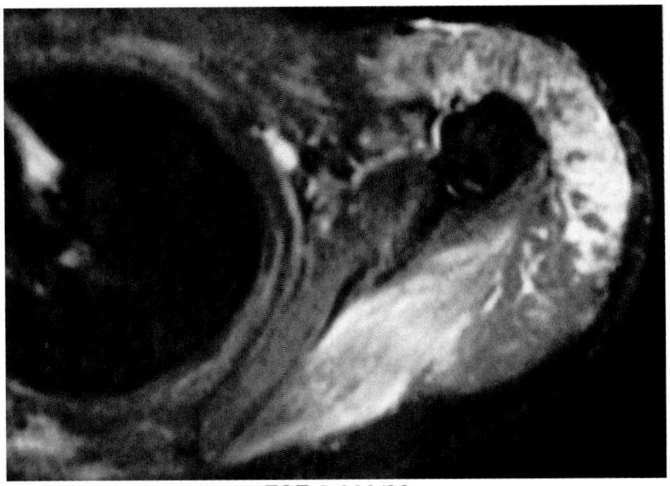

FSE 3,000/80

Figure 11-1

This 15-year-old boy has left shoulder pain, swelling, and weakness. You are shown an axial fast spin-echo, T2-weighted image with fat saturation (Figure 11-1).

57. Which *one* of the following is the MOST likely diagnosis?

    (A) Fascioscapulohumeral muscular dystrophy
    (B) Dermatomyositis
    (C) Plexiform neurofibroma
    (D) Hemangioma
    (E) Fibrosarcoma

QUESTIONS 58 THROUGH 60: MARK YOUR ANSWER SHEET TRUE (T) OR FALSE (F) FOR EACH OF THE RESPONSE CHOICES.

58. Concerning dermatomyositis,

    (A) gadolinium-enhanced imaging is the most sensitive MRI technique for its detection
    (B) the presence of subcutaneous edema helps differentiate it from infectious myositis
    (C) after treatment, abnormalities on MR images persist long after the clinical symptoms have resolved
    (D) patients with clinically active disease rarely have normal MRI studies
    (E) MRI is useful for directing biopsy

59. Concerning plexiform neurofibromas,

    (A) they are virtually pathognomonic of neurofibromatosis type 1
    (B) histologically, neoplastic Schwann cells and matrix displace rather than infiltrate neuronal axons
    (C) retroperitoneal lesions are usually bilateral
    (D) their smooth, noninfiltrating margins help to differentiate them from malignant nerve sheath tumors
    (E) on T2-weighted MR images, they typically have one or multiple "targets," with a low-intensity center and a high-intensity rim

60. Concerning soft tissue hemangiomas of childhood,

    (A) they are the most common tumors of infancy and childhood
    (B) the MRI findings are usually nonspecific
    (C) embolization or surgical management is necessary in most patients
    (D) most arise in striated muscle
    (E) surrounding soft tissue edema is an uncommon finding

Case 12: Questions 61 through 65

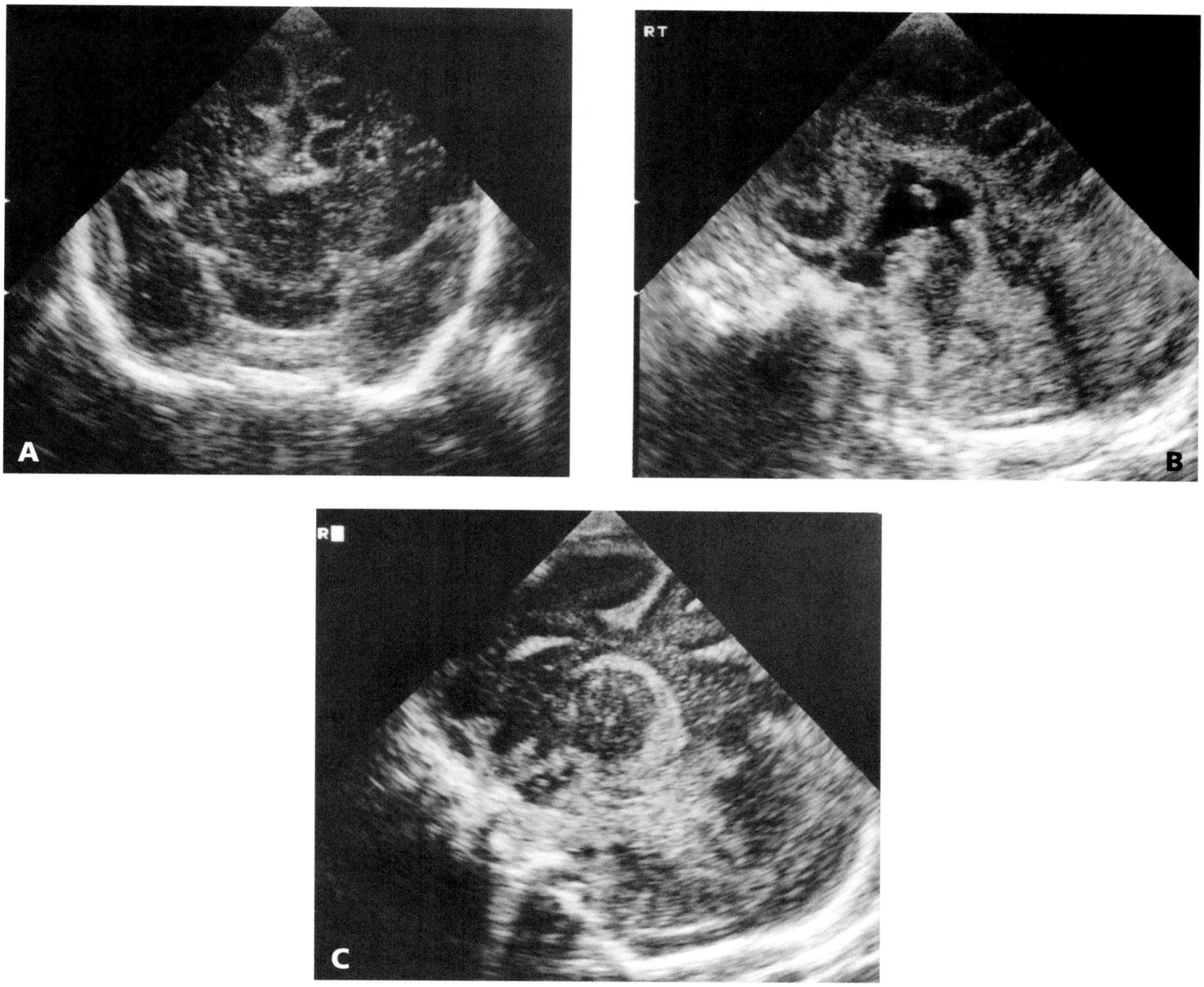

Figure 12-1

This term neonate has a diaphragmatic hernia and severe respiratory distress. Cranial ultrasonography was performed before the initiation of extracorporeal membrane oxygenation. You are shown coronal (A), midline sagittal (B), and right parasagittal (C) sonograms.

QUESTIONS 61 THROUGH 65: MARK YOUR ANSWER SHEET TRUE (T) OR FALSE (F) FOR EACH OF THE RESPONSE CHOICES.

61. The test images demonstrate:

(A) holoprosencephaly
(B) agenesis of the corpus callosum
(C) Chiari II malformation
(D) pachygyria
(E) hypoxic-ischemic encephalopathy

62. Features of semilobar holoprosencephaly include:

(A) agenesis of the anterior portion of the corpus callosum
(B) agenesis of the septum pellucidum
(C) migrational abnormalities of the cerebral cortex
(D) abnormal anterior falx
(E) azygous anterior cerebral artery
(F) cerebellar hypoplasia

63. Anatomic findings associated with agenesis of the corpus callosum include:

(A) colpocephaly
(B) reduced distance between the frontal horns
(C) malpositioned cingulate gyri
(D) inferiorly displaced third ventricle
(E) gray matter heterotopias

64. Concerning the Chiari II malformation,

(A) it is associated with failure of the neural tube to close in nearly all patients
(B) the posterior fossa is usually normal in size
(C) the severity of hydrocephalus often increases after repair of the myelomeningocele
(D) abnormalities of the corpus callosum are present in fewer than 10% of patients

65. Concerning pachygyria,

(A) it is a generalized abnormality of the cerebral cortex
(B) it is characterized by an increased number of gyri
(C) disorganization of neuronal architecture is characteristic
(D) the cortical signal intensity is usually increased on T2-weighted MR images

Case 13: Questions 66 through 69

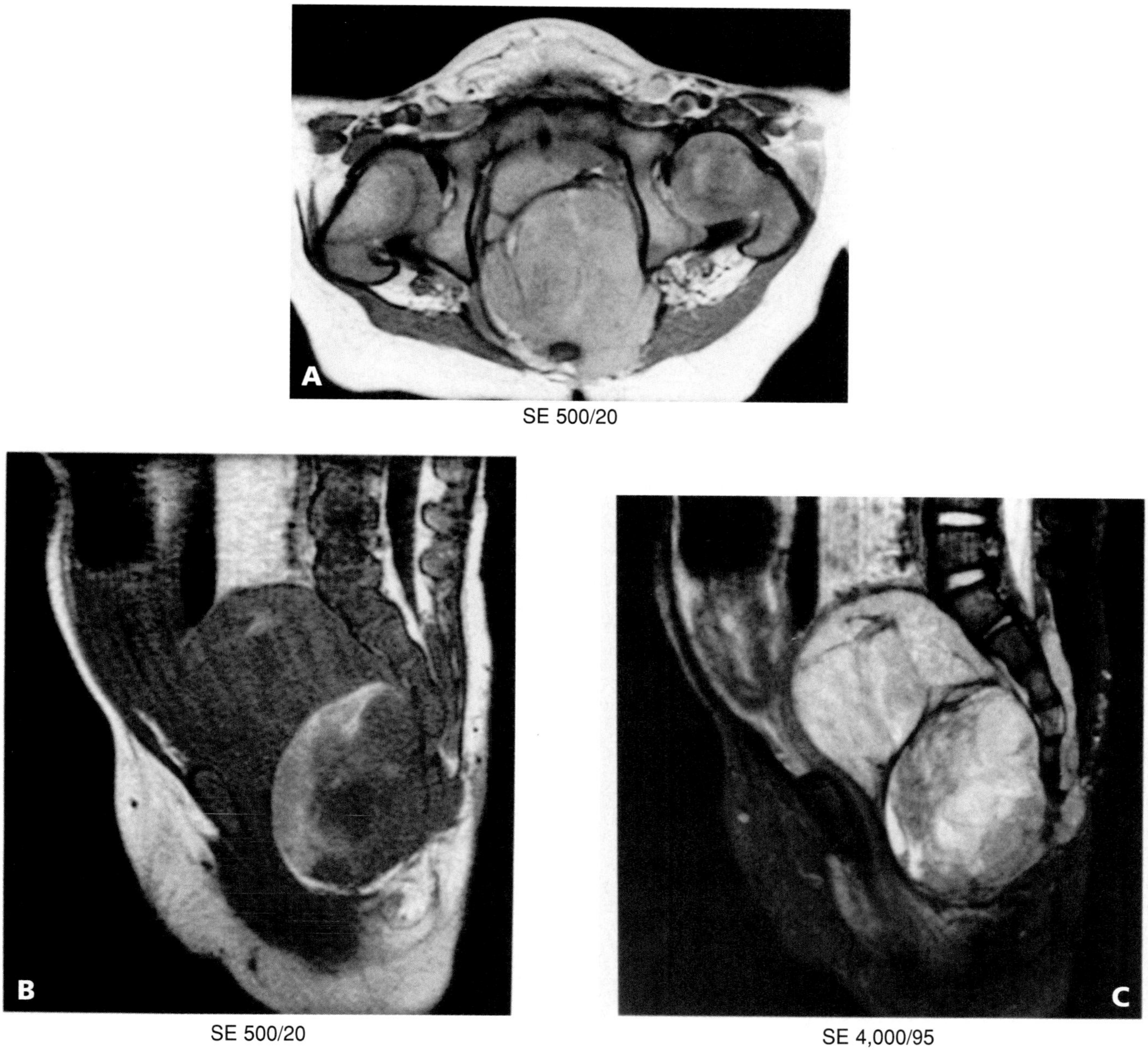

Figure 13-1

This 13-month-old girl has a pelvic mass. You are shown T1-weighted axial (A) and midline sagittal (B) and fat-suppressed T2-weighted sagittal (C) pelvic MR images (Figure 13-1).

66. Which *one* of the following is the MOST likely diagnosis?

    (A) Neuroblastoma
    (B) Rhabdomyosarcoma
    (C) Sacrococcygeal teratoma
    (D) Lymphoma
    (E) Anterior meningocele

QUESTIONS 67 THROUGH 69: MARK YOUR ANSWER SHEET TRUE (T) OR FALSE (F) FOR EACH OF THE RESPONSE CHOICES.

67. Concerning pelvic rhabdomyosarcomas,

    (A) most arise in the presacral region
    (B) central calcification is characteristic
    (C) those arising from the genitourinary tract have a better prognosis than those arising from most other locations
    (D) most are diagnosed in infancy
    (E) radiation therapy is the treatment of choice

68. Concerning sacrococcygeal germ cell tumors,

(A) most are diagnosed at birth
(B) an intrapelvic location favors malignancy
(C) they are predominantly cystic
(D) the highest frequency of malignancy is in children older than 1 year
(E) sacral erosion is typical

69. Features associated with anterior meningocele include:

(A) sacral anomalies
(B) presacral mass
(C) neurofibromatosis type 2
(D) Currarino's triad (imperforate anus, sacral anomaly, presacral mass)
(E) tethered cord

Case 14: Questions 70 through 73

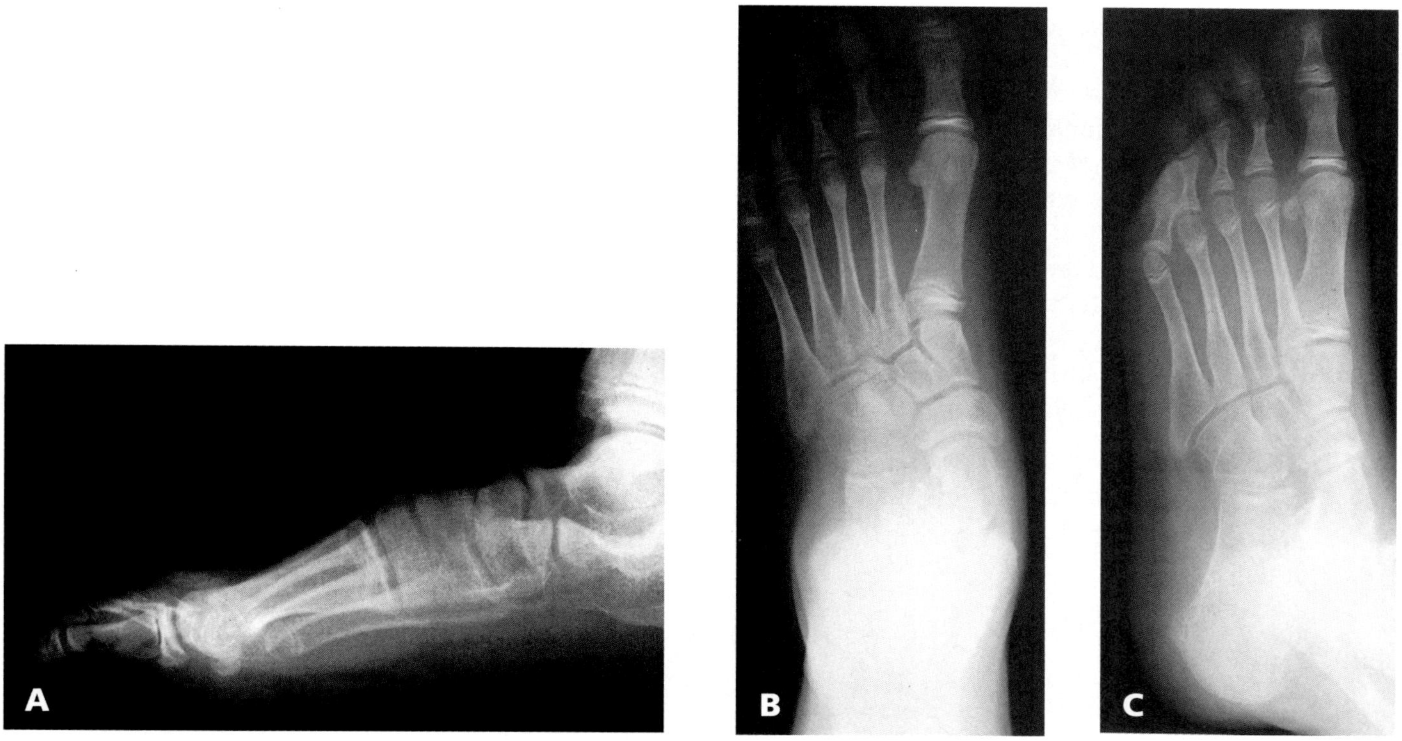

Figure 14-1

This 13-year-old boy has chronic foot pain. You are shown a series of three radiographs of the foot (Figure 14-1).

70. Which *one* of the following is the MOST likely diagnosis?

    (A) Stress fracture
    (B) Nonopaque foreign body
    (C) Tarsal coalition
    (D) Osteochondritis dissecans
    (E) Jones' fracture

QUESTIONS 71 THROUGH 73: MARK YOUR ANSWER SHEET TRUE (T) OR FALSE (F) FOR EACH OF THE RESPONSE CHOICES.

71. Concerning foreign bodies in the feet,

    (A) sonography reliably detects radiolucent foreign bodies
    (B) most nonleaded glass is radiolucent on conventional radiographs
    (C) MRI usually shows findings specific for a foreign body in patients who present with a soft tissue mass
    (D) bone scintigraphy is generally indicated in a patient with a chronic foreign body

72. Concerning tarsal coalition,

(A) most patients are asymptomatic
(B) the most common types involve the calcaneus
(C) in patients with talocalcaneal coalition, fusion most commonly involves the posterior facet
(D) distinguishing osseous from fibrous coalition is important for planning surgical management
(E) fibrous coalitions are delineated better by MRI than by CT

73. Concerning the anatomy of the foot,

(A) the calcaneonavicular joint has three facets
(B) the sinus tarsi separates the anterior and middle facets of the talocalcaneal joint
(C) the talocalcaneal joint is best demonstrated in the axial plane (long axis of the foot)
(D) the calcaneonavicular joint is best demonstrated in the coronal plane (short axis of the foot)

Case 15: Questions 74 through 77

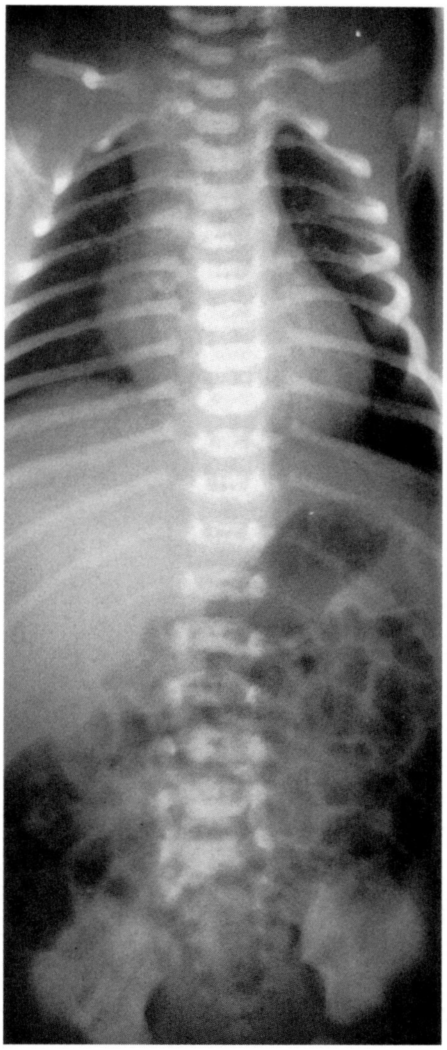

Figure 15-1

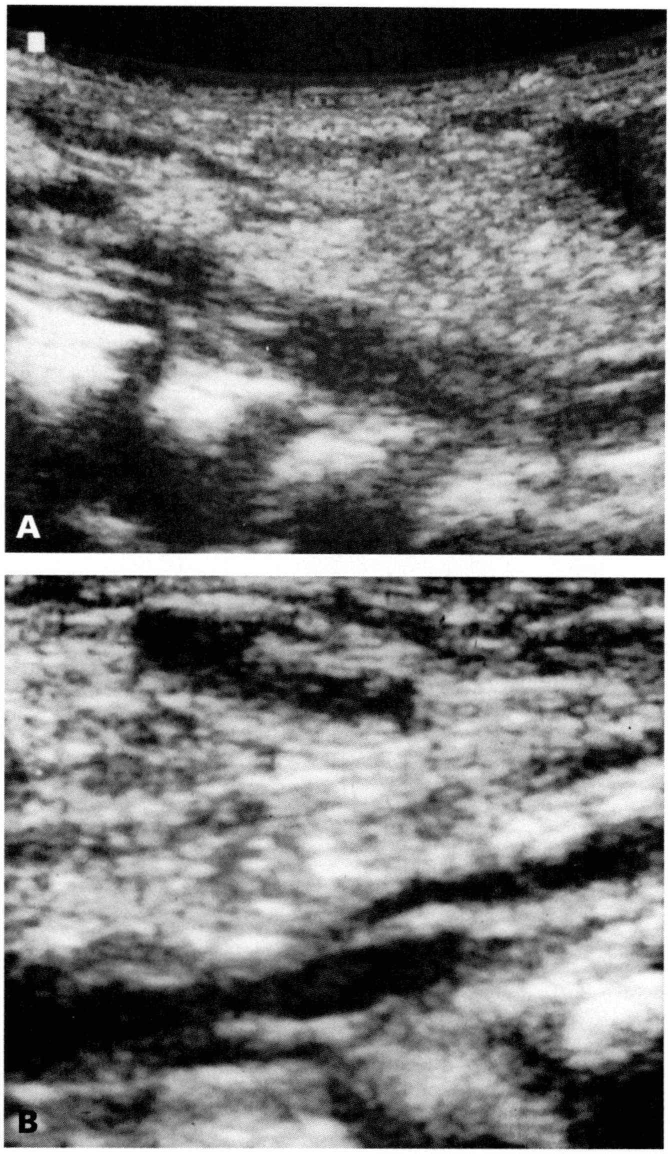

Figure 15-2

This newborn infant has soft tissue fullness of the lower back on physical examination. You are shown a radiograph (Figure 15-1) and three longitudinal sonograms of the spine (Figure 15-2).

74. Which *one* of the following is the MOST likely diagnosis?

(A) Hemangioma
(B) Lipomyelocele
(C) Myelocystocele
(D) Myelomeningocele
(E) Sacrococcygeal teratoma

QUESTIONS 75 THROUGH 77: MARK YOUR ANSWER SHEET TRUE (T) OR FALSE (F) FOR EACH OF THE RESPONSE CHOICES.

75. Concerning lipomyelocele,

(A) it most often occurs in the lower thoracic region
(B) it is invariably associated with cord tethering
(C) surgery is not indicated in asymptomatic patients
(D) vertebral segmentation anomalies are present in nearly all patients
(E) it is synonymous with lipoma of the filum terminale

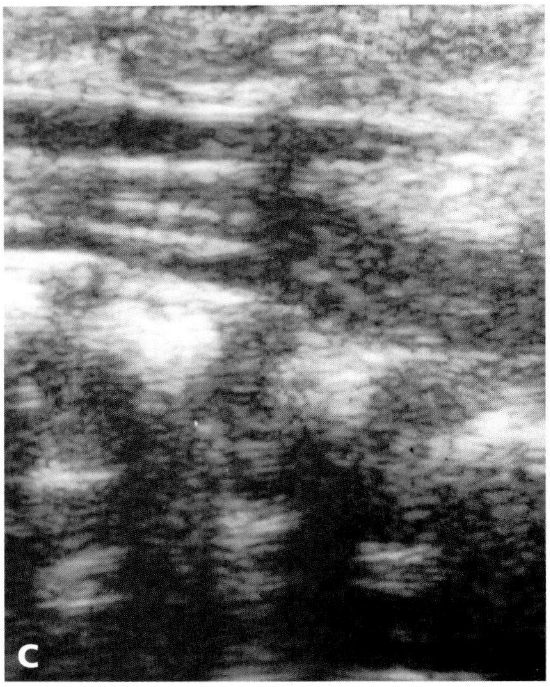

Figure 15-2 (Continued)

76. Concerning myelocystocele,

(A) hydromyelia is present in more than 90% of patients
(B) it most often occurs at the caudal termination of the spinal cord
(C) vertebral anomalies are invariably present
(D) associated cloacal anomalies are present in most patients
(E) the cystocele usually communicates directly with the subarachnoid space

77. Concerning myelomeningoceles,

(A) the dorsal surface of the placode corresponds to the central portion of the spinal canal
(B) about 5% are covered with skin
(C) cord tethering usually occurs as a postoperative complication
(D) the primary role of preoperative imaging is to evaluate the extent of the cord lesion

Case 16: Questions 78 through 81

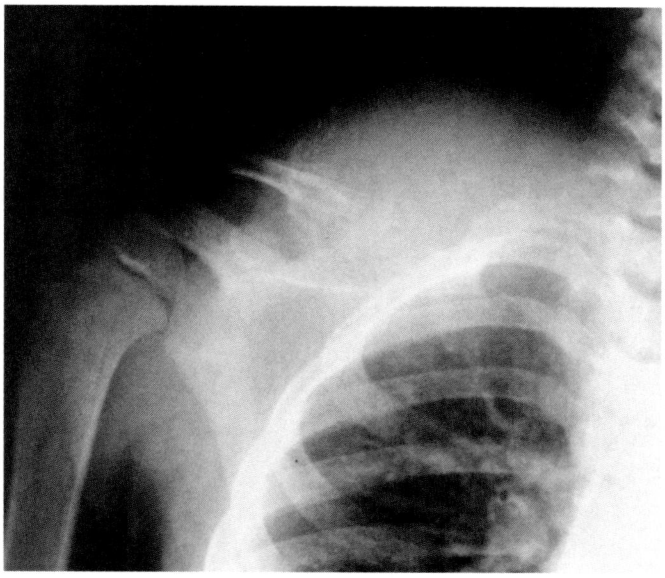

Figure 16-1

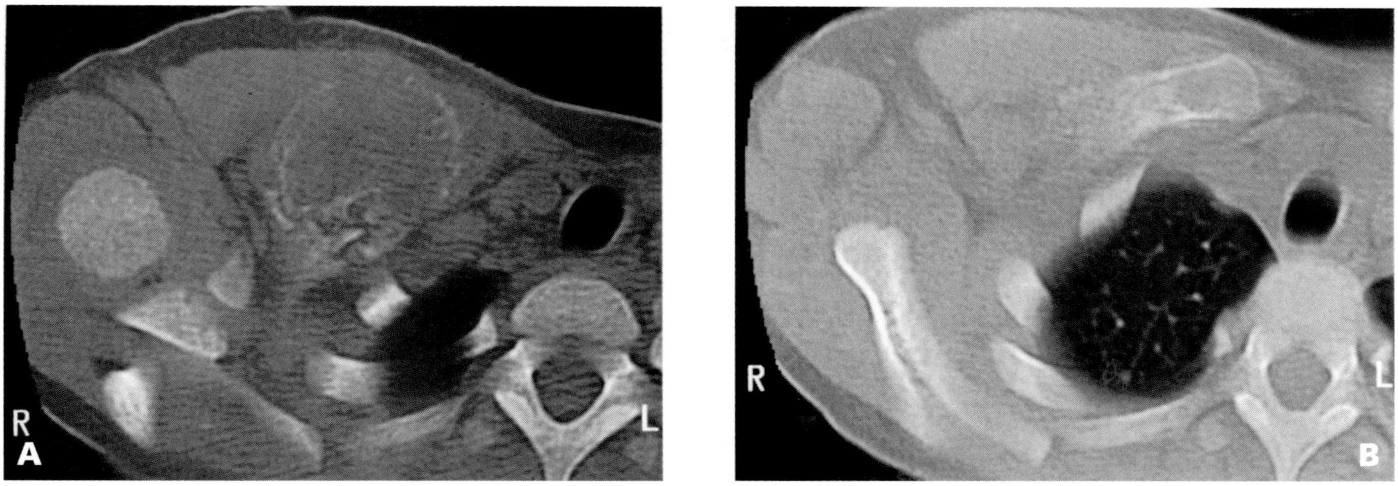

Figure 16-2

This 6-year-old boy was diagnosed with a right clavicular fracture 4 months ago. He has persistent clavicular pain. You are shown an anteroposterior radiograph of the right shoulder region (Figure 16-1) and two axial CT images (Figure 16-2).

78. Which *one* of the following is the MOST likely diagnosis?

   (A) Congenital pseudarthrosis
   (B) Osteomyelitis
   (C) Langerhans cell histiocytosis
   (D) Aneurysmal bone cyst
   (E) Ewing's sarcoma

QUESTIONS 79 THROUGH 81: MARK YOUR ANSWER SHEET TRUE (T) OR FALSE (F) FOR EACH OF THE RESPONSE CHOICES.

79. Concerning congenital clavicular pseudarthrosis,

   (A) it is usually right sided
   (B) it is easily distinguished radiographically from an acute fracture
   (C) it often heals spontaneously
   (D) it is associated with ipsilateral Erb's palsy
   (E) it occurs at any point along the clavicle

80. Concerning clavicular osteomyelitis in children,

(A) most patients are immunodeficient
(B) the clavicle is commonly involved in patients with chronic recurrent multifocal osteomyelitis
(C) the responsible organism is identified in fewer than 30% of patients
(D) radiographs are usually normal

81. Concerning clavicular fracture in children,

(A) the lateral fragment is usually displaced inferiorly
(B) osteolysis is an occasional sequela
(C) in an infant, it strongly suggests child abuse
(D) nonunion is rare
(E) the lateral third is least commonly involved
(F) acromioclavicular joint separation is commonly associated

Case 17: Questions 82 through 85

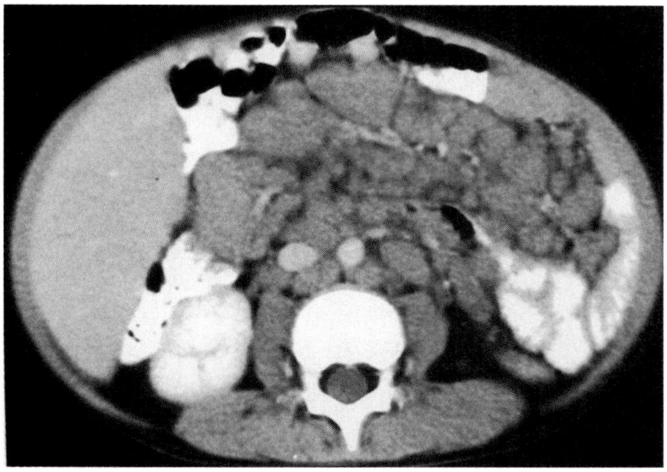

Figure 17-1

This 4-year-old boy has an abdominal mass. You are shown a postcontrast abdominal CT image (Figure 17-1).

82. Which *one* of the following is the MOST likely diagnosis?

    (A) Kawasaki disease
    (B) Tuberculosis
    (C) Chronic granulomatous disease of childhood
    (D) Lymphoproliferative disorder
    (E) Mesenteric adenitis

QUESTIONS 83 THROUGH 85: MARK YOUR ANSWER SHEET TRUE (T) OR FALSE (F) FOR EACH OF THE RESPONSE CHOICES.

83. Concerning lymphoproliferative disorder,

    (A) it occurs most commonly in bone marrow transplant recipients
    (B) the prognosis is more closely related to the cause of the underlying immunodeficiency than to the distribution of the disease
    (C) it is caused by Epstein-Barr virus
    (D) children with congenital B-cell deficiencies are at high risk for its development
    (E) extranodal is more frequent than nodal involvement in the abdomen
    (F) the usual initial treatment is chemotherapy

84. Concerning mesenteric adenitis,

    (A) the diagnosis is usually made by biopsy of affected lymph nodes
    (B) leukocytosis is rarely present
    (C) CT typically shows lymph node enlargement in the large bowel mesentery
    (D) the cause is usually bacterial
    (E) nodal involvement is usually more diffusely distributed than the mesenteric adenopathy seen in patients with appendicitis

85. Concerning diseases that involve the mesentery in children,

    (A) a mass near the root of the mesentery is more likely to be malignant than benign
    (B) the mesentery is involved in more than 50% of children with non-Hodgkin's lymphoma
    (C) cystic lymphangiomas tend to be unilocular
    (D) on CT, mesenteric lymph nodes less than 5 mm in diameter are normal

Case 18: Questions 86 through 89

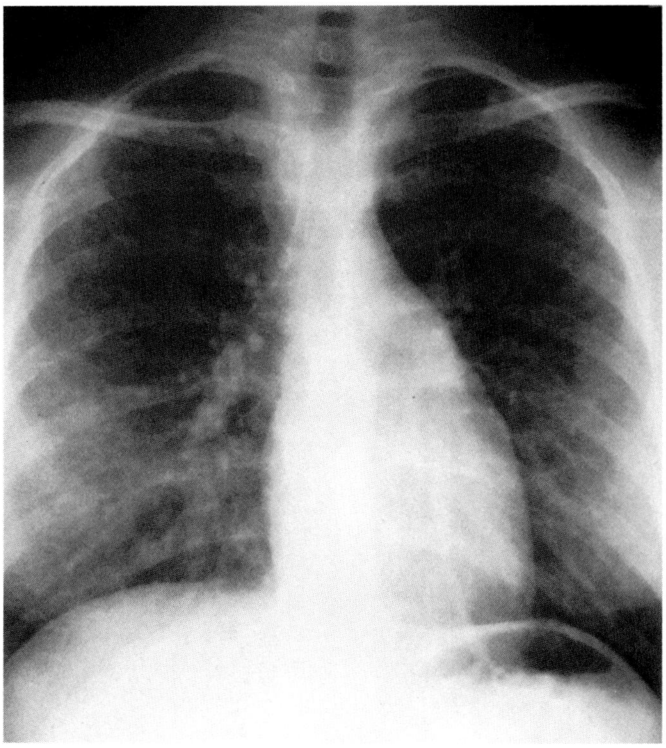

Figure 18-1

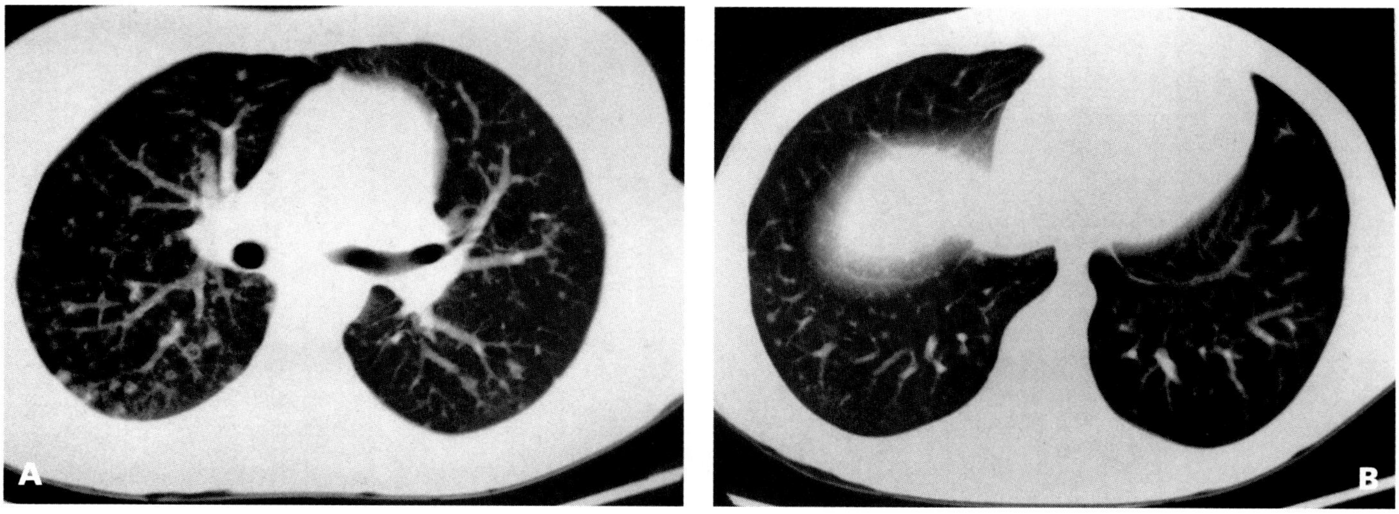

Figure 18-2

This 17-year-old girl had a recent onset of mild exertional dyspnea. You are shown a posteroanterior chest radiograph (Figure 18-1) and two axial CT images (Figure 18-2).

86. Which *one* of the following is the MOST likely diagnosis?

    (A) Prior *Pneumocystis carinii* infection
    (B) Bronchiectasis
    (C) Tuberculosis
    (D) Papillomatosis
    (E) Langerhans cell histiocytosis

QUESTIONS 87 THROUGH 89: MARK YOUR ANSWER SHEET TRUE (T) OR FALSE (F) FOR EACH OF THE RESPONSE CHOICES.

87. Concerning *Pneumocystis carinii* pneumonia in children,

(A) cystic changes are common in acute disease
(B) it usually exhibits a reticulonodular pattern
(C) hilar adenopathy is present in most patients
(D) it is the most common pulmonary disease in children with AIDS
(E) pleural effusions are common

88. Concerning papillomatosis of the airway in children,

(A) it is usually diagnosed at birth
(B) it most often involves the laryngotracheal region
(C) pulmonary involvement occurs in about 5% of patients
(D) it is associated with an increased risk of squamous cell carcinoma
(E) it involutes spontaneously in most patients
(F) pulmonary involvement is characterized by subpleural nodules

89. Disorders associated with cystic lung disease in children include:

(A) Niemann-Pick disease
(B) tuberous sclerosis
(C) von Hippel-Lindau disease
(D) Kawasaki's disease
(E) ciliary dyskinesia syndrome (Kartagener's syndrome)
(F) Ehlers-Danlos syndrome

Case 19: Questions 90 through 93

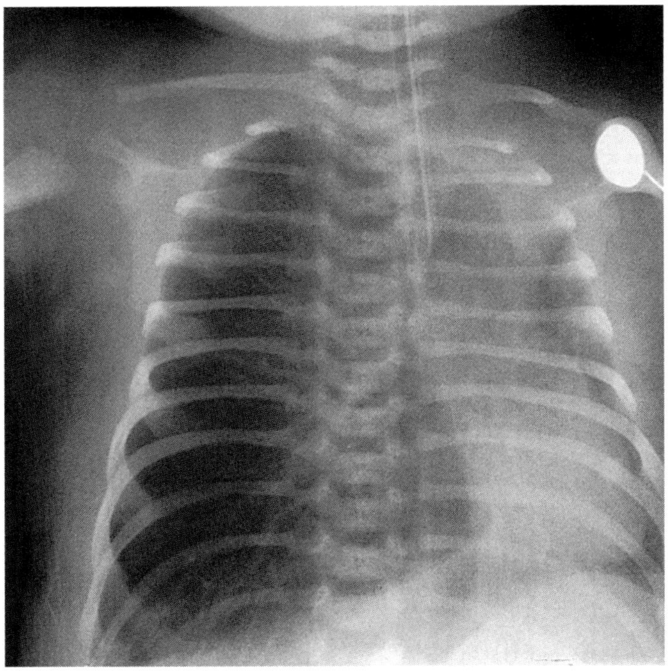

Figure 19-1

This 11-day-old girl had respiratory distress requiring intubation. You are shown an anteroposterior chest radiograph (Figure 19-1).

90. Which *one* of the following is the MOST likely diagnosis?

(A) Pneumothorax
(B) Agenetic lung
(C) Pulmonary sling
(D) Diaphragmatic hernia
(E) Diaphragmatic paralysis

QUESTIONS 91 THROUGH 93: MARK YOUR ANSWER SHEET TRUE (T) OR FALSE (F) FOR EACH OF THE RESPONSE CHOICES.

91. Features associated with pulmonary hypoplasia include:

(A) systemic arterial supply
(B) accessory diaphragm
(C) pulmonary venous drainage to systemic vein
(D) oligohydramnios

92. Concerning congenital diaphragmatic hernia,

(A) it occurs with equal frequency on both sides
(B) ultrasonography helps to distinguish a small one from an eventration
(C) associated malrotation is infrequent
(D) the contralateral lung is nearly always normal
(E) it is synonymous with Bochdalek's hernia

93. Congenital cardiovascular anomalies commonly associated with asymmetrical pulmonary aeration include:

(A) atrioventricular septal defect
(B) Ebstein's anomaly
(C) aberrant right subclavian artery
(D) pulmonary sling
(E) tetralogy of Fallot with absence of the pulmonic valve

Case 20: Questions 94 through 97

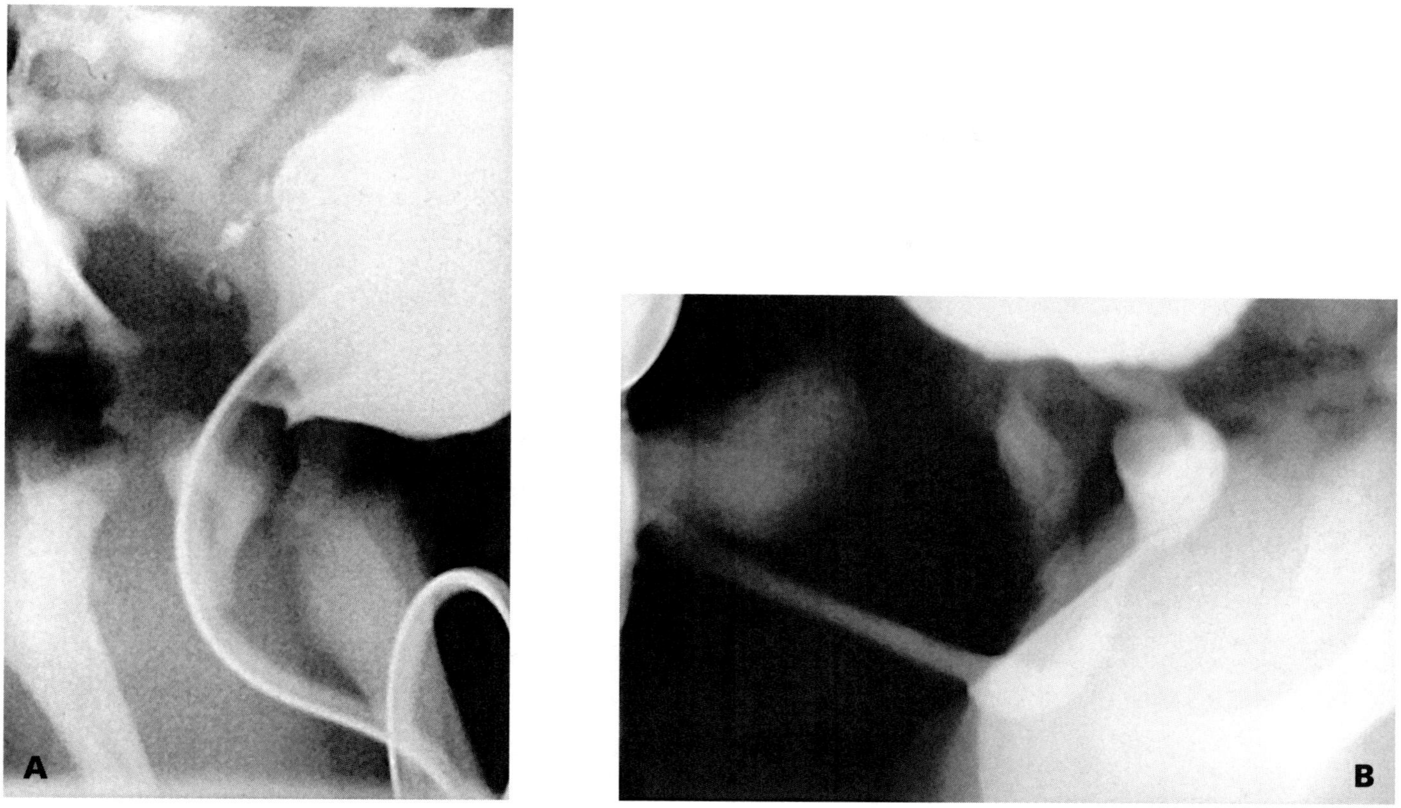

Figure 20-1

This 1-week-old boy has a urinary tract infection. You are shown prevoiding (Figure 20-1A) and voiding (Figure 20-1B) images from a voiding cystourethrogram.

94. Which *one* of the following is the MOST likely diagnosis?

    (A) Posterior urethral valves
    (B) Neurogenic dysfunction of the bladder
    (C) Urethral polyp
    (D) Ectopic ureterocele
    (E) Rhabdomyosarcoma

QUESTIONS 95 THROUGH 97: MARK YOUR ANSWER SHEET TRUE (T) OR FALSE (F) FOR EACH OF THE RESPONSE CHOICES.

95. Concerning posterior urethral valves,

    (A) they are the result of abnormal insertion of the mesonephric ducts
    (B) they rarely occur in phenotypic girls
    (C) nearly all patients have reflux
    (D) they are the most common cause of urinary ascites in neonates
    (E) on ultrasonography, a dilated prostatic urethra is a specific sign

96. Concerning urethral polyps,

(A) they undergo malignant degeneration
(B) they often occur in the posterior urethra
(C) most are pedunculated
(D) they are a cause of prenatally detected hydronephrosis
(E) they mimic urethral diverticula on voiding cystourethrography

97. Concerning ureteroceles,

(A) they are a cause of enuresis
(B) ectopic ones usually are associated with the upper pole ureter of a duplicated system
(C) in boys, ectopic ones are most often associated with nonduplicated systems
(D) they are best demonstrated on cystography when the bladder is maximally distended

Case 21: Questions 98 through 106

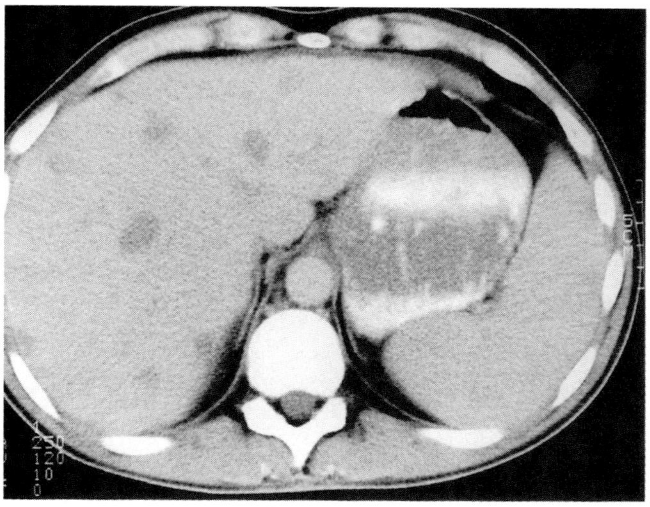

Figure 21-1

This 12-year-old boy had persistent abdominal pain and low-grade fever for 1 week. A contrast-enhanced abdominal CT image was obtained; you are shown an axial image of the liver (Figure 21-1).

QUESTIONS 98 AND 99: MARK YOUR ANSWER SHEET TRUE (T) OR FALSE (F) FOR EACH OF THE RESPONSE CHOICES.

98. Likely explanations for the CT findings include:

    (A) primary hepatic tumor
    (B) metastases
    (C) infection
    (D) ductal dilatation
    (E) unopacified veins

99. In children, features associated more often with the conventional than with the fibrolamellar form of hepatocellular carcinoma include:

    (A) elevated serum alpha-fetoprotein levels
    (B) association with type I glycogen storage disease
    (C) younger mean patient age at diagnosis
    (D) central calcifications
    (E) portal vein invasion

100. Which *one* of the following contrast enhancement phases is BEST for detecting hepatic metastatic disease?

    (A) Arterial phase
    (B) Early portal venous phase
    (C) Late portal venous phase
    (D) Equilibrium
    (E) Late delayed phase

QUESTIONS 101 AND 102: MARK YOUR ANSWER SHEET TRUE (T) OR FALSE (F) FOR EACH OF THE RESPONSE CHOICES.

101. Concerning pyogenic hepatic abscesses in children,

    (A) most are secondary to a source of infection elsewhere in the abdomen
    (B) they are usually solitary
    (C) an air-fluid level is present in most cases
    (D) percutaneous drainage is successful therapy in greater than 80% of cases
    (E) the most common complication of percutaneous drainage is peritonitis

102. Concerning cat scratch disease,

(A) the causative agent is unknown
(B) painful adenopathy is the most common presenting sign
(C) hepatic involvement is present in most patients
(D) biopsy usually is necessary for diagnosis
(E) on sonography, hepatic lesions typically are echogenic
(F) hepatic lesions typically appear as target lesions on postcontrast CT

For each of the numbered infections listed below (Questions 103 through 106), select the *one* lettered feature (A, B, C, D, or E) that is MOST closely associated with it. Each feature may be used once, more than once, or not at all.

103. Amebiasis
104. Candidiasis
105. Echinococcosis
106. Schistosomiasis

(A) diaphragmatic invasion
(B) target lesion on sonography
(C) peripheral hepatic calcification
(D) biliary ductal dilatation
(E) uniformly enhancing lesions on CT

Case 22: Questions 107 through 111

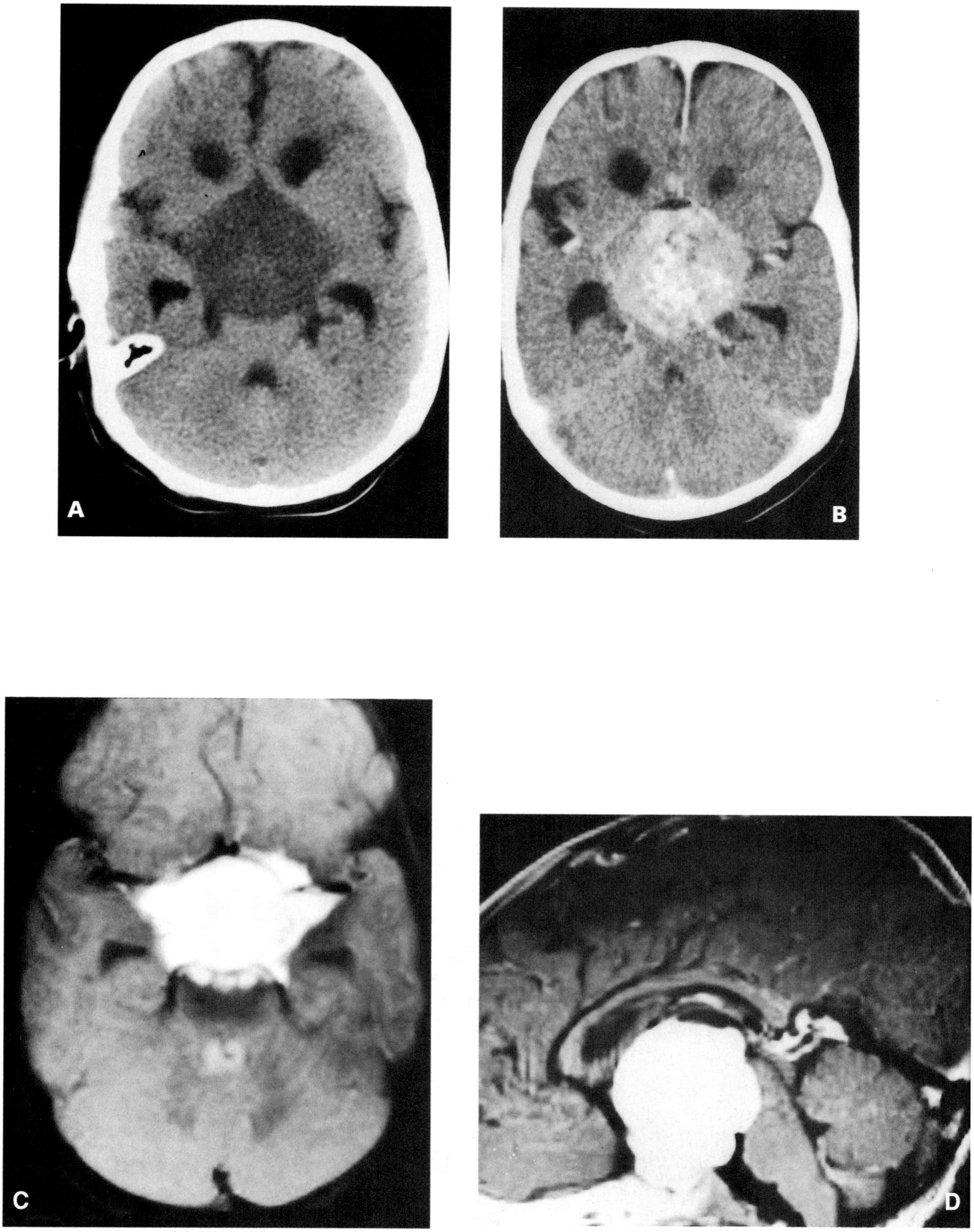

SE 3,000/45 SE 700/20

Figure 22-1

This 7-month-old child has abnormal eye movements and hyperphagia. You are shown axial precontrast (A) and postcontrast (B) CT scans, as well as axial proton-density-weighted (C) and sagittal postcontrast T1-weighted (D) MR images (Figure 22-1).

107. Which *one* of the following is the MOST likely diagnosis?

(A) Langerhans cell histiocytosis
(B) Hypothalamic hamartoma
(C) Craniopharyngioma
(D) Suprasellar germinoma
(E) Hypothalamic-chiasmatic glioma

QUESTIONS 108 THROUGH 111: MARK YOUR ANSWER SHEET TRUE (T) OR FALSE (F) FOR EACH OF THE RESPONSE CHOICES.

108. Concerning intracranial Langerhans cell histiocytosis,

(A) most patients also have extracranial involvement
(B) patients often have precocious puberty
(C) diabetes insipidus is attributable to involvement of the hypothalamic nuclei
(D) an early finding on MRI is thickening of the pituitary stalk
(E) absence of the neurohypophyseal signal on a T1-weighted MR image is a characteristic finding

109. Concerning hypothalamic hamartoma,

(A) it is a congenital lesion
(B) it involves the tuber cinereum
(C) precocious puberty is the usual presenting symptom
(D) gelastic seizures are characteristic
(E) it usually is 1 to 2 cm in diameter
(F) it usually enhances intensely

110. Concerning craniopharyngioma,

(A) it is calcified in about 30% of cases
(B) is usually enhances uniformly
(C) intrasellar involvement occurs in about 10% of cases
(D) leptomeningeal spread is common
(E) it is the most common suprasellar mass in childhood

111. Concerning hypothalamic-chiasmatic glioma,

(A) it is associated with diencephalic syndrome
(B) it is associated with neurofibromatosis type 1
(C) cystic components are seen on MRI in most lesions
(D) enhancement occurs in less than 20% of lesions

Case 23: Questions 112 through 116

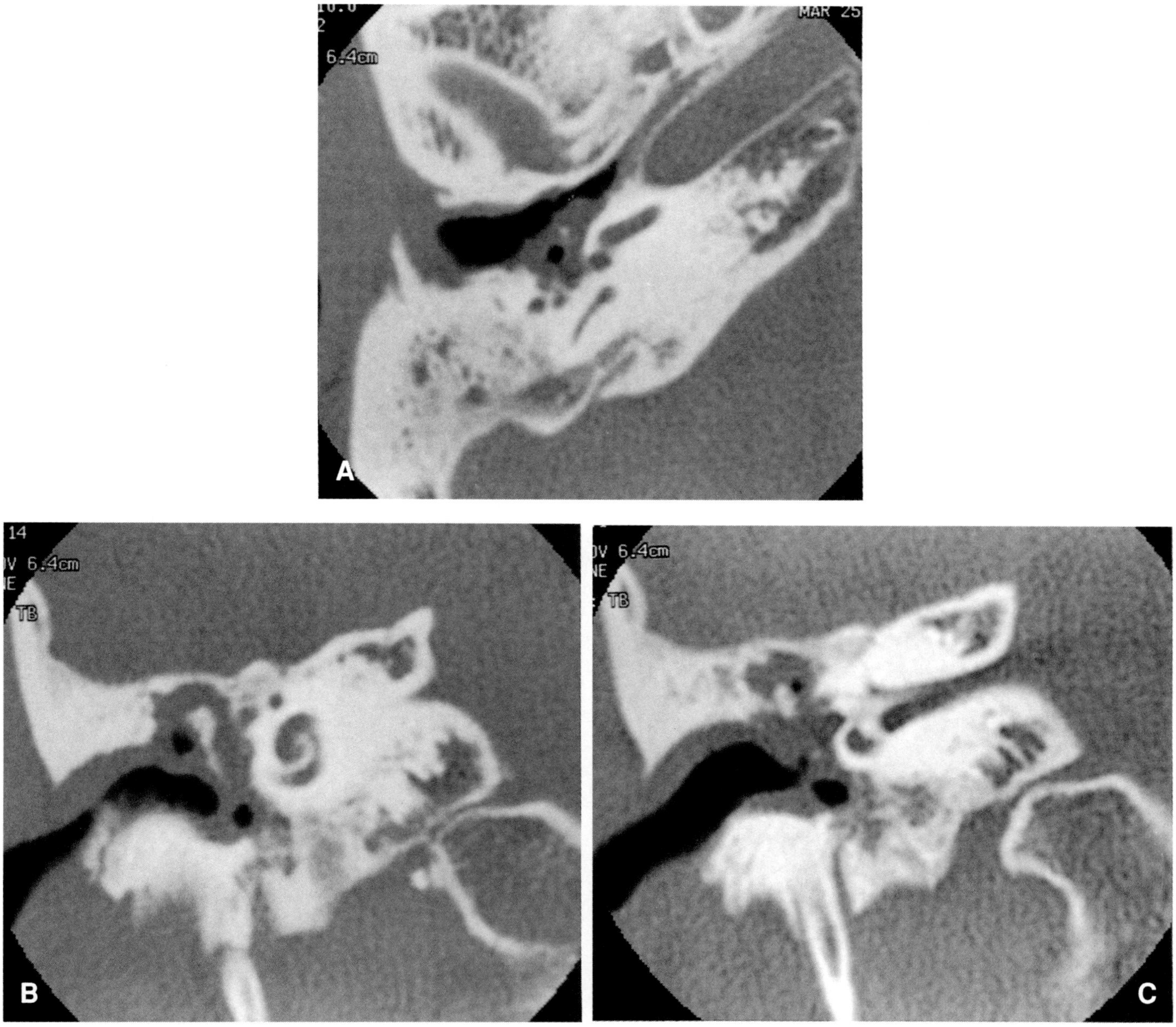

Figure 23-1

This 2-year-old boy has impaired hearing. You are shown a 1-mm axial (A) and contiguous 1-mm direct coronal (B and C) CT images of the petrous bone (Figure 23-1).

112. Which *one* of the following is the MOST likely diagnosis?

    (A) Congenital cholesteatoma
    (B) Acquired cholesteatoma
    (C) Rhabdomyosarcoma
    (D) Langerhans cell histiocytosis
    (E) Cholesterol granuloma

QUESTIONS 113 THROUGH 116: MARK YOUR ANSWER SHEET TRUE (T) OR FALSE (F) FOR EACH OF THE RESPONSE CHOICES.

113. Concerning congenital cholesteatoma,

    (A) it usually appears as an asymptomatic mass behind an intact tympanic membrane
    (B) it usually is diagnosed in the neonatal period
    (C) it usually originates anterior to the malleus
    (D) it is difficult to distinguish from acquired cholesteatoma in most patients

114. Concerning acquired cholesteatoma,

(A) it is associated with chronic suppurative otitis media in most patients
(B) it usually can be diagnosed on physical examination
(C) axial CT images are the most sensitive images for detecting bone destruction
(D) it usually is treated with antibiotics alone

115. Concerning Langerhans cell histiocytosis of the temporal bone,

(A) it represents the most common site of involvement in the skull
(B) it can present clinically as chronic otitis externa
(C) ossicular sclerosis is characteristic
(D) it usually is a component of the chronic multifocal form of Langerhans cell histiocytosis

116. Concerning cholesterol granuloma,

(A) it usually is the result of a viral infection
(B) it usually occurs in children less than 3 years old
(C) physical examination demonstrates a blue tympanic membrane
(D) it is pathologically similar to cholesteatoma
(E) the lesion exhibits high signal intensity on both T1- and T2-weighted images

Case 24: Questions 117 through 120

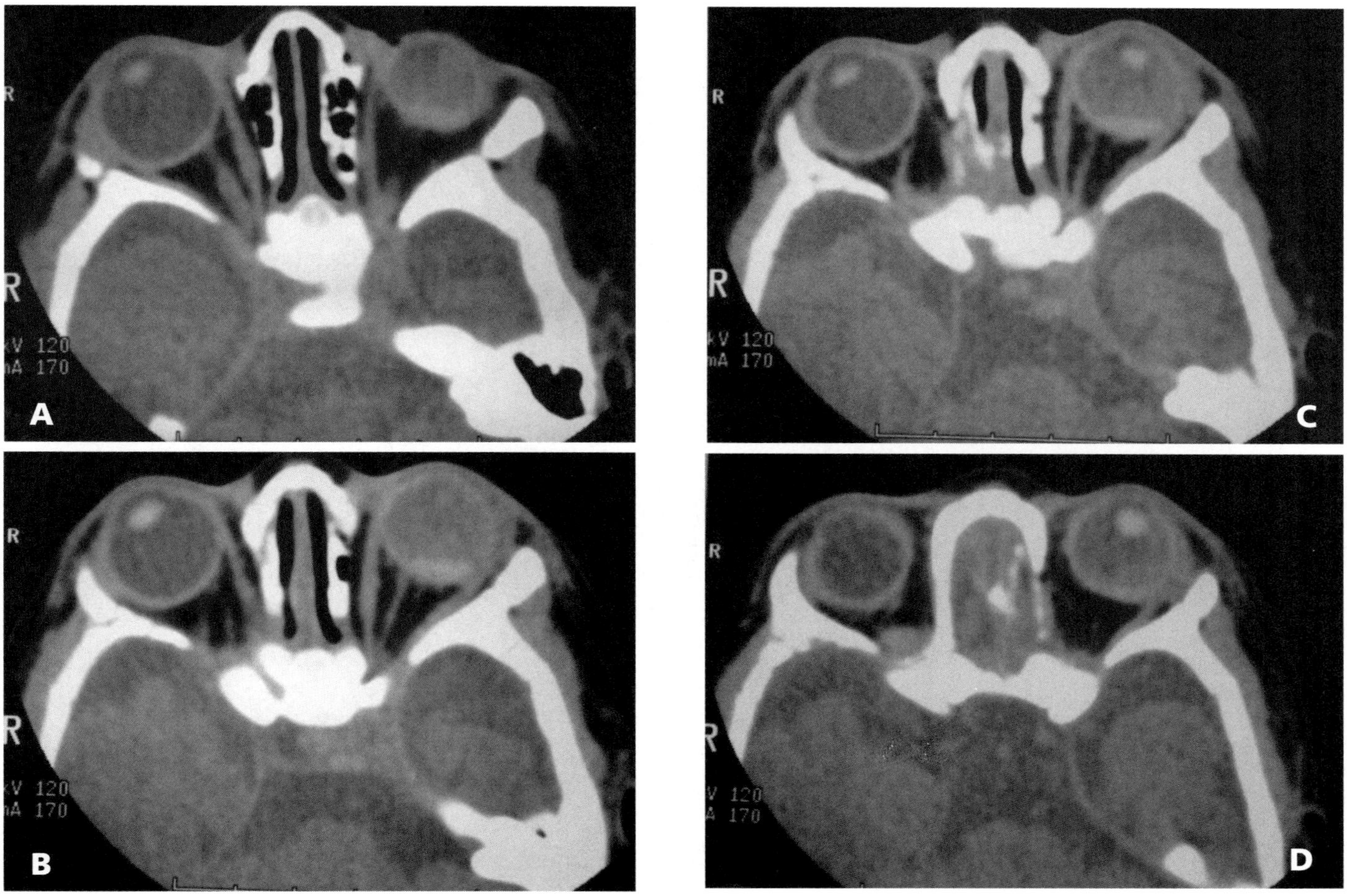

Figure 24-1

This 4-week-old girl has an abnormal left-sided light reflex on physical examination. You are shown postcontrast CT scans of the orbits (Figure 24-1).

117. Which *one* of the following is the MOST likely diagnosis?

(A) Retinoblastoma
(B) Coats' disease
(C) Toxoplasmosis
(D) Coloboma
(E) Persistent hyperplastic primary vitreous

QUESTIONS 118 THROUGH 120: MARK YOUR ANSWER SHEET TRUE (T) OR FALSE (F) FOR EACH OF THE RESPONSE CHOICES.

118. Concerning retinoblastoma,

(A) it is inheritable in approximately 40% of cases
(B) the heritable form is associated with an increased incidence of second primary tumors
(C) it spreads chiefly by direct invasion
(D) leukocoria is characteristic
(E) tumor calcification is identified by CT in about 90% of cases
(F) the trilateral form involves the pituitary gland

119. Concerning Coats' disease

(A) it is a vasculitis
(B) it usually is unilateral
(C) CT demonstrates increased attenuation of the posterior chamber of the globe
(D) the subretinal exudate usually is calcified

120. Concerning coloboma,

(A) it results from lack of closure of the choroidal fissure
(B) it involves only the optic nerve
(C) it is associated with midline intracranial anomalies
(D) on CT, there is bulbous enlargement of the optic nerve at its junction with the globe
(E) it is associated with retinal detachment

Demographic Data Questions

Please answer all of the questions in this section. The data you provide will be used to supply information that will allow you to compare your performance on the examination with that of others at similar levels of training and with similar backgrounds and for purposes of planning continuing education projects. Please answer each question as accurately and as objectively as possible. Please mark the *one* BEST response for each question. Recall, of course, that we do *not* want individual names. Our analyses will reflect only categories and groups; everything will remain completely anonymous, and no attempt will be made to identify any specific individual.

121. The ACR will be evaluating the questions in this examination to determine their degree of difficulty and to determine the success of the examination as an instrument of self-evaluation and continuing education. To assist the ACR, please indicate in which of the following ways you took this examination.

(A) Used reference materials or read the syllabus portion of this book to assist in answering some portion of the examination
(B) Did not use reference materials and did not read the syllabus portion of this book while taking the examination

122. How much residency and fellowship training in Radiology have you completed?

(A) None
(B) Less than 1 year
(C) 1 year
(D) 2 years
(E) 3 years
(F) 4 years
(G) 5 or more years

123. When did you finish your residency training in Radiology?

(A) More than 10 years ago
(B) 5 to 10 years ago
(C) 1 to 5 years ago
(D) Less than 1 year ago
(E) Not yet completed
(F) Radiology is not my specialty

124. Have you been certified by the American Board of Radiology?

(A) Yes
(B) No

125. Have you completed fellowship training in pediatric radiology?

(A) Yes
(B) No

126. Which one of the categories listed below BEST describes the setting of your practice in the immediate past 3 years? (For residents and fellows, in which one did you or will you spend the major portion of your residency or fellowship?)

(A) Community or general hospital—less than 200 beds
(B) Community or general hospital—200 to 499 beds
(C) Community or general hospital—500 or more beds
(D) University-affiliated hospital
(E) Office practice

127. In which one of the following general areas of Radiology do you consider yourself MOST expert?

(A) Breast imaging
(B) Cardiovascular radiology
(C) Chest radiology
(D) Gastrointestinal radiology
(E) Genitourinary radiology
(F) Head and neck radiology
(G) Musculoskeletal radiology
(H) Neuroradiology
(I) Pediatric radiology
(J) Other

128. In which one of the following radiologic modalities do you consider yourself MOST expert?

(A) Computed tomography
(B) General angiography
(C) Interventional radiology
(D) Magnetic resonance imaging
(E) Nuclear radiology
(F) Ultrasonography
(G) Radiation oncology
(H) Other

Pediatric Disease

(Fifth Series)

Test and Syllabus

The Table of Contents is placed in this unusual location so that the reader will not be distracted by information helping to answer the questions before completing the test. A detailed index of the topics considered in this syllabus is provided (beginning on p. 345) for further reference.

Table of Contents

Pediatric Disease

(Fifth Series)

Syllabus

CASE 1

Marta Hernanz-Schulman, M.D.

Extralobar Sequestration

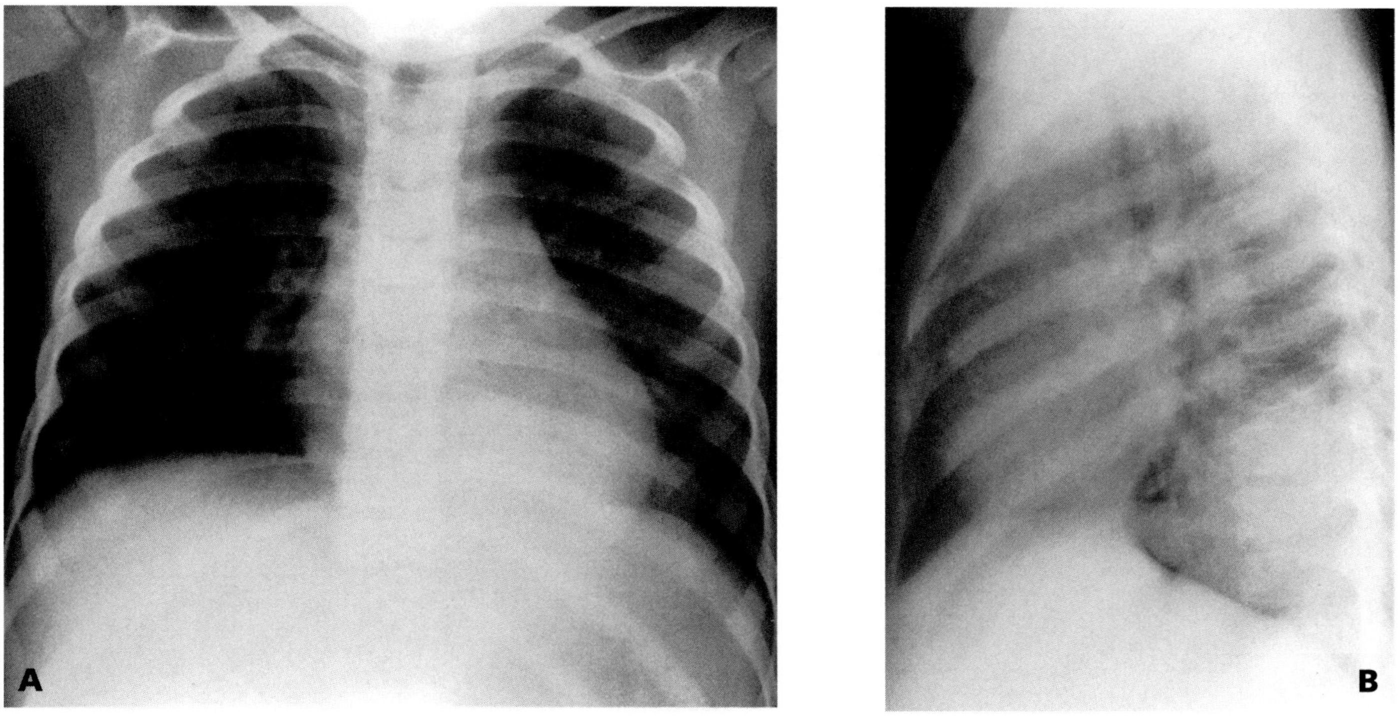

Figure 1-1

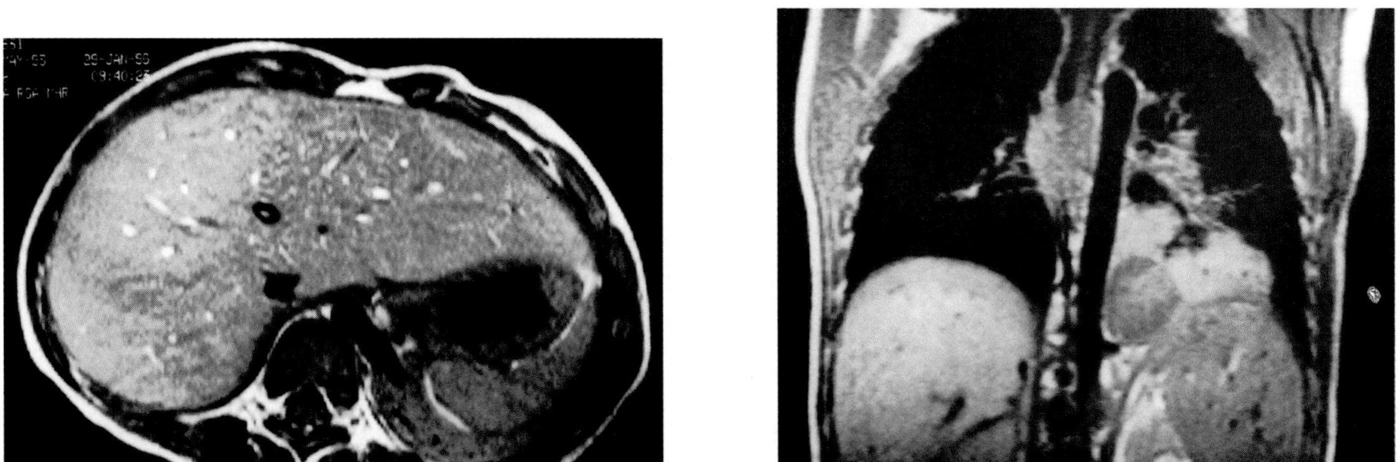

SE 641/15 SE 641/15

Figure 1-2

Question 1

This 7-year-old girl has been treated for pneumonia for 3 weeks and has not responded to antibiotic therapy. You are shown frontal (A) and lateral (B) chest radiographs (Figure 1-1) and axial (A) and coronal (B) T1-weighted MR images (Figure 1-2).

Which *one* of the following is the MOST likely diagnosis?

(A) Lung abscess
(B) Pulmonary blastoma
(C) Infected pulmonary cyst
(D) Bronchopulmonary sequestration
(E) Neuroblastoma

The test patient's chest radiographs (Figure 1-1) demonstrate an opacity at the left base posteriorly that is devoid of air bronchograms (Figure 1-3). The lateral and anterior borders of this lesion are somewhat indistinct but appear circumscribed and outwardly convex, especially on the lateral view, suggesting a masslike lesion. The finding of such a lesion, especially in a posterior basilar segment, should suggest bronchopulmonary sequestration in a patient with repeated episodes of pneumonia confined to the same location or in a patient with a poor response to appropriate antibiotic treatment. The typical location, masslike borders, and association with a recalcitrant febrile illness led to performance of the MRI examination in the test patient. T1-weighted axial and coronal MR images (Figure 1-2) demonstrate a central mass with cystic components, as well as a large systemic artery arising from the descending aorta and supplying the lesion (Figure 1-4). These findings confirm that bronchopulmonary sequestration is the most likely diagnosis (**Option (D) is correct**). The supplying systemic artery is outlined more precisely on an oblique parasagittal T1-weighted image (Figure 1-5) obtained by prescribing a plane paralleling the course of the vessel on the basis of the axial scans.

Lung abscess (Option (A)) can present as a masslike lesion within an area of pneumonia (Figure 1-6A and B). If there has been erosion into the airway, an air-fluid level will be present. If not, imaging studies will demonstrate a fluid-filled cavity (Figure 1-6C). In patients with a pulmonary abscess within normal lung parenchyma, however, a single, large systemic vessel feeding the mass would not be found. Therefore, abscess is an unlikely diagnosis.

Solid pulmonary tumors are usually large masses at presentation and are rare in childhood. Therefore, although a tumor is possible in the test patient, it is a statistically unlikely consideration on the basis of the chest radiographs. The MR images further demonstrate a single large aortic branch supplying this mass, which would render a tumor highly unlikely.

Solid pulmonary neoplasms that occur in children include pulmonary leiomyosarcoma, rhabdomyosarcoma, Askin tumor, and pulmonary blastoma. The symptoms at presentation include cough or pneumonia, although some patients are asymptomatic.

Pulmonary leiomyosarcoma and rhabdomyosarcoma are rare myogenic tumors. Leiomyosarcomas arise in smooth muscle in the pulmonary vasculature or the walls of the tracheobronchial tree. Rhabdomyosarcomas can arise in patients with preexisting cystic disease, such as a cystic adenomatoid malformation or mesenchymal cystic hamartoma. The radiologic ap-

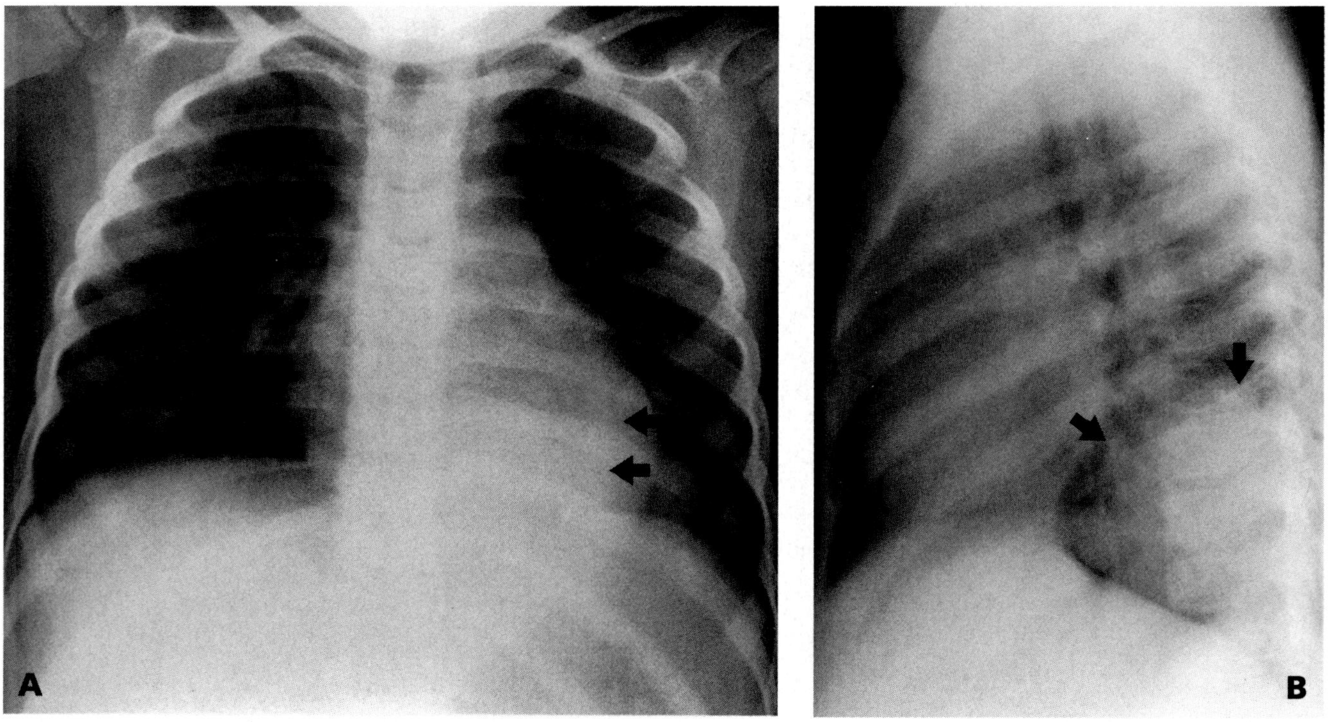

Figure 1-3 (Same as Figure 1-1). Sequestration. Frontal (A) and lateral (B) radiographs of the chest demonstrate a retrocardiac opacity (arrows). On the lateral radiograph, the opacity appears as a mass lesion that lacks air bronchograms.

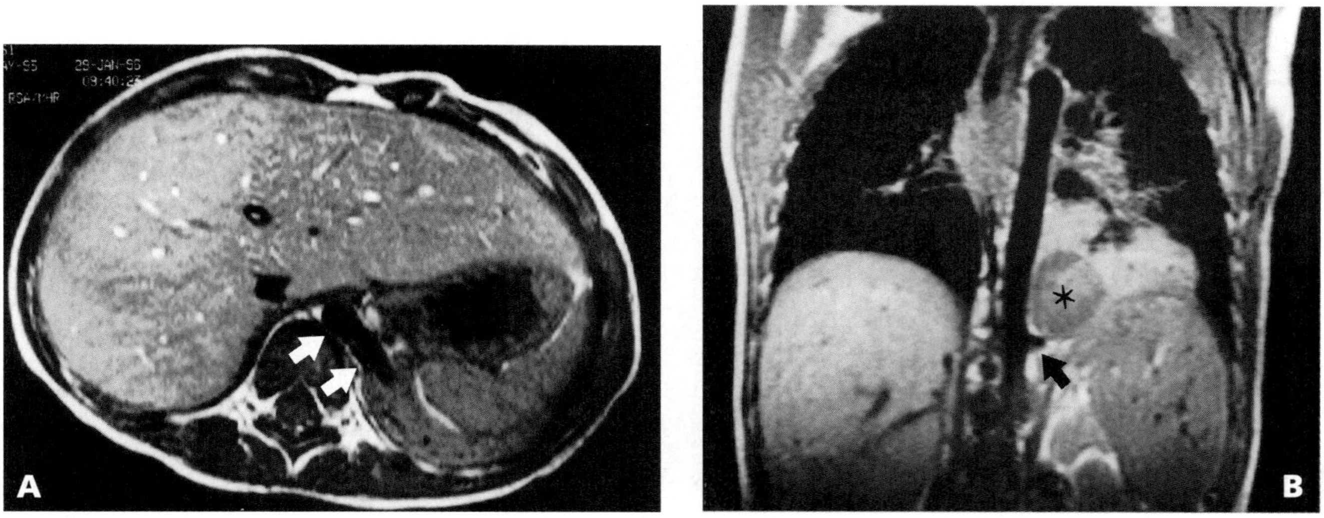

SE 641/15 SE 641/15

Figure 1-4 (Same as Figure 1-2). Sequestration. Axial (A) and coronal (B) T1-weighted images confirm the juxtadiaphragmatic location of the lesion, which is of mixed attenuation, with a lower-intensity cystic area (*) more medially. A large, single feeding artery arises from the juxtacrural portion of the aorta (arrows). Note the similarity in the appearance of the mass on the coronal image and on the frontal chest radiograph (Figure 1-3A).

pearance of rhabdomyosarcomas is similar to that of other pulmonary neoplasms and consists of a large opacity on chest radiographs (Figure 1-7A) that, on further imaging, is demonstrated to be a solid lesion with heterogeneous contrast enhancement (Figure 1-7B and C). The lesion can be associated with spontaneous pneumothorax. The Askin tumor is a highly malignant primitive neuroectodermal tumor that arises in the chest wall; it can grow inwardly and fill the hemithorax, simulating necrotizing pneumonia both clinically and on radiologic imaging. In some patients, the mass appears to be purely parenchymal; more than half will experience local rib erosion. Pulmonary blastoma (Option (B)) consists of mesenchymal and epithelial elements, usually presenting as a large solid mass that can arise in an area of preexisting cystic disease, and may be part of the spectrum of pulmonary mesenchymal cystic sarcoma. It is considered distinct from pulmonary blastoma in adults because of its variable anatomic location, primitive embryonic blastema and stroma, absence of carcinomatous components, and potential for sarcomatous differentiation. The clinical presentation is nonspecific, and children are often treated initially for presumed pulmonary infection. The tumor can be accompanied by pleural effusion and, more rarely, by pneumothorax.

Pulmonary parenchymal cysts are believed to originate as a result of abnormal peripheral bronchial multiplication between weeks 6 and 16 of gestation, resulting in disorganization and separation of distal bronchial generations from the central tracheobronchial tree. The cysts contain air as a result of communication with the normal airways; however, bronchial communication is not invariable, and a noncommunicating cyst can be fluid filled and may be discovered incidentally as an asymptomatic lesion. The abnormal connections lead to susceptibility of the resultant spaces to recurrent infection and to air trapping. An infected cyst typically contains fluid, exhibits an air-fluid level, and has a thickened wall. If obstructed, the cyst can be fluid filled and airless. Continued enlargement of the cyst through air trapping can lead to acute respiratory embarrassment and a tension cyst or pneumothorax at presentation (Figure 1-8). The typical location is within the lung periphery. Pulmonary cysts can be multiple and can affect one or both lungs. Communication with the airway, although not invariable, is usually present; therefore, an airless mass would be atypical. Moreover, there is no systemic vascular supply to a cyst. Consequently, in-

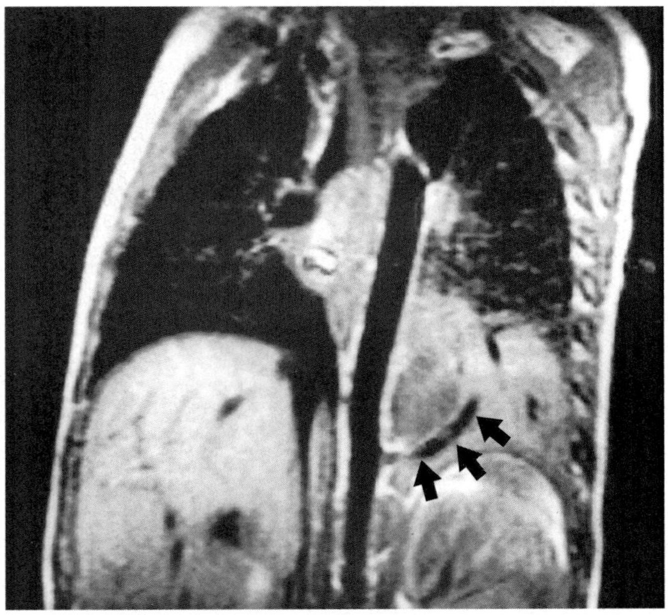

Figure 1-5. Same patient as in Figures 1-1 through 1-4. Sequestration. A parasagittal oblique T1-weighted MR image demonstrates the course of the aortic feeding vessel (arrows) into the sequestered lung segment. The plane of the section in this figure is described by a line drawn along the axis of the feeding artery in Figure 1-4A.

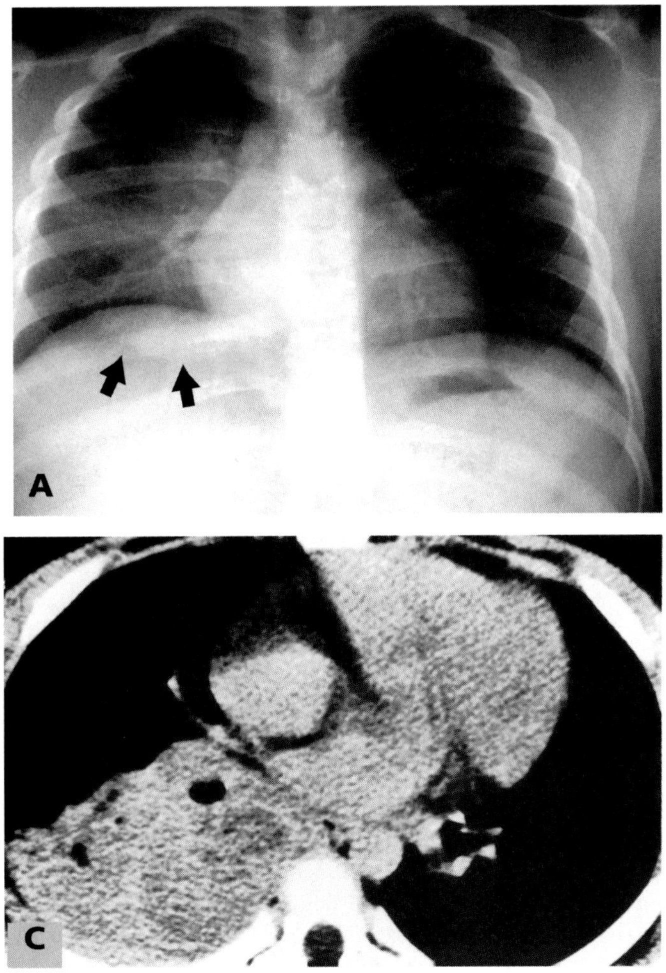

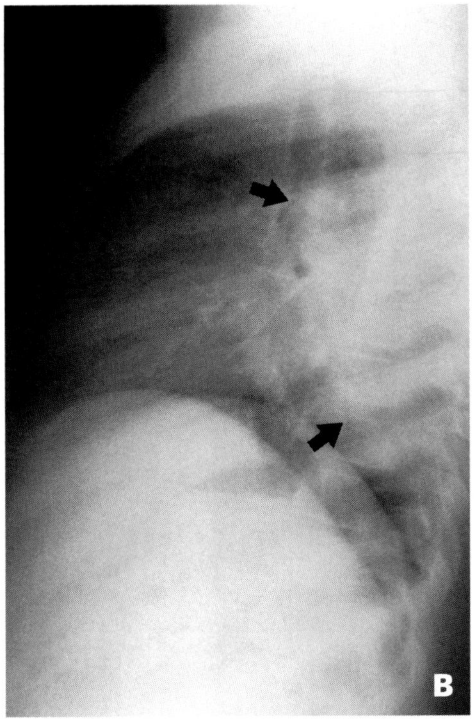

Figure 1-6. Lung abscess. Frontal (A) and lateral (B) radiographs of the chest in a 7-year-old girl with persistent pneumonia involving the superior segment of the right lower lobe show a masslike component at the right base (arrows). (C) An image from a postcontrast CT scan demonstrates a central area of low attenuation with modest but diagnostic mural enhancement, surrounded by consolidated parenchyma. This appearance is consistent with a central abscess without communication with the bronchial tree.

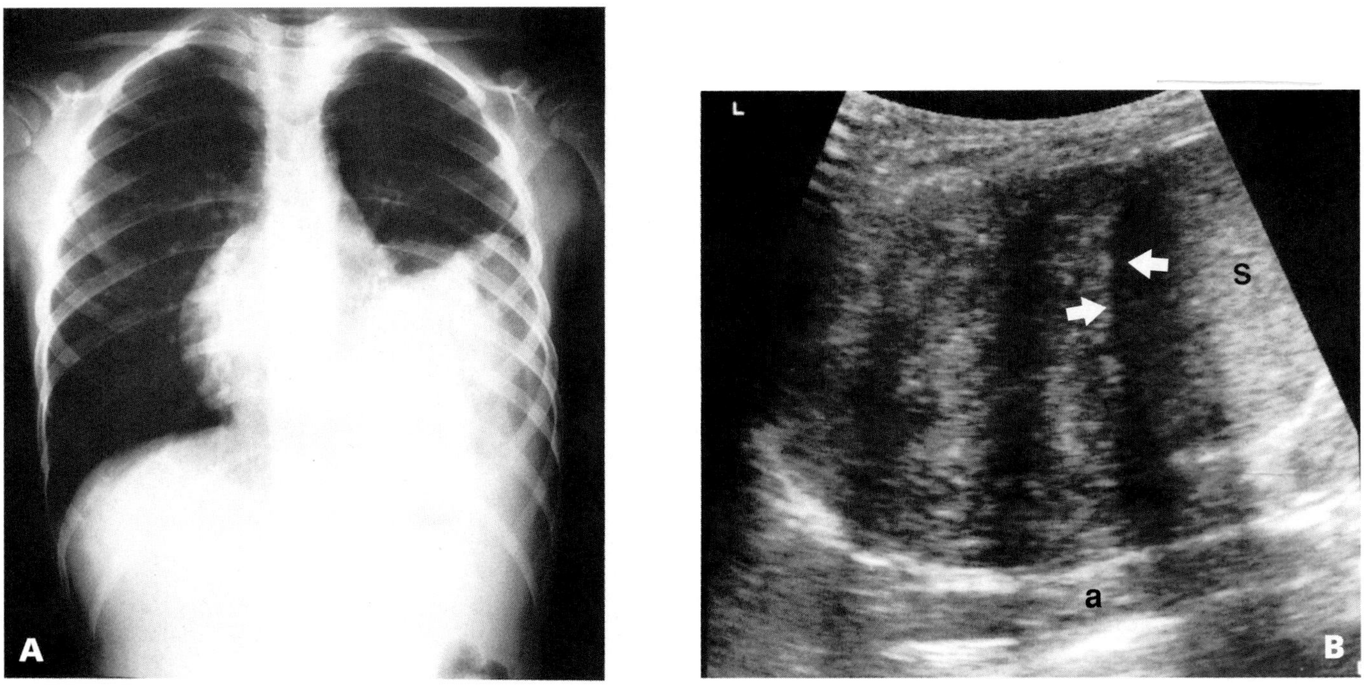

Figure 1-7. Pulmonary rhabdomyosarcoma. (A) A chest radiograph of a 4-year-old girl with cough and fever demonstrates a dense lesion at the left base, devoid of air bronchograms. (B) A left coronal sonogram shows that the lesion is solid, lacking the branching, echogenic bronchial structures typically seen in consolidated parenchyma. There is no pleural effusion. a = aorta; S = spleen. Arrows point to the diaphragmatic interface.

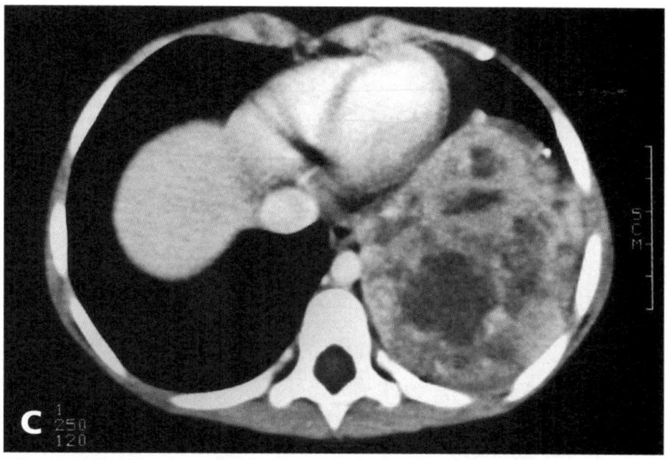

Figure 1-7 (Continued). Pulmonary rhabdomyosarcoma. (C) An image from a postcontrast CT scan confirms the absence of normal pulmonary parenchymal structures. The mass is of heterogeneous attenuation, demonstrating multiple internal areas of necrosis.

fected pulmonary cyst (Option (C)) is not a likely diagnosis in the test patient.

Neuroblastoma (Option (E)) is the most common solid tumor of childhood, and approximately 15% occur in the chest in a paraspinal location. Approximately 30% of thoracic neuroblastomas demonstrate some calcification on conventional radiographs, and rib erosions are often present. However, most thoracic neuroblastomas are not calcified, and rib erosions are not a prerequisite for the diagnosis. Therefore, this entity is a possible diagnosis on the basis of the chest radiographs of the test patient. However, further observations demonstrate that the upper borders of the lesion in the test patient are not well defined, presumably owing to surrounding pneumonitis, whereas the borders of the mediastinal lesion in patients with neuroblastoma are usually well outlined by the air in the adjacent lung (Figure 1-9A and B). Internal cystic components, which are present in the test patient, are not characteristic of paraspinal neuroblastoma, which typically appears as a solid, homogeneous mass on CT or MRI (Figure 1-9C to E). Metastatic pulmonary involvement in patients with neuroblastoma is rare, occurs very late in the disease, and is usually a grave prognostic sign. It is reported in approximately 11% of autopsies, but is rarely documented during life. The vascular supply of thoracic neuroblastoma arises from the systemic circulation, but is derived from parasitization of small, neighboring vessels rather than through a single, large, systemic feeding vessel. Thus, neuroblastoma is an unlikely diagnosis in the test patient.

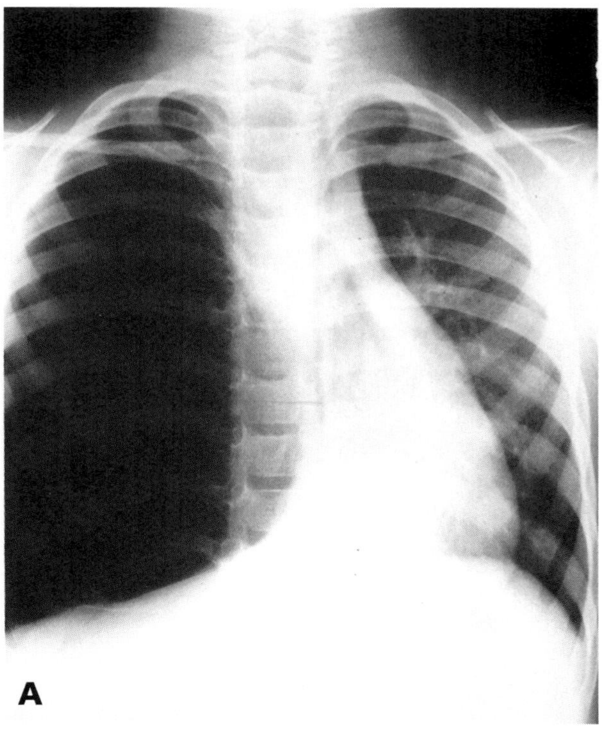

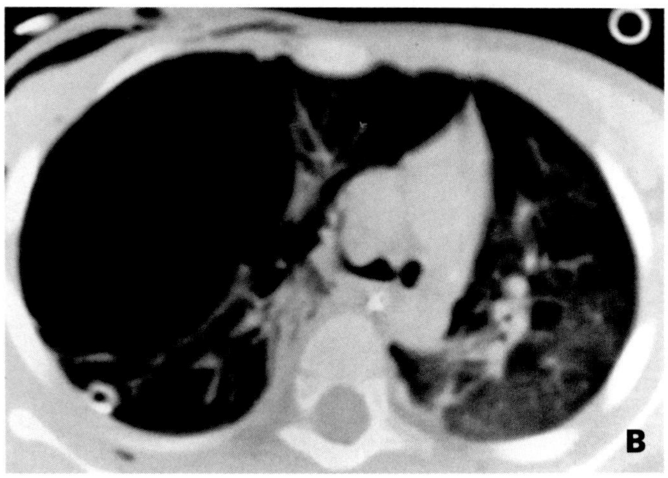

Figure 1-8. Pulmonary cyst. (A) A chest radiograph of a child with severe respiratory distress demonstrates an air-filled tension cyst expanding the right hemithorax, depressing the ipsilateral hemidiaphragm, and producing a contralateral mediastinal shift. (B) A CT scan of the tension cyst demonstrates a large cyst producing a contralateral mediastinal shift. A chest tube placed to treat a coincident pneumothorax (and associated subcutaneous emphysema) is seen posterolaterally.

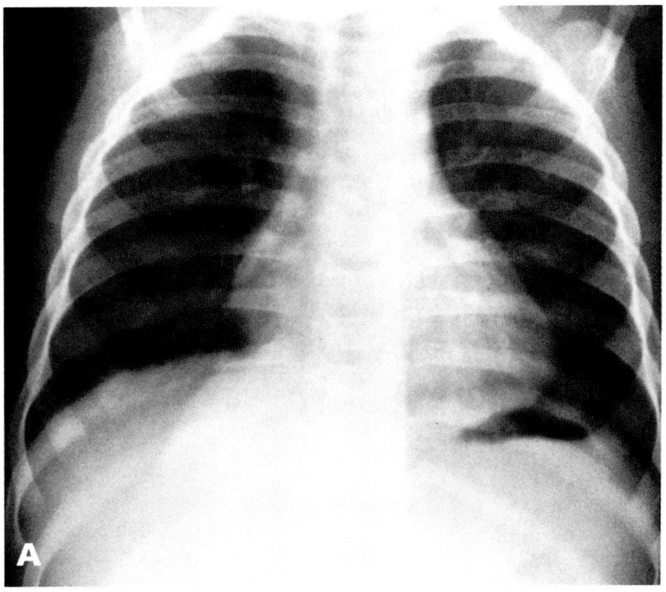

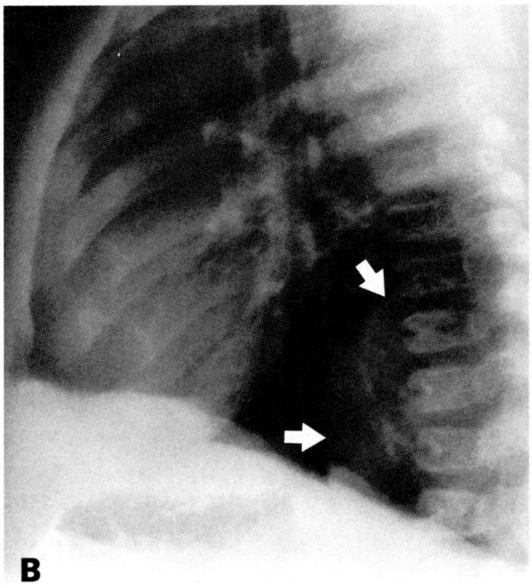

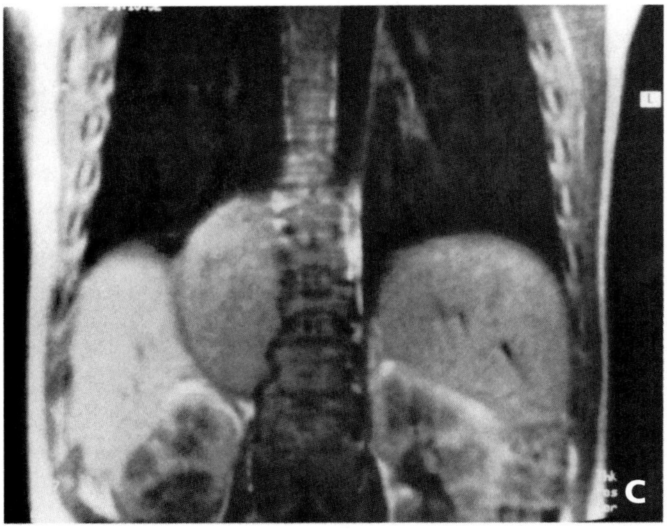

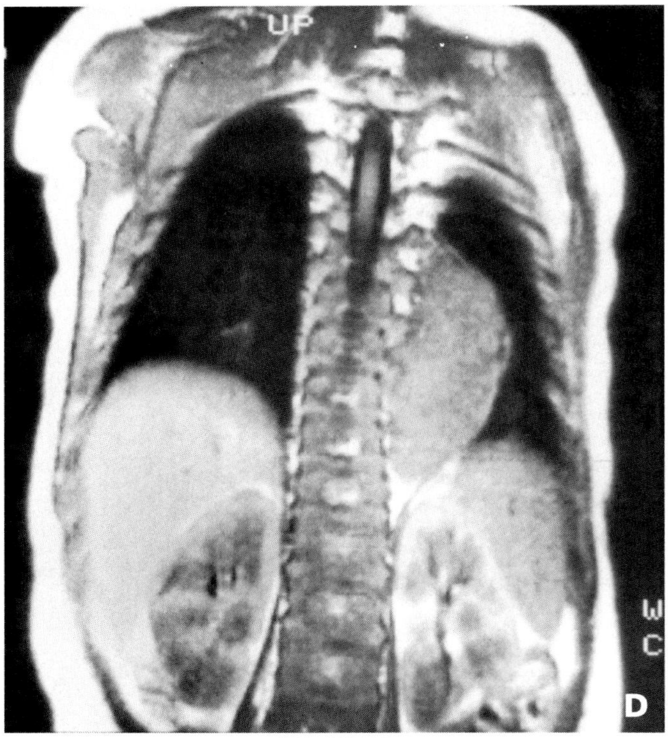

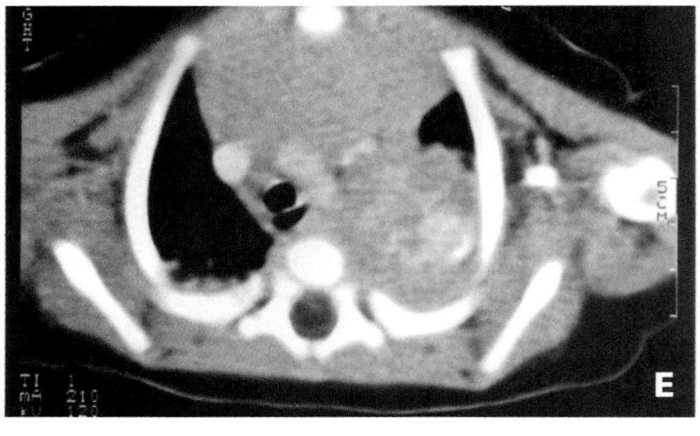

Figure 1-9. Paraspinal neuroblastoma. Frontal (A) and lateral (B) chest radiographs obtained for reasons unrelated to the neuroblastoma demonstrate a mass at the right base. Note the well-defined borders of the posterior lesion (arrows). (C) A coronal T1-weighted MR image demonstrates the solid, homogeneous mass. (D) A coronal MR image of another patient demonstrates a solid, homogeneous left-sided paraspinal neuroblastoma with characteristic interdigitations into the neural foramina. (E) An axial postcontrast CT scan of another patient shows a solid paraspinal mass; high-density areas within the lesion were present on precontrast images and represent calcifications.

Question 2

Concerning lung abscess,

(A) in a neonate, it is usually associated with sepsis
(B) an underlying congenital anomaly is usually present
(C) the diagnosis should be suspected in a patient with pneumonia unresponsive to antibiotic treatment
(D) an air-fluid level is present on CT in virtually all patients
(E) surgical treatment is usually necessary

Primary pulmonary abscesses are defined as those occurring in patients without underlying predisposing conditions, such as cystic fibrosis or immune deficiency. They are believed to be less common than secondary abscesses, which occur in immunocompromised patients, although more recent experience has shown a decline in the latter group, probably secondary to more vigilant monitoring of susceptible children. The age distribution favors younger children (mean age, 8 years), although abscesses can occur at all ages. In infants, although rare, abscesses are usually associated with sepsis (**Option (A) is true**). Abscesses in older children infrequently originate in an underlying congenital anomaly, such as a cystic adenomatoid malformation, but usually occur as a complication of pneumonia or aspiration or distal to an obstructing foreign body (**Option (B) is false**). Recovery of organisms is often confounded by prior antibiotic treatment; however, common blood culture isolates include *Staphylococcus aureus*, *Streptococcus pneumoniae*, *Klebsiella pneumoniae*, and *Escherichia coli*. The lesions are distributed equally in both lungs, although some authors have observed a preponderance in the right lung.

Pulmonary abscess should be considered in a patient of any age in whom a persistent pulmonary opacity devoid of air bronchograms is seen on radiographs after adequate treatment for underlying pneumonia or sepsis (Figure 1-6A and B) (**Option (C) is true**). When an abscess is suspected on the basis of these radiographic findings and clinical course, further imaging, such as CT scanning, should be undertaken to identify the lesion so that appropriate treatment can be instituted. On CT scans, the abscess cavity is of low or similar attenuation relative to the surrounding consolidated parenchyma and, because there is no pulmonary tissue, is devoid of air bronchograms or vascular markings. After the intravenous administration of contrast material, a peripheral ring of increased enhancement is noted around the abscess cavity (Figure 1-6C). There is less enhancement of the surrounding infected pulmonary parenchyma. The abscess cavity may contain an air-fluid level when there is communication with the airway, but this is not a prerequisite for the diagnosis on the basis of either chest radiographs or CT scans (**Option (D) is false**).

The prognosis of lung abscess in children is excellent if it is treated with appropriate intravenous antibiotics. CT- or sonography-guided transthoracic aspiration can be performed to obtain appropriate material for culturing, and percutaneous drainage can expedite complete recovery. Surgical management, such as lobectomy, is reserved for patients for whom medical therapy has not been effective and is seldom required (**Option (E) is false**).

Question 3

Concerning imaging of bronchopulmonary sequestration,

(A) the feeding vessel usually arises from the subdiaphragmatic aorta
(B) identification of systemic arterial supply is pathognomonic for sequestration
(C) angiographic evaluation is usually necessary to delineate the feeding vessel
(D) sonography is a reliable diagnostic technique in neonates
(E) on CT, the feeding vessel enhances at the same time as the aorta

Bronchopulmonary sequestrations are defined as areas of lung tissue without a normal connection to the tracheobronchial tree; approximately 80% of them are supplied by a single vessel and 20% are supplied by several vessels from the systemic circulation, usually the lower thoracic or upper abdominal aorta or its branches. Approximately 80% of sequestrations are intralobar, and the systemic vessel arises from the thoracic aorta in 73% of these (**Option (A) is false**).

Sequestrations are believed to be part of the spectrum of bronchopulmonary foregut malformations and to arise from abnormal or supernumerary budding of the branching tracheobronchial tree, with separation of the resultant segment from the parent bronchus and retention of the primitive systemic arterial supply of the foregut. Extralobar sequestrations are invested with their own pleural envelope, and venous drainage is usually to the systemic circulation. Extralobar sequestrations are located at the left base in approximately 90% of patients, as in the test patient. However, they can also be found in the mediastinum, within the pericardium or diaphragm, or infradiaphragmatically in the retroperitoneum, where the sequestered segment is usually found to have undergone maldevelopment into a cystic adenomatoid malformation.

Intralobar sequestrations lie within the pulmonary parenchyma and lack an intrinsic pleural investment; their venous drainage is usually to the pulmonary circulation. Most intralobar sequestrations are also located at the left base, but approximately 40% are found at the right base.

In as many as 50% of patients, extralobar sequestration is associated with other congenital anomalies, most commonly diaphragmatic hernia, cystic adenomatoid malformation, and bronchogenic cyst. The spectrum of presentation varies greatly, from fetal hydrops to asymptomatic lesions; the latter are especially likely when the sequestration is extrathoracic. In older children and young adults, both intralobar and extralobar types are associated with recurrent infections. Because intralobar sequestrations are most commonly encountered in this older group and associated congenital anomalies are typically absent, some authors have postulated that these are acquired lesions, resulting from recurrent infections leading to obliteration of a normal connection to the tracheobronchial tree and to parasitization of systemic vessels from the inferior pulmonary ligament. However, intralobar sequestration is occasionally found in infants (Figure 1-10), can receive its vascular supply from an infradiaphragmatic branch of the abdominal aorta, and can demonstrate a connection to the gastrointestinal tract, indicating that it, too, is a bronchopulmonary foregut malformation, at least in some cases.

Sequestrations are typically airless, and small or large cysts can be found within the solid internal architecture, reflecting adenomatoid elements or repeated episodes of infection in older children. These cysts can contain serous or mucoid material and are of low attenuation on CT scans (Figure 1-11) or appear as anechoic spaces on sonography. The mucoid material results in high signal intensity on T1-weighted MR images, as in the test patient, and intermediate or high signal intensity on T2-weighted images. Patent communication with the gastrointestinal tract can produce unusual air spaces within the lesion (Figure 1-10).

By definition, sequestrations are pulmonary parenchymal lesions without normal communication with the tracheobronchial tree. In the past, bronchography was used to identify this lack of communication, demonstrating "draping" of normal bronchi around the mass. However, lack of air within any lesion implies effective sequestration from the airway, regardless of etiology, and this invasive and relatively nonspecific modality is no longer believed to be of clinical value.

The preoperative differentiation of sequestration from other congenital cystic lung lesions lies in the identification of the systemic feeding vessel, which is seen in approximately 95% of lesions. However, demonstration of an anomalous artery is not specific for sequestration. Other lung lesions, such as chronic infection or a systemic-pulmonary arteriovenous fistula, can demonstrate systemic arterial supply (**Option (B) is false**). Differentiation between intralobar and extralobar sequestrations preoperatively is unnecessary, and it is probably not possible for intrapulmonary lesions owing to the overlap in venous drainage that can occur between these types of lesions. Before the advent of Doppler sonography, CT, and MRI, the diagnosis of sequestration was made by angiography (Figure 1-12), a procedure that was believed to be mandatory to identify an abdominal feeding artery that could retreat into the abdomen during attempted resection and lead to exsanguination of the patient. However, because pediatric surgeons are aware

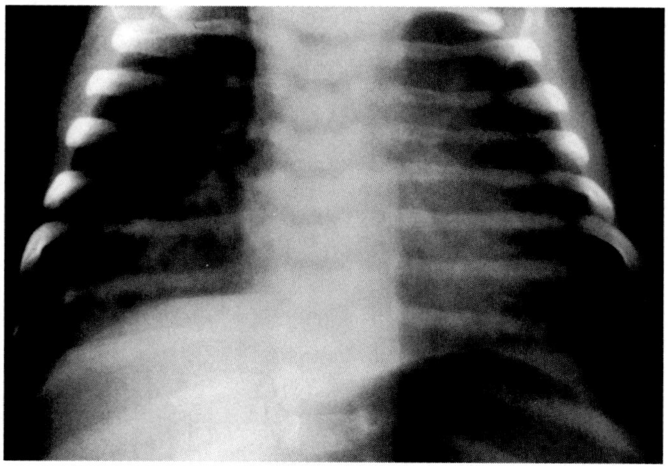

Figure 1-10. Sequestration. A frontal chest radiograph of a 2-month-old infant, obtained for evaluation of a murmur that was later proven to result from a patent ductus arteriosus, demonstrates a right basilar density. Multiple rounded lucencies within the lesion arose from a patent communication with the esophagus, which was demonstrated at surgery.

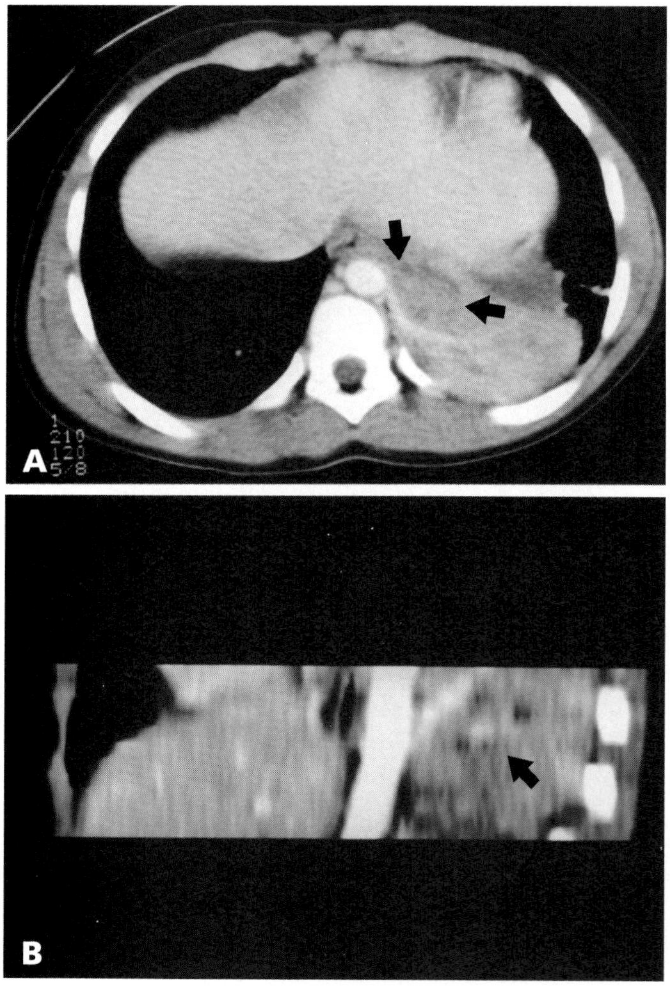

Figure 1-11. Sequestration. (A) A postcontrast CT scan of a 10-year-old girl with pneumonia shows a masslike lesion at the left base. The spiral examination with 5-mm collimation demonstrates the feeding vessel opacifying synchronously with the thoracic aorta. Note the anterior cystic area of lower attenuation (arrows). (B) Parasagittal reconstruction, described by a line drawn along the axis of the feeding artery similar to the method described for Figure 1-5, demonstrates the course of the feeding artery into the sequestration.

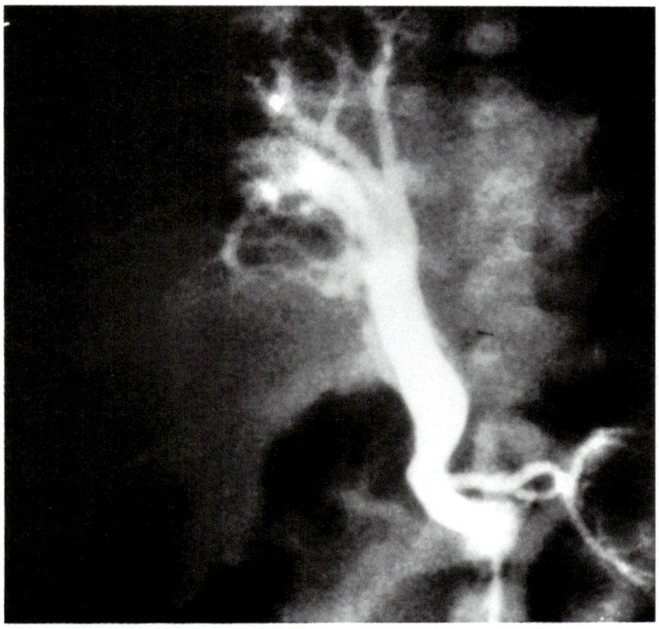

Figure 1-12. Same patient as in Figure 1-10. Seqestration. An angiogram demonstrates a very large feeding vessel arising from the abdominal aorta and extending across the diaphragmatic crura to supply the sequestered lung segment.

of this possibility, abdominal feeding vessels within the pulmonary ligament can be controlled intraoperatively, and angiography is no longer considered necessary. The presence of a feeding vessel can be demonstrated by several less invasive means (**Option (C) is false**).

In infants and young children, Doppler-guided sonography with either the abdomen or the airless sequestration itself as the insonating window will usually successfully demonstrate the feeding vessel (Figure 1-13) (**Option (D) is true**). For older patients or patients in whom interposition of aerated lung prohibits successful sonographic imaging, either CT or MRI should be considered. CT should be performed with bolus contrast agent administration and thin collimation (3 to 5 mm, depending on the patient's age), preferably with spiral technique and coronal reconstruction. The large feeding vessel will opacify at the same time as the aorta (Figure 1-11) (**Option (E) is true**). The advantages of MRI are its multiplanar capability and lack of dependence on optimal timing of the contrast agent bolus; it may therefore prove successful more often than CT in demonstrating the systemic supply to the lesion. T1-weighted images in the axial and coronal planes, supplemented by oblique scans if desired, as in the test patient, are usually sufficient. MRI angiography and TurboFLASH sequences have also been utilized successfully.

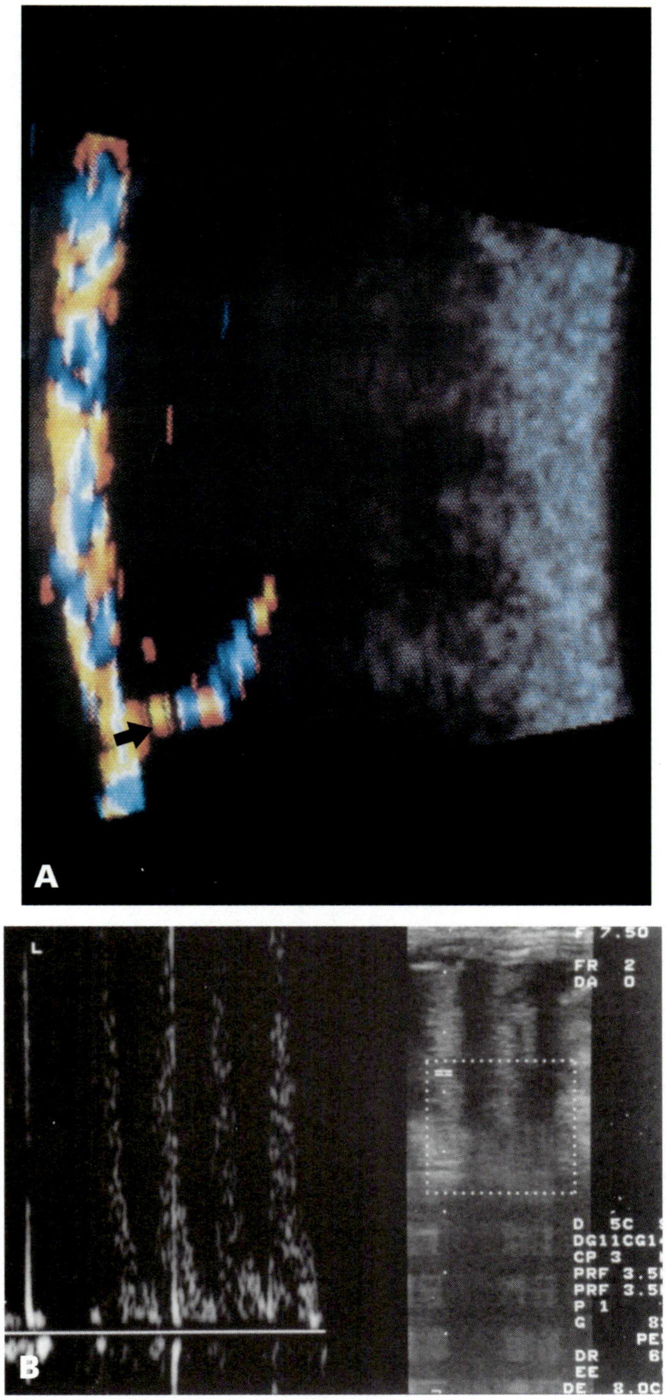

Figure 1-13. Sequestration. A color Doppler angiogram of a newborn infant with an airless left basilar chest mass clearly shows the large subdiaphragmatic aortic feeding vessel. The image was obtained by the left coronal chest approach, with the airless sequestration as the insonating window. (B) Duplex doppler sonogram of a vascular structure within the sequestration demonstrates a systemic arterial signal toward the transducer, indicating flow in a cephalad direction.

Question 4

Concerning thoracic neuroblastoma,

(A) it accounts for about 10% to 15% of all neuroblastomas
(B) it is the most common cause of Horner's syndrome in infancy
(C) opsoclonus-myoclonus at presentation is associated with a poor prognosis
(D) it is less often calcified than abdominal neuroblastoma
(E) the prognosis is better than that of abdominal neuro blastoma

Neuroblastoma is the most common extracranial solid tumor of childhood, accounting for approximately 10% of all childhood cancers. It is slightly more common in boys, with a male/female ratio of approximately 1.2:1. The age distribution is biphasic, with a first incidence peak under 1 year of age and a second peak at 2 to 4 years; 97% of patients are younger than 10 years. Approximately 10% to 15% of neuroblastomas occur in the thorax **(Option (A) is true).**

Clinical manifestations of thoracic neuroblastoma depend partly on the location and size of the lesion. High thoracic lesions involving the stellate ganglion can result in Horner's syndrome (ipsilateral ptosis, miosis, and anhydrosis), but neuro blastoma is an uncommon cause of infantile Horner's syndrome **(Option (B) is false).** In most infants, Horner's syndrome is idiopathic or due to birth trauma. The tumor also may be associated with heterochromia iridis with decreased ipsilateral pigmentation. Pigmentation of the uveal tract is dependent upon an intact sympathetic system; ipsilateral uveal depigmentation can be produced experimentally by excision of the superior cervical ganglion. In children, this association is most often seen in congenital tumors and rarely occurs after 2 years of age. The paraspinal location of these tumors permits growth into the spinal canal through the neural foramina and may lead to symptoms such as pain or paraplegia, although thoracic tumors are often found on chest radiographs taken for other reasons. Large tumors can also cause dysphagia, dyspnea, and repeated respiratory infections.

Paraneoplastic syndromes include hypertension, abdominal distension and watery diarrhea, and opsoclonus-myoclonus. Hypertension occurs in 1% to 5% of patients as a result of abdominal tumors stretching the renal artery, with subsequent activation of the renin-angiotensin system; patients may also undergo episodes of flushing and hypertension as a result of catecholamine release by the tumor. Release of vasoactive intestinal peptide results in abdominal distension and watery diarrhea; this watery diarrhea-hypokalemia syndrome (Werner-Morrison syndrome) is often seen in ganglioneuroblastomas and ganglioneuromas, and therefore it is associated with a good prognosis. Opsoclonus-myoclonus is a syndrome of unknown but possibly autoimmune etiology; neuroblastoma is present in approximately 50% of patients with this syndrome, and approximately 60% of the tumors are present in the thorax. The syndrome may resolve or improve after removal of the primary lesion and is usually responsive to the administration of high-dose corticosteroid or adrenocorticotropic hormone. The tumors that cause this syndrome are usually small, and the prognosis is better than in patients without these associated findings **(Option (C) is false).** Catecholamine neurotransmitters are produced by 90% to 95% of neuroblastomas; the excretion of these neurotransmitters or their metabolites serves as a marker of disease and is of value both in the initial diagnosis and in the monitoring of the disease.

Thoracic tumors can occur in conjunction with intra-abdominal disease. If they are continuous, the dumbbell mass extends through the diaphragmatic hiatus (Figure 1-9A to C). Distinct tumors may occur in some patients with a genetic predisposition to this disease, a germinal mutation that follows an autosomal dominant pattern of inheritance. Approximately 20% of patients with familial neuroblastoma may have bilateral adrenal or multifocal primary tumors. These tumors also tend to occur in younger patients; the median age at diagnosis of these patients is approximately 9 months. It has been estimated that as many as 22% of neuroblastomas may result from a germinal mutation. The initial diagnostic evaluation should include imaging of both the abdomen and the chest by either CT or MRI. Although CT can detect calcifications that are inapparent on MRI, calcifications in thoracic neuroblastomas are present in only approximately 30% of patients, compared with at least 60% of patients with abdominal disease **(Option (D) is true).** MRI is preferable to CT in patients with paraspinal lesions because it more reliably detects extensions into the neural foramina and spinal canal than does CT. On MRI, thoracic neuroblastomas usually show homogeneous signal intensity, similar to or slightly higher than that of muscle on T1-weighted images (Figure 1-9C and D) and higher signal intensity on T2-weighted images, with marked homogeneous enhancement after the administration of gadolinium chelates.

Neuroblastoma exhibits a unique pattern of metastatic spread: to regional and distant lymph nodes, bone marrow, liver, and cortical bone; to the bones of the skull and orbit (Figure 1-14), clinically manifested as periorbital ecchymoses and proptosis; and to the skin, clinically manifested as nontender mobile bluish nodules.

There are several staging systems for neuroblastoma. One system is the Evans system used by the Children's Cancer Study Group. The more recent International Neuroblastoma Staging System (INSS) is based on clinical, imaging, and surgical findings. The INSS can be recognized by its use of arabic numerical designations for staging categories. Stage 1 indicates localized disease, as determined by complete gross excision. Stage 2A denotes localized disease, as determined by incomplete gross excision, but with negative nodes; in stage 2B, ipsilateral nodes are positive. Stage 3 indicates bilateral disease, by virtue of tumor extension across the midline or metastasis to contralateral or bilateral nodes. Stage 4 indicates disease disseminated to distant nodes or organs. Stage 4S indicates disease that would otherwise have been classified as stage 1 or 2, but

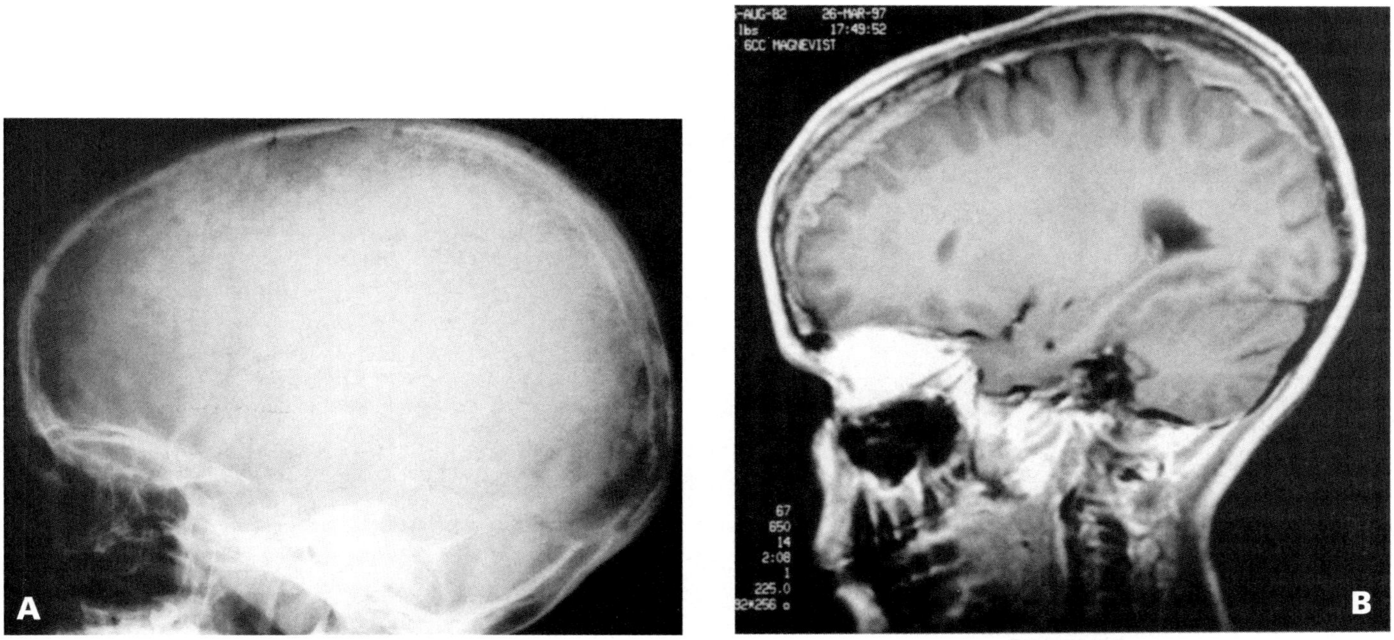

Figure 1-14. Metastatic neuroblastoma. (A) A lateral skull radiograph of a patient with metastatic neuroblastoma demonstrates permeative destruction of skull tables, most marked along the frontal, frontoparietal, and occipital convexities. (B) A parasagittal postcontrast T1-weighted MR image demonstrates multiple enhancing meningeal lesions.

in which distant metastases are limited to skin, liver, and bone marrow (excluding cortical bone).

The prognosis depends on many variables, including age at presentation, staging, site, and histology. Patients who are younger than 1 year at diagnosis have a substantially better prognosis than older children. Spontaneous differentiation into mature ganglioneuroma occurs in approximately 5% of patients, and the majority of these patients are infants. Altogether, more than half of the patients diagnosed with neuroblastoma eventually die of the disease. The overall prognosis for patients with stage 1, 2, and 4S disease is between 80% and 90% 2-year survival; the 2-year disease-free survival rates for patients with stage 3 and 4 disease are 40% and 20%, respectively. Patients with thoracic tumors have a better prognosis than those with abdominal disease, especially tumors originating in the adrenal glands (**Option (E) is true**). Histologically differentiated lesions tend to be associated with localized tumors, and patients with these lesions have a better prognosis than do those with poorly differentiated tumors.

The main methods for the treatment of neuroblastoma are surgery and chemotherapy. Surgery usually is curative for resectable, unilateral tumors (stage 1). Patients with initially unresectable tumors are treated with neoadjuvant chemotherapy followed by surgical resection of residual tumors. Radiation therapy is used for the control of unresponsive, unresectable tumors. Bone marrow transplantation can be used for patients who have a poor long-term prognosis and who have shown initial remission or very good partial remission with chemotherapeutic regimens.

SUGGESTED READINGS

SEQUESTRATION

1. Felker RE, Tonkin IL. Imaging of pulmonary sequestration. AJR 1990; 154:241–249
2. Felson B. The many faces of pulmonary sequestration. Semin Roentgenol 1972; 7:3–16
3. Frush DP, Donnelly LS. Pulmonary sequestration spectrum: a new spin with helical CT. AJR 1997; 169:679–682
4. Gerle RD, Jaretzki A 3d, Ashley C, Berne AS. Congenital bronchopumonary-foregut malformation. Pulmonary sequestration communicating with the gastrointestinal tract. N Engl J Med 1968; 278:1413–1419
5. Hernanz-Schulman M, Johnson JE, Holcomb GW 3rd, Neblett WW 3rd, Heller RM, Ambrosino MM. Retroperitoneal pulmonary sequestration: imaging findings, histopathologic correlation, and relationship to cystic adenomatoid malformation. AJR 1997; 168:1277–1281
6. Hernanz-Schulman M, Stein SM, Neblett WW, et al. Pulmonary sequestration: diagnosis with color Doppler sonography and a new theory of associated hydrothorax. Radiology 1991; 180:817–821
7. Rosado-de-Christenson ML, Frazier AA, Stocker JT, Templeton PA. From the archives of the AFIP. Extralobar sequestration: radiologic-pathologic correlation. RadioGraphics 1993; 13:425–441
8. Stocker JT, Kagan-Hallet K. Extralobar pulmonary sequestration: analysis of 15 cases. Am Soc Clin Pathol 1979; 79:917–925

PULMONARY ABSCESS

9. Asher MI, Spier S, Beland M, Coates AL, Beaudry PH. Primary lung abscess in childhood: the long-term outcome of conservative management. Am J Dis Child 1982; 136:491–494
10. Ball WS Jr, Bisset GS 3d, Towbin RB. Percutaneous drainage of chest abscesses in children. Radiology 1989; 171:431–434
11. Emanuel B, Shulman ST. Lung abscess in infants and children. Clin Pediatr 1995; 34:2–6
12. Groskin SA, Panjcek DM, Ewing DK, et al. Bacterial lung abscess: a review of the radiographic and clinical features of 50 cases. J Thorac Imaging 1991; 6:62–67
13. Johnson JF, Shiels WE, White CB, Williams BD. Concealed pulmonary abscess: diagnosis by computed tomography. Pediatrics 1986; 78:283–286

14. Kaye MG, Fox MJ, Bartlett JG, Braman SS, Glassroth J. The clinical spectrum of *Staphylococcus aureus* pulmonary infection. Chest 1990; 97: 788–792
15. Lee SK, Morris RF, Cramer B. Percutaneous needle aspiration of neonatal lung abscesses. Pediatr Radiol 1991; 21:254–257
16. Tan TQ, Seilheimer DK, Kaplan SL. Pediatric lung abscess: clinical management and outcome. Pediatr Infect Dis J 1995; 14:51–55
17. vanSonnenberg E, D'Agostino HB, Casola G, Wittich GR, Varney RR, Harker C. Lung abscess: CT-guided drainage. Radiology 1991; 178:347–351
18. Yang PC, Luh XT, Lee YC, et al. Lung abscesses: US examination and US-guided transthoracic aspiration. Radiology 1991; 180:171–175

PULMONARY CYSTS

19. Hernanz-Schulman M. Cysts and cystlike lesions of the lung. Radiol Clin North Am 1993; 31:631–649
20. Shanji F, Sachs J, Perkins D. Cystic disease of the lungs. Surg Clin North Am 1988; 68:581–618
21. Stocker J, Madewell JE, Drake RM. Congenital cystic adenomatoid malformation of the lung. Classification and morphologic spectrum. Hum Pathol 1977; 8:155–171

PULMONARY NEOPLASMS

22. Allan BT, Day DL, Dehner LP. Primary pulmonary rhabdomyosarcoma of the lung in children. Report of two cases presenting with spontaneous pneumothorax. Cancer 1987; 59:1005–1011
23. Burge HJ, Novotny DB, Schiebler ML, Delany DJ, McCartney WH. MRI of Askin's tumor. Case report at 1.5 T. Chest 1990; 97:1252–1254
24. Fink IJ, Kurtz DW, Cazenave L, et al. Malignant thoracopulmonary small-cell ("Askin") tumor. AJR 1985; 145:517–520
25. Hartman, GE, Shochat SJ. Primary pulmonary neoplasms of childhood: a review. Ann Thorac Surg 1983; 36:108–119
26. Manivel JC, Priest JR, Watterston J, et al. Pleuropulmonary blastoma. The so-called pulmonary blastoma of childhood. Cancer 1988; 62:1516–1526
27. Saifuddin A, Robertson RJ, Smith SE. The radiology of Askin tumours. Clin Radiol 1991; 43:19–23
28. Senac M Jr, Wood BP, Isaacs H, Weller M. Pulmonary blastoma: a rare childhood malignancy. Radiology 1991; 179:743–746

NEUROBLASTOMA

29. Bousvaros A, Kirks DR, Grossman H. Imaging of neuroblastoma: an overview. Pediatr Radiol 1986; 16:89–106
30. Brodeur GM. Neuroblastoma and other peripheral neuroectodermal tumors. In: Fernbach DJ, Vietti TJ (eds), Clinical pediatric oncology. 4th ed. St. Louis: Mosby-Year Book 1991:437–464
31. Carachi R, Campbell PE, Kent M. Thoracic neural crest tumors. A clinical review. Cancer 1983; 51:949–954
32. Dernevik L, Larsson S. Management of dumbbell tumours. Reports of seven cases. Scand J Thorac Cardiovasc Surg 1990; 24:47–51
33. Dietrich RB, Kangarloo H, Lenarsky C, Feig SA. Neuroblastoma: the role of MR imaging. AJR 1987; 148:937–942
34. George ND, Gonzalez G, Hoyt CS. Does Horner's syndrome in infancy require investigation? Br J Ophthalmol 1998; 82:51–54
35. Halperin DS, Oberhansli I, Siegrist CA. Intrathoracic neuroblastoma presenting with neonatal cardiorespiratory distress. Chest 1984; 85:822–833
36. Jaffe N, Cassady R, Petersen R, Traggis D. Heterochromia and Horner syndrome associated with cervical and mediastinal neuroblastoma. J Pediatr 1975; 87:75–77
37. Koh PS, Raffensperger JG, Berry S, et al. Long-term outcome in children with opsoclonus-myoclonus and ataxia and coincident neuroblastoma. J Pediatr 1994; 125:712–716
38. Kornreich L, Horev G, Kaplinsky C, Ziv N, Grunebaum M. Neuroblastoma: evaluation with contrast enhanced MR imaging. Pediatr Radiol 1991; 21:566–569
39. Merten DF, Gold SH. Radiologic staging of thoracoabdominal tumors in childhood. Radiol Clin North Am 1994; 32:133–149
40. Towbin R, Gruppo RA. Pulmonary metastases in neuroblastoma. AJR 1982; 138:75–78

CASE 2

Donald P. Frush, M.D.

Ganglioneuroma

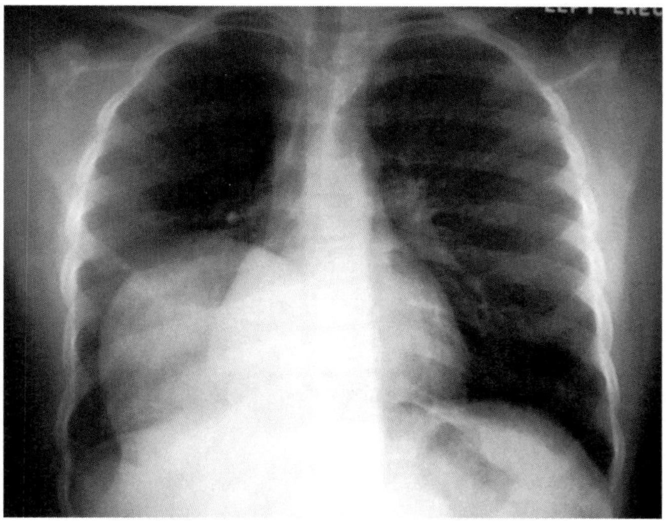

Figure 2-1

Question 5

This 8-year-old girl has right-sided chest pain. You are shown a posteroanterior chest radiograph (Figure 2-1).

Which *one* of the following is the MOST likely diagnosis?

(A) Thymolipoma
(B) Pericardial cyst
(C) Bronchogenic cyst
(D) Askin tumor
(E) Ganglioneuroma

The posteroanterior chest radiograph of the test patient demonstrates a large mass in the lower right chest; the mass does not silhouette or displace the heart (Figure 2-1). The sharp margin indicates that this mass is either pleural or extrapleural. Key findings that can be observed on this frontal radiograph include the widening of the intercostal space between the 10th and 11th ribs (Figure 2-2) and the mild scoliosis at this level. No bone destruction is apparent, however. These features indicate that the mass is posterior mediastinal in location. Of the options listed, ganglioneuroma is the only posterior mediastinal mass (**Option (E) is correct**). The posterior mediastinal location of the mass was confirmed on a lateral chest radiograph (Figure 2-3).

A ganglioneuroma is a benign tumor of ganglion cell origin. This tumor is the differentiated tumor of the neuroblastoma-ganglioneuroblastoma-ganglioneuroma spectrum. Because of the ganglion origin, ganglioneuromas can occur anywhere along the spine, although about 45% of them occur in the posterior mediastinum. Rib spreading and erosion, scoliosis, and vertebral erosion are features that distinguish neurogenic tumors from nonneurogenic masses in the posterior mediastinum. These osseous deformities are most common with neuroblastoma, occurring in up to 45% of patients. Osseous abnormalities do not distinguish the types of neurogenic tumors, although rib destruction is seen only in association with malignant tumors.

Thymic disorders present as anterior mediastinal masses and account for about 6% of all mediastinal masses in children. A thymolipoma (Option (A)) is a rare cause of a thymic mass. A thymolipoma typically contains variable amounts of

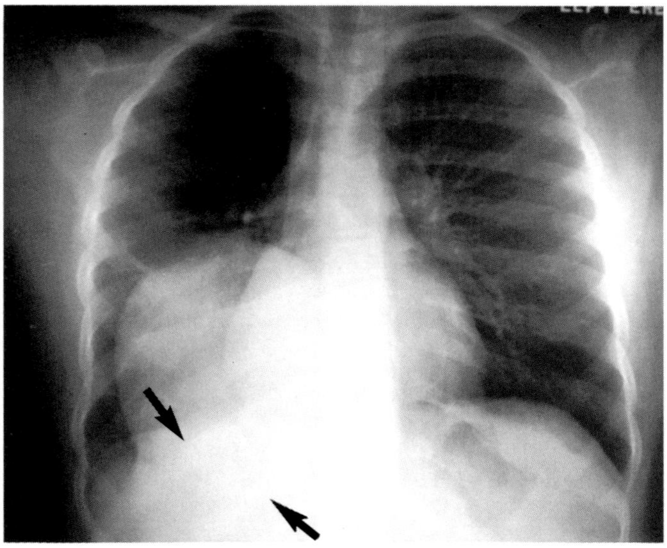

Figure 2-2 (Same as Figure 2-1). Ganglioneuroma. The posteroanterior chest radiograph demonstrates a right posterior mediastinal mass with sharply defined borders. Note the mild associated levoscoliosis and the widening of the intercostal space between the 10th and 11th ribs (arrows).

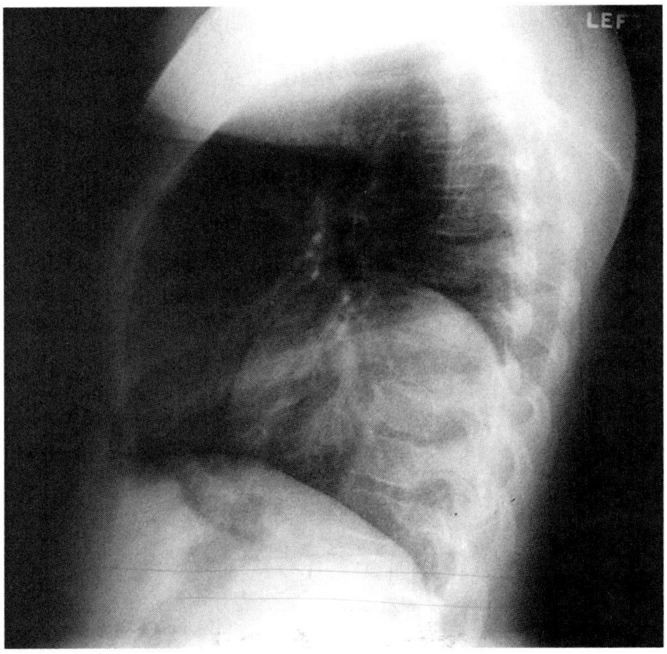

Figure 2-3. Same patient as in Figures 2-1 and 2-2. Ganglioneuroma. A lateral radiograph demonstrates that the mass is centered in the posterior mediastinum. Consequently, the majority of the posterior and inferior margins are inseparable from the posterior chest wall and adjacent diaphragm.

fat, which are well depicted on CT or MRI. Thymolipomas occasionally present as masses in the cardiophrenic sulci or are mistaken for cardiomegaly. Because the right heart margin is not obscured and because of costovertebral involvement, the mass in the test patient is not in the anterior mediastinum.

Pericardial cysts (Option (B)) are typically unilocular and filled with clear fluid and have a mesothelial or endothelial lining. The overall prevalence is 1 in 100,000 patients, but they are extremely rare in children. They can be located in the posterior mediastinum, but most are found relatively anteriorly (Figure 2-4). More than half (50% to 67%) are found at the right cardiophrenic angle; 22% to 38% are found at the left cardiophrenic angle. Although a posterior mediastinal location is possible, rib spreading or erosion is not a characteristic of pericardial cysts.

Pericardial cysts are congenital abnormalities that result from a failure of fusion of fetal pericardial lacunae. They represent up to 7% of mediastinal masses in all age groups. Most patients are asymptomatic, and the cysts are discovered incidentally on chest radiographs. When symptomatic, the cysts cause nonspecific chest pain, cough, or dyspnea. Even when the cysts are large, they rarely affect the heart. Echocardiography, CT, and MRI are all capable of demonstrating the location and fluid-filled characteristics of the cyst adjacent to the heart (Figure 2-5). On CT, the cyst is usually unilocular, with homogeneous water attenuation and a thin wall. In adults, pericardial cysts associated with symptoms or with atypical imaging features are usually removed by either thoracotomy or thoracoscopy. As noted above, pericardial cysts are rare in children. Because other cystic masses are more common, pericardial cysts are often removed.

Pericardial cysts can be quite large, and differentiation from other cystic mediastinal masses and a loculated pleural

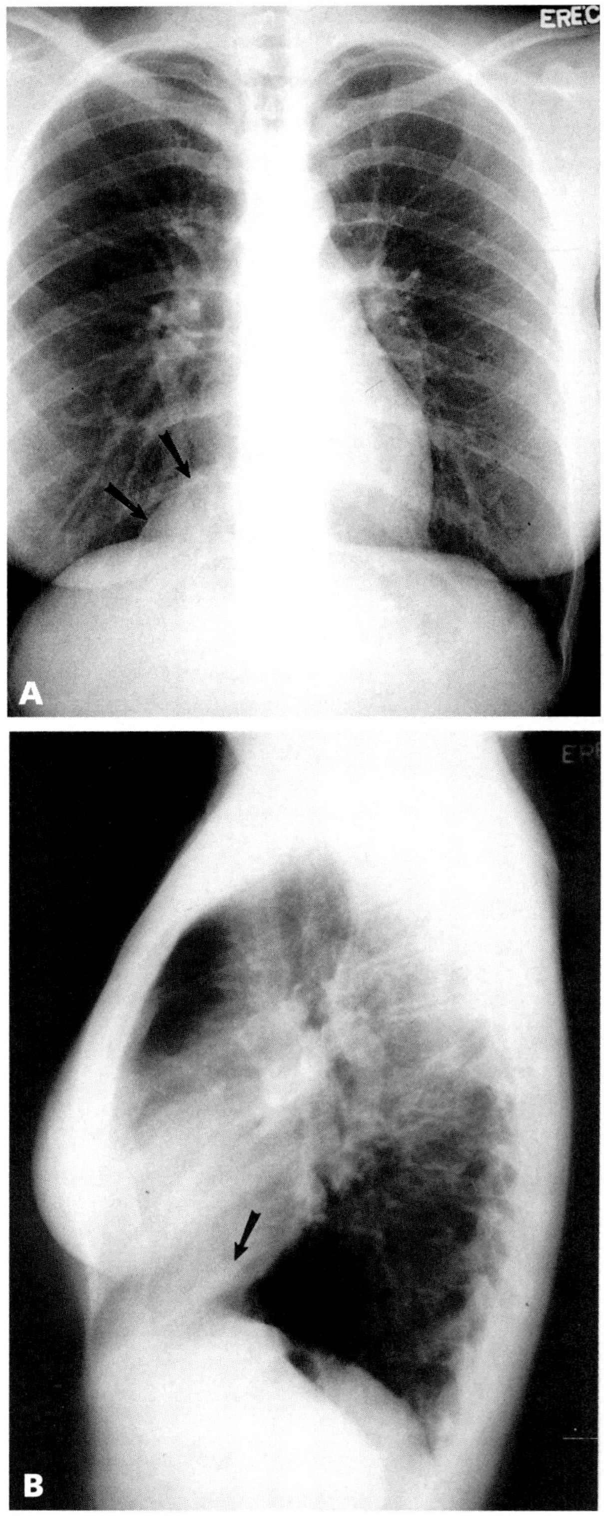

Figure 2-4. Pericardial cyst in a 21-year-old woman. (A) The posteroanterior radiograph shows a well-defined opacity (arrows) located in the right cardiophrenic sulcus. (B) The cyst is more clearly defined as anterior in location on the lateral radiograph (arrow).

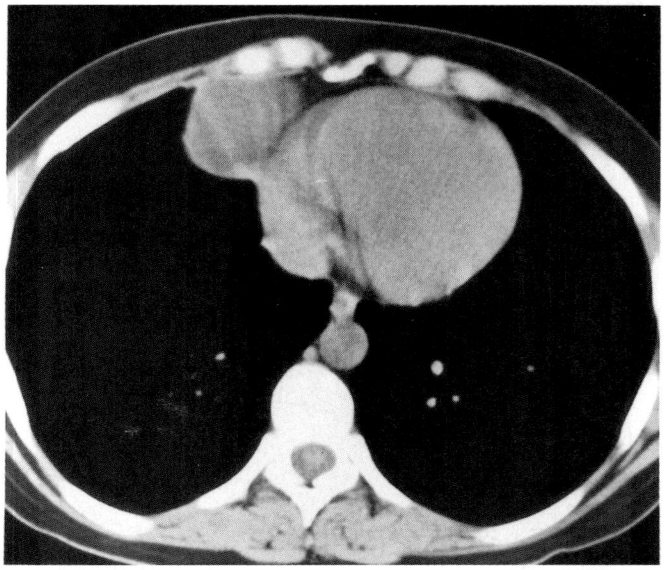

Figure 2-5. Pericardial cyst in a child. This noncontrast CT scan demonstrates a homogeneous, water-attenuation mass adjacent to the right side of the heart.

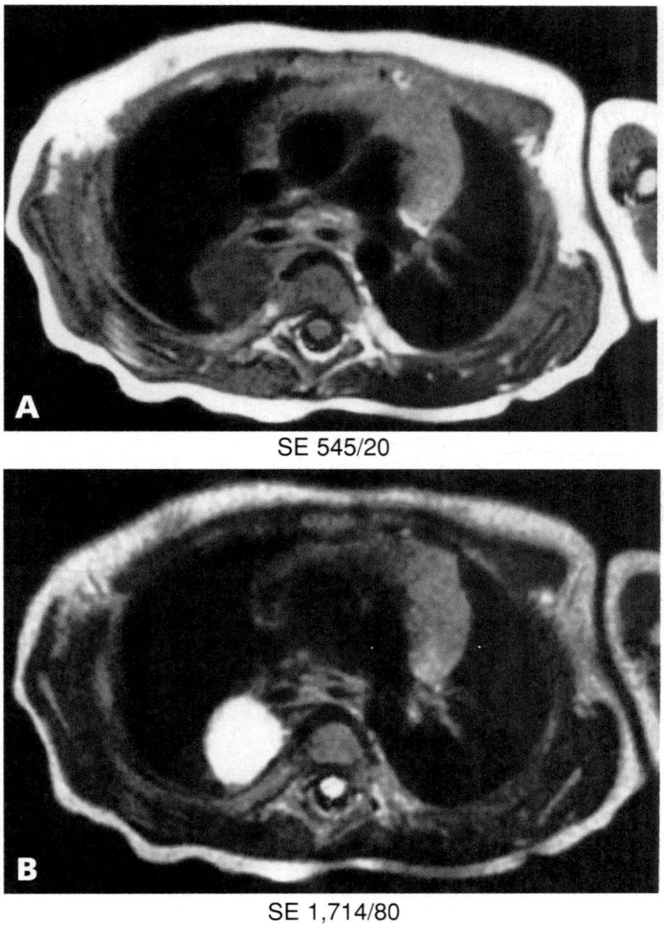

Figure 2-6. Right posterior mediastinal foregut cyst in a 6-month-old girl with wheezing. (A) An axial T1-weighted MR image demonstrates the homogeneous intermediate-intensity mass adjacent to the vertebral body. (B) A T2-weighted MR image with fat saturation shows that the cyst has very high signal intensity.

effusion is sometimes difficult. The differential diagnosis for a cystic mass in this location in a child includes bronchogenic cyst, lymphangioma, teratoma, thymic cyst, and loculated pleural or pericardial fluid. The absence of septations and isolated anterior mediastinal location make a lymphangioma (cystic hygroma) unlikely. A teratoma typically demonstrates mixed fat, fluid, calcium, and soft tissue components.

A bronchogenic cyst (Option (C)) is one of the abnormalities in the spectrum of congenital bronchopulmonary foregut malformations. Other abnormalities that can present as a middle or posterior mediastinal mass in this spectrum are esophageal duplication and neurenteric cysts. These cysts are all foregut malformations and can be difficult to differentiate histologically. Bronchogenic and esophageal duplication cysts arise from the ventral foregut, and neurenteric cysts arise from the dorsal foregut. Foregut cysts account for 10% to 15% of all mediastinal masses, and up to 65% of foregut cysts are bronchogenic cysts. Bronchogenic cysts are lined by respiratory epithelium and contain cartilage. There is no muscular wall, a feature of esophageal duplication cysts. Bronchogenic cysts are found in the mediastinum or lung. The mediastinal location of bronchogenic cysts is more common than the parenchymal location. Carinal and paratracheal locations are most frequent, accounting for approximately 50% of mediastinal cysts. Paraesophageal or posterior mediastinal (Figure 2-6), superior mediastinal, and intrapericardial locations are rare. Even with the infrequent occurrence in the posterior mediastinum, rib displacement is not a feature of a bronchogenic cyst. Therefore, this is an unlikely diagnosis for the test patient.

Symptomatic bronchogenic cysts are related in part to their location in the mediastinum or the lung. Of children with mediastinal bronchogenic cysts, about 30% overall are asymptomatic. Children under the age of 5 who are diagnosed with bronchogenic cysts are almost always symptomatic. Cysts are more often discovered incidentally in older children and adolescents. Approximately 80% of symptomatic children have respiratory symptoms, including cough, dyspnea, respiratory distress, or chest pain. Hilar and more peripheral locations of bronchogenic cysts are also found (Figure 2-7). In 33% of symptomatic patients with parenchymal locations, the symptoms are due to acute infection. Of children with pulmonary bronchogenic cysts, 20% are asymptomatic. Even if there is a strong suspicion that a thoracic mass is a bronchogenic cyst, operative removal is necessary because of the risk of later infection.

On chest radiography, cysts that originate in the lung parenchyma have a nonspecific appearance characteristic of a solid mass or, more rarely, appear as a cavitary lesion with an air-fluid level if there is infection and communication with the airway. A mediastinal bronchogenic cyst is often detected on a chest radiograph or a barium esophagram. Although a paratracheal or subcarinal smooth mediastinal mass demonstrated radiographically in a child is probably a bronchogenic cyst, CT or MRI will provide additional diagnostic information and aid in preoperative planning. On CT, the bronchogenic cyst is a mass that typically has internal contents of soft tissue or water

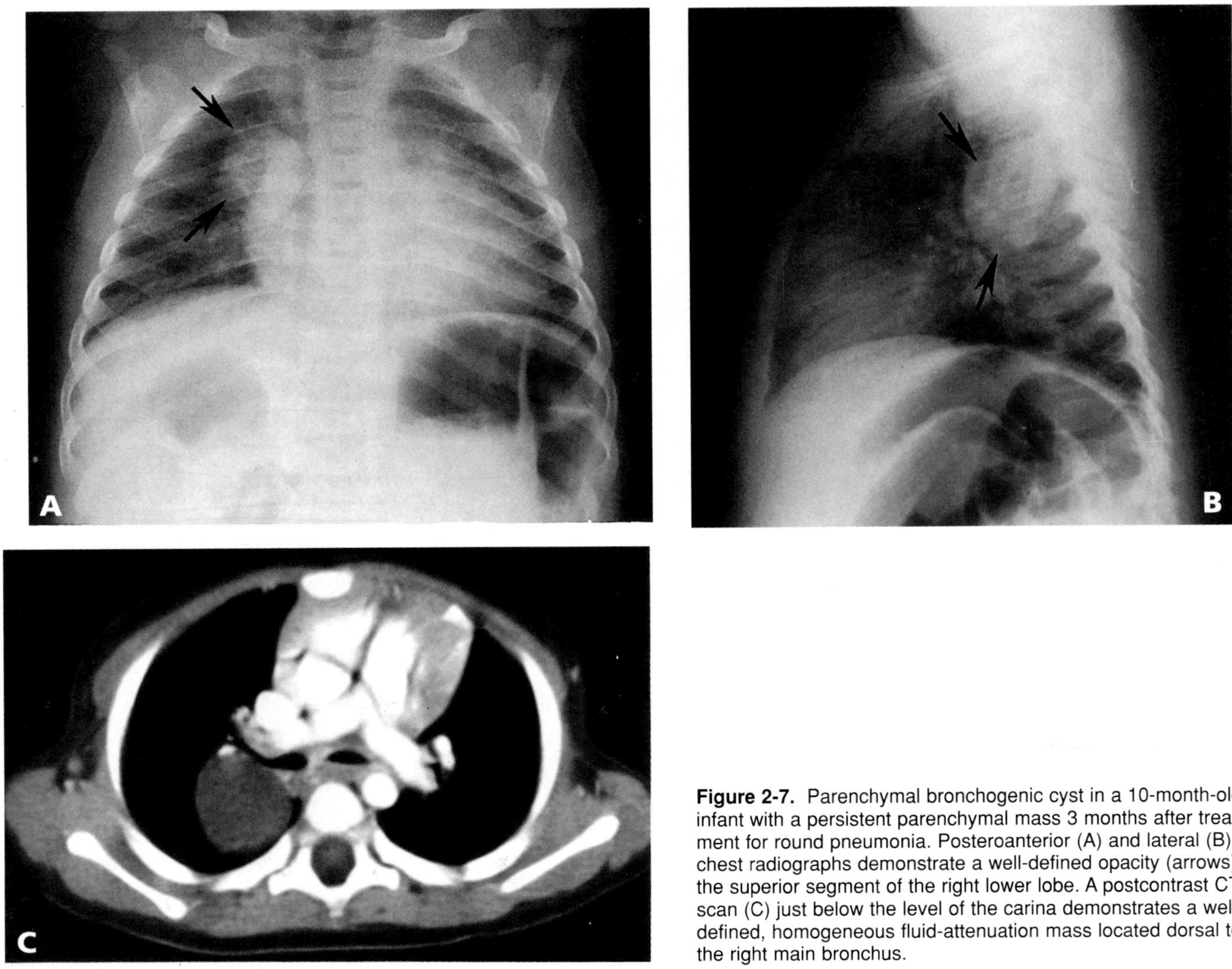

Figure 2-7. Parenchymal bronchogenic cyst in a 10-month-old infant with a persistent parenchymal mass 3 months after treatment for round pneumonia. Posteroanterior (A) and lateral (B) chest radiographs demonstrate a well-defined opacity (arrows) in the superior segment of the right lower lobe. A postcontrast CT scan (C) just below the level of the carina demonstrates a well-defined, homogeneous fluid-attenuation mass located dorsal to the right main bronchus.

attenuation (depending on the fluid content) and is located in the middle or, more rarely, posterior mediastinum. A wall can be present, but there is no calcification. The MRI appearance also depends on the composition of the fluid within the cyst. Increased signal intensity on T2-weighted images is consistently present, but the intensity on T1-weighted images has been reported to range from intermediate to high (greater than fat). This feature may be attributable to proteinaceous or hemorrhagic fluid. There is no advantage of MRI over CT for detection and presurgical planning. The CT or MRI appearance can be identical to that of other mediastinal lesions, most of which are removed.

Formerly referred to as an Askin tumor (Option (D)), the primitive neuroectodermal tumor (PNET) of the chest wall is an aggressive cancer of children and young adults. It usually arises from soft tissue or bone but can, in rare circumstances, originate in the periphery of the lung. PNET is one of the pediatric small round cell tumors, which include neuroblastoma, rhabdomyosarcoma, lymphoma, and Ewing's sarcoma. Differentiation of PNET from Ewing's sarcoma can be difficult and is confirmed only when lobular rosettes, neuronal elements, and neuron-specific enolase are demonstrated. Even then, these two tumors are arguably part of a spectrum of tumors that arise from the neural crest. PNET has been considered a Ewing's sarcoma of the rib or adjacent soft tissue. PNET and Ewing's sarcoma are treated identically.

The chest wall site of origin of Ewing's sarcoma is rare, accounting for less than 7% of all locations. When PNET is present in the chest wall, symptoms are attributable to the mass itself or to a pleural effusion (Figure 2-8), which is usually large at the time of diagnosis. The chest wall PNET presents radiographically as a chest wall mass. Rib destruction is seen in 25% to 63% of patients, but there can be a large soft tissue mass without rib involvement. When adjacent bones are affected, bone destruction or periosteal reaction, rather than displacement, is typical.

Invasion of adjacent soft tissues and bones by PNET is best demonstrated by cross-sectional imaging. On CT, the mass is typically noncalcified, with heterogeneous enhancement (Figure 2-9). On MRI, the signal intensity of the lesion is also heterogeneous because of areas of hemorrhage or necrosis. MRI better depicts the extent of chest wall involvement (Figure 2-10). CT

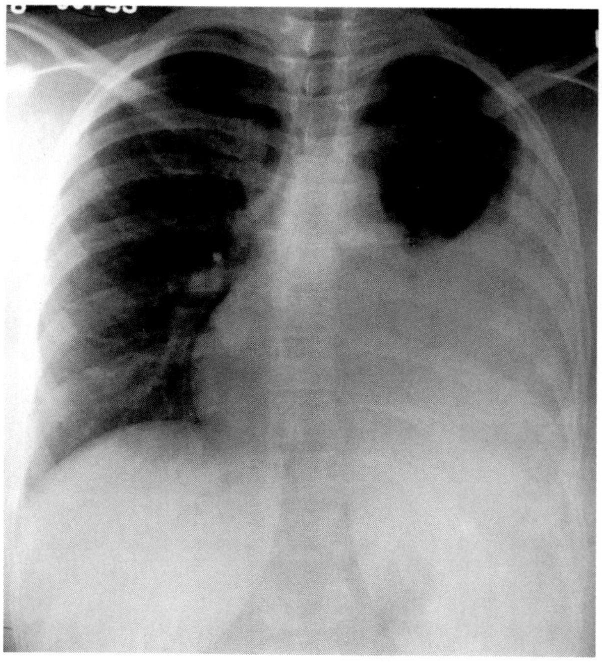

Figure 2-8. Primitive neuroectodermal tumor of the chest wall (Askin tumor) in a 16-year-old girl with left-sided chest pain. A posteroanterior chest radiograph shows a large left pleural effusion.

or MRI is able to detect lung involvement in fewer than one third of patients. Metastases are present in 10% to 38% of patients at the time of presentation. Common sites are bones, lungs, and lymph nodes.

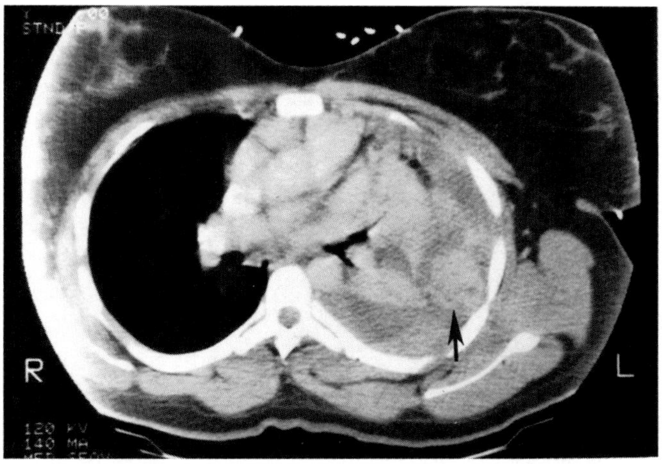

Figure 2-9. Same patient as in Figure 2-8. A postcontrast CT scan distinguishes soft tissue components of the tumor (arrow) from adjacent pleural fluid. No rib destruction was present. Soft tissue attenuation near the hilum is atelectatic lung.

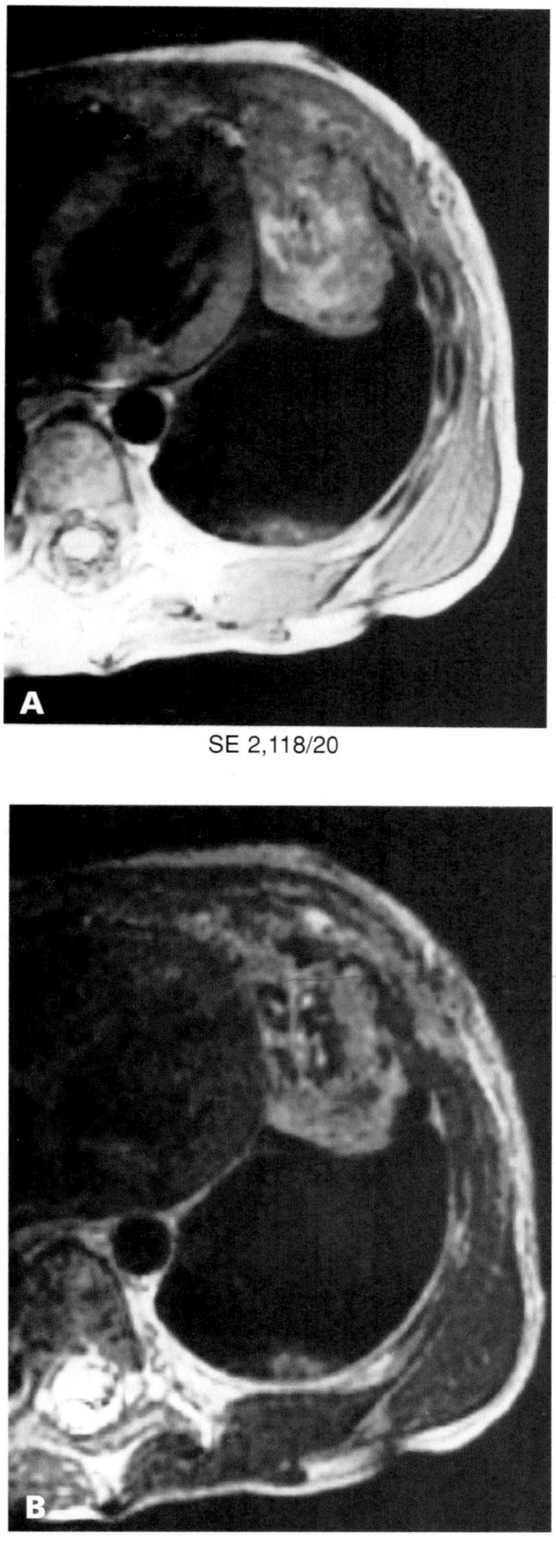

Figure 2-10. Primitive neuroectodermal tumor of the chest wall in a 6-year-old girl. Axial proton-density-weighted (A) and T2-weighted (B) MR images show that the mass has heterogeneous signal intensity and involves the anterior chest wall. The tumor is inseparable from the pericardium as well. The area of increased signal intensity in the posterior lung is atelectasis.

Question 6

Which *one* of the following is the MOST appropriate next study for the evaluation of the test patient?

(A) MRI
(B) CT
(C) Biopsy
(D) Bone scintigraphy
(E) Barium esophagram

Virtually any modality can be used to evaluate mediastinal masses. Evaluation usually begins with detection of a mediastinal mass by chest radiography. Radiography helps determine the presence and location of the mass. This localization in the anterior, middle, or posterior mediastinum is useful for narrowing the differential diagnosis, but further evaluation is almost always necessary. The goals of imaging mediastinal masses are to (1) determine the etiology, (2) define the extent, and (3) evaluate for involvement of contiguous structures (such as vessels, bone, airway, or spinal canal). Since most mediastinal masses are surgically removed, diagnostic imaging should be directed toward preoperative evaluation of the tumor extent and involvement of adjacent structures and spaces. Both CT and MRI can be used to limit the differential diagnosis and aid in preoperative planning.

CT (Option (B)) is well suited for the evaluation of mediastinal masses. First, CT provides information about the composition and size of the mass. It can distinguish among fat, calcification or bone, water-density fluid, air, and soft tissue. Masses of vascular origin (such as a dilated azygos vein, aortic aneurysm, or aortic arch or arch vessel anomaly) can be demonstrated after the intravenous administration of contrast material.

CT is also excellent for demonstrating the involvement of adjacent structures. Tracheal compromise, usually from anterior mediastinal masses, is well demonstrated and is an important piece of preoperative information (Figure 2-11). Atelectasis and air trapping are also easily identified; this information is unavailable with MRI. Involvement of cortical bone (e.g., rib involvement) is well depicted by CT. Esophageal contrast material helps to define the course of the structure relative to a mass but is probably used less frequently in children than adults, given the rarity of esophageal abnormalities, such as cancer, in children.

Overall, spatial resolution is better with CT than with MRI. Because CT is limited to transaxial imaging, neural involvement is not optimally assessed. This is an important operative point since decompressive laminectomy can accompany operative removal of a posterior mediastinal mass. Finally, although spiral CT now affords retrospective overlapping reconstruction for improved anatomic depiction as well as multiplanar and three-dimensional reconstructions (advantages previously available only with MRI), its value for demonstrating neural involvement by posterior mediastinal masses in children has not been proven.

Like CT, MRI is excellent for depicting the presence and size of mediastinal masses in children. In addition to absence of ionizing radiation and only rare need for intravenous contrast material, specific advantages of MRI include multiplanar depiction and excellent soft tissue contrast resolution. Chest wall invasion is better demonstrated by MRI than by CT. Because of both improved contrast resolution and multiplanar depiction, MRI is well suited for imaging of vascular lesions (e.g., aortic aneurysm, pulmonary artery aneurysm, dilatation, or postoperative pseudoaneurysm) or paracardiac tumors (Figure 2-12). For masses in the posterior mediastinum, bone marrow involvement (Figure 2-13), soft tissue contrast differences (Figure 2-14), and spinal involvement (e.g., cord compression) are better depicted by MRI than by CT (Figure 2-15). For these reasons, MRI is the most appropriate imaging modality for the evaluation of posterior mediastinal masses and should be the next study in the test patient (Figure 2-16) **(Option (A) is correct).** Expense, more limited availability, extended imaging times, and increased need for sedation are disadvantages of MRI.

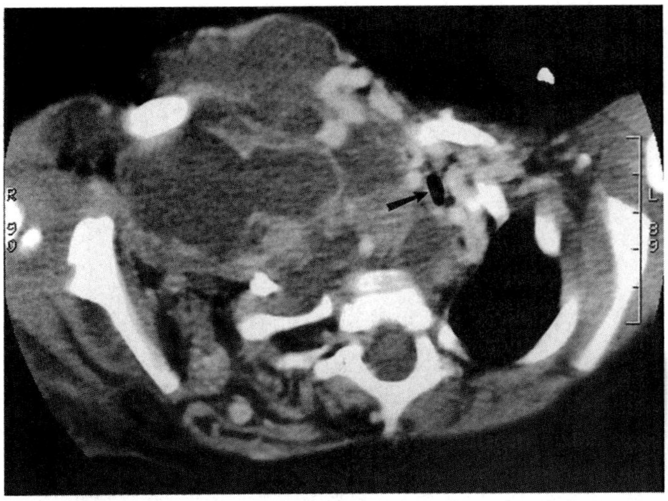

Figure 2-11. Cystic hygroma in an infant with tracheal compression and displacement (arrow). A contrast-enhanced CT scan also reveals involvement of the right chest wall anteriorly, laterally, and posteriorly.

Biopsy of mediastinal masses (Option (C)) can be performed percutaneously or surgically via thoracoscopy, thoracotomy, or sternotomy. Percutaneous aspiration or biopsy is usually performed when there is suspicion of an anterior mediastinal abscess or postoperative fluid collection; recurrent thymic tumor, such as lymphoma or leukemia; or metastasis. Although biopsy can be performed in children with newly diagnosed mediastinal masses, it rarely is done since the majority of isolated mediastinal masses in children are removed. Imaging evaluation in such patients is directed toward defining the extent and adjacent involvement of the tumor for surgical planning. Biopsy is rarely necessary before surgery.

Bone scintigraphy (Option (D)) can demonstrate both the extension of mediastinal masses into adjacent bone and distant osseous metastatic disease. Osteomyelitis and diskitis, which may have an adjacent soft tissue mass, are also demonstrated by bone scintigraphy. However, bone scintigraphy is not the principal modality in establishing the etiology of mediastinal mass-

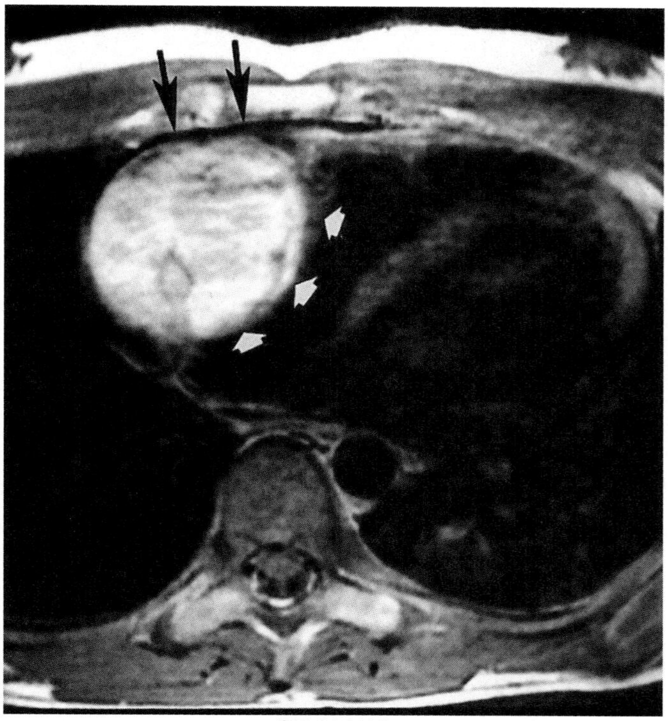

SE 916/15

Figure 2-12. Hemangioma within the pericardial space in an 8-year-old boy. An ECG-gated T1-weighted cardiac MRI examination illustrates a high-signal-intensity mass lying within the pericardium (black arrows). The right atrium and ventricle (white arrows) are effaced at the level of the atrioventricular valve. High T1-weighted signal intensity is likely attributable to slowly flowing blood.

es, since the vast majority do not have osseous involvement.

Lesions within and adjacent to the esophagus can be detected with a barium esophagram (Option (E)). Paraesophageal

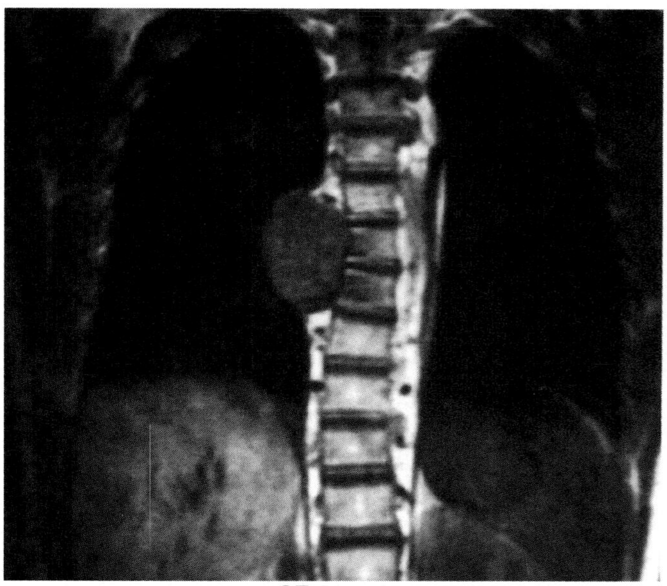

SE 916/13

Figure 2-13. Pheochromocytoma in a 14-year-old girl. A T1-weighted MR image shows homogeneous intermediate signal intensity. This finding is nonspecific. The image also shows the adjacent scoliosis and marrow signal abnormality attributable to infiltration.

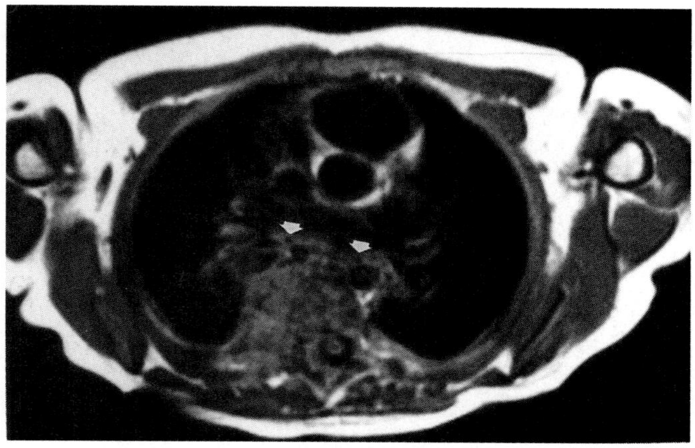

SE 916/13

Figure 2-14. Spinal hemangioma in a 1-year-old child. A T1-weighted axial MR image clearly shows a soft tissue mass in the right paraspinal area with adjacent soft tissue and vertebral involvement. The scattered areas of fat signal intensity, as well as adjacent vessels (arrows), are typical of a hemangioma.

abnormalities include bronchogenic cysts, esophageal duplications, and neurenteric cysts. In addition, contrast studies are useful in the setting of a hiatal hernia or other diaphragmatic hernias or the rare esophageal diverticulum. An esophagram can also demonstrate a dilated esophagus that presents as a mediastinal mass. In such cases, radiography can suggest the etiology if there is an air-fluid level in the course of the esophagus. Strictures in children can be iatrogenic (e.g., tracheoesophageal repair, sclerotherapy for esophageal varices) or inflammatory (e.g., gastroesophageal reflux, chronic granulomatous disease). When a mass is demonstrated initially on radiography to be in the posterior or anterior mediastinum, esophagraphy is not necessary (unless there is a compelling clinical setting for an esophageal etiology) since a more beneficial anatomic display is provided by cross-sectional imaging.

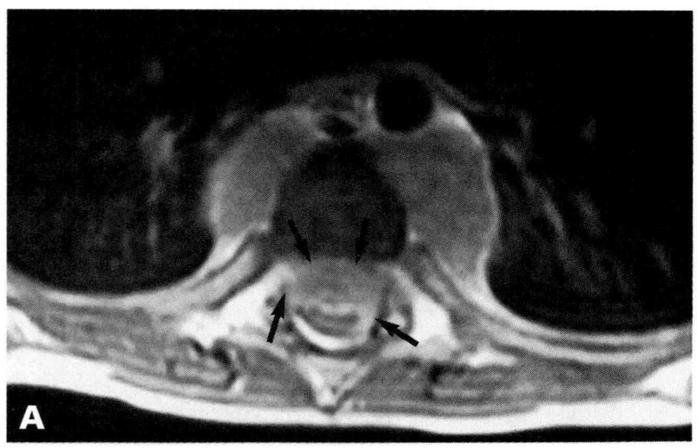

SE 580/12

Figure 2-15. Spinal cord compression caused by a posterior mediastinal undifferentiated sarcoma. This 3-year-old child presented with acute-onset back pain and lower extremity weakness. (A) An axial T1-weighted postcontrast MR image shows a soft tissue mass extending around both sides of the T6 vertebral body, as well into the spinal canal on the left side (arrows).

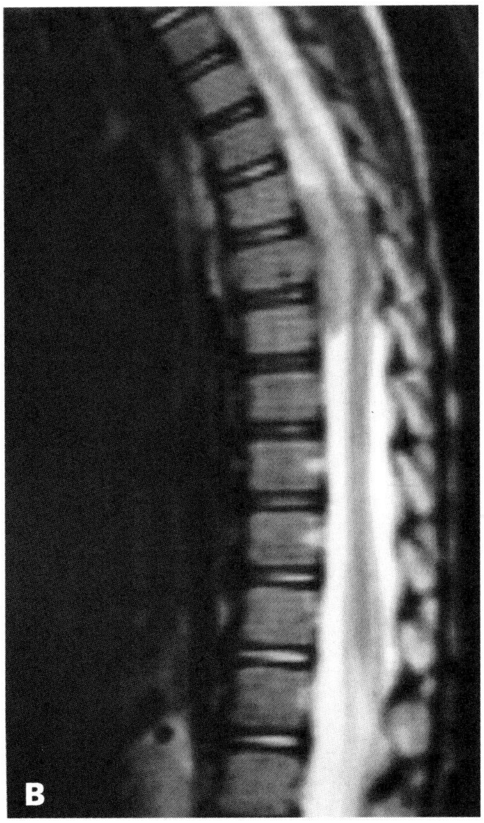

SE 3,600/60

Figure 2-15 (Continued). Spinal cord compression caused by a posterior mediastinal undifferentiated sarcoma. (B) A midline sagittal T2-weighted image of the thoracic spine better illustrates the degree and extent of posterior displacement and compression of the thoracic spinal cord by the tumor. The T6 vertebral body is also compressed.

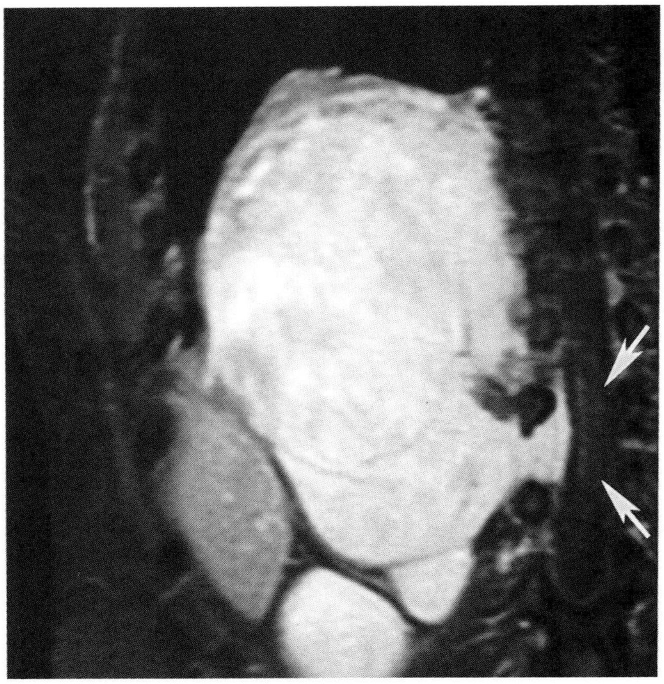

SE 3,000/102

Figure 2-16. Same patient as in Figures 2-1 through 2-3. Ganglioneuroma. A coned-down T2-weighted coronal MR image of the right posterior mediastinum shows the foraminal and intraspinal extent of the mass, with leftward displacement of the cord (arrows). The mass is predominantly of high signal intensity and extends into the posterior sulcus.

Question 7

Concerning posterior mediastinal masses in children,

(A) at least 85% are neurogenic in origin
(B) most patients present with neurologic symptoms
(C) percutaneous biopsy is the preferred method of histologic diagnosis
(D) nerve cell tumors are more common than in adults
(E) they are less common than middle mediastinal masses

The mediastinum contains the extrapleural intrathoracic structures and is bordered by the sternum anteriorly, the vertebral column posteriorly, the thoracic inlet superiorly, and the diaphragm inferiorly. The traditional classification divides the mediastinum into superior, anterior, middle, and posterior compartments based on the lateral radiograph. There have been several different variations for this arbitrary compartmentalization, including, more recently, classification based on CT anatomy, which combines the middle mediastinum and posterior mediastinum into a single compartment. The common principle for each of the variations is to predict the type of mass based on the anatomic structures in or adjacent to the region. The posterior mediastinum includes the intrathoracic area from the posterior chest wall and vertebral bodies (the paravertebral "gutter") as far anteriorly (depending on the classification scheme) as the plane formed by the dorsal tracheal wall. The structures in the posterior mediastinum include the paraspinal nerves (sympathetic and parasympathetic plexuses), blood vessels (e.g., the aorta and azygos vein), esophagus (Figure 2-17), lymph nodes, and mesenchyma. Adjacent structures from which abnormalities that result in masses extending into the posterior mediastinum can arise include the vertebral bodies, costovertebral junction, pleura, and diaphragm.

In children, the mediastinum is the most common location of chest masses. The middle mediastinum is the least frequent site (20%) for mediastinal masses (**Option (E) is false**). Masses in the anterior mediastinum occur at approximately the same frequency as do posterior mediastinal masses. Posterior mediastinal masses account for approximately 40% of all mediastinal masses.

The different posterior mediastinal masses are listed in Table 2-1. Over 85% of posterior mediastinal masses are neurogenic in origin (**Option (A) is true**). Almost all of these neu-

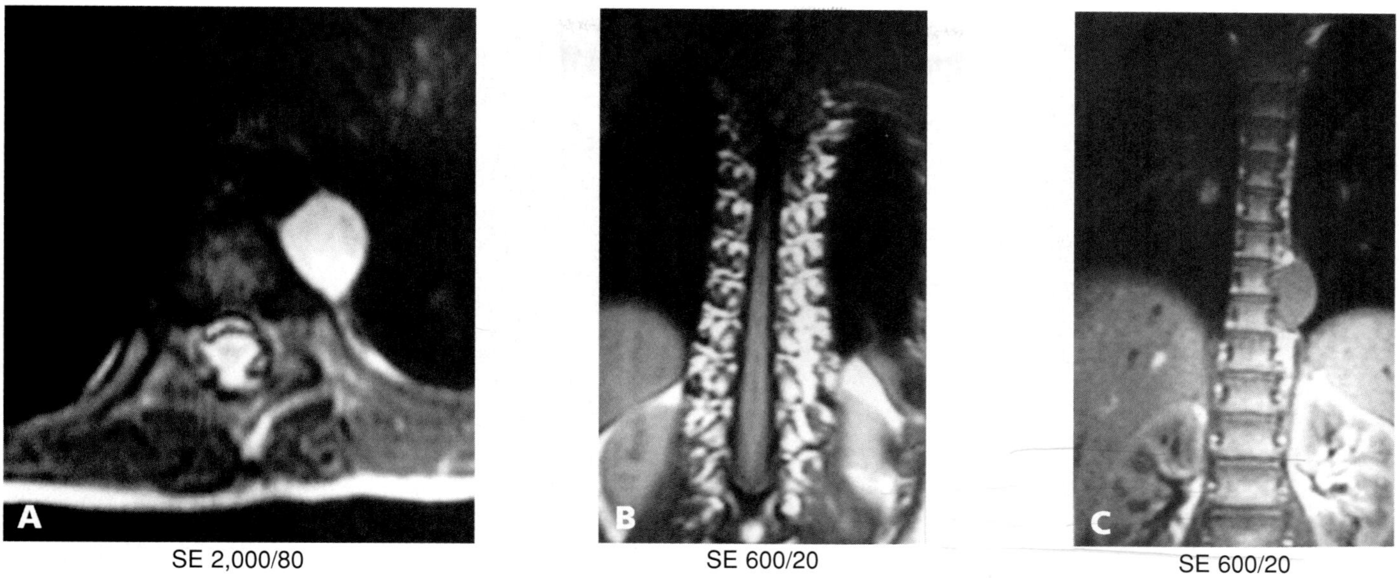

Figure 2-17. Esophageal duplication discovered incidentally on chest radiography in a 2-year-old asymptomatic boy. (A) A T2-weighted axial MR image shows that the cyst is well defined, with homogeneous high signal intensity. The adjacent T9 vertebral body is unaffected. (B and C) Coronal T1-weighted images do not show any involvement of the neural foramina (B) or vertebral bodies (C). The cyst is intermediate in signal intensity.

rogenic tumors arise from the sympathetic ganglia or nerve sheath. The frequency of the different types of tumors depends on the age of the patient. Neurogenic tumors in infants and children almost always arise from the nerve cells (ganglion cells), whereas in adults, nerve sheath tumors predominate (**Option (D) is true**).

For all of the ganglion tumors, symptoms are present in about 75% of patients. Symptoms related to respiratory compromise are the most common. Neurologic symptoms (e.g., spinal cord compression and Horner's syndrome) are less common (**Option (B) is false**). Musculoskeletal symptoms (chest pain or back pain) can also be attributable to large neurogenic tumors in children and adolescents. For masses that are not neurogenic in origin, the clinical history is helpful in establishing the diagnosis. For example, a paraspinal hematoma can be related to trauma or a bleeding disorder, extramedullary hematopoiesis to a hemoglobinopathy, abscess to systemic infection, and adenopathy to diffuse adenopathy in patients with leukemia. For these rare nonneurogenic causes of posterior mediastinal masses, treatment is more often conservative. Usually, the diagnosis of a posterior mediastinal mass is uncertain, and operative removal or biopsy is indicated. Since most masses are removed, percutaneous biopsy plays a limited role in the evaluation of masses (**Option (C) is false**). Suspected recurrent tumor, metastasis, and infection are circumstances in which percutaneous biopsy may be considered.

Table 2-1: Posterior mediastinal masses in children

Location	Name
Neural (>85%)	
Nerve cell (ganglion)	Neuroblastoma (including ganglioneuroblastoma), ganglioneuroma
Nerve sheath	Neurofibroma, benign schwannoma (neurilemmoma), malignant schwannoma
Other (rare)	Paraganglioma (alternate terms: chemodectoma, pheochromocytoma)
Nonneural (<15%)	
Foregut	Bronchogenic cyst, esophageal duplication, neurenteric cyst, esophageal dilatation
Vascular	Aortic aneurysm, azygos or hemiazygos enlargement, hemangioma
Lymphatic	Lymphoma, lymphangioma (cystic hygroma)
Paravertebral	Hematoma, extramedullary hematopoiesis, abscess, metastasis
Diaphragmatic	Bochdalek's hernia, paraesophageal or hiatal hernia, eventration
Other	Mesenchymal tumors (sarcoma, lipoma, fibroma), teratoma, leukemia, nodal infiltration (e.g., Castleman's disease, sarcoid, histoplasmosis)

Question 8

Concerning thymolipomas,

(A) they account for approximately 10% of mediastinal masses
(B) most patients are asymptomatic
(C) they are often associated with myasthenia gravis
(D) large ones simulate pericardial masses
(E) they are typically of homogeneous attenuation on CT

Up to 50% of mediastinal masses are located in the anterior mediastinum. In general, masses in this location include lymphadenopathy, vascular abnormalities (aortic arch anomalies, aneurysm), germ cell tumors, lymphangioma or hemangioma, and thymic abnormalities. Lymphomas, teratomas, and benign thymic enlargement account for 85% of anterior mediastinal masses in children. Thymic enlargement is attributable to either diffuse or focal disease. Rare causes (<1% each) include primary mediastinal lymphangiomas, hemangiomas, thymomas, and thymolipomas (**Option (A) is false**).

Thymolipomas are most common in the second through fourth decades, and one third are discovered by 20 years of age. However, they can occur as early as 2 years of age. Most individuals are asymptomatic (**Option (B) is true**). When symptoms are present, they are nonspecific and include chest pain, upper respiratory infection, dyspnea, and tachypnea. An association of thymolipomas with myasthenia gravis has been reported but is extremely rare (**Option (C) is false**).

Thymolipomas are grossly soft, lobulated, encapsulated masses, which can have a pedicle connecting them to the thymus. They consist of variable proportions of normal thymic tissue and large amounts of adipose tissue (at least 30%) with benign histologic features. When excessive collagenous tissue is also present, the mass is referred to as a thymofibrolipoma.

Thymolipomas are not reliably distinguished from other anterior mediastinal masses by chest radiography. They can be large enough to occupy additional mediastinal compartments although, because they are soft, there is surprisingly little mass effect. An anteroinferior location is seen in 80% of patients, and these tumors are occasionally mistaken for cardiomegaly or a paracardiac mass (**Option (D) is true**). Because of the fat and soft tissue content, both CT and MRI are useful imaging options. In more than 90% of patients, fat and soft tissue are identified by CT in a pattern of whorls and linear stranding or of soft tissue nodules surrounded by fat (**Option (E) is false**). More fat is generally present histologically than is seen by CT (Figure 2-18). Calcification is not a CT feature. MRI likewise demonstrates a mixed pattern of fat and soft tissue.

The differential diagnosis of a fatty mass in the anterior mediastinum in children consists of teratoma, lipoma, focal predominance of mediastinal fatty deposition, fat in a Morgagni hernia, and hemangioma or vascular malformation. Mature teratomas can usually be diagnosed by the presence of an admixture of tissues including fluid-filled spaces, calcification, and soft tissues as well as fat. The presence of viscera or other abdominal tissue and continuity with the abdomen identify a hernia. Cystic spaces in combination with large vessels are more typical of a vascular malformation, which can contain a variable amount of fat. Imaging may not be able to distinguish among these conditions. However, except for lymphoma, anterior mediastinal masses in children are all removed. For thymolipomas, complete excision is curative.

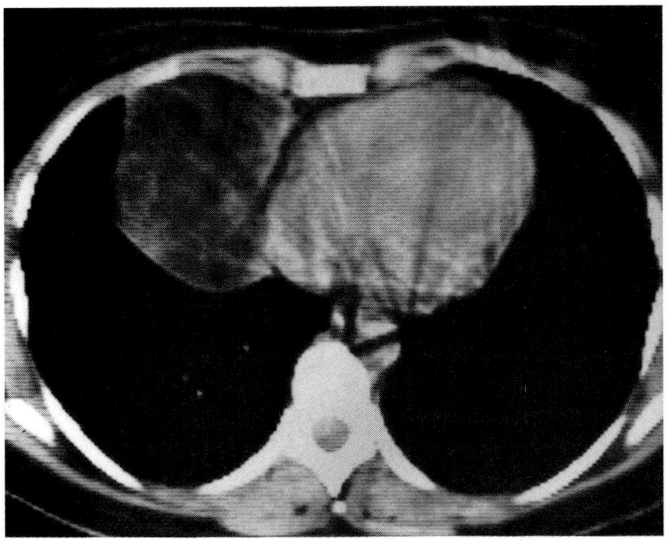

Figure 2-18. Thymolipoma. CT shows a predominantly fatty mass in the right cardiophrenic angle. Soft tissue stranding is noted within the lesion.

Question 9

Concerning ganglioneuroma in children,

(A) it arises from the sympathetic chain
(B) it occurs most often in children younger than 5 years
(C) it is associated with neurofibromatosis type 1
(D) it usually contains calcifications visible by CT
(E) it usually is limited to a single vertebral segment

Ganglion cell tumors include neuroblastoma and ganglioneuroma. Armstong et al. reported that neuroblastomas were diagnosed about seven times more frequently than ganglioneuromas, while Ribet and colleagues reported an approximately equal incidence. The frequency of the different types of ganglion cell tumors in children depends on age. In infants and young children, neuroblastoma is most common. Approximately 50% of all neuroblastomas are detected in the first year of life, and two thirds are diagnosed before the age of 5 years. About 15% of neuroblastomas occur in the chest. Ganglioneuromas are not seen in infancy, and 80% are diagnosed after 5 years of age, with a mean age at diagnosis of about 7 years (**Option (B) is false**). Ganglioneuromas may not be detected until adulthood. Ganglioneuromas are one of the most common of the posterior mediastinal masses. The mass can be an incidental finding or can become evident as a result of symptoms related to mass effect. Presentations include back pain, shortness of breath, and shoulder pain. Neurofibromas are most often found in patients with neurofibromatosis type 1 (von Recklinghausen's disease), but schwannomas and ganglioneuromas are associated with this syndrome as well (**Option (C) is true**).

Ganglioneuromas arise from the ganglion cells in the sympathetic chain (**Option (A) is true**). Histologically, the tumor consists of ganglion cells and axons with a lack of cellular palisading; loose matrix separates cellular fascicles. Ganglioneuromas are usually solitary and well defined, and their growth is very slow. They are generally very large at the time of diagnosis. About 70% occupy 3 to 5 interspaces, and an additional 12% occupy 6 to 10 interspaces (**Option (E) is false**). More than 90% of ganglioneuromas are smooth, whereas thoracic neuroblastomas tend to be lobulated or have indistinct margins. In general, the nerve cell tumors tend to be elongated and have tapered superior and inferior borders. Ganglioneuromas are elongated in 80% of patients; in contrast, the nerve sheath tumors (schwannomas and neurofibromas) are spherical in 50% to 80% of patients.

Calcification is better seen by CT than by radiography (Figure 2-19) and is more typically amorphous than discrete. On CT, calcification is seen less often in patients with ganglioneuroma (20%) than in those with neuroblastoma (40%) (**Option (D) is false**). The attenuation of ganglioneuroma on CT is homogeneous (the attenuation may be less than that of the musculature), with minimal enhancement. The overall signal is similarly homogeneous on MRI. The signal intensity is intermediate on T1-weighted images and very high on T2-weighted images (Figure 2-16). Ganglioneuromas can be indistinguishable from posterior mediastinal tumors, both benign and malignant; therefore, they are surgically removed (Figures 2-20 and 2-21).

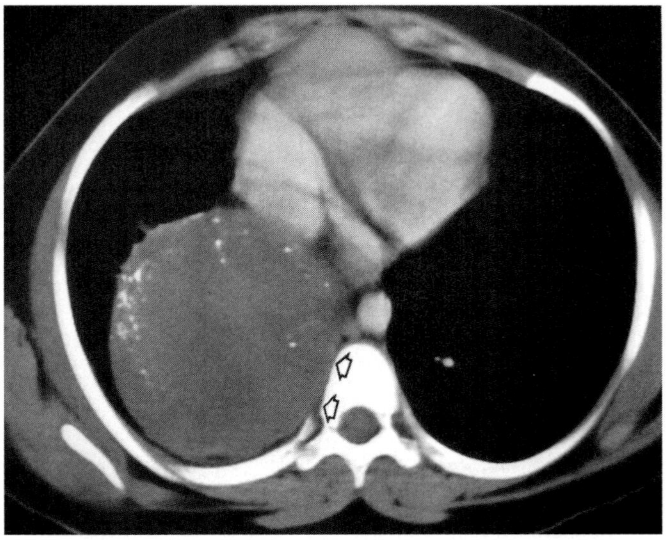

Figure 2-19. Same patient as in Figures 2-1 through 2-3 and 2-16. Ganglioneuroma. A CT scan shows a relatively punctate pattern of peripheral calcifications in a large, sharply defined posterior mediastinal mass. The right and left atria are compressed, and there is subtle erosive flattening of the right aspect of the vertebral body (arrows).

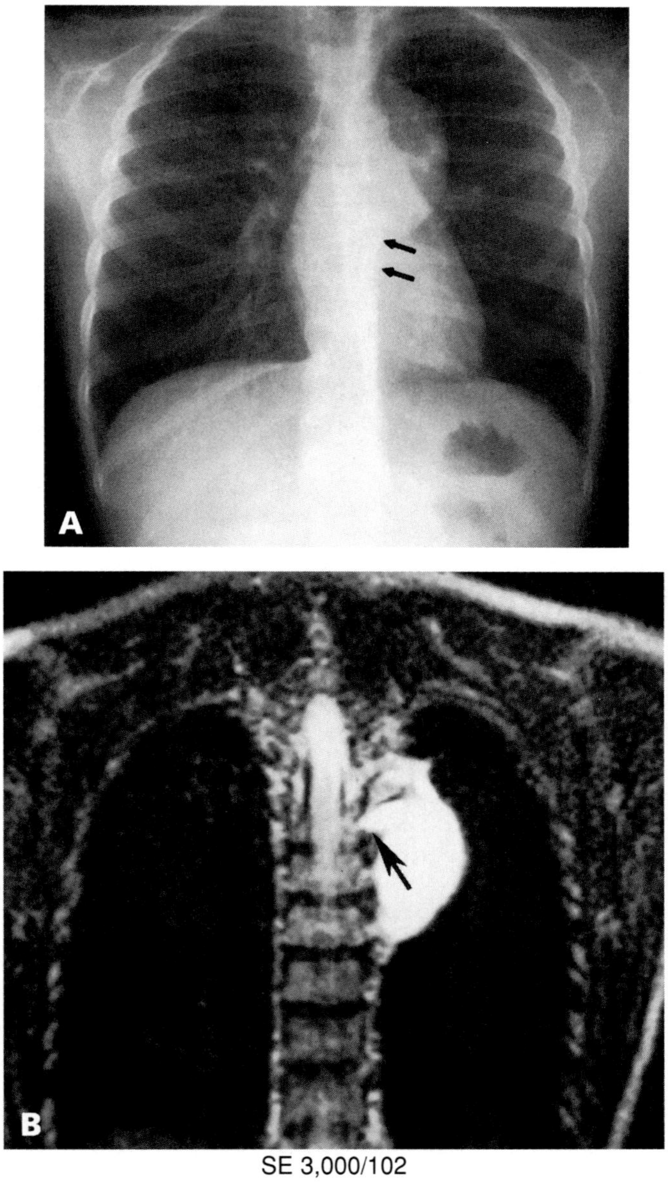

Figure 2-20. Ganglioneuroma in a 6-year-old child. (A) The mass was incidentally discovered on a chest radiograph. This sharply defined ganglion tumor can be seen to be posterior in location because the paraspinal stripe is interrupted (arrows) and the aortic arch and pulmonary outflow tract are not silhouetted. The chest radiographic appearance is nonspecific and can be mimicked by other posterior mediastinal masses. (B) A T2-weighted coronal MR image shows homogeneous high signal intensity, which is a nonspecific finding and can be seen with neurogenic tumors other than ganglioneuroma, as well as with esophageal and bronchogenic cysts. The foraminal involvement (arrow) is seen most often when posterior mediastinal masses are neurogenic in origin. The tapered superior and inferior borders are typical of ganglioneuroma but are also not diagnostic.

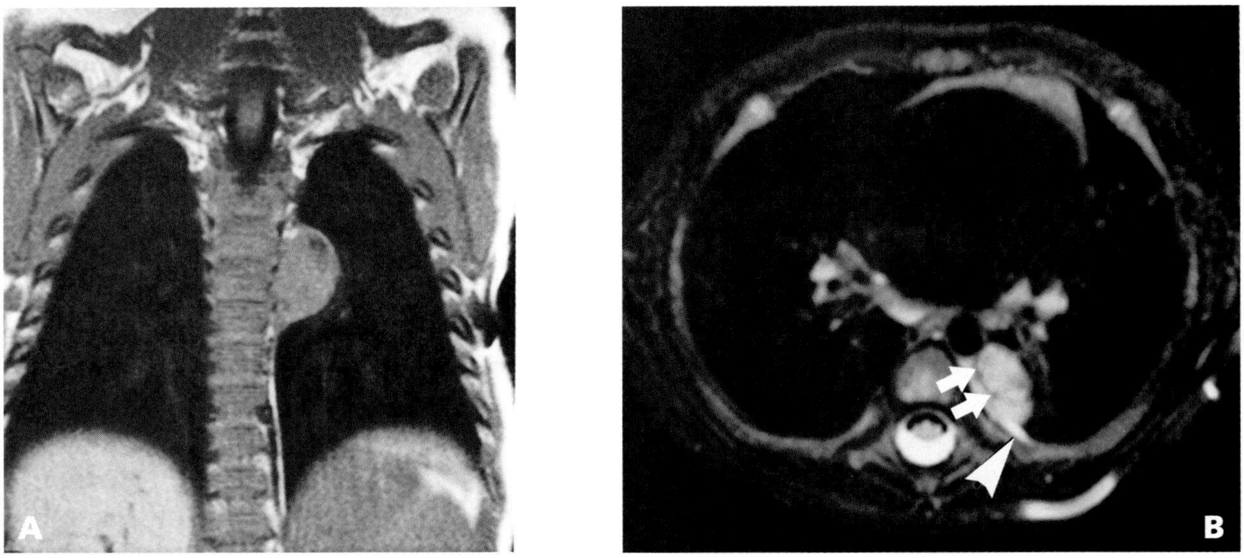

Figure 2-21. Stage 1 neuroblastoma incidentally discovered on a preoperative chest radiograph for tympanostomy tube placement in a 10-month-old infant. (A) This T1-weighted coronal MR image shows the mass to be homogeneous and of intermediate signal intensity. There was no involvement of the neural foramina or spinal canal. (B) The signal intensity of the tumor on this T2-weighted MR image is relatively homogeneous. Septation is present (arrows). Adjacent pleural reaction is also evident (arrowhead). The appearance of this lesion is indistinguishable from that of a benign ganglioneuroma.

SUGGESTED READINGS

GANGLIONEUROMAS

1. Armstrong EA, Harwood-Nash DC, Ritz CR, Chuang SH, Pettersson H, Martin DJ. CT of neuroblastomas and ganglioneuromas in children. AJR 1982; 139:571–576
2. Ichikawa T, Ohtomo K, Araki T, et al. Ganglioneuroma: computed tomography and magnetic resonance features. Br J Radiol 1996; 69:114–121
3. Reed JC, Hallet KK, Feigin DS. Neural tumors of the thorax: subject review from the AFIP. Radiology 1978; 126:9–17
4. Ribet ME, Cardot GR. Neurogenic tumors of the thorax. Ann Thorac Surg 1994; 58:1091–1095

THYMOLIPOMAS

5. Moran CA, Rosado-de-Christenson M, Suster S. Thymolipoma: clinical pathologic review of 33 cases. Mod Pathol 1995; 8:741–744
6. Moran CA, Zeren H, Koss MN. Thymofibrolipoma. A histologic variant of thymolipoma. Arch Pathol Lab Med 1994; 118:281–282
7. Rosado-de-Christenson ML, Pugatach RD, Moran CA, Galobardes J. Thymolipoma: analysis of 27 cases. Radiology 1994; 193:121–126

PERICARDIAL CYSTS

8. Abad C, Rey A, Feijoo J, Gonzalez G, Martin-Suarez J. Pericardial cyst. Surgical resection in two symptomatic cases. J Cardiovasc Surg 1996; 37: 199–202
9. Ravitch MM. Mediastinal cysts and tumors. In: Welch KJ, Randoph JG, Ravitch MM, O'Neill JA, Rowe MI (eds), Pediatric surgery. Chicago: Year Book Medical Publishers; 1986:602–617
10. Satur CM, Hsin MK, Dussek JE. Giant pericardial cysts. Ann Thorac Surg 1996; 61:208–210
11. Sugita T, Yasuda R, Magara T, Nishikawa T, Katsuyama K, Hanaoka J. Pericardial cyst in the midline position. J Cardiovasc Surg 1994; 35:87–88

BRONCHOGENIC CYSTS

12. LeBlanc J, Guttentag AR, Shepard JA, McLoud TC. Imaging of mediastinal foregut cysts. Can Assoc Radiol J 1994; 45:381–386
13. Ribet ME, Copin MC, Gosselin B. Bronchogenic cysts of the mediastinum. J Thorac Cardiovasc Surg 1995; 109:1003–1010
14. Ribet ME, Copin MC, Gosselin BH. Bronchogenic cysts of the lung. Ann Thorac Surg 1996; 61:1636–1640
15. Suen HC, Mathisen DJ, Grillo HC, et al. Surgical management and radiological characteristics of bronchogenic cysts. Ann Thorac Surg 1993; 55: 476–481

ASKIN TUMOR

16. Faber LP, Somers J, Templeton AC. Chest wall tumors. Curr Probl Surg 1995; 32:661–747
17 Shamberger RC, Tarbell NJ, Perez-Atayde AR, Grier HE. Malignant small round cell tumor (Ewing's-PNET) of the chest wall in children. J Pediatr Surg 1994; 29:179–185
18. Winer-Muram HT, Kauffman WM, Gronemeyer SA, Jennings SG. Primitive neuroectodermal tumors of the chest wall (Askin tumors): CT and MR findings. AJR 1993; 161:265–268

POSTERIOR MEDIASTINAL MASSES

19 Azarow KS, Pearl RH, Zurcher R, Edwards FH, Cohen AJ. Primary mediastinal masses. A comparison of adult and pediatric populations. J Thorac Cardiovasc Surg 1993; 106:67–72
20. Kawashima A, Fishman EK, Kuhlman JE, Nixon MS. CT of posterior mediastinal masses. RadioGraphics 1991; 11:1045–1067
21. King RM, Telander RL, Smithson WA, Banks PM, Han MT. Primary mediastinal tumors in children. J Pediatr Surg 1982; 17:512–520
22. Merten DF. Diagnostic imaging of mediastinal masses in children. AJR 1992; 158:825–832
23. Saenz NC, Schnitzer JJ, Eraklis AE, et al. Posterior mediastinal masses. J Pediatr Surg 1993; 28:172–176

IMAGING EVALUATION OF MEDIASTINAL MASSES

24. Andersson T, Lindgren PG, Elvin A. Ultrasound guided tumor biopsy in the anterior mediastinum. An alternative to thoracotomy and mediastinoscopy. Acta Radiol 1992; 33:423–426
25. Armstrong EA, Harwood-Nash DC, Ritz CR, Chuang SH, Petterson H, Martin DJ. CT of neuroblastomas and ganglioneuromas in children. AJR 1982; 139:571–576
26. Aronberg DJ, Glazer HS, Sagel SS. MRI and CT of the mediastinum: comparisons, controversies, and pitfalls. Radiol Clin North Am 1985; 23: 439–448

27. Bisset GS III. Pediatric thoracic applications of magnetic resonance imaging. J Thorac Imaging 1989; 4:51–57
28. Siegel MJ, Jamroz GA, Glazer HS, Abramson CL. MR imaging of intraspinal extension of neuroblastoma. J Comput Assist Tomogr 1986; 10: 593–595
29. Siegel MJ, Nadel SN, Glazer HS, Sagel SS. Mediastinal lesions in children: comparison of CT and MR. Radiology 1986; 160:241–244

CASE 3

John R. Sty, M.D.

Thyroid Aplasia

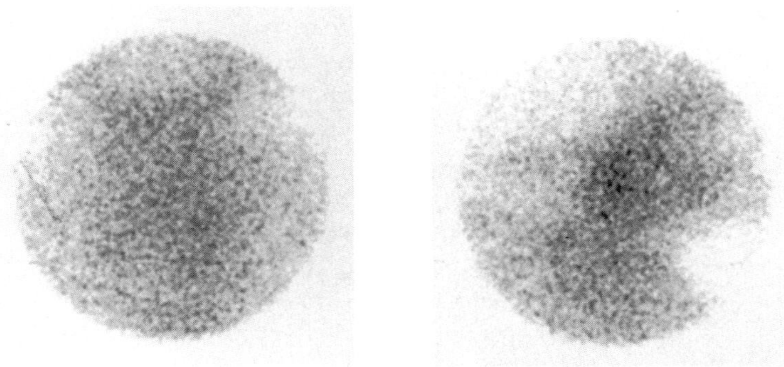

Figure 3-1

Question 10

This 2-day-old girl has neonatal hypothyroidism diagnosed on the basis of a screening thyroxine measurement. A fetal sonogram had shown multiple ovarian cysts. You are shown anterior and right lateral Tc-99m pertechnetate thyroid scintigrams (Figure 3-1).

Which *one* of the following is the BEST explanation for the scintigraphic and clinical findings?

(A) Peroxidase deficiency
(B) Thyroid aplasia
(C) Lingual thyroid
(D) Turner's syndrome
(E) Treatment of maternal hyperthyroidism

The anterior and right lateral pinhole images of the neck (Figure 3-1) in this hypothyroid newborn girl show no accumulation of Tc-99m pertechnetate in the thyroid. There is also marked diminution of salivary gland activity. Although there are many causes of neonatal hypothyroidism (Table 3-1), the differential diagnosis in the test patient includes only disorders that cause the absence of thyroid visualization.

Thyroid morphology and function can be evaluated by scintigraphy with Tc-99m pertechnetate. The dose of Tc-99m pertechnetate is approximately 5 mCi/1.73 m^2 of body surface area, with a minimum dose of 1 mCi. Tc-99m in the form of sodium pertechnetate is trapped in the thyroid gland in the same manner as iodide; however, it is not organified. Pinhole gamma camera images of the thyroid are obtained 30 minutes after intravenous injection of tracer. Since pertechnetate is concentrated in the salivary glands of normal patients and secreted into saliva, it is useful to ask a patient who is able to cooperate to swallow a small amount of water before imaging to wash away esophageal activity.

Thyroid dysgenesis refers to a developmental defect of thyroid morphogenesis. There are three main types: aplasia, hy-

Table 3-1: Causes of neonatal hypothyroidism

Dysgenesis
Aplasia
Hypoplasia
Ectopia
Dyshormonogenesis
Iodine deficiency
Maternal effects
Antithyroid medication
Iodine excess
Maternal antithyroid antibodies
Deficiency of thyrotropin-releasing hormone

poplasia, and ectopia. The physical findings are frequently subtle or absent in 70% of newborns with thyroid dysgenesis, and the abnormality is most often detected on routine neonatal screening. However, some newborns will have clinical manifestations of hypothyroidism, which include respiratory distress, noisy breathing, feeding problems, intermittent cyanosis, persistent neonatal jaundice, and umbilical hernias. Thyroid scintigraphy with Tc-99m pertechnetate in patients with thyroid aplasia fails to demonstrate functional thyroid tissue. The absence of Tc-99m pertechnetate accumulation in the test images makes thyroid aplasia the best diagnosis (**Option (B) is correct**).

The radiologic manifestations in infants and older children with hypothyroidism include normal or slightly retarded bone age, delayed skeletal maturation and long bone growth in the postnatal period, epiphyseal dysgenesis, increased bone density, poor cortical bone differentiation, congenital vertebral anomalies, thickening of the precervical soft tissues, and mild cardiomegaly.

Fetal ovarian cysts are also associated with hypothyroidism. In addition, ovarian cysts are associated with cystic fibrosis, McCune-Albright syndrome, ovarian hyperstimulation syndrome, polycystic ovarian syndrome, and polysplenia syndrome. In these conditions, cysts usually develop in childhood and adolescence.

Thyroid scintigraphy will demonstrate some degree of activity in the thyroid in patients with the other conditions listed in Question 10. Scintigraphy in patients with thyroid ectopia typically demonstrates a round or oval area of uptake of Tc-99m pertechnetate in the midline of the neck (Figure 3-2). The ectopic gland can be lingual (Option (C)), sublingual, or perilaryngeal. Mediastinal or lateral cervical locations are very rare. Functional thyroid tissue may be identified in more than one location, most commonly the lingual and sublingual areas.

Dyshormonogenesis is a less frequent cause of neonatal hypothyroidism (representing about 10% of cases) and is defined as an abnormality of one or more of the enzymes involved in the pathway of thyroid hormone synthesis and secretion. The enzymatic defect is frequently a hereditary trait. The most common defect is thyroid peroxidase deficiency (Option (A)), which results in a failure of oxidation of iodide ion necessary for organification. Hence, iodide is trapped but not organified, and the perchlorate washout test is positive. When enzymatic defects are present in the synthetic pathway beyond the point of organification, the perchlorate washout test is negative. Scintigraphy with Tc-99m pertechnetate in patients with dyshormonogenesis demonstrates a thyroid gland in the normal location. Because of thyrotropin (TSH) stimulation, the gland is usually enlarged and the lobes develop a convex appearance laterally (Figure 3-3). The isthmus is often well visualized, in contrast to the normal gland, and the pyramidal lobe can be enlarged. In some patients, however, the gland is not appreciably enlarged scintigraphically or clinically. Therefore, a normal-appearing thyroid image does not exclude dyshormonogenesis.

Turner's syndrome (Option (D)) is characterized by a relatively short stature, small mandible, webbed neck, and transient lymphedema of the hands and feet in infancy. The chest is shield shaped, with widely spaced, hypoplastic nipples. The syndrome is associated with autoimmune disorders, hypothyroidism (20% of adult women), diabetes mellitus, inflammatory bowel disease, Addison's disease, and thyroiditis. Small cysts within the thyroid can be identified by sonography in adolescent patients. However, thyroid scintigraphy and neonatal thyroid screening tests are normal. In addition, there is ovarian dysgenesis, not ovarian cysts, as in the test patient.

Maternal use of antithyroid medication for hyperthyroidism (Option (E)) does not significantly affect thyroid morphology in the neonate. Propylthiouracil and methimazole are the antithyroid agents that are most frequently used to treat hyperthyroidism. These agents can cross the placenta and affect thyroid metabolism in the fetus by decreasing organification and impairing the coupling reaction. However, the trapping of Tc-99m pertechnetate is unaffected by these drugs. Visualization of the thyroid gland with Tc-99m pertechnetate is dependent only on the iodide trapping mechanism. Thyroid scintigraphy in this circumstance usually demonstrates a thyroid gland in its proper location. It can appear normal in size and uptake or can be en-

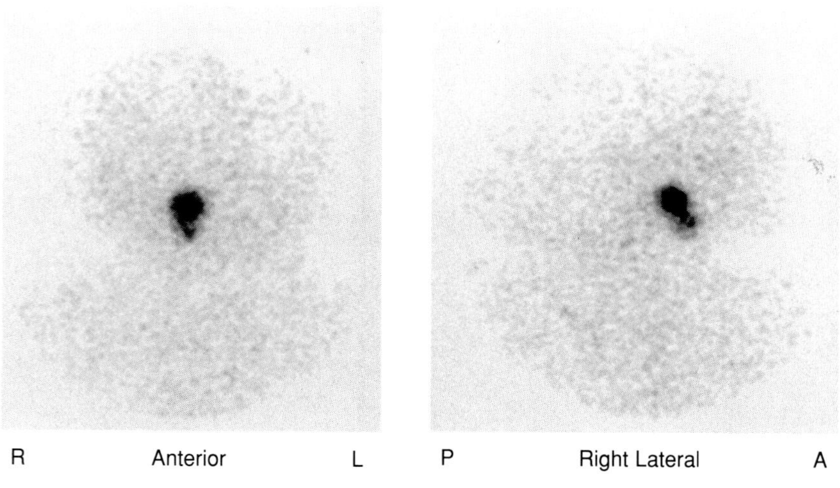

Figure 3-2. Thyroid ectopia. Anterior and right lateral Tc-99m pertechnetate scintigrams of the neck show radiopharmaceutical uptake in a small, rounded lingual thyroid.

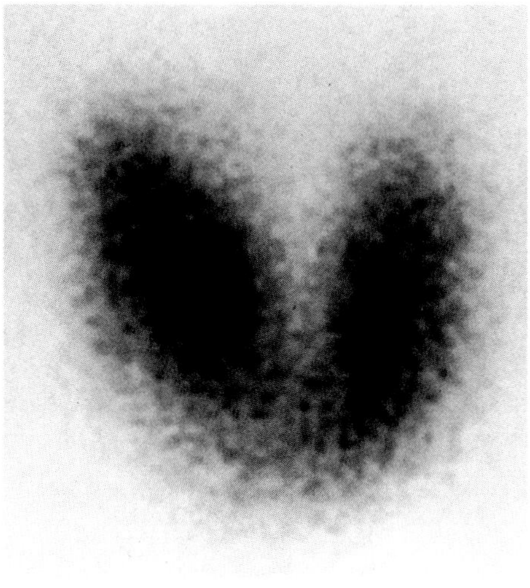

Figure 3-3. Dyshormonogenesis. An anterior Tc-99m pertechnetate scintigram of the neck in a hypothyroid newborn shows an enlarged thyroid gland with a rounded contour.

larged and have increased uptake (if the drugs have caused fetal hypothyroidism and resultant increased fetal secretion of TSH).

Before treatment for neonatal hypothyroidism is begun, a specific anatomic and functional diagnosis should be confirmed with thyroid scintigraphy and other thyroid function tests. Once the diagnosis of hypothyroidism is confirmed by the findings of low serum thyroid hormone levels and a high serum TSH level, it is mandatory to confirm the etiology, severity, and prognosis of the disease. Since aplastic cretinism and other severe forms of congenital hypothyroidism require a lifetime of thyroid hormone replacement therapy, it is important to distinguish patients with these conditions from patients with mild or transient disease and from those with dyshormonogenesis as early as possible.

Despite prompt initiation of therapy, children with thyroid aplasia can have a slightly higher frequency of intellectual retardation and other sequelae than children with other causes of congenital hypothyroidism; this situation is presumably secondary to insufficient thyroid function *in utero.* Children with an ectopic thyroid gland have a much lower frequency of intellectual retardation with proper therapy.

Question 11

Concerning neonatal hypothyroidism,

(A) it is due to thyroid dysgenesis in approximately 80% of patients
(B) it is clinically evident at birth in most patients
(C) elevated serum thyroglobulin levels are typical in infants with aplasia
(D) dyshormonogenesis is most often inherited as an autosomal recessive trait
(E) deafness is associated with thyroid dysgenesis

The overall incidence of neonatal hypothyroidism from all causes is approximately 1 per 4,000 births. Thyroid dysgenesis is the most common cause of neonatal hypothyroidism, accounting for approximately 80% of all cases (**Option (A) is true**). Thyroid dysgenesis refers to a developmental structural defect in the thyroid gland. There are three main types: aplasia, hypoplasia, and ectopia. Aplasia accounts for about 25% of cases, and ectopia accounts for about 75%; hypoplasia is rare. There is an unexplained greater incidence in girls than in boys.

Physical findings are notably absent in most newborns with hypothyroidism attributable to dysgenesis (and hence in most cases of neonatal hypothyroidism), and the biochemical alterations are most often detected on routine neonatal screening tests (**Option (B) is false**). Thyroid hormone levels are decreased and TSH levels are increased. The laboratory abnormalities tend to be more marked in patients with thyroid aplasia than in those with thyroid ectopia. The serum thyroglobulin level is low or undetectable in children with thyroid aplasia (**Option (C) is false**), reflecting the fact that no thyroid tissue is present. Thyroglobulin is a highly specific biochemical marker for functioning thyroid tissue.

Dyshormonogenesis accounts for approximately 15% of all cases of neonatal hypothyroidism. It is caused by the absence or abnormal function of one or more enzymes involved in the pathway of thyroid hormone synthesis and secretion. The enzymatic defect is usually hereditary and is most often inherited as an autosomal recessive trait (**Option (D) is true**). A family history is sometimes present. As noted above, the most common enzyme abnormality is a thyroid peroxidase deficiency. An enlarged thyroid gland can be present at birth, occurring with or without hypothyroidism.

Four types of congenital goiters related to enzymatic defects have been described. Type I goiters involve a defect in iodide transport, probably secondary to an alteration in the synthesis of cell surface proteins necessary for transport. Type II goiters are associated with several defects in iodination mechanisms within the thyroid. One involves the absence of the enzyme peroxidase, necessary for the organification of iodine. Another defect, which is inherited as an autosomal recessive trait, appears to involve peroxidase deficiency and is associated with deaf mutism, a complex known as Pendred's syndrome. A third defect, associated with abnormal peroxidase, allows sufficient compensation for maintenance of a euthyroid state. Type

III goiters are found in patients with dehalogenase defects. Although the precise biochemical abnormality is unclear, patients have complete or partial lack of dehalogenation of monoiodotyrosine and diiodotyrosine released by the breakdown of thyroglobulin. Monoiodotyrosine and diiodotyrosine are excreted in the urine, resulting in a state of relative iodine deficiency. Type IV goiters are associated with defects in the synthesis of thyroglobulin.

Deafness is associated with dyshormonogenesis (specifically with Pendred's syndrome), not with dysgenesis (**Option (E) is false**). The clinical manifestations of Pendred's syndrome include congenital perceptive hearing loss, goiter (euthyroid or hypothyroid), and thyroid carcinoma later in life. The radiologic manifestations include a goiter and the Mondini defect, which is a malformation of the cochlea. Partial aplasia results in 1.5 coils instead of the normal 2.5 to 2.75 coils, with the middle and apical coils sharing a common cochlea.

Questions 12 through 15

For each of the numbered thyroid abnormalities listed below (Questions 12 through 15), select the *one* lettered pattern of Tc-99m pertechnetate scintigraphic findings and laboratory data (A, B, C, D, or E) that is MOST closely associated with it. Each lettered pattern may be used once, more than once, or not at all.

12. Aplasia
13. Chronic lymphocytic thyroiditis
14. Dyshormonogenesis syndrome
15. Graves' disease

	Scintigraphy	*Serum thyroxine*	*Serum thyrotropin*
(A)	Nonvisualization of the thyroid	Increased	Decreased
(B)	Nonvisualization of the thyroid	Decreased	Increased
(C)	Normal	Normal	Normal
(D)	Enlarged thyroid	Increased	Decreased
(E)	Enlarged thyroid	Decreased	Increased

Thyroid scintigraphy in patients with thyroid aplasia fails to demonstrate functional thyroid tissue. Thyroid hormone levels are decreased and TSH levels are increased (**Option (B) is the correct answer to Question 12**). The laboratory abnormalities tend to be more marked in patients with thyroid aplasia than in patients with thyroid ectopia. The serum thyroglobulin level is reported to be undetectable in children with thyroid aplasia. It is important that scintigraphic images include the oropharynx and upper neck, as well as the upper portion of the chest, so that thyroid tissue in an ectopic location can be detected. Children with thyroid aplasia require a lifetime of thyroid hormone replacement therapy. Despite prompt initiation of such therapy, these children have a slightly higher frequency of intellectual retardation, presumably secondary to insufficient thyroid function *in utero.*

Scintigraphy in patients with thyroid ectopia typically demonstrates a round or oval area of uptake of Tc-99m pertechnetate in the midline of the neck. An ectopic thyroid gland is most often lingual, sublingual, or perilaryngeal. Mediastinal and lateral cervical locations are uncommon. Functional thyroid tissue may be identified in more than one location. As noted above, thyroid hormone deficiency and elevation of the TSH level are usually less marked in patients with thyroid ectopia than in those with aplasia. Intellectual development is normal if appropriate replacement therapy is given. Unusual cases do occur in which the ectopic gland is capable of secreting sufficient quantities of thyroid hormone so that routine neonatal screening blood test results are within normal limits. Such patients present with signs of ectopia later in childhood or even in adulthood, when the hyperstimulated gland enlarges, causing a mass with or without local symptoms at the base of the tongue or in the upper neck. Once the diagnosis of ectopia is established, lifetime thyroid hormone replacement is required to prevent further enlargement of the ectopic gland and associated symptoms.

As its name implies, chronic lymphocytic thyroiditis is a chronic inflammatory disease of the thyroid gland characterized by lymphocytic infiltration; this condition is also known as Hashimoto's disease. The condition is thought to be caused by an autoimmune process. It is the most common form of thyroid disease in children and adolescents. It has been estimated to occur in 1% to 5% of all children. It is a common cause of acquired hypothyroidism in childhood, is more prevalent in females, and is more frequent in adults than in children. A family history of thyroid disorders is common. The incidence is increased in patients with chromosomal disorders, including Turner's, Down's, and Klinefelter's syndromes. There is also an association with other autoimmune diseases, including anemias, rheumatoid arthritis, systemic lupus erythematosus, and Jorgenson's syndrome, and with other endocrine disorders, including Addison's disease, hypoparathyroidism, and diabetes mellitus. There is a slightly increased frequency of lymphocytic thyroiditis in patients with thyroid neoplasia, particularly papillary carcinoma. The thyroid gland is typically enlarged in patients with chronic lymphocytic thyroiditis. Early in the disease, thyroxine levels in serum are normal, but as the disease progresses to hypothyroidism, the thyroxine levels eventually decrease. The TSH levels then correspondingly increase (**Option (E) is the correct answer to Question 13**).

Scintigraphy in patients with dyshormonogenesis typically demonstrates a normally located thyroid gland. Because of TSH stimulation, the gland is usually enlarged. Despite the presence of hypothyroidism, Tc-99m pertechnetate uptake is usually increased secondary to TSH stimulation. The scintigraphic findings in patients with dyshormonogenesis are thus identical to those in patients with neonatal Graves' disease; correlation with thyroid hormone levels is required for the differentiation. In patients with thyroid dyshormonogenesis, there typically is an increase in the TSH level in serum and a decrease in the thyroxine level in serum (**Option (E) is the correct answer to Question 14**).

Graves' disease is the most common cause of hyperthyroidism in children. It is an autoimmune disorder characterized by the presence of thyroid-stimulating immunoglobulins. The normal thyroid regulatory mechanisms are overridden by the stimulatory immunoglobulins in patients with Graves' disease. Both thyroxine and triiodothyronine are secreted at increased rates, and triiodothyronine secretion is often disproportionately increased. Typically, the levels of both of these hormones in serum are increased. TSH levels in serum are markedly decreased (**Option (D) is the correct answer to Question 15**).

TSH measurements are useful in the diagnosis of hyperthyroidism. The development of immunometric assays has increased the sensitivity of TSH measurements; TSH levels below the normal range can readily be quantified. In those types of hyperthyroidism that arise independently of TSH secretion, increased circulating levels of thyroid hormones inhibit pituitary TSH secretion. Thus, in hyperthyroidism caused by mechanisms other than TSH hypersecretion, circulating TSH levels are low.

The clinical findings in patients with Graves' disease include diffuse thyroid gland enlargement, thyrotoxicosis, infiltrative ophthalmopathy, and, rarely, infiltrative dermopathy. The term "diffuse toxic goiter" refers to the clinically apparent thyroid gland enlargement with thyrotoxicosis secondary to Graves' disease. Ophthalmopathy occurs secondary to edema and lymphocytic infiltration of the extraocular muscles and orbital connective tissues. The ophthalmopathy can parallel the clinical course of the thyrotoxicosis or can run an independent course that is unaffected by treatment of the thyrotoxicosis.

Metabolism of iodine by the thyroid gland is markedly increased in patients with Graves' disease, which is reflected by increased radionuclide uptake values. If iodine turnover is very rapid, early radioiodine uptake values are markedly increased and the 24-hour uptake values may be normal. The uptake of Tc-99m pertechnetate is also increased.

I-123 or Tc-99m pertechnetate scintigraphy demonstrates diffuse enlargement of the thyroid gland, with a uniform distribution of the radiopharmaceutical. Uptake in a pyramidal lobe occurs in about 40% of patients with Graves' disease. The thyroid scan is occasionally helpful in excluding other causes of thyrotoxicosis, such as uninodular or multinodular toxic goiter, in which tracer uptake is not uniform. Also, in patients with subacute thyroiditis and concurrent hyperthyroidism (attributable to release of thyroid hormone from the inflamed gland), there is markedly reduced tracer uptake on scintigraphy, and thyroid uptake values are typically very low.

Question 16

Concerning neonatal Graves' disease,

(A) it results from transplacental transfer of maternal thyroid-stimulating immunoglobulins
(B) it is associated with premature suture closure
(C) it is associated with mental retardation
(D) Tc-99m pertechnetate thyroid images appear similar to those of infants with peroxidase deficiency
(E) it occurs in 50% of infants of mothers with Graves' disease

Neonatal Graves' disease usually results from transplacental passage of maternal thyroid-stimulating immunoglobulins to the fetus (**Option (A) is true**). Maternal levels of thyroid-stimulating immunoglobulins must be extremely high (more than five times control values) to produce clinical disease in the infant. Neonatal hyperthyroidism is a rare abnormality. It has been reported in approximately 1% of infants born to mothers with a history of Graves' disease (**Option (E) is false**) and rarely in children of mothers with chronic lymphocytic thyroiditis. Maternal thyroid-stimulating immunoglobulins can cause neonatal thyrotoxicosis despite the absence of maternal hyperthyroidism. This occurs when the maternal thyroid has been rendered unresponsive to thyroid-stimulating immunoglobulins by previous ablative therapy or by concurrent chronic thyroiditis.

The first manifestation of neonatal Graves' disease may be fetal tachycardia, with heart rates greater than 160/minute in the third trimester. Many of the affected infants are born prematurely. Thyrotoxic symptoms in neonates are usually evident within hours after birth. However, the clinical findings can be delayed for 2 to 10 days when the newborn's thyroid hormone synthesis remains suppressed by antithyroid drugs taken by the mother. The clinical findings can be delayed for 4 to 6 weeks as a result of transplacental passage of TSH receptor-blocking antibodies along with thyroid-stimulating immunoglobulins.

The symptoms of thyrotoxicosis include irritability, tremor, flushing, hyperactivity, gastrointestinal dysfunction (weight loss, vomiting, diarrhea, ferocious appetite, or, less commonly, difficulty feeding), and cardiac dysfunction (tachycardia, other arrhythmias, or congestive heart failure). Thyromegaly is common and can produce airway obstruction. Hepatosplenomegaly associated with jaundice and hypoprothrombinemia are occasionally present. The mortality rate in affected neonates is approximately 15%. Later problems include craniosynostosis (**Option (B) is true**), ophthalmopathy, and mental retardation (**Option (C) is true**). Mental retardation often occurs in association with craniosynostosis. Cross-sectional imaging of the central nervous system can show developmental abnormalities, which include ventriculomegaly, widening of the interhemispheric fissure, and an exaggerated gyral pattern.

Scintigraphy with Tc-99m pertechnetate in patients with neonatal hyperthyroidism demonstrates diffuse enlargement of the thyroid gland. I-123 or Tc-99m pertechnetate uptake values are in the hyperthyroid range. The high thyroid hormone levels and low serum TSH levels allow neonatal hyperthyroidism to be differentiated from neonatal goiter attributable to dyshormonogenesis. The scintigraphic images in patients with these two conditions appear the same (**Option (D) is true**).

SUGGESTED READINGS

THYROID DYSGENESIS

1. al-Jurayyan NA, el-Desouki MI. Transient iodine organification defect in infants with ectopic thyroid glands. Clin Nucl Med 1997; 22:13–16
2. Arnold MB, Arulananthani K, Bapat V. Characteristics of infantile hypothyroidism discovered on neonatal screening. J Pediatr 1984; 104: 539–544
3. Brooks PT, Archard ND, Carty HM. Thyroid screening in congenital hypothyroidism: a review of 41 cases. Nucl Med Commun 1988; 9:613–617
4. Czernichow P, Schlumberger M, Pomarede R, Fragu P. Plasma thyroglobulin measurements help determine the type of thyroid defect in congenital hypothyroidism. J Clin Endocrinol Metab 1983; 56:242–245
5. De Bruyn R, Ng WK, Taylor J, et al. Neonatal hypothyroidism: comparison of radioisotope and ultrasound imaging in 54 cases. Acta Paediatr Scand 1990; 79:1194–1198
6. Delange F. Neonatal screening for congenital hypothyroidism: results and perspectives. Horm Res 1997; 48:51–61
7. Farriaux JP, Dhondt JL. Thyroid scanning, ultrasound and serum thyroglobulin in determining the origin of congenital hypothyroidism. Am J Dis Child 1988; 142:1023–1024
8. Fisher DA. Thyroid physiology in the fetus and newborn: current concepts and approaches to perinatal thyroid disease. In: New MI, Fiser RH (eds), Diabetes and other endocrine disorders during pregnancy and in the newborn. New York: Alan R. Liss; 1976:221–233
9. Horlick M, Goldfarb CR, Schoeneman M, Ongseng F, Lee J. The role of imaging in neonatal hypothyroidism. Am J Dis Child 1988; 142:1139
10. Jafri SZ, Bree RL, Silver TM, Ouimette M. Fetal ovarian cysts: sonographic detection and association with hypothyroidism. Radiology 1984; 150:809–812
11. LeFranchi S. Congenital hypothyroidism: etiologies, diagnosis, and management. Thyroid 1999; 7:735–740
12. Macchia PE, Felice MD, Lauro RD. Molecular genetics of congenital hypothyroidism. Curr Opin Genet Dev 1999; 9:289–294
13. Price DA, Ehrlich RM, Walfish PG. Congenital hypothyroidism. Clinical and laboratory characteristics in infants detected by neonatal screening. Arch Dis Child 1981; 56:845–851
14. Singh A. Impaired trapping of Tc-99m pertechnetate in the salivary glands of patients with congenital hypothyroidism. Clin Nucl Med 1990; 15:257–259
15. Van Vliet G. Neonatal hypothyroidism treatment and outcome. Thyroid 1999; 1:79–84
16. Verelst J, Chanoine JP, Delange F. Radionuclide imaging in primary permanent congenital hypothyroidism. Clin Nucl Med 1991; 16:652–655
17. Wells RG, Sty JR. Diagnostic imaging for pediatric diseases: Thyroid scintigraphy. In: Miller JH, Gelfand MJ (eds), Pediatric nuclear imaging. Philadelphia: WB Saunders; 1994:45–64
18. Willi SM, Moshang T Jr. Diagnostic dilemmas. Results of screening tests for congenital hypothyroidism. Pediatr Clin North Am 1991; 38:555–566

DYSHORMONOGENESIS

19. Cone L, Oates F, Vazquez R. Congenital hypothyroidism: diagnostic scintigraphic evaluation of an organification defect. Clin Nucl Med 1988; 13: 419–420
20. de Vijlder JJ, Ris-Stalpers C, Vulsma T. Inborn errors of thyroid hormone biosynthesis. Exp Clin Endocrinol Diabetes 1997; 4:32–37
21. Fisher DA. Second International Conference on Neonatal Thyroid Screening: progress report. J Pediatr 1983; 102:653–654
22. Fisher DA, Klein AH. Thyroid development and disorders of thyroid function in the newborn. N Engl J Med 1981; 304:702–712
23. Heyman S, Crigler JF Jr, Treves S. Congenital hypothyroidism: ^{123}I thyroidal uptake and scintigraphy. J Pediatr 1982; 101:571–574
24. Kim EE, Domstad PA, Choy YC, DeLand FH. Avid thyroid uptake of [Tc-99m] sodium pertechnetate in children with goitrous cretinism. Clin Pediatr (Phila) 1981; 20:437–439
25. O'Connor MK, Freyne PJ, Cullen MJ. Low-dose radioisotope scanning and quantitative analysis in the diagnosis of congenital hypothyroidism. Arch Dis Child 1982; 57:490–494
26. Schoen EJ, dos Remedios LV, Backstrom M. Heterogeneity of congenital primary hypothyroidism: the importance of thyroid scintigraphy. J Perinat Med 1987; 15:137–142
27. Sfakianakis GN, Ezuddin SH, Sanchez JE, Edison M, Cleveland W. Pertechnetate scintigraphy in primary congenital hypothyroidism. J Nucl Med 1999; 40:799–804
28. Wells RG, Sty JR, Duck SC. Technetium 99m pertechnetate thyroid scintigraphy: congenital hypothyroid screening. Pediatr Radiol 1986; 16: 368–373

CHRONIC LYMPHOCYTIC THYROIDITIS

29. Fisher DA, Oddie TH, Johnson DE, Nelson JC. The diagnosis of Hashimoto's thyroiditis. J Clin Endocrinol Metab 1975; 40:795–801
30. Maceri DR, Sullivan MJ, McClatchney KD. Autoimmune thyroiditis: pathophysiology and relationship to thyroid cancer. Laryngoscope 1986; 96:82–86
31. Reiter EO, Root AW, Rettig K, Vargas A. Childhood thyromegaly: recent developments. J Pediatr 1981; 99:507–518
32. Set PA, Oleszczuk-Raschke K, von Lengerke JH, Brämswig J. Sonographic features of Hashimoto thyroiditis in childhood. Clin Radiol 1996; 5:167–169
33. UCLA conference. Autoimmune thyroid diseases—Graves' and Hashimoto's. Ann Intern Med 1978; 88:379–391
34. Winter J, Eberlein WR, Bongiovanni AM. The relationship of juvenile hypothyroidism to chronic lymphocytic thyroiditis. J Pediatr 1966; 69: 709–718

NEONATAL HYPERTHYROIDISM

35. Polak M. Hyperthyroidism in early infancy: pathogenesis, clinical features and diagnosis with a focus on neonatal hyperthyroidism. Thyroid 1998; 12:1171–1177
36. Roti F, Minelli R, Salvi M. Clinical review 80: management of hyperthyroidism and hypothyroidism in the pregnant woman. J Clin Endocrinol Metab 1996; 81:1679–1682
37. Zimmerman D. Fetal and neonatal hyperthyroidism. Thyroid 1999; 7: 727–733

CASE 4

John R. Sty, M.D.

Enteric Duplication

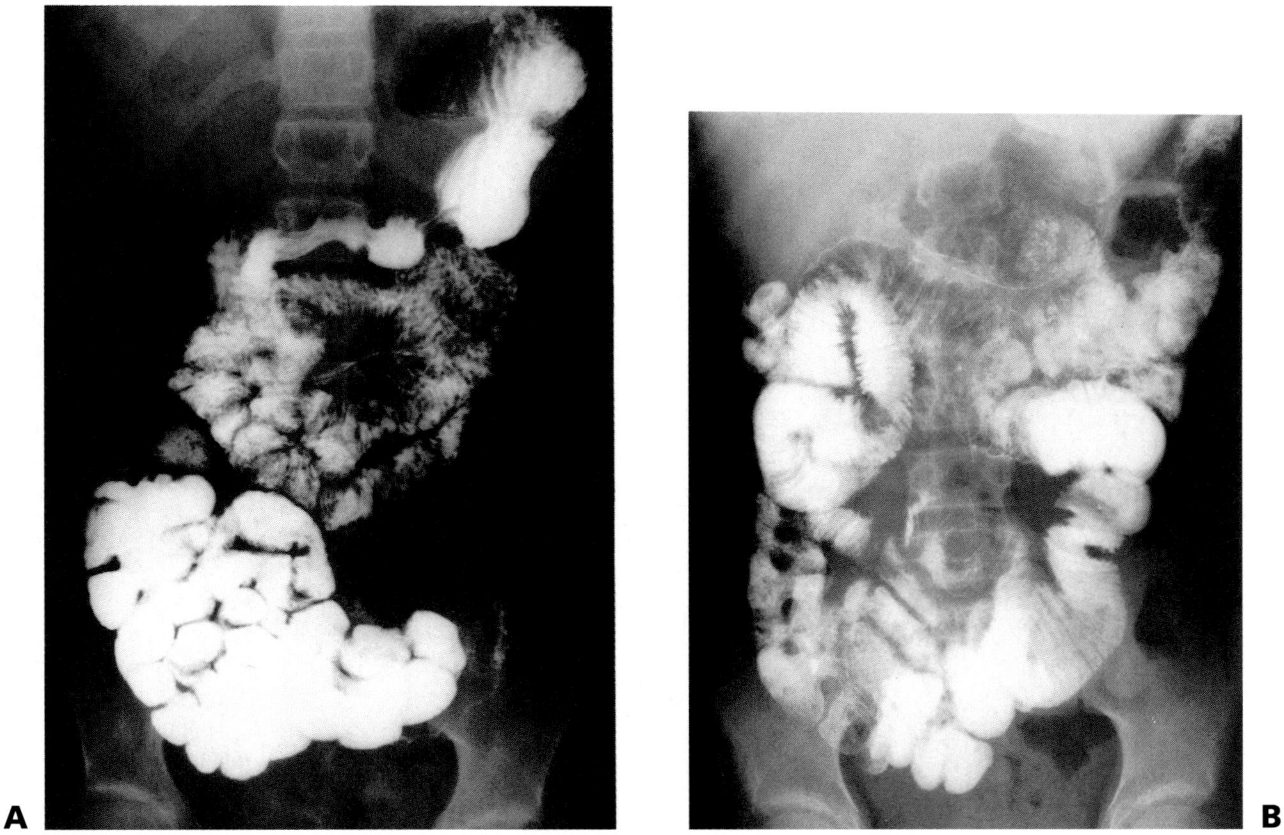

Figure 4-1

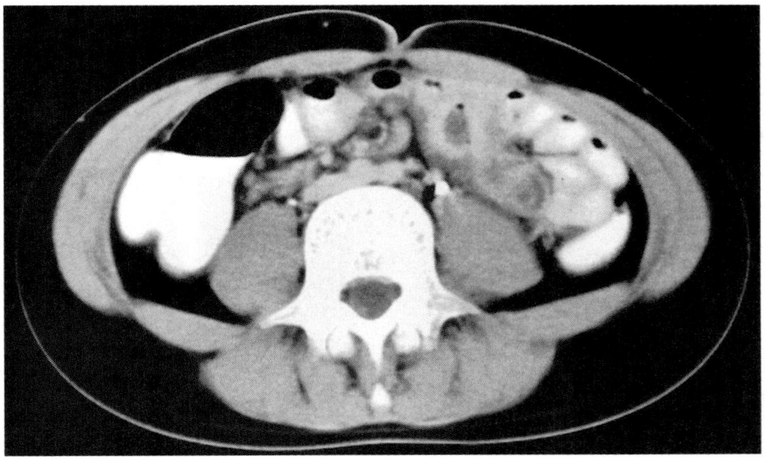

Figure 4-2

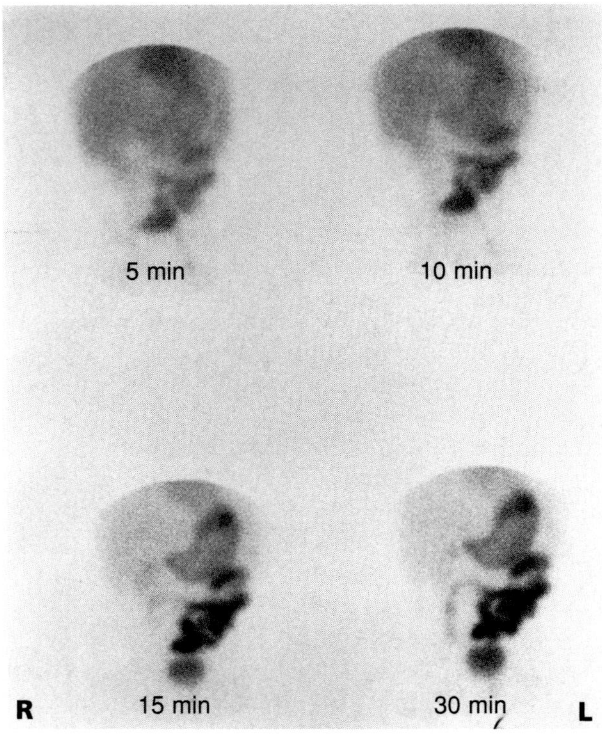

Figure 4-3 (See page 42)

Question 17

This 14-year-old boy has a history of intermittent abdominal pain and guaiac-positive stools. You are shown abdominal radiographs obtained 60 minutes (Figure 4-1A) and 90 minutes (Figure 4-1B) after the ingestion of barium and a postcontrast CT image (Figure 4-2).

The diagnoses that should be considered include:

(A) regional enteritis
(B) intussusception
(C) B-cell lymphoma
(D) Henoch-Schönlein purpura
(E) enteric duplication

Anteroposterior radiographs of the abdomen obtained 60 and 90 minutes after the ingestion of barium (Figure 4-1) show separation of small bowel loops in the lower abdomen and midabdomen, a focally dilated segment of small bowel with a plicated fold pattern, and a narrowed segment of small bowel in the left upper quadrant. Barium is noted within the colon. There is no evidence of a complete bowel obstruction (Figure 4-4). Figure 4-2 is a CT scan through the midabdomen obtained after administration of oral and intravenous contrast agents. The CT scan shows a tubular structure in the left abdomen between the psoas muscle and adjacent anterior small bowel loops; the structure has enhancing walls and low-attenuation contents, including a small amount of air (Figure 4-5). This appearance could represent either intrinsic disease of the bowel wall (e.g., inflammation, hemorrhage, or tumor) or

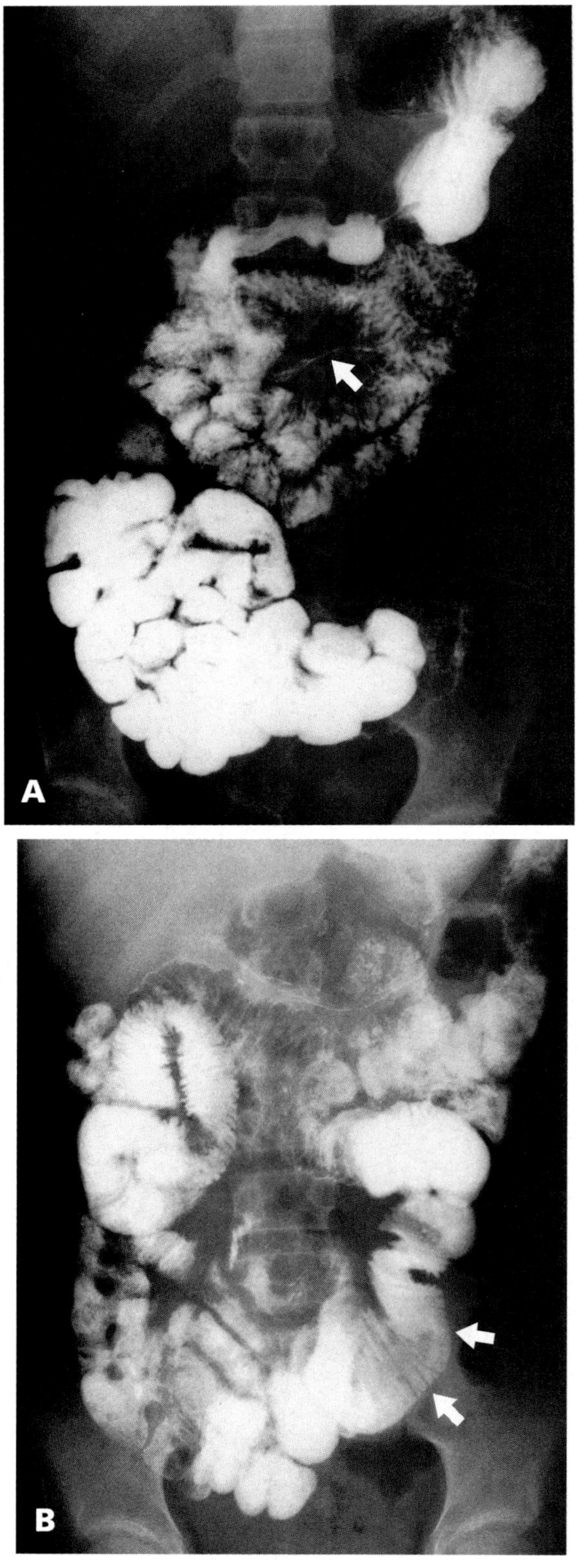

Figure 4-4 (Same as Figure 4-1). Enteric duplication. (A) A 60-minute radiograph of the abdomen during a small bowel examination shows separation of loops of small bowel in the midabdomen. There is a narrowed segment of small bowel in the left upper abdomen (arrow). (B) A 90-minute radiograph of the abdomen during a small bowel examination shows separation of loops of small bowel, with a focally dilated segment (arrows) having a plicated fold pattern.

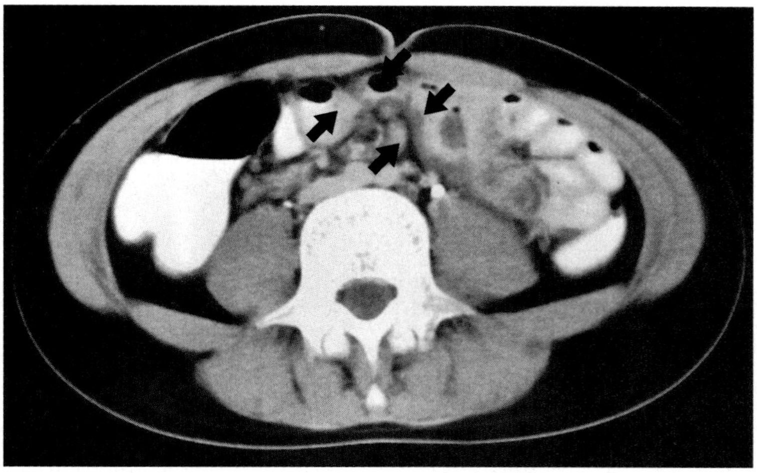

Figure 4-5 (Same as Figure 4-2). Enteric duplication. A CT image through the midabdomen after administration of oral and intravenous contrast agents shows an enhancing tubular structure (arrows) in the left abdomen, between the psoas muscle posteriorly and bowel loops anteriorly. This mass contains a small amount of gas. Its wall is thick, homogeneous, and not sharply defined.

an extrinsic mass contiguous with or adherent to the bowel wall. The imaging findings, consistent with small bowel wall thickening and inflammation, as well as the clinical findings in the test patient, are certainly compatible with a diagnosis of early regional enteritis **(Option (A) is true).**

Regional enteritis (Crohn's disease) is a disease of unknown etiology with a prolonged and unpredictable course characterized by discontinuous and asymmetric involvement of bowel. It is associated with recurring episodes of diarrhea, abdominal pain, low-grade fever, weight loss, anorexia, occult blood loss, and anemia. This process most commonly involves the small bowel. The terminal ileum is involved alone or in combination with other segments in more than 80% of patients. However, small bowel disease with a normal terminal ileum is found in up to 20% of patients at presentation.

Barium examination of the upper gastrointestinal tract and small bowel detects diseases and demonstrates the classic pathologic changes of regional enteritis in over 75% of cases. Blunting, flattening, distortion, straightening, or thickening of the mucosal folds of the small intestine may be the first manifestations of regional enteritis demonstrated on a small bowel examination (Figure 4-6). The radiographic appearance is attributable to submucosal edema and secretions on the mucosal surface of the intestine. A nodular pattern caused by more focal submucosal edema and localized inflammation can develop. Early in the course of the disease, the contour of the bowel is irregular but the wall is usually pliable. Ulcerations are not uncommon in patients with regional enteritis. Aphthoid ulcers are early lesions and correspond to mucosal erosions and edematous mounds up to 3 mm in diameter and 2 mm in depth. In order of decreasing frequency, they appear in the colon, duodenum, stomach, and esophagus. Ulcerations early in the disease are interspersed with normal mucosa.

Later in the disease, additional radiographic findings develop. The mucosal ulcerations frequently advance and fuse with each other in a linear fashion and, with intervening edematous mucosa, produce an ulceronodular pattern that results in a cobblestone appearance. Skipped areas are typical because of discontinuous involvement of the bowel. Sinus tracts, fistulas, and bowel destruction develop. There is fatty thickening or retraction of the mesentery. Loops of bowel can be separated, because of massive proliferation of mesenteric fat or lymphadenopathy, or they may display a concentric shape (the omega sign). The term "creeping fat" has been used to describe the appearance of fatty infiltration of the mesentery. Ultimately, fibrosis and scarring can result in pseudodiverticula, which are bulging areas of normal wall opposite a scarred wall; rigid, featureless bowel; long- or short-segment strictures with obstruction; and foreshortening of bowel. Many of these lesions appear at the mesenteric side of the small bowel. More proximally, dilated loops caused by incomplete chronic bowel obstruction can occur.

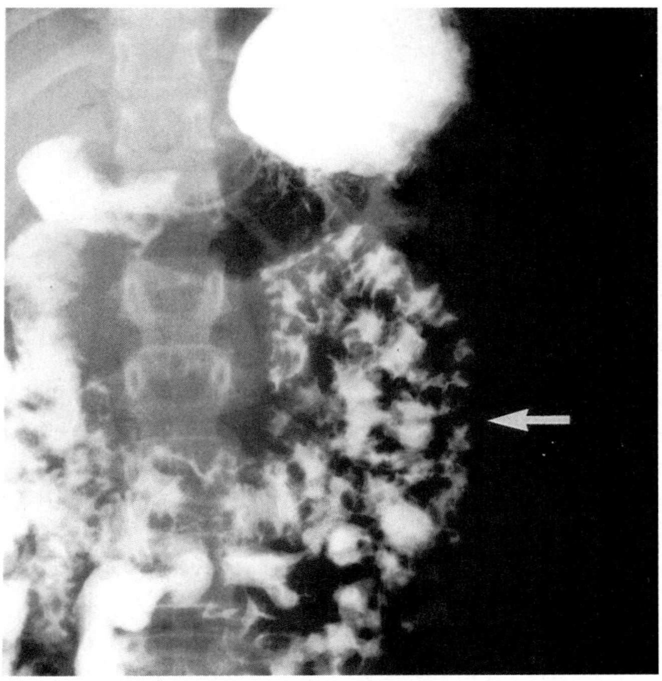

Figure 4-6. Regional enteritis. A 45-minute delayed radiograph from a small bowel examination shows blunting, distortion, and thickening of the mucosal fold pattern (arrow), characteristic of acute regional enteritis.

CT is more accurate than standard radiographs and barium enema for determining the full extent of intestinal abnormalities, especially for detecting extraintestinal complications such as abscesses (Table 4-1). A CT scan of a patient with regional enteritis will show thickening of the bowel wall. Normal bowel wall, if distended, is usually less than 2 to 3 mm thick. The mean diameter of the bowel wall in patients with early regional enteritis is between 5 and 6 mm (Figure 4-7). The intestinal lumen is typically surrounded by an inner low-density ring, secondary to edematous mucosa, and an outer ring of soft tissue thickening. This thickening, which occurs in up to 65% of patients, is observed most frequently in the terminal ileum, but other portions of the small bowel, colon, duodenum, stomach, and esophagus also can be affected. The inflamed mucosa and serosa at times will show enhancement after bolus intravenous administration of contrast medium, and the intensity of enhancement correlates with the clinical activity of disease. Other CT findings include increased mesenteric fat, soft tissue inflammation (characterized by soft tissue stranding), adenopathy in small bowel mesentery, fistula, and abscess (Figure 4-8).

CT provides useful information about intra- and extraluminal involvement with disease. However, meticulous attention to detail and technique is required. Complete bowel opacification must be achieved. An unopacified loop of intestine can be misdiagnosed as a mass, lymph node, or abscess. It is also necessary to have the bowel opacified to measure the wall thickness accurately. CT does not replace the small bowel barium examination for diagnosis, but is a powerful adjunct, especially for detecting complications. It can provide additional information in about 25% of symptomatic patients. Usually, fistulas and abscesses are the most frequent, important discovery. Another role for CT in patients with regional enteritis is guidance for percutaneous abscess drainage.

Abdominal sonography also has been found useful in de-

Table 4-1: Complications of regional enteritis

Category
Primary bowel abnormality
Fistula (30%)
Enteroenteric (most frequent between ileum and cecum)
Enterocutaneous (rectum to skin, rectum to vagina)
Perineal fistula, sinus tract
Intramural sinuses
Abscess
Toxic megacolon
Small bowel obstruction
Extraintestinal manifestations
Fatty liver
Gallstones
Sclerosing cholangitis
Cancer
Urolithiasis
Arthritis
Erythema nodosum
Uveitis

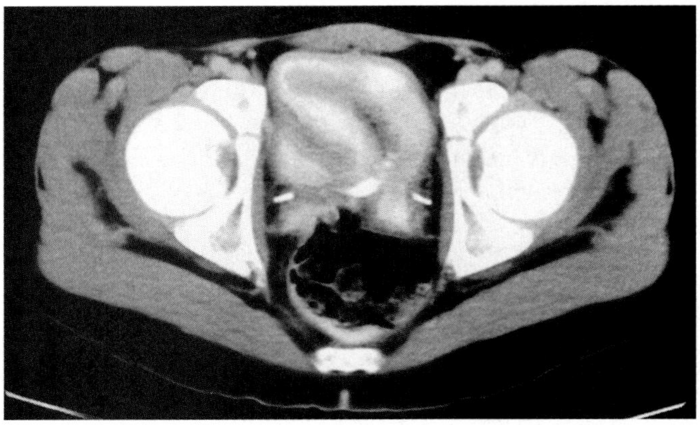

Figure 4-7. Regional enteritis. A CT image through the pelvis demonstrates irregularly thickened bowel wall as a result of the inflammatory changes of regional enteritis.

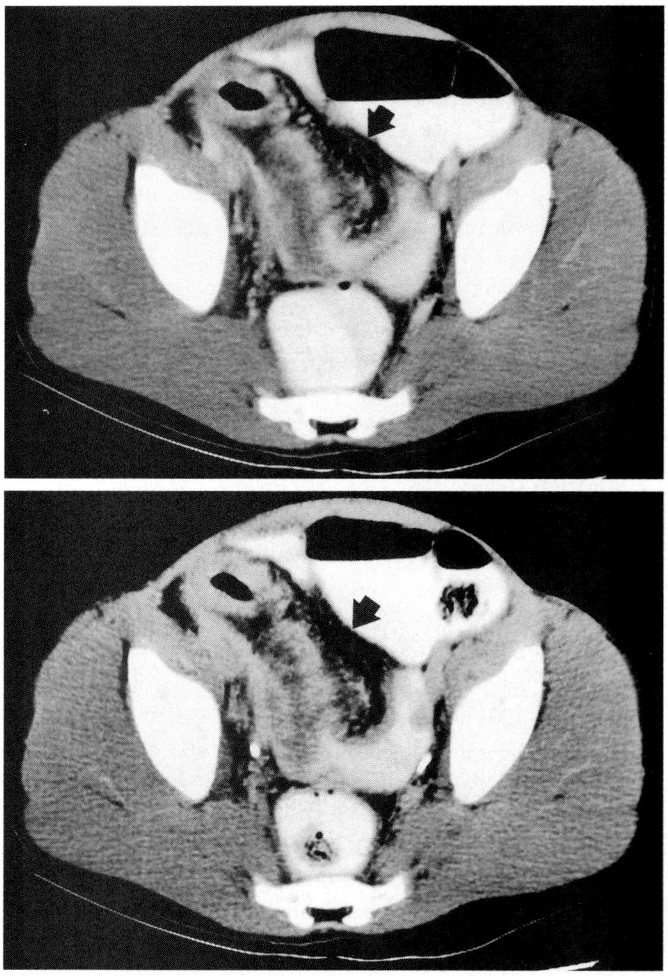

Figure 4-8. Regional enteritis. Two CT images of a 14-year-old girl demonstrate a thickened bowel wall. The bowel loops are separated by infiltrating fat within the mesentery (creeping fat) (arrows).

tection and follow-up of inflammatory bowel disease. The bowel has a bull's-eye appearance on cross-sectional images, produced by a sonolucent mantle (attributable to the thickened muscular wall) surrounding dense central mucosal echoes. Longitudinally, it appears as an elongated tubular structure with a thickened hypoechoic wall surrounding bright central mucosal echoes (Figure 4-9). Other sonographic findings include diminished peristalsis, diminished compressibility, decreased mobility, prestenotic bowel dilatation, and thickening of the mesentery. Sonography is also useful for detecting abscesses in patients with regional enteritis. An abscess can be differentiated from a loop of thickened bowel by the presence of a thick, hypervascular wall. Thickened bowel has a hypoechoic, hypovascular wall.

Sonography can also be potentially useful in separating acute-phase (inflammation) from chronic-phase (transmural fibrosis) disease by demonstrating mural stratification (i.e., visualization of distinct mucosal, submucosal, and muscularis propria layers). Stratification indicates that transmural fibrosis has not occurred and that medical therapy may be successful in reversing the edema and inflammation of the bowel wall. Even a small decrease in bowel wall thickness often produces a dramatic increase in the cross-sectional luminal area and resolution of obstruction.

Intussusception represents a common abdominal emergency of early childhood, leading to acquired bowel obstruction. Approximately 40% of intussusceptions occur in children between 3 and 9 months of age, 50% occur in children younger than 1 year, and 75% occur in children younger than 2 years. Blood in the stool (typically characterized as "currant jelly" in appearance) is present in 75% of patients. More than 75% of intussusceptions are ileocolic.

Standard abdominal radiographs are normal in 25% of children with intussusception. Radiographs, if positive, can show a small bowel obstruction, a soft tissue mass, a reduction in the length of the colon, absence of gas in the cecum or ascending colon or both, and a small bowel gas pattern in the cecal region (Figure 4-10). An antegrade small bowel examination will show a coiled-spring pattern or beaklike, abrupt narrowing of the barium column, demonstrating a central channel. CT shows multiple concentric rings (usually three concentric cylinders). The central cylinder represents the lumen plus the wall of the intussusception; the middle cylinder represents the crescent of mesenteric fat; and the outer cylinder represents the returning intussusceptum plus the intussuscipiens. CT also can show a proximal bowel obstruction and a lead mass, such as a duplication or tumor (Figure 4-11). The age of the test patient, the absence of any of the specific imaging signs of intussusception, and the absence of evidence for high-grade bowel obstruction on the barium and CT studies exclude intussusception from further consideration (**Option (B) is false**).

B-cell lymphoma is the most common cancer of the gastrointestinal tract in childhood. It occurs in the distal ileum, cecum, appendix, and proximal ascending colon. Lymphomatous involvement of the stomach or duodenum in children is unusual. Non-Hodgkin's lymphoma involves the gastrointestinal tract in approximately 10% to 20% of affected children. This disease is often widely disseminated at the time of presentation. Patients can present with blood loss, weight loss, and anorexia. Abdominal pain is common, and variable degrees of

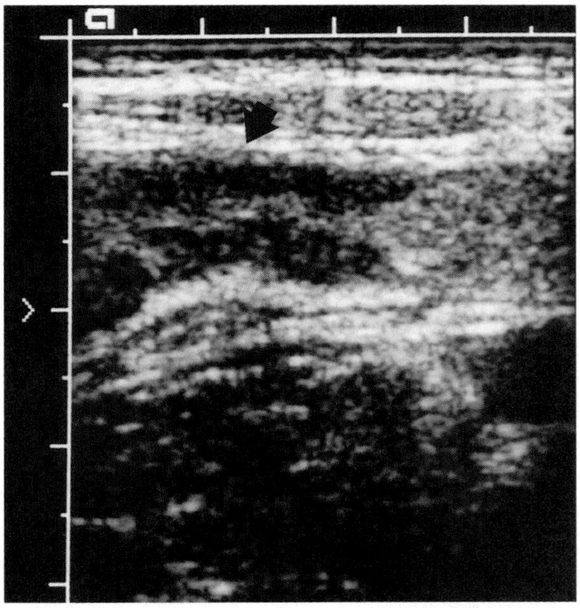

Figure 4-9. Acute regional enteritis in a 12-year-old boy. A longitudinal sonogram shows an elongated tubular segment of bowel. There is a thickened hypoechoic wall surrounding a narrowed lumen. The echogenic linear structure represents mucosa. This segment of bowel is the terminal ileum (arrow).

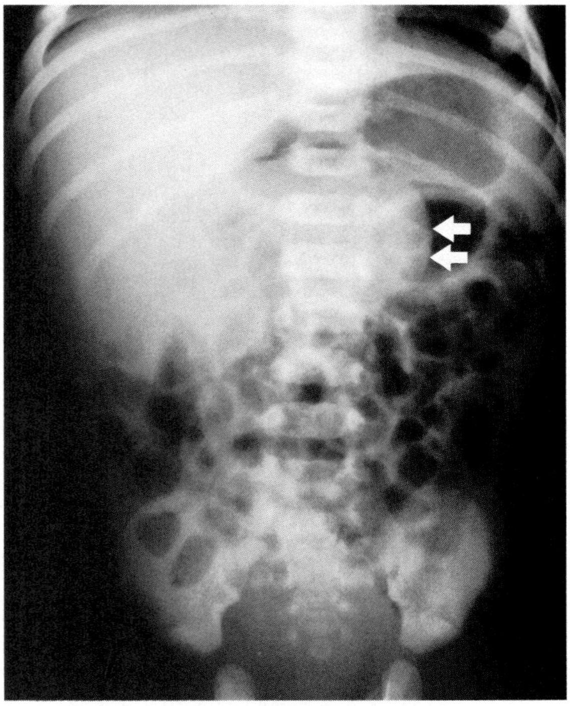

Figure 4-10. Intussusception. An abdominal radiograph shows a soft tissue mass (the intussusceptum) (arrows) in the transverse colon surrounded partially by air.

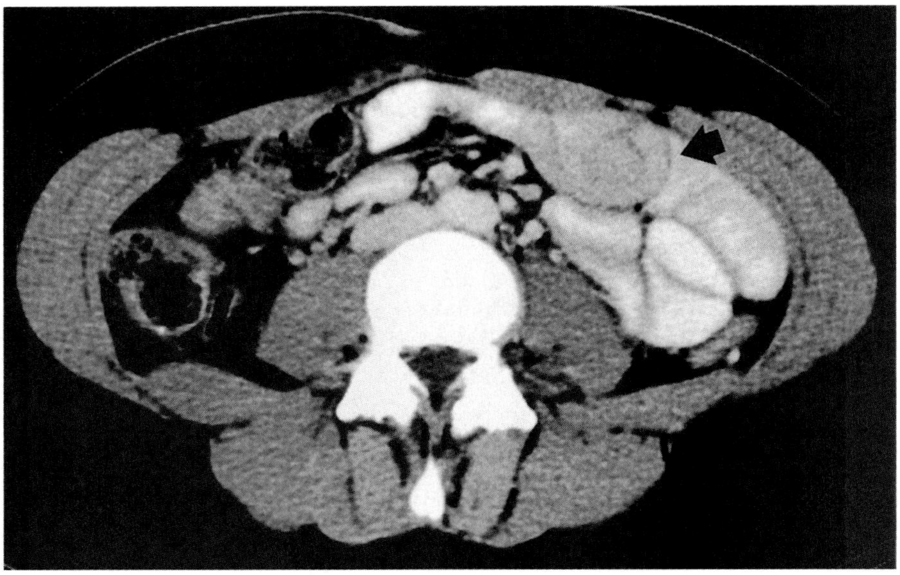

Figure 4-11. Intussusception. A CT image of a 17-year-old girl with intermittent abdominal pain shows a concentric ring appearance (arrow) as well as the intussusceptum and intussuscipiens. At surgery a small benign polyp was identified in the small bowel.

intestinal obstruction may be related to encroachment of the mass on the bowel lumen or, occasionally, to intussusception. A large palpable abdominal mass is common, occurring in more than 50% of children with this disease. Most often the lymphomatous process spreads circumferentially throughout the submucosa of the intestine.

On barium studies, small bowel lymphoma can take the form of an infiltrative process or a polypoid mass. The infiltrative variety causes marked thickening of the bowel wall (Figure 4-12). There also may be aneurysmal dilatation of the bowel lumen owing to the replacement of the muscular layers by tumor tissue (Figure 4-13). Barium is frequently stagnant in these adynamic dilated segments. The infiltrating pattern of lymphoma in the gastrointestinal tract usually involves a segment of bowel wall more than 10 cm long.

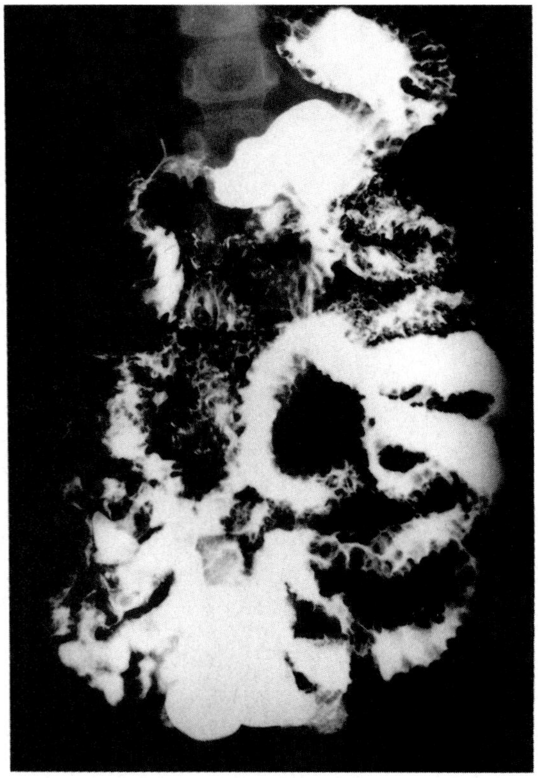

Figure 4-12. Lymphoma. A 45-minute delayed radiograph of the abdomen during a small bowel examination shows extensive nodularity of the entire small bowel as a result of lymphoma. Note the wide separation of bowel loops, indicating wall thickening.

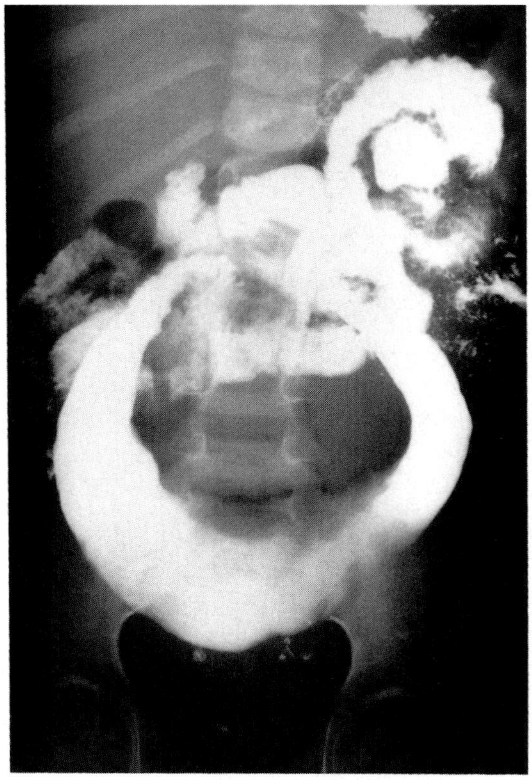

Figure 4-13. Lymphoma. A 90-minute radiograph of the abdomen during a small bowel examination shows separation of loops of intestine with aneurysmal dilatation of one long segment.

The polypoid type of lymphoma can produce nodular defects, with or without ulceration, on the small bowel examination. It occasionally results in intussusception or a sprue-like pattern. When there is mesenteric or retroperitoneal adenopathy, multiple extraluminal masses are identified displacing or separating bowel loops. These masses also can engulf and encase adjacent loops of intestine (Figure 4-14).

CT findings for bowel lymphoma include a wall thickness of more than 1 cm, aneurysmal dilatation, polypoid masses with exophytic extension, and mesenteric and retroperitoneal adenopathy (Figure 4-15). The exophytic characteristics of lymphoma and the mesenteric and retroperitoneal adenopathy are better appreciated on CT scans than on barium examinations. Because lymphoma can thicken the bowel wall and cause a variety of imaging findings, it should be included in the differential diagnosis of the test patient (**Option (C) is true**).

On rare occasions, regional enteritis and non-Hodgkin's lymphoma of the gastrointestinal tract cannot be distinguished, causing a diagnostic dilemma. Both entities have a predilection for the terminal small bowel and cause thickening of the bowel wall. In some patients with lymphoma, small fistula tracts can extend into the neoplastic mass and, rarely, abscesses or perforations develop, further mimicking regional enteritis.

Henoch-Schönlein (anaphylactoid) purpura is a diffuse vasculitis. In most children, it appears as purpura associated with joint pain and occasionally with nephritis. The gastrointestinal tract is frequently involved; bowel manifestations occur before the more diagnostic dermatologic findings become evident in about 10% of patients. Intramural hemorrhage results from capillary damage, and perivascular inflammation can involve both large and small bowels. On a barium examination, the small intestine can show symmetric thickened folds (i.e., a stack-of-coins appearance) or nodular impressions (i.e., thumbprinting). Loops of intestine can become separated. An area of bowel wall bleeding can act as a lead point for intermittent intussusception. In addition, luminal narrowing can occur as a result of bowel wall thickening attributable to bleeding (Figures 4-16 and 4-17). CT and ultrasonography demonstrate bowel wall thickening and intussusception if present (Figures 4-18 and 4-19). The presence of appar-

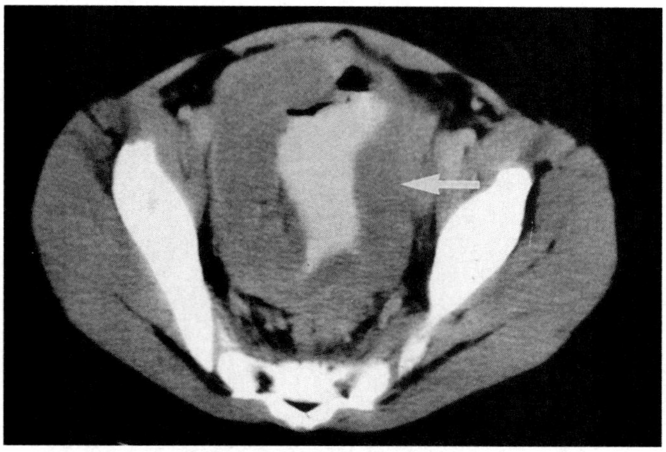

Figure 4-15. Lymphoma. A CT image through the pelvis after oral and intravenous contrast agent administration shows a long segment of small bowel (arrow) with wall thickening of more than 3 cm.

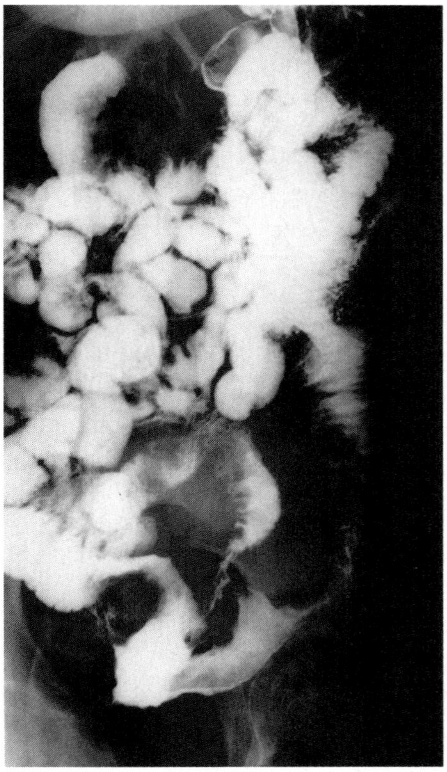

Figure 4-14. Lymphoma. A 60-minute radiograph of the abdomen during a small bowel examination shows separation of intestinal loops, segments where there is narrowing of the intestinal lumen, and other, dilated segments, with loss of the normal intestinal fold patterns.

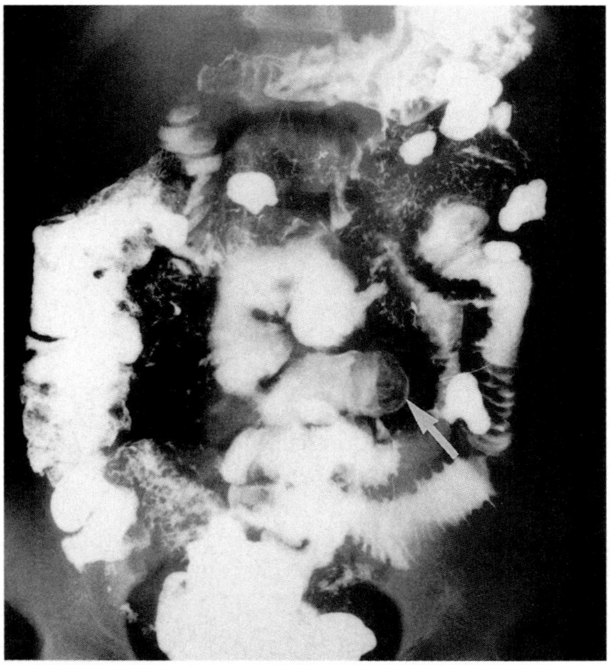

Figure 4-16. Henoch-Schönlein purpura. A 4-hour delayed abdominal radiograph during a small bowel examination shows separation of intestinal loops, symmetric thickened folds, and an associated intussusception (arrow).

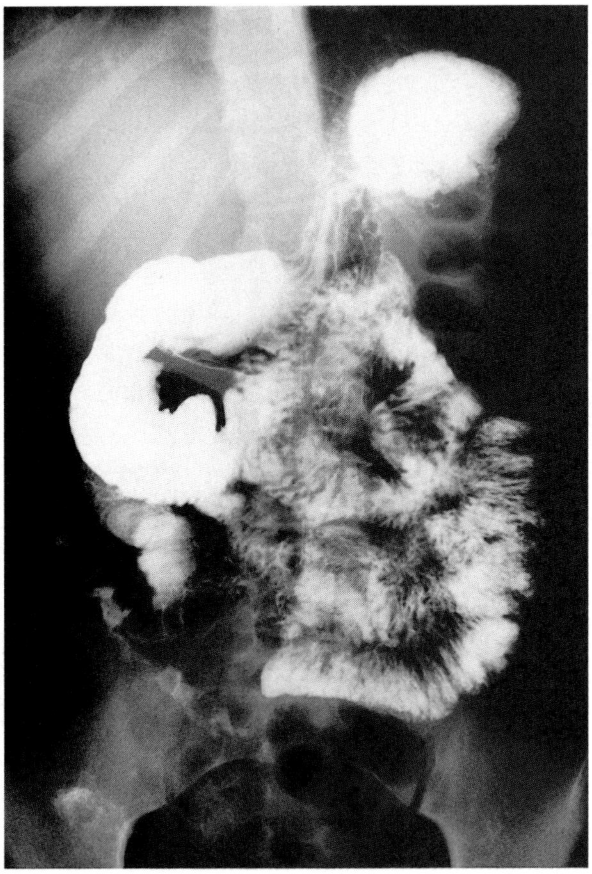

Figure 4-17. Henoch-Schönlein purpura. A small bowel examination of a 12-year-old girl shows dilatation of the duodenum secondary to a more distal hemorrhage in the bowel wall. The ileum is thickened and nodular, and loops of small bowel are separated.

ent bowel wall thickening in the test patient makes Henoch-Schönlein purpura a possible diagnosis (**Option (D) is true**).

Gastrointestinal duplications can be either spherical or tubular. They can arise anywhere from the tongue to the anus, but the distal ileum is the most frequent location, followed by the distal esophagus, stomach, and duodenum. Approximately

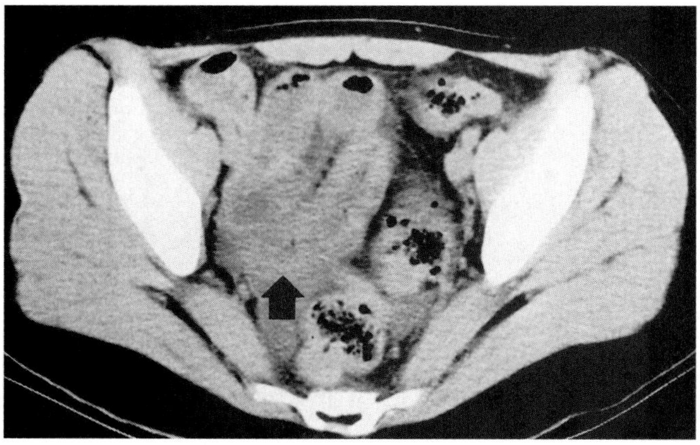

Figure 4-18. Henoch-Schönlein purpura. A nonenhanced CT image through the pelvis shows a moderately thickened small bowel wall (arrow) secondary to hemorrhage. There is no evidence of creeping fat or an inflammatory abnormality.

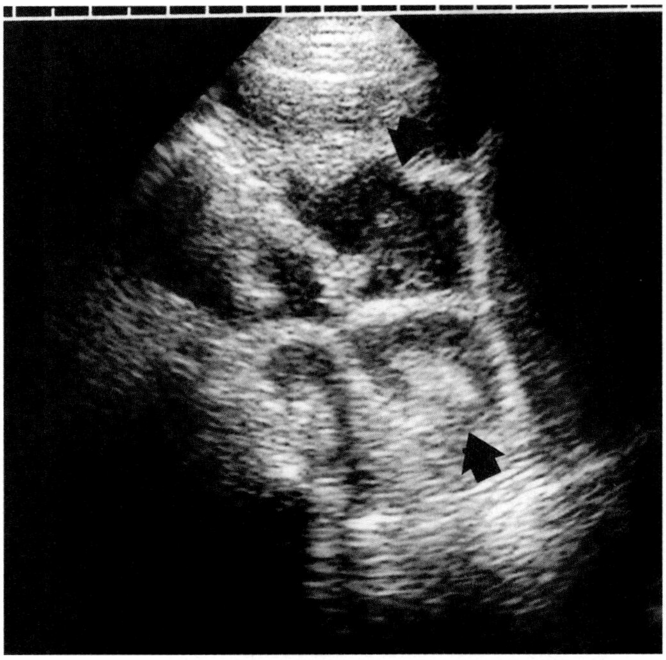

Figure 4-19. Henoch-Schönlein purpura. A sonogram of the right lower quadrant shows echogenic mucosa surrounded by thickened hypoechoic bowel walls. This segment of bowel is the terminal ileum (arrows).

50% of patients with duplications of the small intestine present with abdominal pain attributable to partial or complete bowel obstruction. An abdominal mass is palpable in about 20% of patients; this is more common in infants. Gastrointestinal hemorrhage or intussusception is seen in about 10% of patients. Chronic, intermittent abdominal pain is a frequent complaint in older children.

Radiographic findings of duplication include an intestinal obstruction, most often attributable to volvulus, and a soft tissue mass; barium studies show displacement or compression of bowel loops (Figures 4-20, 4-21, and 4-22). Duplications rarely fill with contrast medium. CT shows a spherical or tubular mass with a well-defined wall (Figure 4-23). This mass is usually unilocular, but a multilobular or septated mass is occasionally identified. The lumen may contain gas, blood, or fluid. Associated findings include thickening of adjacent bowel wall and mesentery secondary to inflammatory changes. Because duplication can cause a mass adjacent to bowel, as well as thickened bowel loops, this diagnosis must be considered in the test patient (**Option (E) is true**).

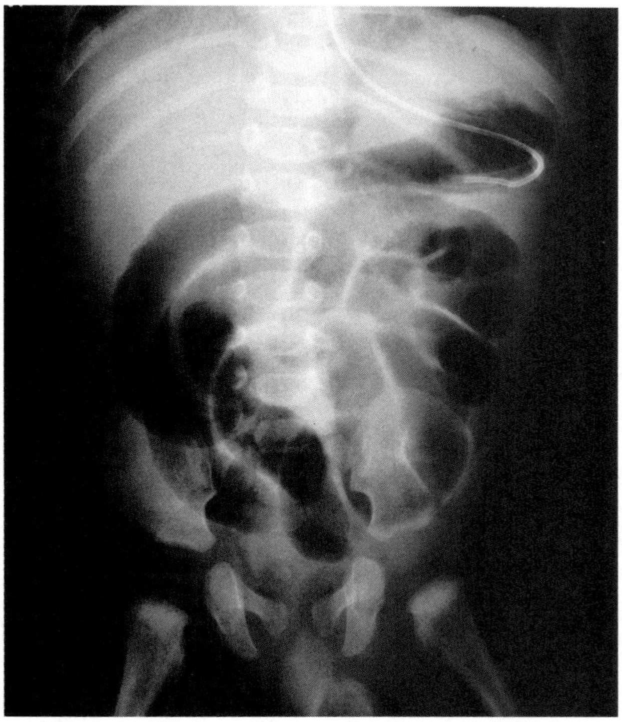

Figure 4-20. Enteric duplication. An abdominal radiograph shows a nasogastric tube in the stomach and multiple dilated featureless loops of small bowel in a 1-month-old boy. The findings indicate small bowel obstruction, but the cause is not identified. This was an intestinal obstruction due to volvulus from a small bowel duplication.

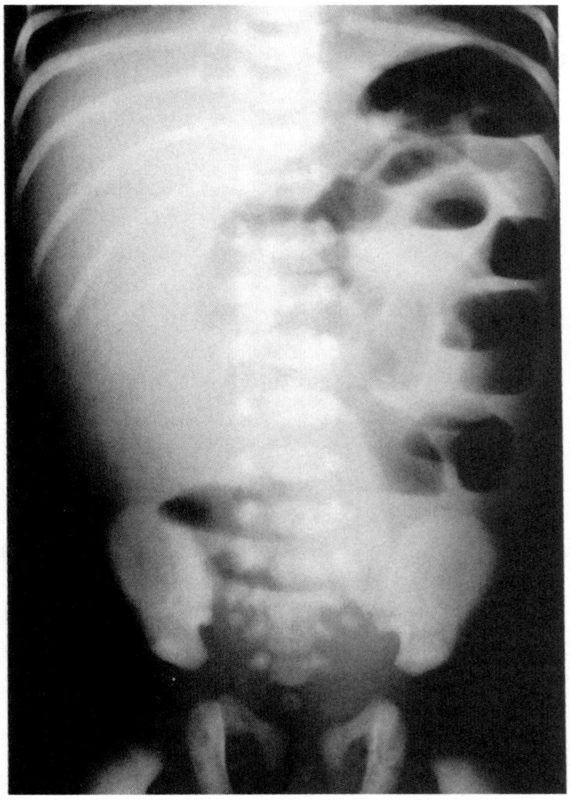

Figure 4-21. Duplication. This newborn boy presented with a bowel obstruction attributable to an ileal duplication. The upright radiograph shows air-fluid levels and distension of small bowel, indicating a small bowel obstruction. The etiology cannot be determined from the radiograph.

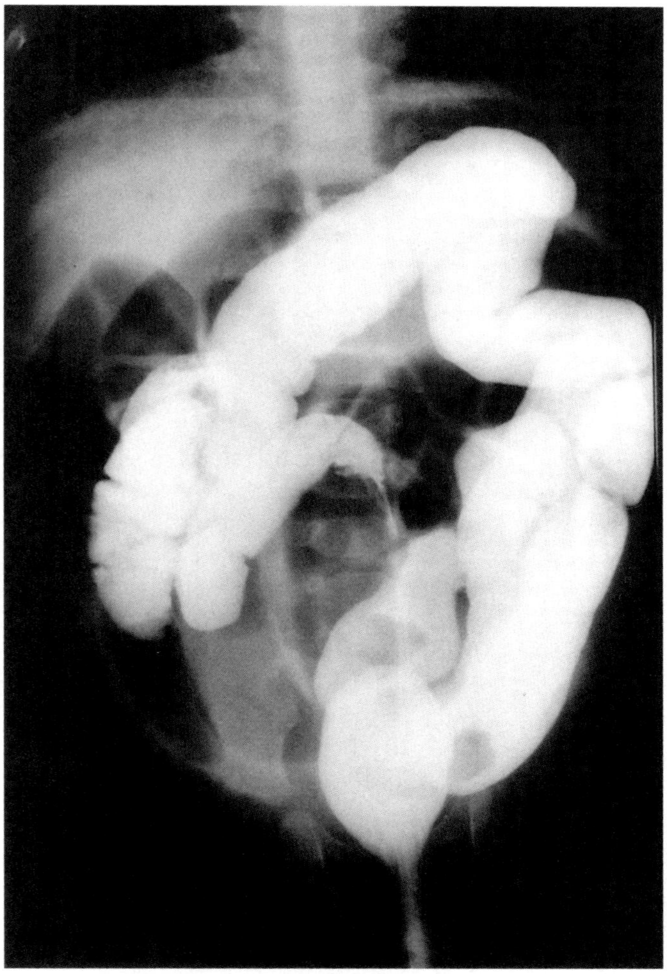

Figure 4-22. Duplication. A water-soluble enema shows a normal colon with extrinsic compression of the ileal lumen. A mass effect caused by the duplication situated between the ileum and the sigmoid colon is also present.

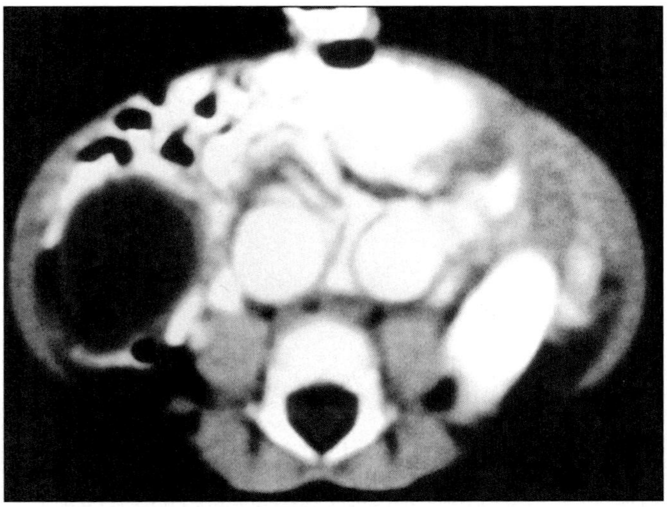

Figure 4-23. Duplication. A CT image shows a fluid-filled mass with a thin wall obstructing the terminal ileum and displacing bowel. This finding represents an ileal duplication. An umbilical hernia is also present.

Question 18

The patient then underwent abdominal imaging with Tc-99m pertechnetate. You are shown sequential anterior images (Figure 4-3) (see page 34).

Which *one* of the following is the MOST likely diagnosis?

(A) Regional enteritis
(B) Intussusception
(C) B-cell lymphoma
(D) Henoch-Schönlein purpura
(E) Enteric duplication

The sequential Tc-99m pertechnetate abdominal images of the test patient (Figure 4-3) show progressive accumulation of radiopharmaceutical in a long tubular structure (Figure 4-24). The radiopharmaceutical concentrating in the tubular structure appears simultaneously with the appearance of gastric mucosa, and thus the tubular structure could not be filling by translocation of activity secreted into gastric contents. The duodenum and proximal jejunum would be seen sequentially after the stomach and before the tubular structure if the latter were filling from above.

Preoperative detection of ectopic gastric mucosa is facilitated by Tc-99m pertechnetate abdominal imaging. The specificity of this test is greater than 95% for detection of ectopic gastric mucosa. Pertechnetate ions accumulate in the mucous cells of the gastric mucosa and subsequently are secreted into the lumen of the stomach, duplication, or Meckel's diverticulum. Mucous cells normally secrete fluid that is similar to an ultrafiltrate of plasma to which mucus has been added. Histologically identical mucous cells are found in the mucosa of the small intestine, but they are less abundant, and the secretory rate is lower than that of gastric mucosa cells. Parietal cells do not specifically accumulate pertechnetate ions and, consequently, are not essential for a positive Tc-99m pertechnetate study.

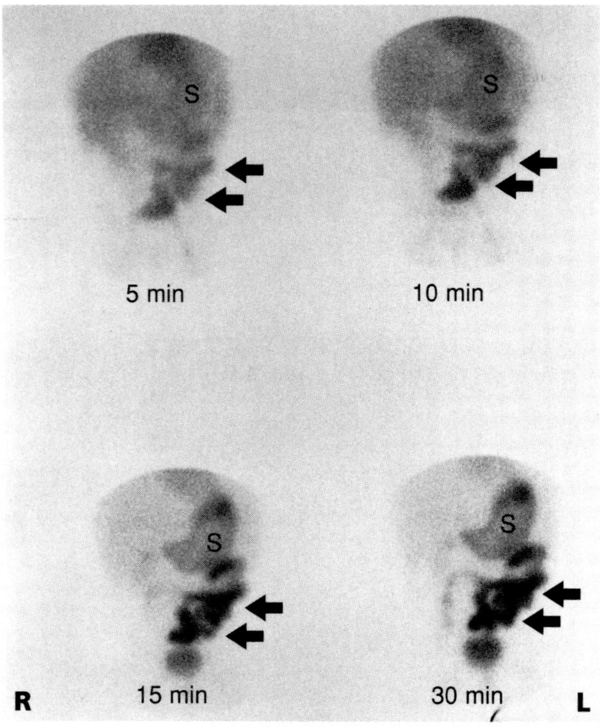

Figure 4-24 (Same as Figure 4-3). Enteric duplication. Sequential anterior images obtained after injection of Tc-99m pertechnetate demonstrate progressive accumulation of tracer (arrows) in a long segment of what appears to be small bowel in the left abdomen but actually represents a long duplication paralleling the bowel. The uptake in the duplication occurs simultaneously with the uptake in the stomach (S).

Ectopic gastric mucosa that accumulates Tc-99m pertechnetate can be easily recognized by Tc-99m pertechnetate abdominal imaging because of the high contrast against a relatively low-activity background. In general, the radiopharmaceutical uptake in the ectopic gastric mucosa appears simultaneously with that in the stomach. However, there is less gastric mucosa in the Meckel's diverticulum or duplication than in the stomach, and therefore the intensity of uptake in the stomach is frequently greater. The abnormal accumulation of radiopharmaceutical usually persists during the study. Occasionally, the activity decreases with time because of translocation of the secreted tracer into more distal bowel or because of dilution.

Of the lesions in the differential diagnosis, only small bowel duplication contains ectopic gastric mucosa. Gastric mucosa is found in at least 15% of small bowel duplications. Consequently, enteric duplication is the most likely diagnosis **(Option (E) is correct).**

The diagnosis of duplication in the test patient was confirmed at surgical exploration. The entire duplication was removed. Histologic examination demonstrated gastric, pancreatic, and colonic mucosae.

The radiographic findings in the test patient are readily understood once the diagnosis is known. The gastrointestinal barium examination (Figure 4-1) demonstrated the presence of a duplication with narrowing of the normal bowel lumen, as well as displacement of bowel loops. The duplication itself did not fill with barium. There was no specific characterization of the duplication with this examination. CT (Figure 4-2) showed a tubular structure with minimally enhancing walls and low-attenuation contents. A small amount of air also was identified within this tubular mass. These findings are suggestive of an intestinal duplication. The Tc-99m pertechnetate abdominal images (Figure 4-3) showed that the tubular mass that displaced intestinal loops contained gastric mucosa. These images definitively identified the abnormality as a duplication preoperatively.

A number of factors can influence the detectability of ectopic gastric mucosa. A false-negative diagnosis can result if Tc-99m pertechnetate imaging is performed within 24 hours of a barium gastrointestinal study, because the photons are attenuated by the barium. Potassium perchlorate also can cause a false-negative result because it will competetively inhibit the uptake of the radiopharmaceutical. Finally, a large urine-filled bladder that contains radiopharmaceutical can mask a small duplication or Meckel's diverticulum adjacent to the bladder.

There are several causes of false-positive diagnoses. These include isolated mural rests of ectopic gastric mucosa, which can occur anywhere in the gastrointestinal tract. Although they are usually small and clinically not significant, they are occasionally large enough to be detected by abdominal imaging. Whether these lesions could lead to small bowel ulcerations and subsequent bleeding is open to clinical debate.

Inflammation of the gastrointestinal tract secondary to regional enteritis, ulcerative colitis, or other disorders can be associated with increased uptake of Tc-99m pertechnetate as a result of hyperemia. Hemangiomas also can be visualized with Tc-99m pertechnetate because of their increased blood volume. However, during the course of the examination, inflammatory lesions and hemangiomas become less intense with time (Figure 4-25).

Tc-99m pertechnetate imaging in patients with regional enteritis (Option (A)), intussusception (Option (B)), B-cell lymphoma (Option (C)), or Henoch-Schönlein purpura (Option (D)) will either be normal or show findings more consistent with inflammation than with ectopic gastric mucosa. Therefore, they are not likely diagnoses in the test patient.

If the clinical presentation suggests Meckel's diverticulum or small bowel duplication and routine Tc-99m pertechnetate abdominal imaging is normal, a repeat study after administration of pentagastrin, cimetidine, or glucagon may provide additional information. Pentagastrin enhances gastric secretion directly; cimetidine, a potent histamine H2-receptor antagonist, inhibits the secretion of pertechnetate from mucous cells into the gastrointestinal lumen; and glucagon, an intestinal antiperistaltic agent, improves the quality of images by decreasing bowel peristalsis. The combined pharmacologic effects of these drugs potentially would lessen the dilution of tracer at the site of ectopic gastric mucosa.

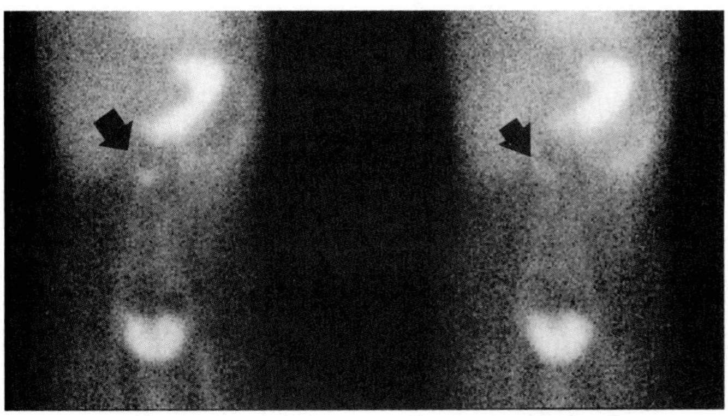

Figure 4-25. Hemangioma. This 2-year-old boy presented with gastrointestinal bleeding attributable to a duodenal hemangioma. The 10-minute Tc-99m pertechnetate image shows a focal area of abnormal activity in the transverse portion of the duodenum (arrow). A small amount of radiopharmaceutical is present distally. The 20-minute image shows less activity in the lesion (arrow) and more activity in the bowel. Surgery confirmed a hemangioma of the duodenum. Bleeding was found at the site of the lesion.

In addition to Tc-99m pertechnetate abdominal imaging, Tc-99m sulfur colloid imaging and Tc-99m erythrocyte imaging have been used for detection and localization of gastrointestinal bleeding, with excellent results. These scintigraphic techniques appear to be more sensitive than angiography for the detection of active bleeding; however, they are limited in that they do not define the etiology or the precise anatomic location of bleeding. Nonetheless, scintigraphic bleeding studies are useful as a guide to endoscopy or as a screening test for arteriography in the management of acute gastrointestinal bleeding.

With Tc-99m sulfur colloid imaging, the lower two thirds of the abdomen is imaged with a gamma camera. If there is active bleeding into the lumen of the gastrointestinal tract, a small volume of injected radiopharmaceutical will extravasate at the bleeding site whereas a larger portion will be extracted from the circulation by the reticuloendothelial system of the liver and spleen. Because of the rapid clearance of the radiopharmaceutical from the vascular system by the liver and spleen, high contrast is eventually obtained between the site of bleeding and the background activity in the abdomen caudal to the liver and spleen. Gastrointestinal bleeding of as little as 0.1 mL/minute can be detected. Because of the intense uptake of Tc-99m sulfur colloid in the liver and spleen, this technique is not useful in evaluating the cause of upper gastrointestinal tract bleeding.

Gastrointestinal bleeding also can be evaluated with the use of Tc-99m erythrocytes. With this technique, the liver and spleen do not interfere with visualization of bleeding in the upper abdomen to the same degree as they do in Tc-99m sulfur colloid imaging. Also, since the radiopharmaceutical remains in the blood pool, continuous or sequential imaging can be performed over a 4- to 6-hour period to detect intermittent bleeding.

Questions 19 through 23

For each of the numbered causes of rectal bleeding listed below (Questions 19 through 23), select the *one* lettered age range (A, B, C, or D) that is MOST closely associated with it. Each lettered age range may be used once, more than once, or not at all.

19. Necrotizing enterocolitis
20. Intussusception
21. Meckel's diverticulum
22. Juvenile polyps
23. Regional enteritis

(A) birth to 1 month
(B) 1 month to 3 years
(C) 3 to 6 years
(D) 6 to 18 years

Necrotizing enterocolitis is a pathologic condition seen almost exclusively in low-birth-weight infants (**Option (A) is the**

correct answer to Question 19). The etiology is ischemia, usually as a complication of the respiratory distress syndrome. Clinically, affected neonates have bloody stools, diarrhea, abdominal distension, and retained feedings. Standard radiographs can show absence of bowel loops in the right lower quadrant; featureless, persistently dilated loops of small intestine; pneumatosis; fluid levels; ascites; portal air; or pneumoperitoneum (Figure 4-26).

Full-term infants also can present with gastrointestinal bleeding. This may be in the form of hematemesis or hematochezia or both. Radiographic investigation in this clinical subset is seldom helpful because surgical etiologies are very uncommon. The cause of bleeding in full-term infants is usually medical rather than surgical. Medical causes of blood in the gastrointestinal tract include swallowed maternal blood, hemorrhagic disease of the newborn, disease processes that cause intestinal hypoperfusion, anal fissures, and colitis. Colitis in this age range is attributable to allergic conditions, infections, or Hirschsprung's disease. However, more than 40% of gastrointestinal bleeding in full-term infants is unexplained and ceases spontaneously. Bleeding in these patients is most likely attributable to stress ulceration. Most medical causes of bleeding in full-term infants are diagnosed by clinical and laboratory examinations and require no imaging evaluation.

Full-term neonates with Hirschsprung's disease occasionally present with bloody stools as a result of enterocolitis. The usual history is delayed passage of meconium. Of normal infants, 95% will pass meconium within 48 hours of birth, whereas 95% of infants with Hirschsprung's disease fail to pass meconium by 48 hours. The usual evaluation for the condition is a barium enema examination (Figure 4-27) and a suction biopsy.

The usual causes of rectal bleeding in infants (1 month to 3 years) are anal fissures, intussusception, inflammation, stress ulceration, and Meckel's diverticulum. The diagnosis will depend on whether the patient has minimal bleeding or severe blood loss.

Minimal blood loss is seen in infants with anal fissures, intussusception, or inflammation. Severe bleeding is usually caused by stress ulceration or Meckel's diverticulum. The diagnosis of an anal fissure is made by clinical evaluation. Intussusception is suspected when there is a history of a well child with acute abdominal pain, "currant jelly" stools, and a palpable mass. Standard radiographs of the abdomen may show a mass with or without evidence of bowel obstruction (Figure 4-10). Bleeding attributable to intussusception and Meckel's diverticulum (Figure 4-28) is most common in the age range from 1 month to 3 years (**Option (B) is the correct answer to Questions 20 and 21**).

Colitis is another cause of bleeding in patients 1 month to 3 years of age. Bloody diarrhea in a patient without fever suggests the clinical diagnosis of colitis caused by milk protein or soybean allergy. If fever is present, the colitis is usually attributable to an infection. Endoscopy can be used to identify inflammation and obtain stool cultures. Barium studies of the colon are generally not needed for diagnosis. However, if a barium

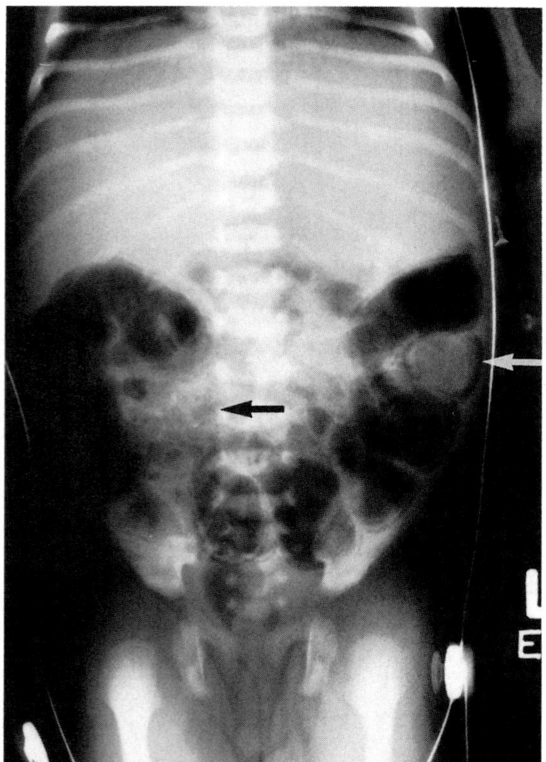

Figure 4-26. Necrotizing enterocolitis. An abdominal radiograph demonstrates pneumatosis of the small bowel and colon (arrows).

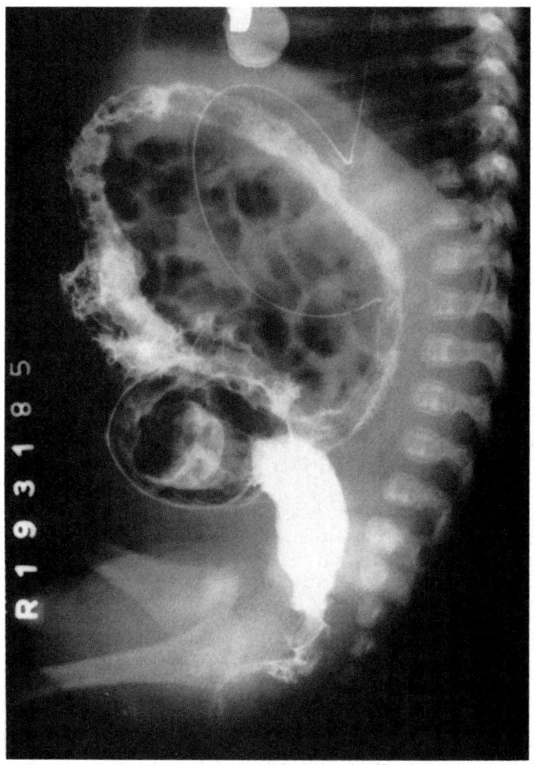

Figure 4-27. Hirschsprung's disease. A lateral radiograph of the abdomen following a barium enema examination in a newborn with Hirschsprung's disease demonstrates a nodular and ulcerative pattern in a narrowed and foreshortened colon with necrotizing colitis.

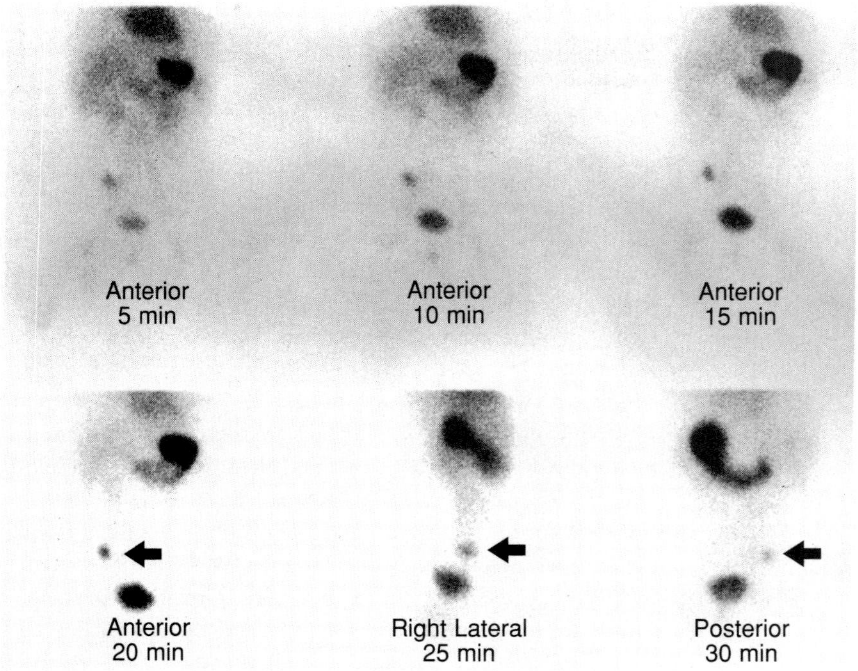

Figure 4-28. Meckel's diverticulum. A series of Tc-99m pertechnetate abdominal images show a focal region of radiopharmaceutical uptake (arrows) in the right lower quadrant. The abnormal focus appears at the same time as the stomach. This finding is characteristic of Meckel's diverticulum containing ectopic gastric mucosa.

enema is performed, stool cultures should be obtained first, since barium inhibits the growth of many organisms.

Juvenile polyps, varices, and ulcers represent the most common causes of rectal bleeding in children in the age range of 3 to 6 years (**Option (C) is the correct answer to Question 22**). Minimal rectal bleeding is the usual presentation of juvenile polyps, which are also referred to as retention or inflammatory polyps. These polyps are thought to be secondary to inflammation or a primary hamartomatous process. Approximately 80% of polyps are located within the reach of a sigmoidoscope. They are usually solitary, but 25% of patients have two or more. There is no known inheritance, nor are there any extraintestinal manifestations. Pathologically, a juvenile polyp is a benign, pedunculated lesion with a preponderance of connective and inflammatory elements overlying a glandular component. The stalk is frequently covered by normal colonic mucosa, but the surface is often denuded and ulcerated because of mechanical trauma. Juvenile polyps often undergo spontaneous amputation with regression of the stalk.

Bright red rectal bleeding is the characteristic presenting feature of a child with a juvenile polyp. The bleeding is usually painless, intermittent, and minimal. Rarely, it is quite profuse. In some patients the bleeding is occult, leading to iron deficiency anemia. Juvenile polyps occasionally have a long stalk that predisposes to intussusception. Other presenting features include prolapse of a pedunculated polyp through the anus, diarrhea, and tenesmus; these are likely to occur with a very low-lying polyp.

Any patient suspected of having colonic polyps should be evaluated by an air contrast barium enema (Figure 4-29). A juvenile polyp is demonstrated as a polypoid lesion projecting into the bowel lumen. They are most common in the rectum and sigmoid, but can occur anywhere in the colon. Most range

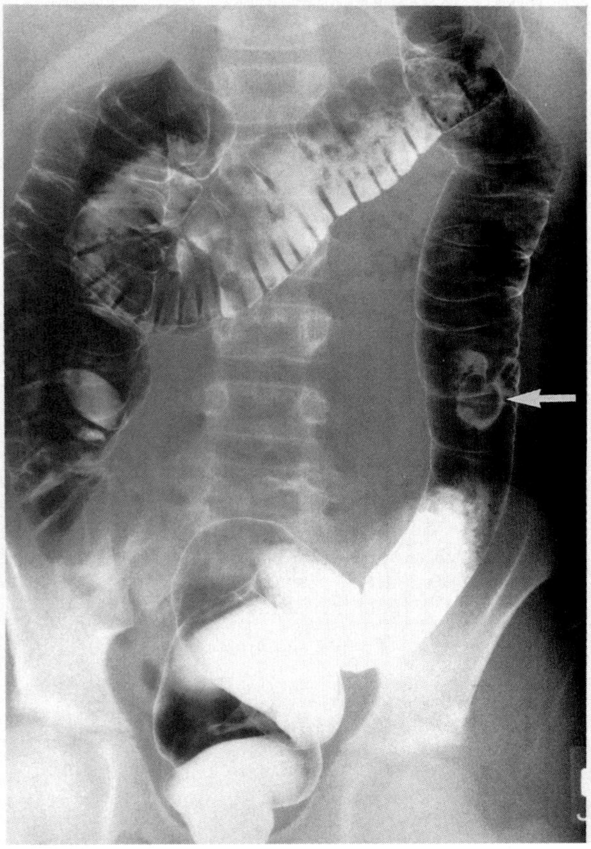

Figure 4-29. Juvenile polyp. A radiograph from an air contrast colon examination shows a polyp with a stalk in the descending segment (arrow).

in diameter from a few millimeters to 2 cm, have a smooth surface, and are usually attached to the bowel wall by a short pedicle. The differential diagnosis of juvenile polyps includes several polyposis syndromes (Table 4-2).

Regional enteritis, or Crohn's disease, is the most common chronic inflammatory small bowel disease in childhood. Of all patients with regional enteritis, 25% present during childhood; the peak incidence is in young adults. The incidence of regional enteritis in children younger than 17 years is about 6 in 10,000. It is rare in children younger than 5 years and occurs most often in children between 6 and 18 years of age (**Option (D) is the correct answer to Question 23**).

Question 24

Extraintestinal manifestations of regional enteritis include:

(A) gallstones
(B) sclerosing cholangitis
(C) urolithiasis
(D) retroperitoneal fibrosis
(E) hypertrophic osteoarthropathy

Extraintestinal complications develop in approximately 30% of patients with inflammatory bowel disease (Table 4-1). The most common serious complications of extraintestinal inflammatory bowel disease occur in the liver and biliary tract. These complications, with the exception of fatty infiltration of the liver, usually do not correlate with disease activity, duration, or severity.

Fatty liver is found in approximately 30% to 40% of patients with inflammatory bowel disease and can be caused by fat malabsorption, hyperalimentation, sepsis, protein-losing enteropathy, malnutrition, or drug therapy. CT is an excellent means of showing hepatic steatosis noninvasively. On CT, fat produces decreased attenuation of the hepatic parenchyma.

There is an increased prevalence of cholelithiasis in patients with regional enteritis (**Option (A) is true**). Bile is normally produced by hepatocytes, modified by biliary ducts, and both modified and stored in the gallbladder. Bile salts are formed in the liver from cholesterol and are then conjugated with either glycine or taurine. The conjugated bile salts are eliminated via the biliary system into the gastrointestinal tract; approximately 75% of the bile salts are then reabsorbed from the terminal ileum without bacterial alteration. The remaining bile salts are deconjugated by bacterial enzymes within the small intestine. The unconjugated portion is reabsorbed from the terminal ilium, returned to the liver via the portal system, and reconjugated with glycine or taurine. Under normal circumstances, the rate of synthesis of bile salts equals the rate of their elimination in the feces. This rapid and efficient recycling is essential for normal fat absorption.

Ileal dysfunction secondary to regional enteritis or surgery can result in inadequate absorption of bile salts from the intestinal tract. This results in depletion of the hepatic bile salts and decreases the bile salt content within excreted bile. The liver has a limited ability to change cholesterol to bile salts in order to reestablish normal levels. However, cholesterol continues to be secreted by hepatocytes into bile. This results in the excretion of bile salts supersaturated with cholesterol and finally in cholesterol gallstones. Risk factors for developing calculi include older patient age, longer duration of disease, and previous intestinal resection.

Table 4-2: Polyposis syndromes

Syndrome	Inheritance[a]	Type of Polyps[b]	Location of Polyps[c]	Risk of Malignancy
Juvenile polyps	None	Juv.	C	None
Juvenile polyposis coli	AD	Juv.	C	None
Familial polyposis coli	AD	Aden.	C, SB, ST	High
Gardner's syndrome	AD	Aden.	C, SB, ST	High
Turcot's syndrome	AR (?)	Aden.	C	High
Peutz-Jeghers syndrome	AD	Ham.	SB, C, ST	Low
Cronkhite-Canada syndrome	None	Juv.	ST, C, SB	None
Generalized gastrointestinal juvenile polyposis	AD	Juv.	SB, C	None

[a] AD, autosomal dominant; AR, autosomal recessive.
[b] Juv., juvenile; Aden., adenomatous; Ham., hamartoma.
[c] C, colon; SB, small bowel; ST, stomach.

About 30% to 50% of patients with regional enteritis eventually develop gallstones. Sonography is the primary means of detecting gallstones, while CT is superior for detecting choledocholithiasis.

Sclerosing cholangitis, which can be primary or secondary, is an uncommon disease in children. The primary idiopathic form can occur at any age and usually presents with hepatosplenomegaly and/or jaundice. The secondary form is associated with inflammatory bowel disease, both regional enteritis and ulcerative colitis (**Option (B) is true**).

Sclerosing cholangitis can affect the intrahepatic or extrahepatic biliary system or both. Histologically, there is a chronic obliterative fibrotic inflammation. The common bile duct is almost always involved; the intrahepatic and extrahepatic ducts are involved in 60% to 85% of patients; and the cystic duct is involved in about 10% to 20% of patients. Ultrasonography, CT, transhepatic cholangiography, endoscopic retrograde cholangiopancreatography, and biliary scintigraphy are all useful in the diagnosis (Figures 4-30 through 4-32). Ultrasonography shows brightly echogenic portal triads, and the intrahepatic biliary system has thickened echogenic walls with irregular dilatation and narrowing. CT shows focal dilatation, pruning, and beading of the intrahepatic bile ducts in more than 80% of patients. The larger ducts can show diffuse wall thickening. Frequently, the ducts also show contrast enhancement, which is characteristic of this disease. Complications of sclerosing cholangitis, such as secondary portal hypertension attributable to biliary cirrhosis and cholangiocarcinoma, also are well seen by CT scanning.

Transhepatic cholangiography usually demonstrates multifocal ductal strictures, usually at bifurcations, along with skip regions containing normal-caliber or slightly dilated ducts. Other findings include uniform obstruction of the peripheral radicles ("pruned-tree" appearance) or pseudodiverticula of the biliary system or both. Biliary scintigraphy with Tc-99m iminodiacetic acid agents shows delayed hepatic clearance and multiple areas of retained radiopharmaceutical in the distribution of the intrahepatic biliary tree. The gallbladder is not visualized in 25% to 75% of patients.

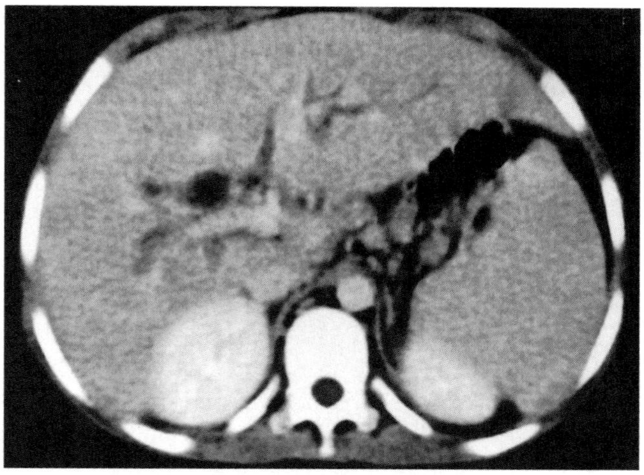

Figure 4-31. Sclerosing cholangitis. This 16-year-old boy presented with fever and right upper abdominal pain. Diagnostic evaluation revealed the etiology to be sclerosing cholangitis. A CT image of the upper abdomen with intravenous contrast material shows irregular dilatation of the intrahepatic biliary duct. The walls are slightly thickened and minimally enhanced.

Inflammatory bowel disease is the underlying disorder in about 65% of cases of secondary sclerosing cholangitis. Sclerosing cholangitis is much more common in patients with ulcerative colitis than in those with regional enteritis. Approximately 2% of patients with inflammatory bowel disease will develop sclerosing cholangitis. The remainder of patients with secondary sclerosing cholangitis have diseases such as cirrhosis, chronic active hepatitis, pancreatitis, retroperitoneal fibrosis, Peyronie's disease, Riedel's thyroiditis, hypothyroidism, and orbital pseudotumor.

Urolithiasis and hydronephrosis are important renal complications of inflammatory bowel disease (**Option (C) is true**).

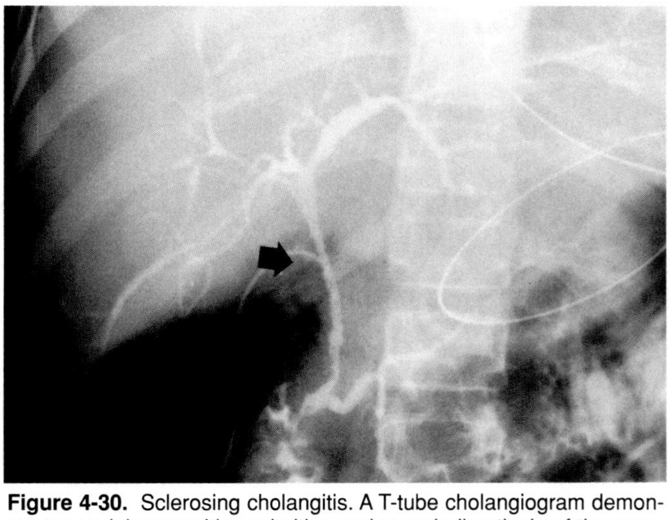

Figure 4-30. Sclerosing cholangitis. A T-tube cholangiogram demonstrates nodular mural irregularities and pseudodiverticula of the common bile duct (arrow). The intrahepatic biliary system shows the typical "pruned-tree" appearance of sclerosing cholangitis.

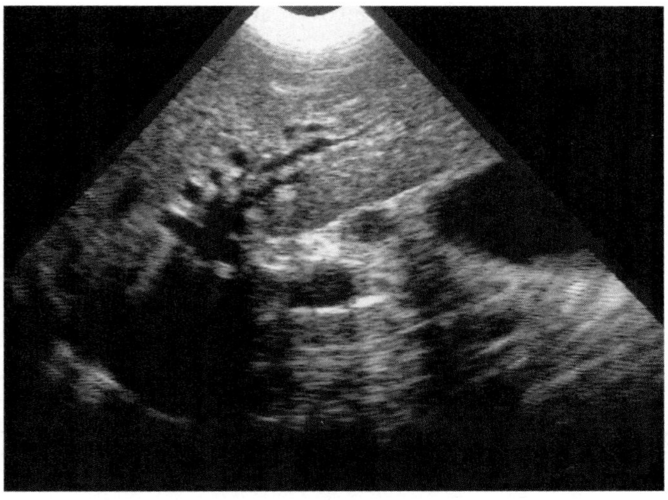

Figure 4-32. Same patient as in Figure 4-31. Sclerosing cholangitis. A sonogram shows brightly echogenic biliary duct walls with irregular dilatation.

Oxalate and uric acid stones occur in the majority of cases. The urolithiasis is probably attributable to the interruption of the enterohepatic circulation of bile salts. The exact pathophysiologic mechanisms that lead to oxalate renal stones are not known, but several have been postulated. (1) Bacteria deconjugate the increased amounts of glycine-conjugated bile salts passing into the colon. The excess glycine in the colon is further converted to glyoxalate by bacterial mechanisms, absorbed from the colon, transported to the hepatocytes, and converted to oxalate, with subsequent hyperoxaluria. (2) Malabsorbed fatty acids decrease the amount of intraluminal calcium available for binding with dietary oxalate. This facilitates abnormal oxalate absorption, leading to hyperoxaluria and nephrolithiasis. (3) Unabsorbed bile salts increase the permeability of the colon to oxalate and lead to secondary hyperoxaluria.

Calculous disease of the urinary tract is found in up to 6% of adults and 5% to 6% of children with regional enteritis. Oxalate stones can be detected by radiography or sonography. Urate stones are best seen by sonography. Hydronephrosis can also develop in patients with regional enteritis as a result of calculous disease or extrinsic compression of the ureter by abscess, phlegmon, or creeping fat.

Retroperitoneal fibrosis is uncommon in children and is not associated with inflammatory bowel disease (**Option (D) is false**). Retroperitoneal fibrosis can be either primary or secondary. The primary form represents approximately 60% of cases. It is most probably an autoimmune disease, with antibodies to ceroid leading to systemic vasculitis associated with fibrosis. The mean age of patients is 30 to 65 years. The secondary form is caused by drugs such as methysergide, phenacetin, hydralazine, ergotamine, methyldopa, amphetamine, and lysergic acid diethylamide (LSD). Tumors such as lymphomas, carcinoids, and retroperitoneal metastases are also associated with this condition. Connective tissue disease occasionally results in retroperitoneal fibrosis.

The imaging findings are characteristic. Urographic findings in patients with retroperitoneal fibrosis include delayed excretion of contrast medium with unilateral (20%) or bilateral (68%) hydronephrosis, displacement of the middle one third of the ureter, and narrowing of the ureters at the L4-L5 level. The obstruction in patients with retroperitoneal fibrosis often appears minimal despite clinical renal failure. This suggests that the obstruction is related to interference with the normal peristaltic activity of the ureter rather than to mechanical obstruction. This hypothesis is further supported by histologic examination of the ureters, which often demonstrates edema and inflammation but rarely shows fibrosis. Sonographic, CT, and MRI findings are those of a well-defined retroperitoneal mass centered over the sacral promontory. The mass surrounds the aorta and inferior vena cava circumferentially and extends laterally to entrap the ureters, with obliteration of tissue planes. Variable degrees of hydronephrosis and hydroureter are sometimes present. Retroperitoneal fibrosis is hypoechoic on sonography. On CT, retroperitoneal fibrosis has an attenuation value equal to that of muscle on unenhanced images. During the early, vascular stage of the disorder, CT shows enhancement, whereas in the late, avascular stage, enhancement is absent. On MRI, retroperitoneal fibrosis generally has low signal intensity on T1-weighted images and variable intensity on T2-weighted images depending on the stage of the disease. In the early, inflammatory stage of retroperitoneal fibrosis, there is high signal intensity on T2-weighted images, reflecting the presence of capillaries with leaking epithelial junctions and a high fluid content within the tissues. In the late, fibrous stage of the disease, there is characteristic low signal intensity on T2-weighted images, consistent with fibrosis with a low fluid content. Following steroid treatment, the signal intensity of the tissue edema in the early stage of disease can decrease on T2-weighted images. Thus, MRI may be able to assess the response to therapy.

Hypertrophic osteoarthropathy is uncommon in the pediatric population. Two categories are recognized, a primary or idiopathic form and a secondary form associated with an underlying cause. There are multiple causes, but hypertrophic osteoarthropathy is most often associated with pulmonary disease. Cystic fibrosis is the most common cause, although bronchiectasis and metastatic tumors are also causes. Rarely, hypertrophic osteoarthropathy is the presenting sign of underlying disease. Other associated conditions include biliary atresia, chronic inflammatory bowel disease (**Option (E) is true**), congenital heart disease, Hodgkin's disease, and immunodeficiency syndromes. Secondary hypertrophic osteoarthropathy can be encountered in children as young as 1 year of age.

Clinically, patients present with clubbing of the fingers or toes and arthropathy. The radiographic findings are those of periosteal new bone formation. Periosteal new bone is usually symmetric and limited to the diaphyses. It can appear smooth or laminated, and it is sometimes associated with thickening of the adjacent cortex. The most common sites, in decreasing order of frequency, include the radius and ulna, tibia and fibula, humerus and femur, metacarpals and metatarsals, and proximal and middle phalanges.

Bone scintigraphy is also a useful diagnostic modality to determine the presence of disease, and it can show disease before radiographic changes are apparent. The scintigraphic findings consist of increased accumulation of radiopharmaceutical in the diaphysis (Figure 4-33).

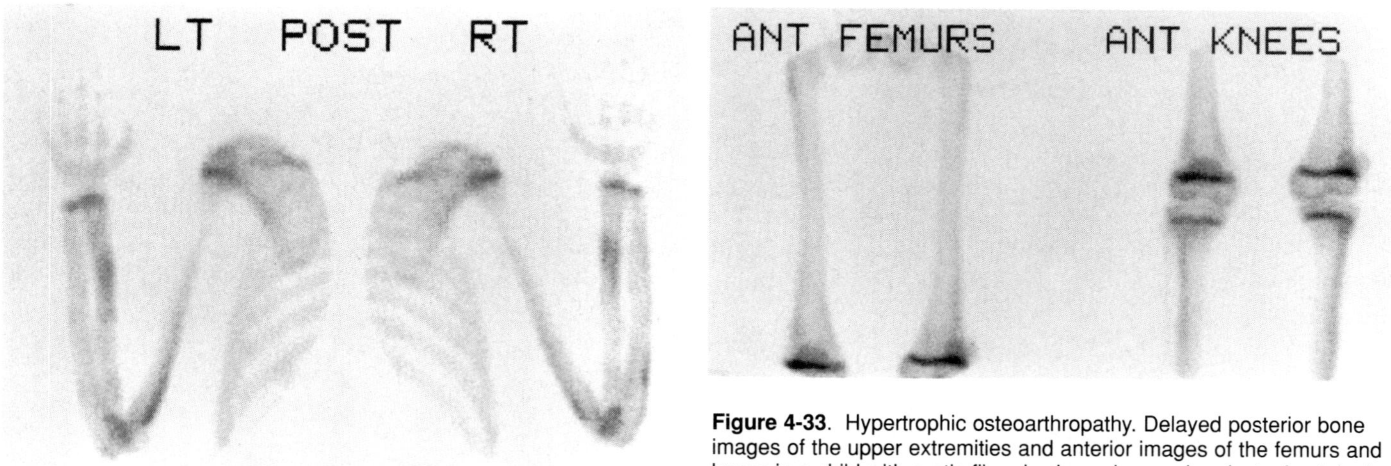

Figure 4-33. Hypertrophic osteoarthropathy. Delayed posterior bone images of the upper extremities and anterior images of the femurs and knees in a child with cystic fibrosis show abnormal periosteal uptake in the long bones.

Question 25

Concerning Henoch-Schönlein purpura,

(A) the renal findings on ultrasonography are similar to those of acute glomerulonephritis
(B) associated hydronephrosis is usually attributable to an intramural hematoma of the ureter
(C) testicular involvement occurs in about 50% of patients
(D) skin manifestations resemble erythema nodosum
(E) hydrops of the gallbladder is characteristic

Henoch-Schönlein purpura is a small-vessel vasculitis that affects children between the ages of 3 and 10 years. Boys are affected more often than girls. The disease is usually preceded by an upper respiratory tract infection 1 to 3 weeks before the onset of the clinical syndrome. The clinical manifestations relate to the skin, joints, gastrointestinal tract, and kidneys.

The disease usually begins with an acute, symmetric, erythematous, macular rash. It frequently starts around the malleoli of the ankles but eventually extends over the dorsal surfaces of the legs, buttocks, and ulnar surfaces of the arms. It frequently spares the trunk. The purpura can recur over several months. The skin manifestations do not resemble erythema nodosum (**Option (D) is false**).

The urinary tract abnormalities in patients with Henoch-Schönlein purpura are sometimes transient and can escape detection unless frequent examination of the urinary sediment is performed. Micro- or macroscopic hematuria is found in 25% of patients, and proteinuria is found in 25% to 75%. Clinical signs of renal involvement can follow or coincide with the appearance of purpura, but they rarely antedate it. Renal involvement is more common in patients with recurrent attacks of purpura and in patients with abdominal manifestations. Nephritis due to Henoch-Schönlein purpura is usually a self-limited disease, but is occasionally complicated by severe hypertension and chronic renal insufficiency.

The cortical and medullary regions of the kidney, as well as the calyxes and vessels, can be differentiated by sonography. Alterations in echogenicity within these regions provide important clues to the pathologic process. Abnormal cortical echogenicity is defined as an echotexture equal to or greater than that of the liver or spleen. Increased cortical echogenicity and increased renal size are seen in 5% of patients with Henoch-Schönlein purpura (Figure 4-34). The medulla of the kidney increases in size, as does the cortex. These findings are similar to those of acute glomerulonephritis (**Option (A) is true**). Renal biopsy will be needed to distinguish glomerulonephritis from Henoch-Schönlein purpura and to predict the outcome. Most patients with Henoch-Schönlein purpura will have a normal renal sonogram, however.

Since Henoch-Schönlein purpura is an acute inflammatory angiitis that involves small arterioles and capillaries, it can result in bleeding into the urothelium of the ureter and bladder. This results in intramural hematomas that can obstruct the ureteral lumen, leading to hydronephrosis (Figure 4-35). Although fibrosis is a sequela of hemorrhage, it is rare. Hydronephrosis is more likely to be attributable to an intramural hematoma (**Option (B) is true**).

Testicular involvement has been found in 5% to 10% of patients with Henoch-Schönlein purpura (**Option (C) is false**). Genital involvement can be the primary manifestation or can be preceded by involvement of other organs. Henoch-Schönlein purpura of the scrotum presents as painful scrotal swelling, typically in association with a purpuric rash. The pain can be severe enough to mimic orchitis or torsion. Sonography typically shows a normal-sized testis, enlarged epididymis, and scrotal skin thickening. Hyperemia of the epididymis and scrotal soft tissues is noted on color flow Doppler imaging. Radionuclide scrotal scintigraphy can also be useful in differentiating the hyperemia caused by vasculitis from ischemic torsion. If the clinical diagnosis is in doubt, surgical exploration is mandatory because torsion can occur simultaneously with Henoch-Schönlein purpura.

Acute distension of the gallbladder without associated anomalies, calculi, or acute inflammation has been identified

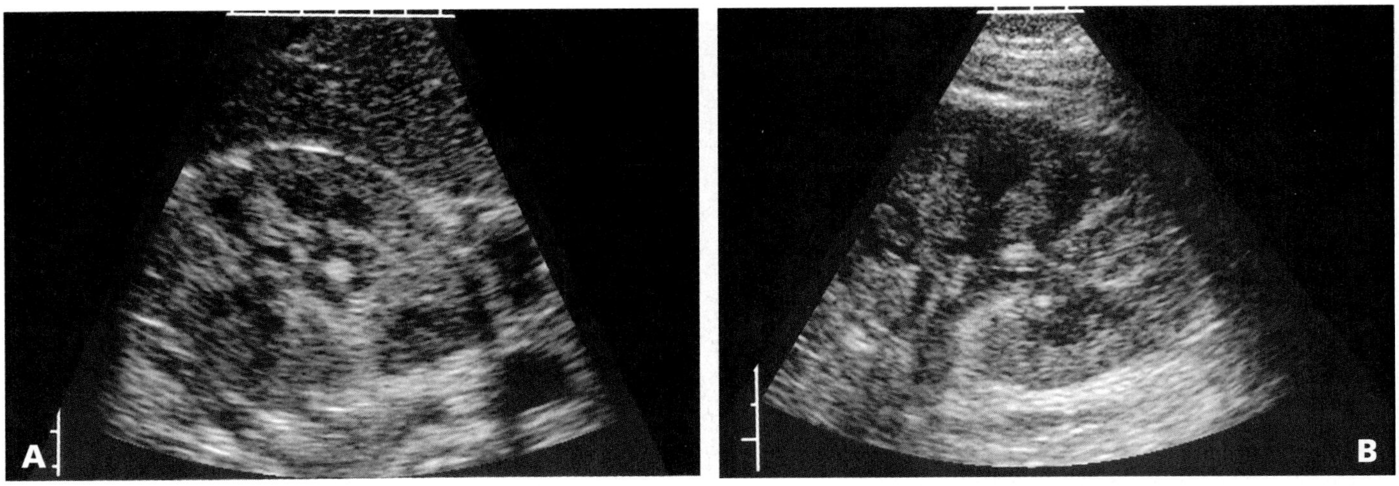

Figure 4-34. Henoch-Schönlein purpura. Longitudinal (A) and transverse (B) sonograms in a 12-year-old girl show a renal length two standard deviations greater than normal. The echogenicity of the renal cortex is higher than that of the liver, and the size of the medullary portion of the kidney is increased. These findings are similar to those seen in acute glomerulonephritis.

in children with upper respiratory tract infection, gastroenteritis, leptospirosis, sepsis, burns, ascariasis, typhoid fever, and mucocutaneous lymph node syndrome (Kawasaki disease). Hydrops of the gallbladder is not a characteristic finding of Henoch-Schönlein purpura (**Option (E) is false**).

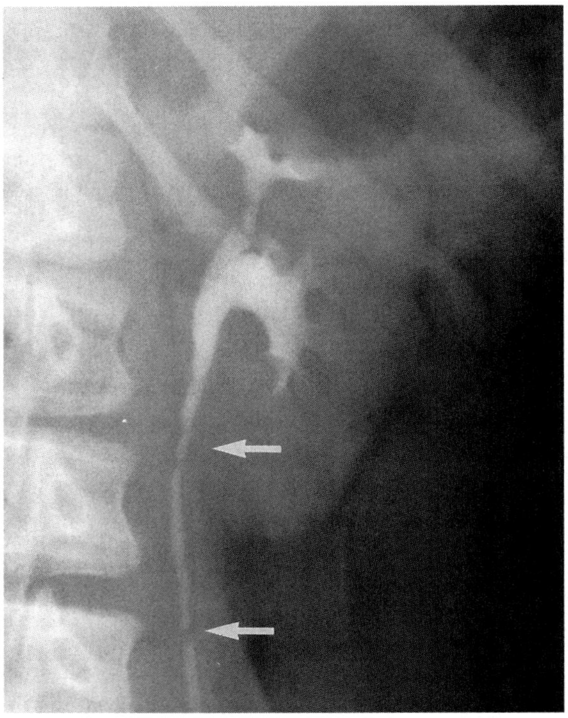

Figure 4-35. Henoch-Schönlein purpura. An 8-minute urogram of the left kidney and proximal ureter shows the beaded appearance (arrows) of the upper ureter from bleeding into the uroepithelium as a result of Henoch-Schönlein purpura.

SUGGESTED READINGS

ENTERIC DUPLICATION

1. Berrocal T, Lamas M, Gutieérrez J, Torres I, Prieto C, del Hoyo ML. Congenital anomalies of the small intestine, colon, and rectum. RadioGraphics 1999; 19:1219–1236
2. Bissler JJ, Klein RL. Alimentary tract duplications in children: case and literature review. Clin Pediatr 1988; 27:152–157
3. Bower RJ, Sieber WK, Kiesewetter WB. Alimentary tract duplications in children. Ann Surg 1978; 188:669–674
4. Brown RL, Azizkhan RG. Gastrointestinal bleeding in infants and children: Meckel's diverticulum and intestinal duplication. Semin Pediatr Surg 1999; 8:202–209
5. Ildstad ST, Tollerud DJ, Weiss RG, Ryan DP, McGowan MA, Martin LW. Duplications of the alimentary tract. Clinical characteristics, preferred treatment, and associated malformations. Ann Surg 1988; 208: 184–189
6. Rossi P, Gourtsoyiannis N, Bezzi M, et al. Meckel's diverticulum: imaging diagnosis. AJR 1996; 166:567–573
7. Seibert JJ, Williamson SL. Gastrointestinal scintigraphy. In: Miller JH, Gelfand MJ (eds), Pediatric nuclear imaging. Philadelphia: WB Saunders; 1994:157–182
8. Winter PF. Sodium pertechnetate Tc-99m scanning of the abdomen. Diagnosis of an ileal duplication cyst. JAMA 1977; 237:1352–1353
9. Yousefzadeh DK, Bickers GH, Jackson JH Jr, Benton C. Tubular colonic duplication—review of 1876–1981 literature. Pediatr Radiol 1983; 13: 65–71

REGIONAL ENTERITIS

10. Balan V, LaRusso NF. Hepatobiliary disease in inflammatory bowel disease. Gastroenterol Clin North Am 1995; 24:647–669
11. Bartram CI, Halligan S. Radiological investigation of chronic inflammatory bowel disease in childhood. Baillieres Clin Gastroenterol 1994; 8: 101–119
12. Charron M, del Rosario JF, Kocoshis S. Use of technetium-tagged white blood cells in patients with Crohn's disease and ulcerative colitis: is differential diagnosis possible? Pediatr Radiol 1998; 28:871–877
13. Gore RM, Balthazar EJ, Ghahremani GG, Miller FH. CT features of ulcerative colitis and Crohn's disease. AJR 1996; 167:3–15
14. Guillaumin E, Jeffrey RB Jr, Shea WJ, Asling WC, Goldberg HI. Perirectal inflammatory disease: CT findings. Radiology 1986; 161: 153–157
15. Hoffman AD. The child with diarrhea. In: Hilton SVW, Edwards DK III (eds), Practical pediatric radiology. Philadelphia: WB Saunders; 1994: 239–285

16. Horton KM, Corl FM, Fishman EK. CT evaluation of the colon: inflammatory disease. RadioGraphics 2000; 20:399–418
17. Hyams J, Markowitz J, Treem W, Davis P, Grancher K, Daum F. Characterization of hepatic abnormalities in children with inflammatory disease. Inflamm Bowel Dis 1995; 1:27–33
18. Jabra AA, Fishman EK, Taylor GA. Crohn disease in the pediatric patient: CT evaluation. Radiology 1991; 179:495–498
19. Jabra AA, Fishman EK, Taylor GA. CT findings in inflammatory bowel disease in children. AJR 1994; 162:975–979
20. James S, Balfe DM, Lee JK, Picus D. Small-bowel disease: categorization by CT examination. AJR 1987; 148:863–868
21. Kohn A, Cerro P, Millie G, De Angelis E, Prantera C. Prospective evaluation of transabdominal bowel sonography in the diagnosis of intestinal obstruction in Crohn's disease: comparison with plain abdominal film and small bowel enteroclysis. Inflamm Bowel Dis 1999; 5:153–157
22. Low RN, Francis JR, Politoske D, Bennett M. Crohn's disease evaluation: comparison of contrast-enhanced MR imaging and single-phase helical CT scanning. J Magn Reson Imaging 2000; 11:127–135
23. Marteau P. Inflammatory bowel disease. Endoscopy 2000; 32:131–137
24. Schwerk WB, Beck K, Raith M. A prospective evaluation of high resolution sonography in the differential diagnosis of inflammatory bowel disease. Eur J Gastroenterol Hepatol 1992; 4:173–182
25. Siegel MJ, Evans SJ, Balfe DM. Small bowel disease in children: diagnosis with CT. Radiology 1988; 169:127–130
26. Simpkins KC, Gore RM. Multiorgan involvement in Crohn disease. In: Gore RM, Levin MS, Laufer I (eds), Textbook of gastrointestinal radiology. Philadelphia: WB Saunders; 1994:2660–2681
27. Stringer DA. Pediatric gastrointestinal imaging. Toronto: BC Decker; 1986:286–296
28. Willis JS, Lobis IF, Denstman FJ. Crohn disease: state of the art. Radiology 1997; 202:597–610
29. Zeman RK. The role of noninvasive screening in suspected sclerosing cholangitis. Abdom Imaging 1995; 20:113–114

INTUSSUSCEPTION

30. Campbell JB. Contrast media in intussusception. Pediatr Radiol 1989; 19:293–296
31. Daneman A, Alton DJ, Lobo E, Gravett J, Kim P, Ein SH. Patterns of recurrence of intussusception in children: a 17-year review. Pediatr Radiol 1998; 28:913–919
32. del-Pozo G, Albillos JC, Tejedor D, et al. Intussusception in children: current concepts in diagnosis and enema reduction. RadioGraphics 1999; 19:299–319
33. DiFiore JW. Intussusception. Semin Pediatr Surg 1999; 8:214–220
34. Hadidi AT, El Shan N. Childhood intussusception: a comparative study of nonsurgical management. J Pediatr Surg 1999; 34:304–307
35. Reijnen JA, Joosten HJ, Festen C. Intussusception in children 5–15 years of age. Br J Surg 1987; 74:692–693
36. Stephenson CA, Seibert JJ, Strain JD, Glasier CM, Leithiser RE Jr, Iqbal V. Intussusception: clinical and radiographic factors influencing reducibility. Pediatr Radiol 1989; 20:57–60
37. Wayne ER, Campbell JB, Burrington JD, Davis WS. Management of 344 children with intussusception. Radiology 1973; 107:597–601

B-CELL LYMPHOMA

38. Dodd GD. Lymphoma of the hollow abdominal viscera. Radiol Clin North Am 1990; 28:771–783
39. Goodman P, Raval B. Omental cakes in American Burkitt lymphoma. Computed tomography demonstration. Clin Imaging 1989; 13:117–118
40. Hamrick-Turner JE, Saif MF, Powers CI, Blumenthal BI, Royal SA, Iyer RV. Imaging of childhood non-Hodgkin lymphoma: assessment by histologic subtype. RadioGraphics 1994; 14:11–28
41. Miller JH, White L. Lymphoma. In: Miller JH (ed), Imaging in pediatric oncology. Baltimore: Williams & Wilkins; 1985:427–448
42. Thomas CR Jr, Share R. Gastrointestinal lymphoma. Med Pediatr Oncol 1991; 19:48–60

HENOCH-SCHÖNLEIN PURPURA

43. Ben-Sira L, Laor T. Severe scrotal pain in boys with Henoch-Schönlein purpura: incidence and sonography. Pediatr Radiol 2000; 30:125–128
44. Connolly B, O'Halpin D. Sonographic evaluation of the abdomen in Henoch-Schönlein purpura. Clin Radiol 1994; 49:320–323
45. Khan AV, Williams TH, Malek RS. Acute scrotal swelling in Henoch-Schönlein purpura syndrome. Urology 1997; 10:139–144
46. Loh HS, Jalan OM. Testicular torsion in Henoch-Schönlein syndrome. Br Med J 1974; 2:96–97
47. Melloul MM, Garty BZ. Radionuclide scrotal imaging in anaphylactoid purpura. Clin Nucl Med 1993; 18:298–301
48. O'Regan S, Robitaille P. Orchitis mimicking testicular torsion in Henoch-Schönlein's purpura. J Urol 1981; 126:834–835
49. Siskind BN, Burrell MI, Pun H, Russo R Jr, Levin W. CT demonstration of gastrointestinal involvement in Henoch-Schönlein syndrome. Gastrointest Radiol 1985; 10:352–354
50. Slovis T, Sty JR, Haller JO. Imaging of the pediatric urinary tract. Philadelphia: WB Saunders; 1989:163–180

NECROTIZING ENTEROCOLITIS

51. Buonomo C. The radiology of necrotizing enterocolitis. Radiol Clin North Am 1999; 37:1187–1198
52. Hsueh W, Caplan MS, Tan X, MacKendrick W, Gonzalez-Crussi F. Necrotizing enterocolitis of the newborn: pathologic concepts in perspective. Pediatr Dev Pathol 1998; 1:2–16
53. Maalouf EF, Fagbemi A, Dugan PJ, et al. Magnetic resonance imaging of intestinal necrosis in preterm infants. Pediatrics 2000; 105:510–514

POLYPS

54. Desai DC, Neale KF, Talbot IC, Hodgson SV, Phillips RK. Juvenile polyposis. Br J Surg 1995; 82:14–17
55. Harned RK, Buck JL, Sobin LH. The hamartomatous polyposis syndromes: clinical and radiologic features. AJR 1995; 164:565–571
56. Longo WE, Touloukian RJ, West AB, Ballantyne GH. Malignant potential of juvenile polyposis coli. Report of a case and review of the literature. Dis Colon Rectum 1990; 33:980–984

RETROPERITONEAL FIBROSIS

57. Amis ES Jr. Retroperitoneal fibrosis. Urol Radiol 1990; 12:135–137
58. Arrive L, Hricak H, Tavares NJ, Miller TR. Malignant versus nonmalignant retroperitoneal fibrosis: differentiation with MR imaging. Radiology 1989; 172:139–143
59. Kottra JJ, Dunnick NR. Retroperitoneal fibrosis. Radiol Clin North Am 1996; 34:1259–1275
60. Rubenstein WA, Gray G, Auh YH, et al. CT of fibrous tissues and tumors with sonographic correlation. AJR 1986; 147:1067–1074
61. Sherman C, Winchester P, Brill PW, Mininberg D. Childhood retroperitoneal fibrosis. Pediatr Radiol 1988; 18:245–247

CASE 5

John R. Sty, M.D.

Acute Osteomyelitis

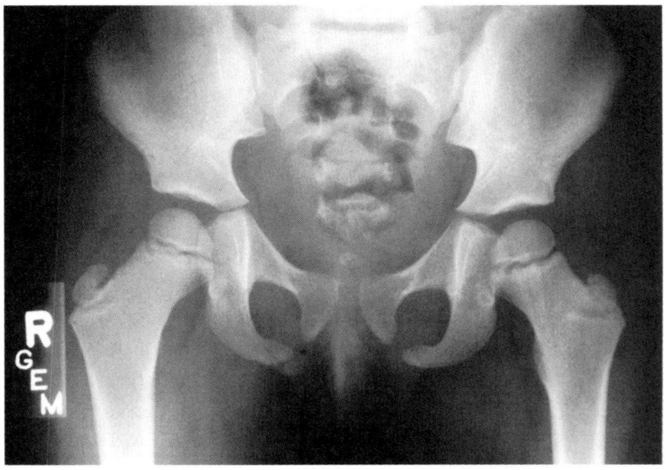

Figure 5-1

Question 26

This 4-year-old boy has acute limp, thigh swelling, and fever. You are shown an anteroposterior radiograph (Figure 5-1) and immediate (A) and delayed (B) Tc-99m methylene diphosphonate scintigrams (Figure 5-2).

Which *one* of the following is the MOST likely diagnosis?

(A) Leukemia
(B) Metastatic neuroblastoma
(C) Legg-Perthes disease
(D) Osteomyelitis
(E) Transient synovitis

Figure 5-1 shows deep swelling of the tissues of the upper right thigh (Figure 5-3), but no osseous abnormality is evident. The proximal right femur is not displaced. An immediate (blood-pool-phase or tissue-phase) Tc-99m methylene diphosphonate (MDP) image (Figure 5-2A) shows a photon-deficient region in the area of the right hip joint and the femoral neck, representing a large joint effusion (Figure 5-4A). The delayed conventional scintigrams and magnified pinhole collimator

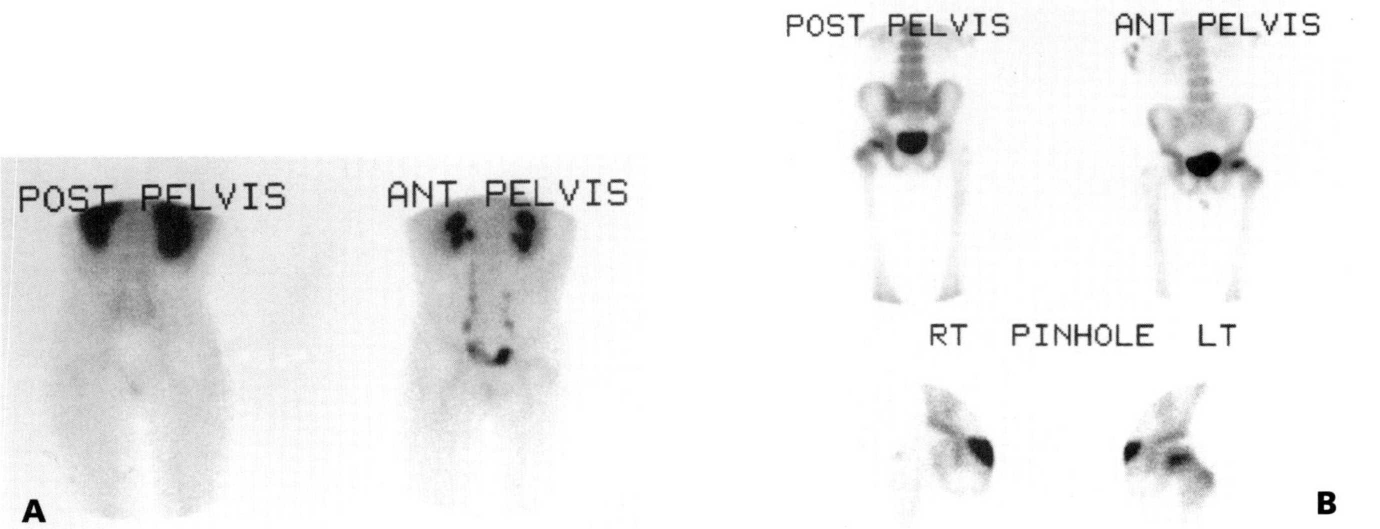

Figure 5-2

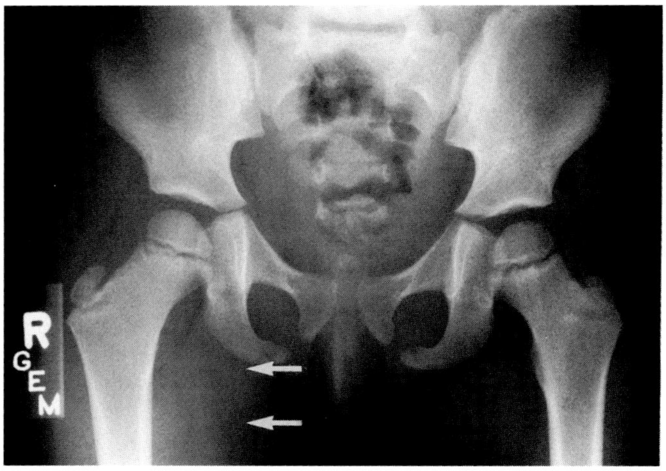

Figure 5-3 (Same as Figure 5-1). Acute osteomyelitis. An anteroposterior radiograph of the pelvis demonstrates more prominent soft tissues (arrows) in the right proximal thigh than in the left. No osseous destructive lesions are seen.

scintigrams (Figure 5-2B) show a photon-deficient right femoral head, growth plate, metaphysis, and neck (Figure 5-4B). No other abnormalities are demonstrated. Osteomyelitis is the most likely explanation for these radiographic and scintigraphic findings **(Option (D) is correct).** The patient's clinical history of acute limp, thigh swelling, and fever is also quite consistent with this diagnosis.

Acute hematogenous osteomyelitis is generally regarded as a disease of infants and children. Hematogenous osteomyelitis usually begins in the metaphysis. The infecting organisms gain access to the bone via the nutrient arteries. The terminal arterial branches of the nutrient arteries form loops (loop capillaries) immediately adjacent to the growth plate. Arterial blood then passes into venous sinusoids in the intramedullary portion of the metaphysis. Blood flow in this region is slow and turbulent, allowing the infecting organisms to implant and proliferate.

As the organisms proliferate, an acute exudative process develops in the intramedullary portion of the metaphysis. The intraosseous pressure is increased by edema and vascular spasm, leading to slowing of blood flow and eventual thrombosis of the sinusoids, arterioles, and venules. Some bone necrosis occurs in all patients.

The elevated intraosseous pressure found in patients with osteomyelitis contributes to the dissemination of the infecting organisms through the interstices of endosteal bone. Longitudinal spread from the metaphysis can occur through the medullary cavity into the diaphysis. With lateral extension, the infection can penetrate the cortex and produce a subperiosteal fluid collection. Extension through the periosteum can then lead to infection of the deep soft tissues. Depending on the site of the joint capsule attachment in relation to the metaphysis, cortical disruption may reach the joint space. The capsule of the hip attaches below the metaphysis of the femur; therefore, when metaphyseal infection of the proximal femur ruptures through the cortex, a secondary hip joint infection results. More frequently, joint fluid associated with adjacent osteomyelitis represents a sympathetic effusion, caused by reactive synovitis.

In older infants and children, the relatively avascular growth plate serves as a barrier to the extension of infection into the epiphyseal ossification center. However, the physes of infants younger than 12 months have vascular communications that can allow infection to extend through the physes into the epiphyseal ossification center and subsequently into the adjacent joint. During fetal life, perichondrial vessels progress toward the end of the cartilaginous anlagen, turning back when they reach the unossified cartilaginous end of the bone. Late in gestation and in the first 6 to 12 months after birth, the growing cartilage is established but is not yet limited by bone on the epiphyseal side. Some vessels at the surface of the metaphysis penetrate the growth plate to supply the epiphysis. At their terminal extent, these vessels form large venous lakes that are similar to the metaphyseal sinusoids. This architecture affords a

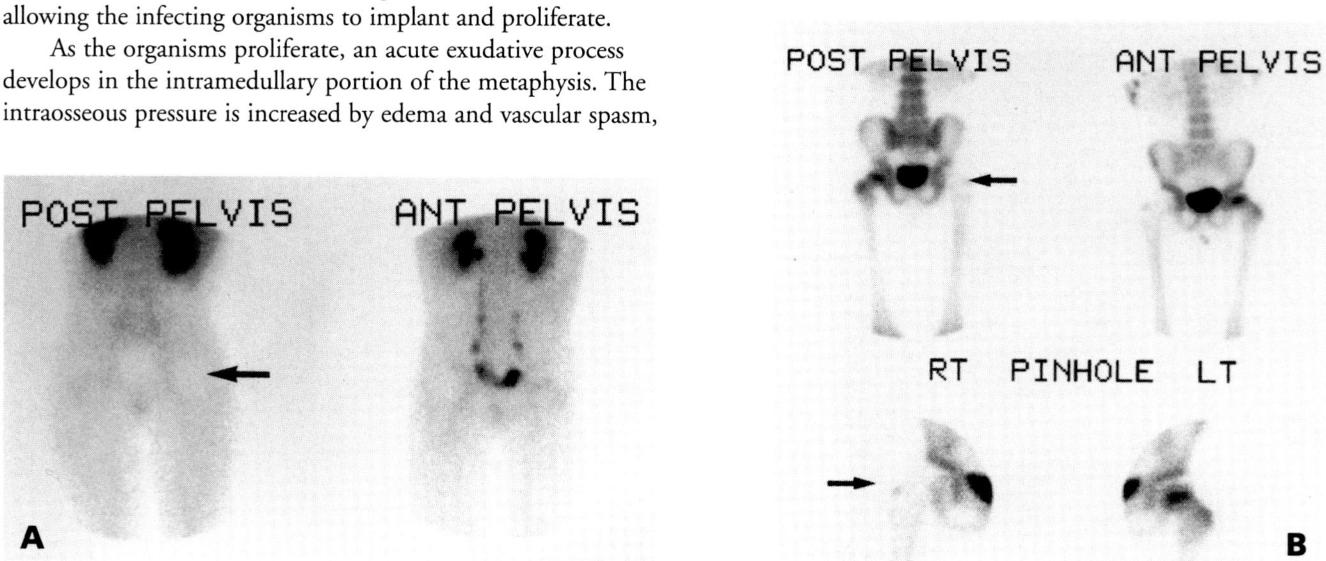

Figure 5-4 (Same as Figure 5-2). Acute osteomyelitis. (A) Immediate posterior and anterior Tc-99m MDP scintigrams of the hips and pelvis demonstrate a photon-deficient area in the region of the right hip (arrow), consistent with an effusion. (B) Delayed posterior and anterior scintigrams and magnified anterior pinhole-collimated images of both hips show a large area of absent tracer uptake (arrows) in the right femoral head, growth plate, metaphysis, and neck.

vascular connection between the metaphyses and the epiphyses and explains the increased frequency of epiphyseal and articular infections in infants of this age.

Between the age of approximately 1 year and the time when the growth plates (physes) fuse, the childhood vascular pattern (as opposed to the fetal pattern described above) is present at the ends of tubular bones. Apart from the vessels found in a narrow fringe at the periphery of the cartilage, capillaries on the metaphyseal side of the growth plate are the terminal ramifications of the nutrient artery. It is here that the vessels turn in acute loops to drain into the sinusoidal veins that occupy the intramedullary portion of the metaphysis. This is therefore a region of sluggish and turbulent blood flow. The epiphyseal blood supply is distinct from that of the metaphysis; the physis serves as a barrier through which vessels do not pass. These anatomic features explain why hematogenous ostemyelitis usually affects the metaphysis and spares the epiphysis in children beyond infancy.

In adolescence, after closure of the epiphyseal growth plate, metaphyseal vessels progressively penetrate the remaining cartilaginous structures, thereby reestablishing a vascular connection between the metaphysis and the epiphysis. Blood in the nutrient vessels can reach the end of the bone through large anastomosing channels, and organisms in these vessels can gain access to the ends of bones and adjacent articular surfaces and joints.

Imaging plays an important role in the diagnosis of acute osteomyelitis. The radiographic signs associated with acute infection may be detected as early as 3 days after the onset of symptoms. These early findings, combined with appropriate clinical and laboratory information, suggest the diagnosis. Early diagnosis and treatment are imperative for favorable long-term outcomes and for prevention of complications, such as leg length discrepancy, angular bone deformity, and ankylosis.

Local soft tissue abnormalities are the initial radiographic indicators of bone infection. In general, there is deep soft tissue swelling with displacement and obliteration of adjacent fat planes. These areas of soft tissue swelling are usually adjacent to the site of metaphyseal infection and do not directly involve the soft tissues adjacent to the diaphysis or the joint. On high-quality radiographs, infection can be detected on days 1 to 3 of illness if careful attention is paid to evaluating the soft tissues. Additional radiographic changes become apparent 4 or 5 days later as metaphyseal inflammation and edema increase. The osseous structures still remain radiographically normal, but the inflammatory process enlarges the muscles adjacent to the site of bone infection. The swelling can extend for a considerable distance from the metaphysis, causing a loss of the muscle and subcutaneous tissue planes. An effusion can develop in the joint. Edema develops in the subcutaneous tissues and is indicated by thickening and increased visualization of the subcutaneous vessels and lymphatics.

Radiographs usually do not detect bone lysis until a lesion is 1 cm in diameter or has destroyed more than 30% of the bone matrix. These findings develop between 10 and 14 days after the onset of infection. Bone lysis is manifested as a radiolucency, initially focal and subsequently confluent, in the infected bone. This process is more rapid in neonates because of their soft spongiosa. The localized metaphyseal lucency rapidly progresses to a pattern of irregular bone destruction. There is frequent extension into the metaphyseal cortex and subperiosteum; periosteal new bone formation is identified at this time. In some patients with osteomyelitis who are given appropriate antibiotic therapy early in the course of the illness, radiographic abnormalities never develop.

Bone scintigraphy is quite sensitive for the early detection of hematogenous osteomyelitis. Three-phase or combined immediate (blood-pool) and delayed radionuclide bone imaging is necessary to detect and distinguish among osteomyelitis, septic arthritis, and cellulitis. Radionuclide bone imaging has a 95% sensitivity and a 90% specificity for the diagnosis of osteomyelitis, in contrast to the radiologic examination, which has a 35% sensitivity and a 90% specificity. The classic appearance of osteomyelitis on bone scintigraphy is that of a well-defined region of avid uptake on both early and delayed images (Figure 5-5). The lesion is typically metaphyseal and often has a somewhat characteristic "flame" shape. Occasionally, the focal area of increased uptake in the bones is superimposed on a larger region of diffuse uptake as a result of generalized soft tissue hyperemia. Bone scintigraphy becomes positive as early as 24 hours after the onset of symptoms. Therefore, scintigraphically detectable abnormalities are seen significantly earlier than radiographic changes. When the diagnosis of osteomyelitis is made early in the disease by bone scintigraphy and the patient is treated with antibiotics, radiographs can remain normal throughout the illness.

In addition to the typical avid radionuclide uptake pattern seen in patients with osteomyelitis, another pattern, resulting in a photopenic region on tissue-phase and delayed imaging, can be found. This occurs in patients in whom the infectious process is severe enough to cause increased marrow pressure and thus interfere with the blood supply to the metaphysis, ultimately causing compression of the microvascular circulation and ischemia. Secondary thrombophlebitis of the diaphyseal or medullary vessels can also cause ischemia. The radiopharmaceutical is not delivered to the bone in the presence of ischemia, and focally reduced activity is visible scintigraphically. This phenomenon has been termed "cold osteomyelitis." Infarctive osteomyelitis has a poorer prognosis than the more classic radionuclide-avid osteomyelitis. Table 5-1 lists common and uncommon etiologies of photon-deficient abnormalities seen on radionuclide bone imaging.

Infarctive osteomyelitis is sometimes a difficult scintigraphic diagnosis. In addition to the photon-deficient region attributable to marrow ischemia, an extended pattern of increased activity in the soft tissues can result from reactive hyperemia. The increased activity in the soft tissues can cause difficulty in recognizing the photon-deficient region in bone (Figure 5-6).

Cross-sectional imaging is useful in patients with subacute

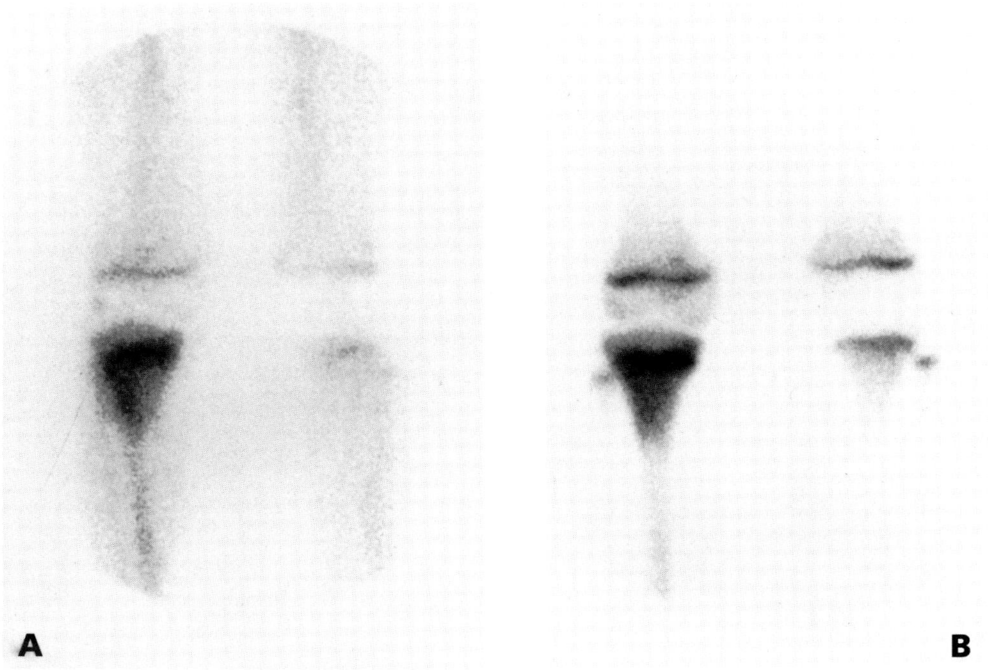

Figure 5-5. Osteomyelitis. (A) An anterior early (tissue-phase) image of the knees of a child shows a flame-shaped region of avid radiopharmaceutical uptake in the metaphysis of the right tibia. (B) An anterior delayed bone image of the knees shows intense accumulation of radiopharmaceutical in the same region.

or chronic infection or with disease in regions of complex osseous anatomy. MRI is very sensitive in the detection of increased water content attributable to edema. In bone, edema results in homogeneous decreased marrow signal intensity relative to that of normal marrow on T1-weighted imaging sequences and increased signal intensity on T2-weighted and fat suppression sequences. Cortical destruction is visualized as an interruption in the normal black stripe (low signal intensity) of the cortex. Reactive bone formation appears as areas of low signal intensity. MRI is also quite sensitive in demonstrating extension of infection into the adjacent soft tissues. Soft tissue extension appears as abnormal increased signal intensity on T2-weighted images (Figure 5-7). A subperiosteal abscess is well demonstrated on MRI as a hyperintense fluid collection on T2-weighted and fat suppression images (Figure 5-8).

CT is also capable of showing marrow infiltration and edema, both of which increase the attenuation of marrow relative to that of normal fatty marrow. It is also an excellent imaging modality for the detection of a sequestrum (a devitalized bone segment). This finding indicates that surgical debridement is necessary. The CT appearance of a sequestrum is that of an isolated segment of bone in a region of lytic destruction. The sequestrum usually has higher attenuation than does adjacent vascularized bone. Potential complications of osteomyelitis that can be seen by CT include subperiosteal abscess, intraosseous abscess, adjacent cellulitis or abscess, and pathologic fracture, although abscess and cellulitis are better shown by MRI (Figure 5-9).

Leukemia (Option (A)) is not a likely diagnosis in the test patient. Most children with leukemia present with systemic signs and symptoms. Bone pain is present at the time of diagnosis in only 20% of patients. Typically, the pain is periarticular and migratory. The symptoms of leukemia can be confused with those of acute rheumatic fever or rheumatoid arthritis. There may be fever, an elevated sedimentation rate, spleno-

Table 5-1: Etiologies of photon-deficient lesions

Common lesions	Uncommon lesions
Bone infection/joint effusion	Cancer
Osteochondritis dissecans	Leukemia
Sickle cell crisis	Neuroblastoma
Legg-Perthes disease	Ewing's sarcoma
Bone cyst	Langerhans cell histiocytosis
Reflex sympathetic dystrophy	Gaucher's disease
Radiation therapy	Orthopedic hardware
Acute fracture	

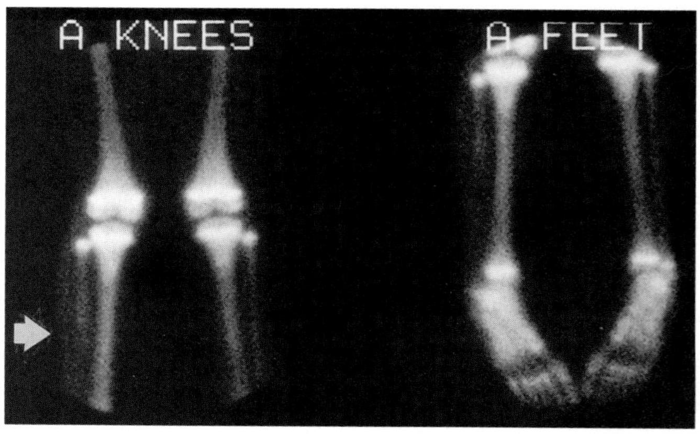

Figure 5-6. This 5-year-old boy had a limp and fever. Delayed scintigrams show the absence of tracer accumulation in the distal right fibula. Note the extended uptake within the soft tissues (arrow).

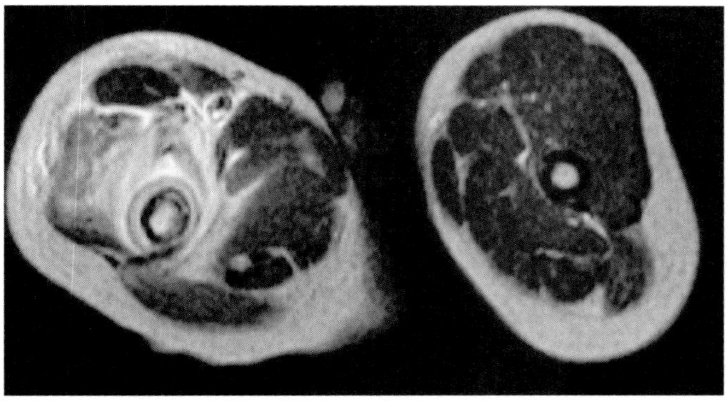

SE 2,750/80

Figure 5-7. Osteomyelitis with soft tissue extension of infection. This 5-year-old boy had fever, thigh swelling, and inability to move the hip. An axial T2-weighted MR image of the upper femur shows a high signal intensity within the muscles secondary to edema. The cortex of the femur is interrupted and shows linear tracts of fluid. A halo of abnormal signal represents subperiosteal accumulation of pus.

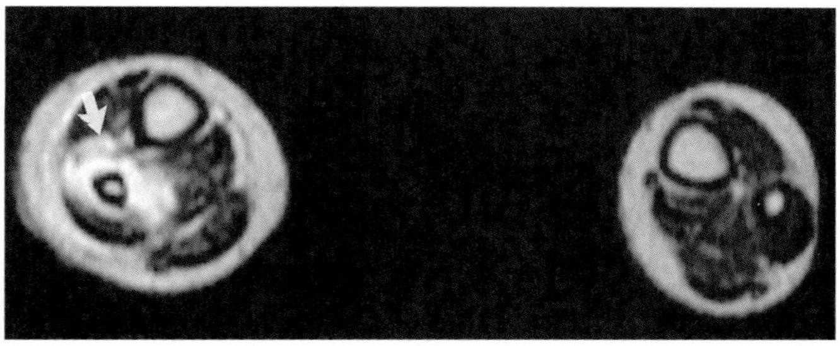

SE 2,750/80

Figure 5-8. Osteomyelitis with subperiosteal abscess. This 5-year-old boy had fever and a limp. Bone scintigraphy (not shown) demonstrated photon-deficient osteomyelitis of the fibula. An axial T2-weighted MR image through the midportion of the lower legs shows increased signal intensity because of a subperiosteal abscess and tissue edema (arrow).

megaly, and, occasionally, lymphadenopathy. Approximately 40% of children with leukemia present with radiographic or scintigraphic abnormalities. However, there is usually no evidence of deep or superficial soft tissue swelling without an underlying bone abnormality on radiographs.

Bone scintigraphy is not typically used to diagnose leukemia, but children with fever and unexplained musculoskeletal complaints may be referred for scintigraphy, which can demonstrate unifocal, multifocal, and diffuse abnormalities before radiographic abnormalities are apparent. Radionuclide bone imaging in children with leukemia usually shows multifocal regions of abnormal increased uptake of radiopharmaceutical involving the axial and appendicular skeleton. The typical pattern is intense uptake localized to the metaphyseal regions and minimally increased uptake in the diaphyses. Joint effusions are uncommon. During blast crises, bone scintigraphy shows marked diffuse abnormality. Approximately 75% of children with acute leukemia have abnormal scintigraphic findings at diagnosis (Figure 5-10). Only half of these patients have positive radiographs. False-negative scans do occur. Photon-deficient abnormalities can be produced by marrow packing, which compromises blood flow. The soft tissue swelling, the radiographically normal osseous structures, and the large hip joint effusion in the test patient make leukemia an unlikely diagnosis.

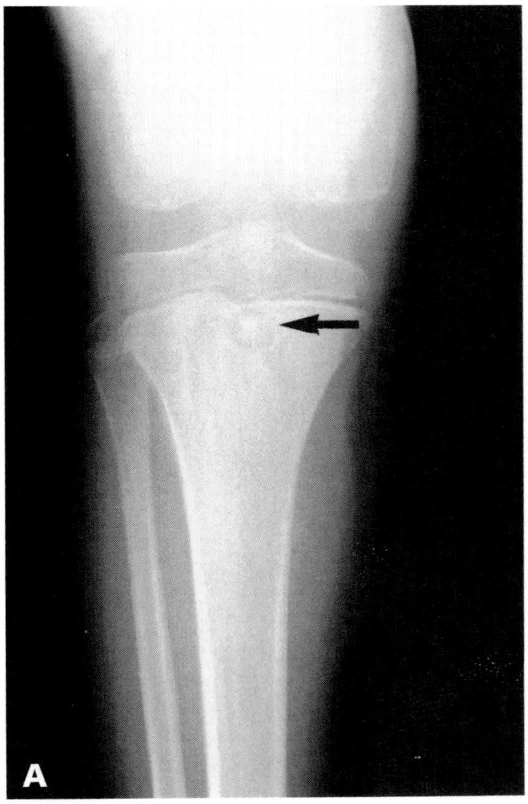

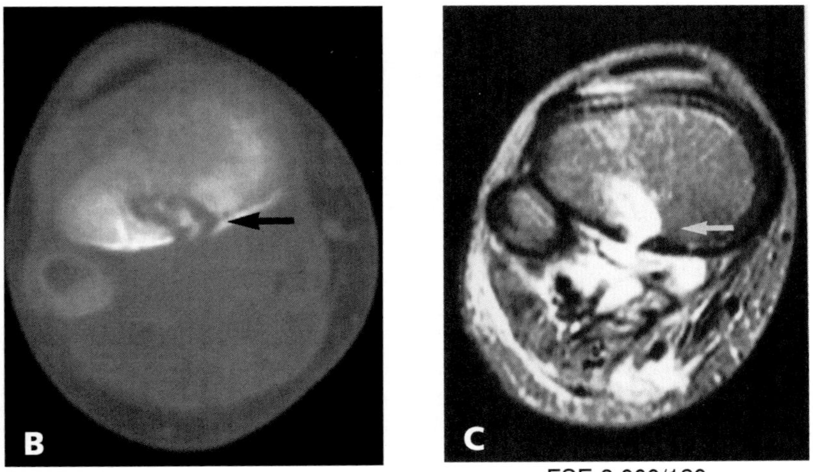

FSE 3,000/120

Figure 5-9. Chronic osteomyelitis. (A) A standard anteroposterior radiograph of the knee demonstrates a lytic tibial metaphyseal lesion (arrow) with a central sequestrum. (B) An axial CT scan at bone-window settings demonstrates a destructive proximal right tibial lytic lesion containing a dense sclerotic segment of bone. There is destruction of the posterior cortex (arrow). (C) An axial T2-weighted MR image shows the high-signal-intensity abnormality of chronic osteomyelitis (arrow) with continuity of the inflammatory process through the disrupted posterior tibial cortex into the adjacent soft tissues.

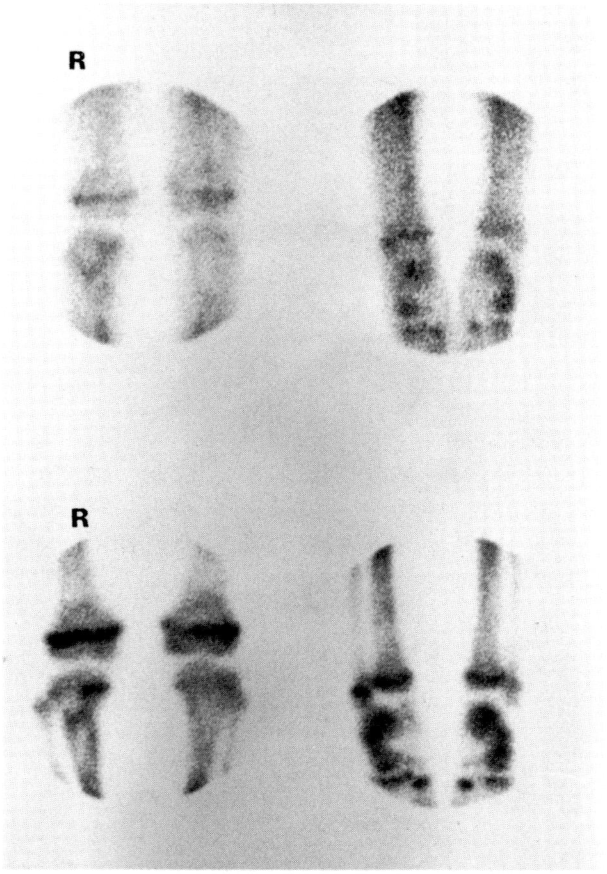

Figure 5-10. Acute lymphocytic leukemia. The top two images are tissue-phase scintigrams, and the bottom two images are delayed scintigrams. There is heterogeneous uptake (both abnormally increased and focally photon deficient) in the metadiaphyses of the femurs and tibias as a result of marrow packing.

Neuroblastoma (Option (B)) typically appears as a palpable abdominal mass and is associated with neurologic symptoms, bone pain, orbital ecchymosis, and proptosis, as well as manifestations related to excessive catecholamine production. Bone marrow aspiration is positive for tumor involvement in up to 70% of children older than 1 year. The skeletal system represents the most common site of hematogenous metastases, which occur rapidly and are widespread. Bone scintigraphy has a greater overall sensitivity than standard radiography in the detection of skeletal metastases. Bone scintigraphy is positive in 15% of patients in whom skeletal radiographic surveys are completely negative. Also, more lesions are found by skeletal scintigraphy than by radiography in 35% of patients who undergo both procedures. In most cases, bone scintigraphy shows metastases that are bilateral and nearly symmetric and often involve the calvarium. False-negative results may occur with metaphyseal metastases adjacent to growth plates. Photopenic lesions occur occasionally. A solitary lesion is a distinctly uncommon sintigraphic pattern in metastatic neuroblastoma.

The characteristic skeletal abnormality in patients with osseous metastatic disease from neuroblastoma is a lytic permeative lesion with indistinct margins. The metaphyses are the most common site of involvement. In the vast majority of patients, the bony metastases are bilateral and nearly symmetric. Soft tissue swelling can occur but is nearly always associated with bone disease. Joint effusions are rare. The presence of unifocal disease, the soft tissue edema, and the normal bone radiography with the joint effusion in the test patient make metastatic neuroblastoma an unlikely diagnosis.

Legg-Perthes disease (Option (C)) refers to idiopathic ischemic necrosis of the femoral head. Ischemic necrosis of bone can be related to a number of pathophysiologic mechanisms. Interruption of blood supply to the bone can result from acute thrombosis, trauma, an underlying vascular abnormality, or an osseous disorder. Any process that increases intramedullary pressure in the bone, such as pyogenic infection, diminishes local blood supply and can result in ischemic necrosis.

The radiographic findings in patients with bone necrosis vary somewhat according to the site of involvement, the age of the patient, and the etiology. Nevertheless, the pathophysiologic changes produced by ischemic necrosis lead to well-defined stages in an orderly sequence. The earliest change consists of ischemia and death of cellular components of the bone. Later stages include revascularization, reossification, and resorption of dead bone. The diagnosis of Legg-Perthes disease can be difficult in the early stages.

Radiographically, the appearance of acutely infarcted bone is indistinguishable from that of normal viable bone. However, skeletal scintigraphy is highly sensitive and specific for the demonstration of acute ischemic necrosis, showing decreased accumulation of bone-seeking radiopharmaceutical. In patients with Legg-Perthes disease, the femoral head is photopenic (Figures 5-11 and 5-12). A small effusion can be present, but large effusions are rare. Soft tissues are usually normal. The involvement of the metaphysis and the large joint effusion in the test patient exclude Legg-Perthes disease as the cause of the pain. In addition, Legg-Perthes disease clinically is not associat-

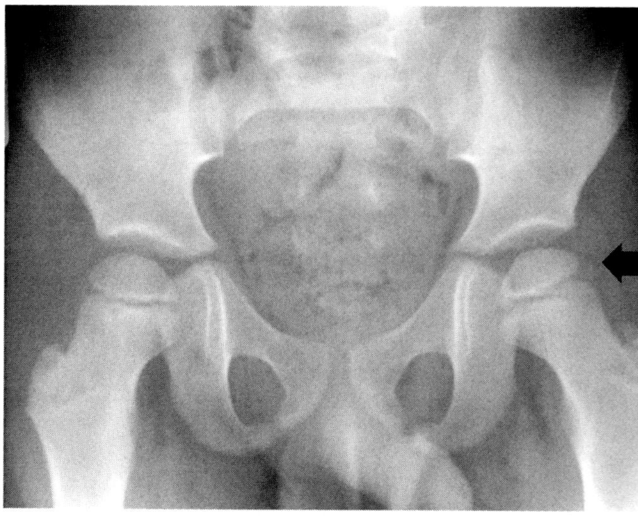

Figure 5-11. Legg-Perthes disease. This 4-year-old boy had several months of intermittent mild left hip pain. A radiograph of the pelvis shows a normal right hip. The left hip shows 3 mm of lateral displacement. The left femoral head is slightly smaller than the right, and there is minimal sclerosis (arrow).

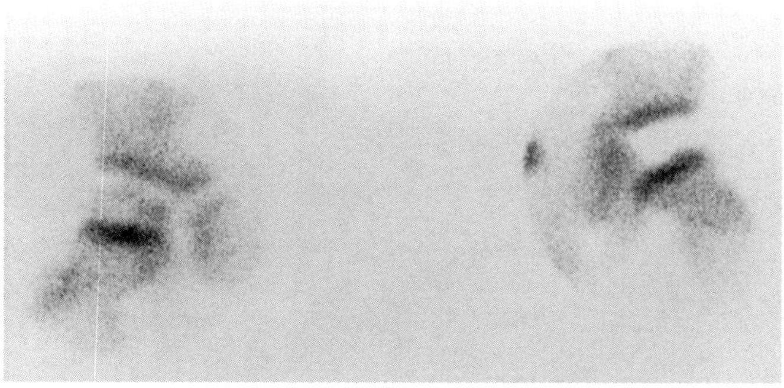

Figure 5-12. Same patient as in Figure 5-11. Legg-Perthes disease. Pinhole images of the hips show a normal right hip. The left hip shows a photon-deficient area in the femoral head. Note the increased accumulation of tracer in the acetabulum, growth plate, and proximal femoral neck. This pattern is typical of Legg-Perthes disease.

ed with soft tissue swelling and fever. The typical child with Legg-Perthes disease has an insidious onset of mild hip or knee pain, provoking an antalgic limp. Most patients are not evaluated with diagnostic imaging until symptoms have been present for more than 1 month. There are no systemic symptoms or signs, and initially the condition may be indistinguishable clinically from transient synovitis of the hip.

Transient synovitis (Option (E)), also called toxic synovitis or irritable hip, most often affects children in the age range of 5 to 10 years who present with hip or knee pain and a limp. Infection, trauma, and allergy have been considered as possible etiologies for this benign condition. More than 60% of patients with transient synovitis have a history of upper respiratory tract infection within 2 weeks of the appearance of hip symptoms. A large percentage of patients have elevated viral antigen titers or positive throat cultures for beta-hemolytic streptococci. A history of injury is present in more than 10% of patients. A small to moderate sterile joint effusion is present. Synovial biopsy shows nonspecific inflammatory changes.

Sonography is the method of choice for detecting joint fluid in the hip in children. The transducer is placed over the anterior aspect of the hip oriented in the longitudinal axis of the femoral neck. The distance from the anterior capsule to the bone is normally less than 3 mm. Sonography is more sensitive than standard radiography for detecting joint effusion. However, there are no reliable sonographic features that permit distinction of pyarthrosis from a sterile joint effusion. If septic arthritis is suspected clinically, the hip must be aspirated regardless of the findings on imaging studies. If the results of the aspiration yield sterile fluid, the diagnosis of transient synovitis is made by exclusion. However, adjacent osteomyelitis may cause a hip joint effusion. In the appropriate clinical circumstances, bone scintigraphy or MRI would exclude the diagnosis of osteomyelitis as the etiology of the hip effusion.

Radiographs of most children with transient synovitis are normal. Slight lateral subluxation of the hip is identified in some patients. A hip that is displaced more than 2 mm laterally on radiographs should be considered abnormal. Displacement is measured medially, between the femoral metaphysis and the "teardrop" of the acetabulum. Unfortunately, hip displacement is nonspecific and can occur in any disease associated with a hip joint effusion.

The displacement of fat planes adjacent to the hip has been described as a radiographic indicator of hip joint effusion. However, anatomic studies indicate that the fat planes change more with the position of the leg than with distension attributable to joint fluid. Joint asymmetry is a more reliable sign in children than is displacement of fat planes. There are no radiographic bone changes at presentation in children with transient synovitis.

Bone scintigraphy is normal in many patients with mild transient synovitis. When bone scintigraphy is abnormal, various patterns are identified. First, there may be normal tissue-phase images and slightly increased periarticular activity on delayed images; this finding is best demonstrated on high-quality pinhole images. Second, there may be a photon-deficient region in the area of the hip on the tissue-phase images; this is attributable to fluid in the hip joint. The delayed images are normal or show a slight increase or decrease in the periarticular accumulation of bone-seeking radiopharmaceutical. In patients with a large tense hip joint effusion, the femoral head or the growth plate can show decreased or absent accumulation of bone-seeking radiopharmaceutical owing to increased intra-articular pressure and vascular tamponade. This pattern is not specific; identical findings can occur in patients with trauma or septic arthritis. Although the photopenia of the femoral head and physis in the test patient could be attributable to transient synovitis, the soft tissue swelling on the radiograph and the photopenia in the metaphysis on bone scintigraphy make this diagnosis unlikely.

Avascular necrosis has been found in 1% to 2% of patients following transient synovitis. The time interval between the synovitis and the avascular necrosis is 3 to 6 months. The etiology is believed to be ischemia secondary to joint effusion and increased intracapsular pressure.

Question 27

Concerning skeletal manifestations of childhood leukemia,

(A) the transverse radiolucent metaphyseal bands represent leukemic infiltration
(B) the metadiaphyseal lesions mimic those seen in patients with metastatic neuroblastoma
(C) skeletal radiographs are abnormal in about 40% of patients
(D) the signal intensity in long bones is slightly higher than normal on T1-weighted MR images
(E) necrosis is a sequela of treatment

Acute lymphocytic leukemia (ALL) accounts for more than 80% of all childhood leukemias, acute myelogenous leukemia accounts for 10%, and a variety of uncommon histologic forms account for the remaining 10%. Most children with ALL present with systemic signs and symptoms. Bone pain is present at the time of diagnosis in 20% of children, and radiographic skeletal abnormalities occur in 40% (**Option (C) is true**). The most common radiographic manifestation of skeletal involvement by ALL in childhood is osteoporosis, in which there is diffuse demineralization of the long bones and spine. This finding is most obvious in the spine and is probably attributable to leukemia in the bone marrow rather than to leukemic changes of the cortical bone. Vertebral compression fractures can occur. These can be seen in patients with diffuse demineralization or with discrete skeletal lesions.

Submetaphyseal lucent bands are seen in approximately 40% of children with ALL (Figure 5-13). The lucent bands, historically referred to as leukemic lines, represent osteopenia, not leukemic infiltration, at the most rapidly growing portion of long bones, the area adjacent to the growing cartilage (**Option (A) is false**). These bands are commonly identified in the distal femur, proximal tibia, proximal humerus, vertebral bodies, and iliac crest and are typically uniform and regular across the entire width of the metaphysis. They are sharply demarcated from the normally ossified or slightly osteoporotic diaphysis. Cortical bone is preserved early in the disease.

Destructive lesions of the long bones are a later finding and occur at the metadiaphyses. They are most probably secondary to infiltration of the bone by leukemic cells. The typical appearance of leukemic involvement is that of multiple, small, oval or spherical osteolytic lesions, representing destruction of the spongiosa and later of the cortex. This finding is identified in 40% to 60% of patients. Pathologic fractures can occur. The radiographic findings seen with leukemia can also be seen in patients with any of the small round cell tumors of childhood, such as metastatic neuroblastoma, with which it can be confused clinically and radiologically (Figure 5-14) (**Option (B) is true**).

Periosteal reaction also occurs in patients with leukemia. It can be smooth, laminated, or, rarely, sunburst in appearance. This reaction is attributable to cortical penetration by sheaths of leukemic cells into the subperiosteum. This finding is seen in 10% to 25% of patients. The common sites of periosteal reaction are the areas of the greatest blood supply: the metaphysis of the distal femur, the proximal tibia, and the proximal humerus. The short tubular bones of the hands and feet are rarely involved.

The use of MRI in imaging childhood leukemias is limited, but it plays a potential role in monitoring the course of re-

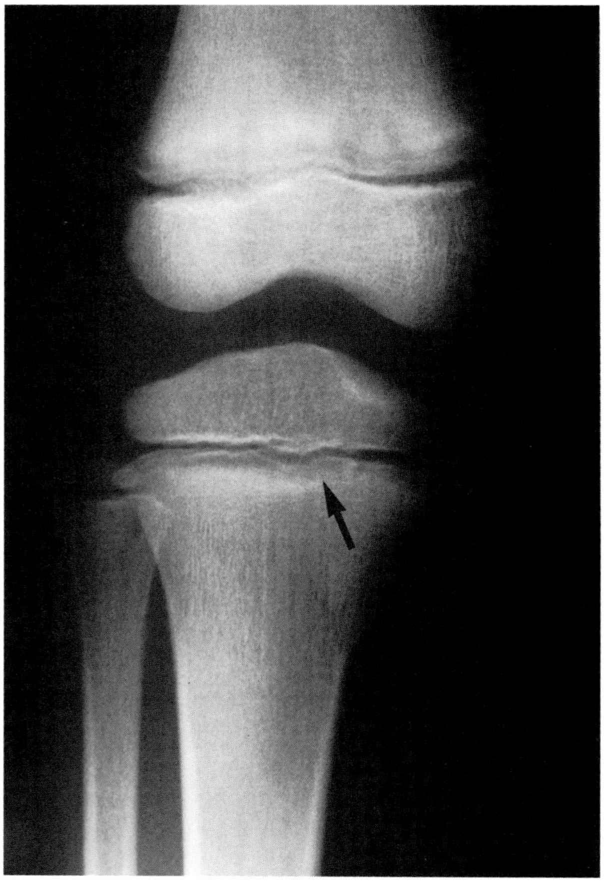

Figure 5-13. Acute lymphocytic leukemia. An anteroposterior radiograph of the right knee shows a submetaphyseal lucent band (arrow).

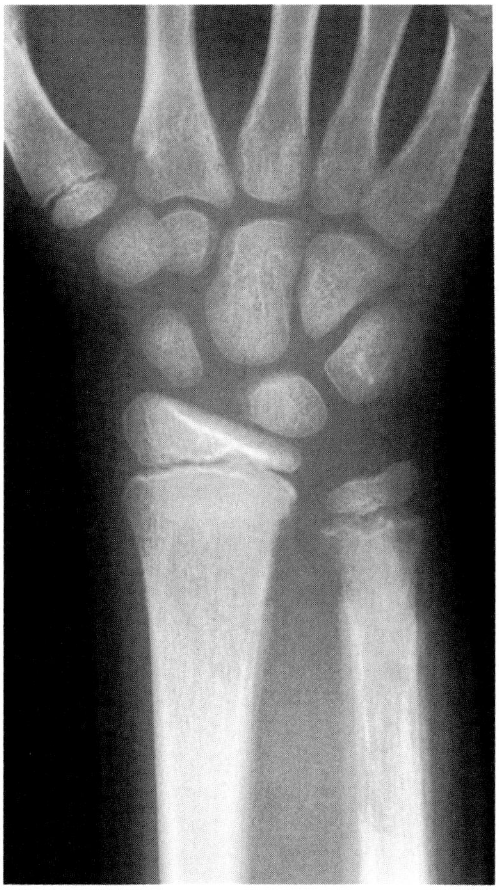

Figure 5-14. Acute lymphocytic leukemia. An anteroposterior radiograph of the wrist shows a lytic permeative lesion in the metadiaphysis of the distal radius and ulna. Both bones show periosteal reaction.

lapse and the complications of treatment in these patients. Leukemic infiltration of bone marrow is usually homogeneous, widespread, and nearly symmetric. On T1-weighted images, leukemic marrow has a low signal intensity because of replacement of normal marrow fat by cells (**Option (D) is false**). On T2-weighted images, the signal intensity is increased and is equal to that of subcutaneous fat (Figure 5-15). The appearance of leukemia can mimic that of hematopoietic marrow on T1- and T2-weighted images. Short-tau inversion-recovery (STIR) or fat-suppressed images can be helpful in distinguishing between these conditions.

In many cases, detection of the pathologic process is obscured by the presence of a strong signal from neighboring fatty tissue. In such cases, suppression of the fat signal improves conspicuity. The signal from fat can be suppressed in a number of ways, such as inversion-recovery techniques (e.g., STIR), in which the signal from fat is nullified; preliminary saturation of the magnetic moments from fat; and selective excitation of the signal from water. Marrow infiltration typically produces increased signal intensity on STIR images, as well as on T2-weighted and fat-suppressed images; however, other diseases, such as edema, necrosis, and hemorrhage, can produce the same findings.

Osteonecrosis of the femoral head and distal femoral metaphysis can be seen at the time of diagnosis of leukemia owing to marrow packing or can occur later as a sequela of treatment with steroids or chemotherapy (**Option (E) is true**). These complications can be evaluated by conventional radiography, skeletal scintigraphy, or MRI, although MRI is considered the most sensitive method for detecting osteonecrosis (Figure 5-16). Consequently, in a leukemic patient undergoing therapy, bone pain could be attributable to recurrent leukemia or to treatment-related osteonecrosis. Acute avascular necrosis can be differentiated from recurrent leukemic lesions on MRI. On T1-weighted MR images, there is usually a well-defined hypointense lesion attributable to marrow edema in the proximal or distal femoral metaphysis if osteonecrosis is present. On T2-weighted images, necrosis appears as a high-intensity lesion with a well-marginated, low-intensity rim. In patients with leukemia, the marrow shows diffuse hypointensity on T1-weighted images and hyperintensity on T2-weighted images.

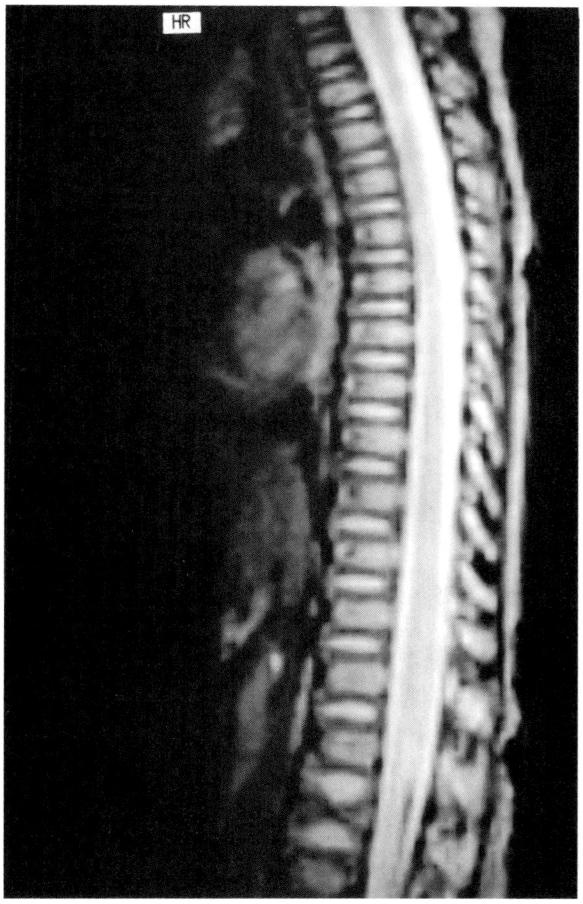

FSE 3,100/120

Figure 5-15. Acute lympocytic leukemia. This 6-year-old boy had back pain and a peripheral blood count indicating leukemia. A sagittal T2-weighted MR image shows multiple regions of vertebral body collapse. The marrow signal intensity is increased and is equal to that of subcutaneous fat. The vertebral body collapse and abnormal signal intensity are typical of leukemia.

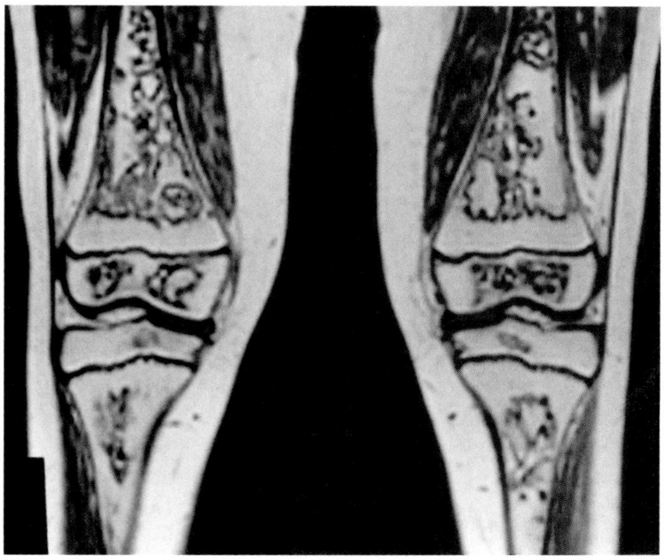

SE 2,750/80

Figure 5-16. Osteonecrosis associated with leukemia. This 11-year-old boy developed bone pain during remission of acute lymphocytic leukemia. A coronal T2-weighted MR image shows necrosis appearing as high-signal-intensity lesions with well-marginated low-intensity rims.

Question 28

Concerning skeletal manifestations of neuroblastoma,

(A) about 30% of children present with bone pain
(B) sutural widening is secondary to cerebral metastases
(C) the diaphyses are the most common site of osseous metastases
(D) cortical metastasis is a unique feature of stage 4S disease
(E) bone scintigraphy is less sensitive than I-131 metaiodobenzylguanidine scintigraphy for diagnosis of bone marrow involvement

Neuroblastoma is the most common extracranial solid malignant tumor in childhood. It usually originates from the sympathetic nervous system. The most frequent primary site is the adrenal gland, and more than 70% of the tumors arise within the abdomen. Neuroblastoma can occur anywhere along the sympathetic nervous system. Extra-abdominal sites include the head and neck (5%), thorax (20%), and pelvis (5%). By the time most children are seen, they are symptomatic. Approximately 90% of children have a palpable mass, and 70% have other findings, including bone pain, opsoclonus, diarrhea, or lower-extremity weakness, as a result of metastases or paraneoplastic syndromes. A total of 25% of cases occur during the first year of life, 50% occur in children younger than 2 years, and 75% occur in children younger than 4 years.

Bone pain is common in patients with metastatic neuroblastoma; it is attributable to marrow packing, bone destruction, and pathologic fractures. Metastatic disease to the marrow and skeletal system causes pain in about 30% to 40% of patients at presentation (**Option (A) is true**). The skeletal system represents the most common site of hematogenous metastasis of neuroblastoma in children older than 1 year. In order of frequency, neuroblastoma in the older child metastasizes to bones, regional lymph nodes, liver, dura, and lungs. The characteristic skeletal abnormality in metastatic neuroblastoma is a lytic permeative lesion. In the appendicular skeleton, the metaphyses represent the most common site of involvement (**Option (C) is false**). In most patients, the osseous metastases are bilateral and nearly symmetric. In addition to lytic lesions, metastases in long bones can produce periosteal reaction, sclerotic lesions, and metaphyseal lucencies. Cortical bone destruction indicates extension of the metastatic tumor into adjacent soft tissues. Periosteal reaction can be single-layered or multilayered. It occasionally shows a sunburst appearance. Periosteal reaction usually occurs with underlying metadiaphyseal bone changes. It rarely occurs with no visual radiographic abnormality in the underlying bone. Osteosclerotic metastases are rare. Sclerotic regions are most often identified during therapy and are attributed to the reparative process (Figure 5-17).

Metastases to the skull usually involve the calvaria and orbits. Radiographic evidence of separation or widening of the cranial sutures is not an uncommon finding when there are extradural (skull, dural, and leptomeningeal) metastases. Cerebral metastases are uncommon and are not the principal cause of sutural widening (**Option (B) is false**). In general, sutural widening does not occur unless there is radiographic or bone scintigraphic evidence of metastatic skull lesions (Figures 5-18 and 5-19). Skull involvement is often quite diffuse, with patchy areas of abnormal accumulation of bone-seeking radiopharmaceutical. Metastasis to the orbit is a classic feature of metastatic neuroblastoma. Orbital involvement usually occurs via direct extension of metastatic lesions from the osseous structures. There are unusual cases in which metastatic neuroblastoma infiltrates orbital soft tissue structures. Metastatic orbital neuroblastoma is bilateral in more than 40% of cases. There are instances in which exophthalmos attributable to metastatic disease is the initial clinical presentation of neuroblastoma with a primary lesion located in the abdomen. Standard radiographs may be normal or may demonstrate permeative osseous destruction. Osseous metastases frequently result in expansile lesions that protrude into the orbit and cause proptosis. These masses typically remain confined by the periosteum and, therefore, protrude into the extraconal space, but do not invade soft tissue structures of the orbit. On CT, the extraconal mass of a metastatic neuroblastoma usually has a relatively high attenuation and may have ill-defined borders. Extension into the preseptal space does not usually occur except in advanced disease, a feature that aids in the differentiation of this entity from rhabdomyosarcoma. Bone-window images show permeative destruction. MRI in cases of orbital metastatic neuroblastoma demonstrates obliteration of the marrow space in the orbital walls by low-signal-intensity material on T1-weighted images. Extraconal orbital metastatic deposits typically produce a low signal intensity on T1-weighted

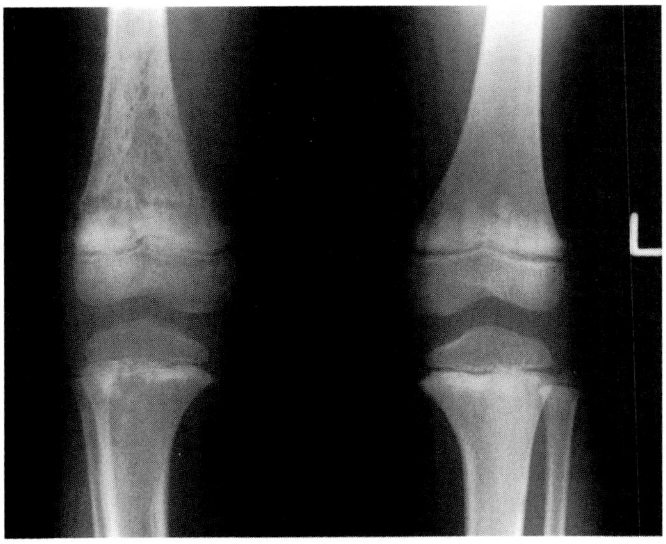

Figure 5-17. Metastatic neuroblastoma. An anteroposterior radiograph of the knees shows bilateral metastatic disease. The right distal femur shows a lytic permeative metadiaphyseal abnormality with cortical bone destruction and a pathologic fracture. The right tibial metaphysis and left distal femur demonstrate the rare osteosclerotic metastatic pattern of disease.

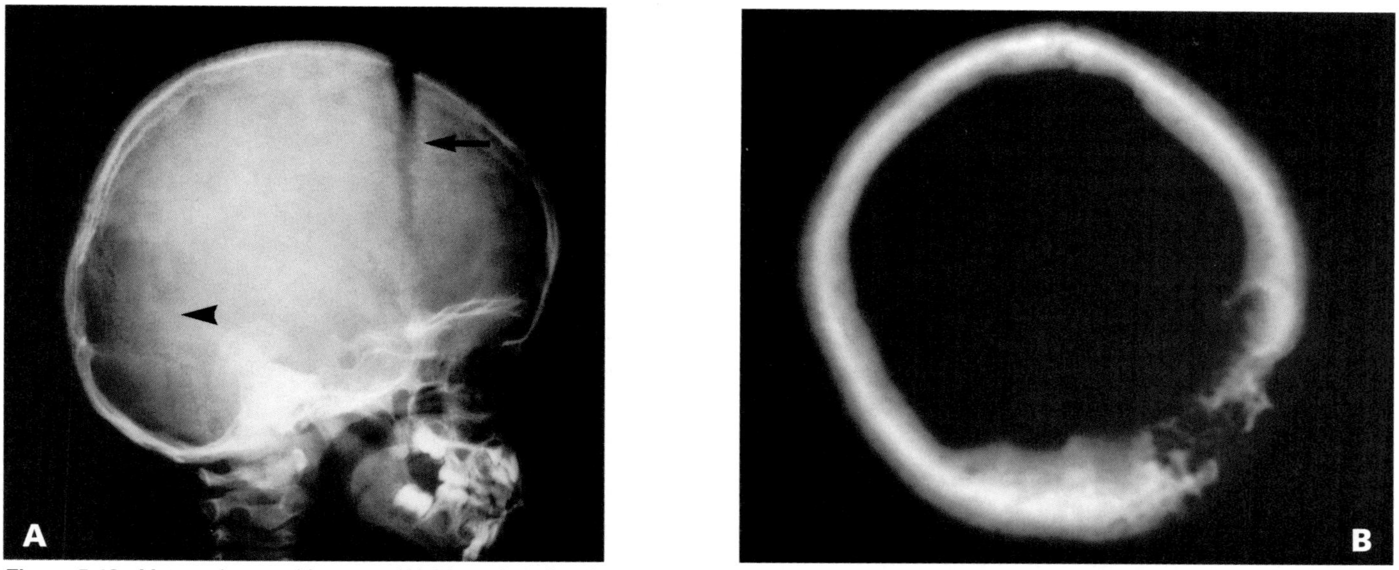

Figure 5-18. Metastatic neuroblastoma. (A) A lateral skull radiograph shows widening of the coronal suture (arrow) and a lytic abnormality in the occipital bone (arrowhead) secondary to metastatic neuroblastoma. (B) An axial CT scan filmed in bone windows demonstrates a destructive lesion in the occipital bone secondary to metastatic neuroblastoma.

images and a high signal intensity on T2-weighted images. T2-weighted sequences are best suited for the differentiation of tumor deposits from normal structures and for the detection of invasion of normal orbital components.

Several staging systems for neuroblastoma exist. The Evans system is based on radiologic findings. Stage I tumors are confined to the organ or structure of origin. Stage II tumors extend beyond the organ or structure of origin but do not cross the midline. Regional lymph nodes on the homolateral side can be involved. Stage III tumors extend beyond the midline. Bilateral regional lymph nodes can be involved. Stage IV indicates remote disease involving the skeletal system, organs, soft tissues, or distant lymph node groups. Stage IVS is classified as a stage I or II primary lesion in a child under 1 year of age who also has distant metastases in the liver, skin, or bone marrow but no radiographic evidence of bone metastases on a skeletal survey.

The more recently developed International Staging System combines imaging and surgical findings. Stage 1 is defined as neuroblastoma confined to the area of origin, complete gross excision with or without microscopic residual disease, and identifiable ipsilateral and contralateral lymph nodes that are negative microscopically. Stage 2A is defined as unilateral tumor with incomplete gross excision; involvement of lymph nodes and liver is the same as in stage 1. Stage 2B is defined as unilateral tumor with complete or incomplete gross excision and with positive ipsilateral regional lymph nodes. Identifiable contralateral lymph nodes are negative microscopically. In stage 3 disease, the tumor infiltrates across the midline with or without regional lymph node involvement; alternatively, there is a unilateral tumor with contralateral regional lymph node involvement or a midline tumor with bilateral regional lymph node involvement. Stage 4 is defined as dissemination of the tumor to distant lymph nodes, bones, bone marrow, liver, or other organs (except as defined in stage 4S). Stage 4S is a localized primary tumor as defined for stage 1, 2A, or 2B with dissemination limited to the liver, skin, or bone marrow. Metastases to bones are specifically excluded (**Option (D) is false**), but metastatic sites such as the pleura, pancreas, and peritoneum, not in the original classification, are now allowed.

The initial evaluation for osseous metastatic disease in patients with neuroblastoma should be bone scintigraphy followed by conventional radiographic examination of abnormal areas. Bone scintigraphy gives negative results in only about

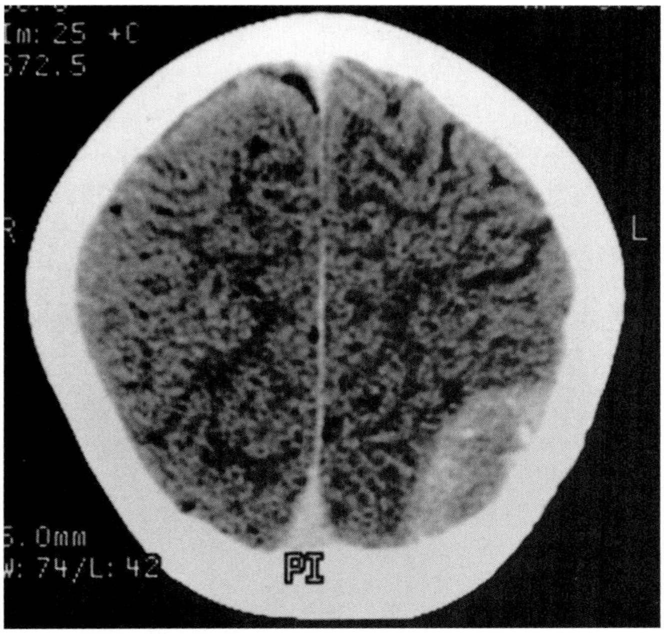

Figure 5-19. Metastatic neuroblastoma. CT scans demonstrate an extradural metastatic lesion attributable to neuroblastoma.

5% of the patients for whom conventional radiographs are positive. Conversely, bone scintigraphy is positive in 15% of patients for whom radiographic skeletal surveys are completely negative. Bone scintigraphy shows more lesions than does conventional radiography in 35% of patients. However, bone scintigraphy does not demonstrate metastatic disease confined to the marrow; there must be an osseous component. Abnormal osteogenesis or vascularity must be present for bone scintigraphy to produce positive results.

I-131 metaiodobenzylguanidine (MIBG) and I-123 MIBG are imaging agents for the diagnosis of tumors originating from neural crest cells. MIBG is a physiologic analog of norepinephrine and guanethidine. Scintigraphy with radiolabeled MIBG is highly accurate in the detection of both primary and metastatic neural crest tumors.

Radiolabeled MIBG is administered intravenously and undergoes specific uptake and storage by the adrenal gland, sympathetic autonomic nervous system, and tumors derived from these tissues. A significant fraction of uptake into these tissues is by means of a specific, high-affinity sodium- and energy-dependent type I anion uptake system. MIBG may be stored within the intravesicular hormone storage system in adrenal medullary and pheochromocytoma cells. The tissues that lack the specific type I uptake mechanism may show a degree of nonspecific uptake, but retention is transient and this "background" activity significantly decreases over time. Specific uptake by medullary tumors is frequently demonstrable within 24 hours after administration. Most of the injected activity is excreted unchanged in the urine; 60% is eliminated within 24 hours, and more than 90% is excreted by 4 days. The normal I-131 MIBG scintigram reveals uptake in the salivary glands, nasopharynx, heart, liver, and urinary bladder. These tissues have sympathetic innervation (salivary glands, nasopharynx, and heart) or are involved in the metabolism and excretion of the tracer (liver and bladder) (Figure 5-20).

Both I-131 and I-123 MIBG have been used for neuroblastoma imaging. I-131 MIBG concentrates in foci of neuroblastoma in moderate to high concentrations, allowing imaging of primary neuroblastoma in the adrenal gland or along the adrenergic sympathetic chain. Recurrent abdominal masses may be imaged, and metastases may be located in bone, bone marrow, lymph node, soft tissue, and liver. Whole-body imaging of neuroblastoma with I-131 MIBG has been effective in studies performed at numerous pediatric centers. The sensitivity of I-131 MIBG for the detection of the primary neuroblastoma is slightly greater than 90%. I-131 MIBG has a sensitivity of 70% or greater for the detection of skeletal metastases. The specificity of positive findings in the extraosseous as well as the osseous structures is nearly 100%. In addition to identifying isolated marrow metastatic disease, MIBG imaging demonstrates cortical deposits (Figure 5-21). MIBG scintigraphy is a better method for characterizing the extent of metastatic tumor than are radiography and bone scintigraphy. These last two examination techniques indicate only bone destruction or repair. MIBG scintigraphy can show evidence of bone or

Figure 5-20. Normal I-131 metaiodobenzylguanidine (MIBG) scintigraphy. This 7-year-old boy had a thoracic neuroblastoma resected 4 years earlier. Follow-up I-131 MIBG scintigrams show normal uptake in the salivary glands, nasopharynx, heart, liver, and urinary bladder.

bone marrow involvement when other imaging studies and bone marrow aspiration yield normal results (**Option (E) is true**). Even when bone scintigraphy or bone marrow aspiration shows that bone or bone marrow is involved, I-131 MIBG imaging often demonstrates that the infiltration of bone and bone marrow is far more extensive than was previously appreciated.

MIBG scintigraphy can also demonstrate residual tumor when CT or sonographic results for the same region are normal and when urinary catecholamine laboratory test results are negative. In one report, 18 MIBG studies were performed in patients with known tumor; the I-131 MIBG examination demonstrated more areas of involvement than the combination of CT, bone scintigraphy, and radiography in 10 of the patients. I-131 MIBG studies showed less involvement than did the other studies in four patients and demonstrated identical involvement in two patients. The results of I-131 MIBG scintigraphy have been shown to return to normal more quickly than those of bone scintigraphy in children who have undergone bone marrow transplantation.

I-123 MIBG may prove more useful than the I-131 agent in the evaluation of neuroblastoma. The physical properties of I-123 greatly favor its use instead of the I-131 agent. The optimal postadministration timing of I-123 MIBG scintigraphy,

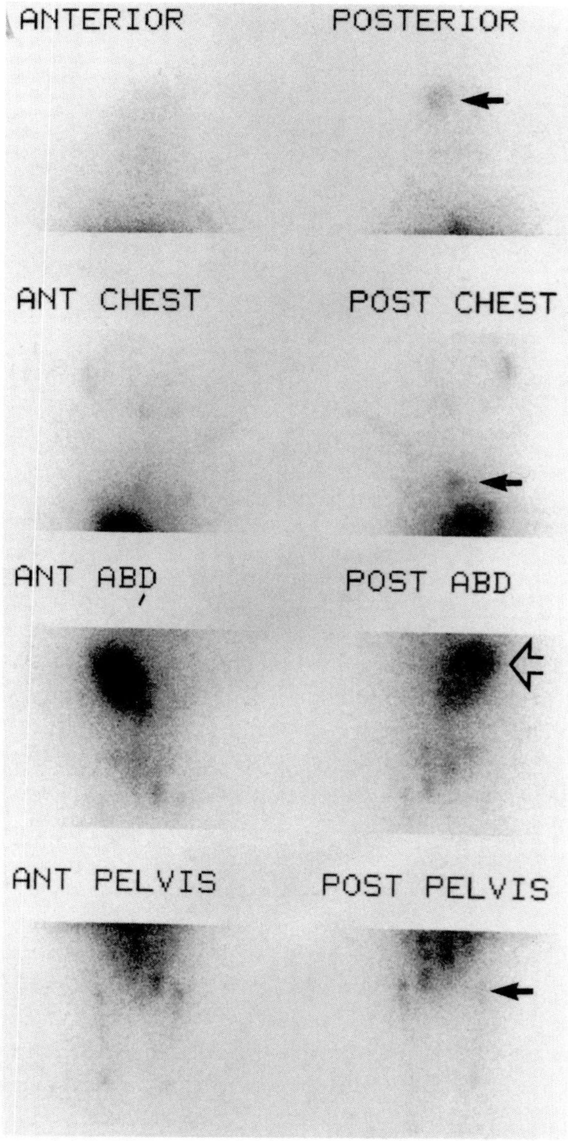

Figure 5-21. Metastatic neuroblastoma. Anterior and posterior I-131 MIBG images of a child with metastatic neuroblastoma show lesions in the left occipital bone, thoracic spine, and femurs (solid arrows) as well as the pelvic bones. The large region of uptake in the right flank (open arrow) is the primary tumor.

however, has not been fully established. The biologic half-life of MIBG in neural crest tumors is longer than its whole-body half-life, and this factor must be taken into account in the determination of optimal imaging protocols. As the tissue background activity falls, pathologic accumulation of MIBG becomes more prominent. The 13-hour physical half-life of I-123 is therefore potentially a limiting factor when delayed images are needed. On the other hand, because of the 159-keV photon energy of I-123 and the increased activity of I-123 MIBG that can be administered, early I-123 MIBG images will have better spatial resolution and information density (at a lower radiation dose) than those obtained with I-131 MIBG.

Somatostatin receptor scintigraphy (with In-111 pentetreotide) has also been used in the pediatric population to detect and evaluate the extent of metastatic neuroblastoma. Various tumors, classically specified as either neuroendocrine or non-neuroendocrine, contain large numbers of somatostatin receptors, which enable in vivo localization of the primary tumor and metastases by scintigraphy with the radiolabeled somatostatin analog octreotide. More than 80% of patients with neuroblastoma have receptor sites in the tumor and will have positive somatostatin receptor scintigraphic studies. In-111 pentetreotide imaging is also useful as a prognostic indicator. Patients with somatostatin receptor-positive neuroblasts seem to survive longer than those with receptor-negative ones.

MRI also is playing an increasing role in the detection of marrow metastases. In a recent study, the multi-institutional Radiology Diagnostic Oncology Group compared the relative accuracies of CT and MRI in staging of children with neuroblastoma. The authors reported that MRI had accuracy comparable to that of the combination of CT and bone scintigraphy for detection of stage 4 disease.

On T1-weighted images, marrow infiltration attributable to neuroblastoma produces focal or diffuse areas of low signal intensity. On T2-weighted and fat-suppressed images, focal metastases are characteristically relatively bright in signal intensity, reflecting increased water content attributable to hypercellularity. Occasionally, neuroblastoma will induce an osteoblastic reaction with bone production. In these cases, focal decreased signal will be seen on all pulse sequences.

Question 29

Concerning Legg-Perthes disease,

(A) most patients have normal radiographs at the time of presentation
(B) bilateral involvement occurs in fewer than 10% of patients
(C) widening of the joint space is related to thickening of the cartilage
(D) bone scintigraphy typically demonstrates a photopenic growth plate
(E) MRI is essential for assessing the response to treatment in most patients

Legg-Perthes disease most often affects children between the ages of 4 and 8 years. The average age at diagnosis is 6 years. It is rare among blacks. A striking retardation of skeletal maturation is found in affected children of both sexes, with the bone age frequently being less than the chronologic age by 2 standard deviations. Siblings of children with Legg-Perthes disease also have retarded skeletal maturation. Legg-Perthes disease is associated with congenital anomalies of the urinary tract and with inguinal hernias. Bilateral disease is present in fewer than 10% of patients (**Option (B) is true**). If bilateral ischemic necrosis of the proximal femoral epiphyseal ossification centers is present, conditions other than Legg-Perthes disease, such as sickle cell disease, steroid-induced osteonecrosis, or hypothyroidism, must be considered. Multiple epiphyseal dysplasia may produce similar radiographic findings, but this disease also is associated with an increased incidence of Legg-Perthes disease.

Legg-Perthes disease is the result of avascular necrosis of the proximal femoral epiphyseal ossification center. The major blood supply to the proximal femoral epiphyseal ossification center arises from the superior and inferior retinacular arteries, which are branches of the medial circumflex femoral artery. Branches of the lateral circumflex femoral artery supply the greater trochanter, the anterior aspect of the femoral neck, and a small segment of the anterior aspect of the uppermost femoral epiphyseal ossification center. These vessels course along the femoral neck within the periosteum. The blood supply to the femoral head during growth is vulnerable between the ages of 4 and 7 years because the retinacular arteries represent the only important vascular route to the femoral epiphyseal ossification center, whereas a double vascular supply exists at younger ages (metaphyseal and retinacular arteries) and at older ages (foveal and retinacular arteries). In adolescence and adulthood, three groups of vessels supply the proximal femur (foveal, retinacular, and metaphyseal arteries). Because of this fragile vascular blood supply, relatively minor abnormalities can result in femoral head ischemia.

Initially, an ischemic episode of undetermined etiology causes the entire proximal femoral epiphyseal ossification center to become avascular. Enchondral ossification of the epiphyseal cartilage temporarily ceases, while the articular cartilage, which is nourished by synovial fluid, develops. Normal growth of the bony epiphyseal ossification center ceases as a result of the ischemic insult. Because the articular cartilage remains viable, it continues to proliferate, resulting in cartilaginous enlargement. The enlarged cartilage leads to widening of the joint space (**Option (C) is true**). This thick cartilage is more obvious on the medial and lateral aspects of the femoral head. Small areas of necrosis can occur in the deepest layers of the articular cartilage. Some authors have suggested that synovial swelling or effusions cause the increased measurement of the joint space, but arthrography and MRI have shown that there is no true subluxation or large synovial fluid collections under pressure in most patients. There is a definite increase in the thickness of the acetabular cartilage, and there is an overgrowth of the cartilage in the femoral head (Figure 5-22). These two radiolucent structures appear to shift the observable epiphyseal ossification center laterally, without any actual increase in the medial joint space.

The blood supply to the femoral epiphyseal ossification center is ultimately reestablished by invasion of vascular granulation tissue, which replaces the epiphyseal marrow. The revascularization begins from the periphery and progresses centrally; resorption of avascular bone and the production of new immature bone occur simultaneously. Because new bone is deposited on the remaining old bone trabeculae, there is an overall increase in bone mass, which accounts in part for the increased

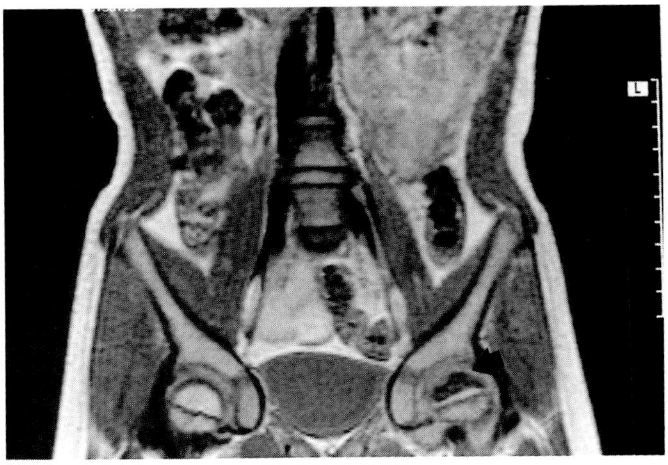

FSE 3,000/12

Figure 5-22. Legg-Perthes disease. This 7-year-old boy has Legg-Perthes disease of the left hip. A proton-density-weighted coronal MR image of the pelvis shows an increase in the thickness of the acetabular cartilage and an overgrowth of cartilage in the femoral head. This overgrowth of cartilage is responsible for the increased joint space measurement on standard radiographs (not shown).

radiographic density seen in the revascularization phase.

In the revascularization stage, the subchondral area of the femoral epiphyseal ossification center becomes extremely susceptible to minor injury. The result is a pathologic fracture. This fracture is painful and frequently radiographically demonstrable. Patients most often present at this stage. Therefore, most children have abnormal radiographs at presentation (Figure 5-23) (**Option (A) is false**).

Other radiographic signs of Legg-Perthes disease in the revascularization stage include a femoral epiphyseal ossification center that is smaller or more flattened than that on the contralateral side, sclerosis of the femoral head, slight widening of the joint space, ipsilateral bone demineralization, and rarefaction of the lateral and medial metaphyseal regions of the neck. Resorption and reossification follow revascularization. The late radiographic signs include delayed ossification of the femoral head, a radiolucent crescent line representing the subchondral fracture, femoral head fragmentation, femoral neck cysts, coxa magna, and coxa plana (Figure 5-24).

Bone scintigraphy with Tc-99m MDP has been extremely valuable in the diagnosis of ischemic necrosis. Positive bone scintigraphy occurs at least 1 month before radiographic changes. The sensitivity and specificity of scintigraphy for diagnosis are 98% and 95%, respectively. The characteristic scintigraphic appearance of Legg-Perthes disease is an absence of tracer accumulation in the femoral capital epiphysis. This is usually best demonstrated on anterior and frog-leg lateral pinhole views. Unlike the situation with femoral head ischemia secondary to joint effusion, activity in the growth plate is preserved in patients with Legg-Perthes disease; in fact, there is often increased activity (**Option (D) is false**). The growth plate is not involved with the ischemic event and can be hyperemic because of recruitment vascularity and metabolic changes.

The size of the photopenic defect probably corresponds to

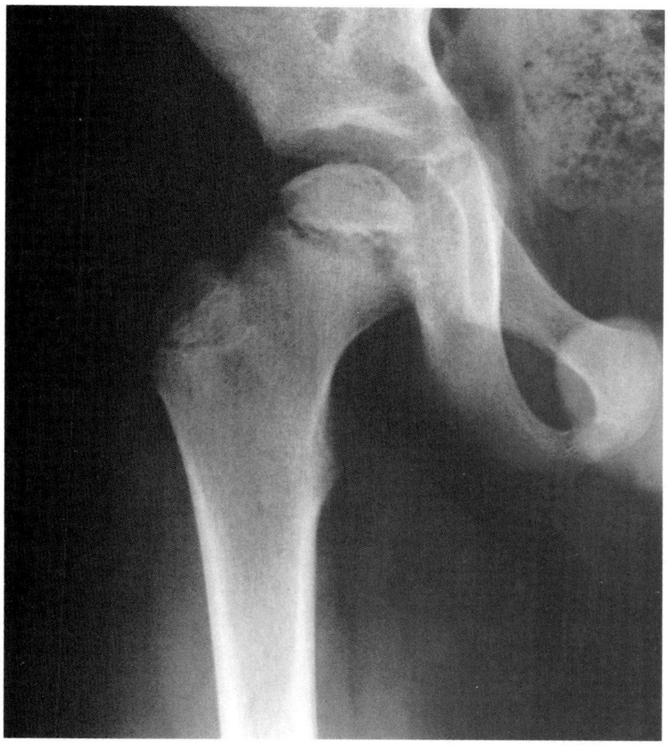

Figure 5-23. Legg-Perthes disease. An anteroposterior radiograph of the right hip shows a somewhat flattened and sclerotic femoral head. A radiolucent line below the articulating surface of the femoral head can be identified. The radiolucent line is the subchondral fracture that is the cause of the painful presentation of Legg-Perthes disease.

the extent of the subchondral fracture. When increased activity is demonstrated in the growth plate, new bone appears relatively early radiographically, but when the increased activity is present in the growth plate and metaphyseal regions, radiographic improvement takes at least twice as long. Bone scintigraphy usually becomes normal approximately 1 year after presentation. Early revascularization of the femoral head is identified scintigraphically by the appearance of the lateral column or a band of activity in the most lateral aspect of the femoral epiphyseal ossification center (Figure 5-25). The increased activity seen on bone scintigraphy during the revascularization phase appears approximately 4 to 6 months before radiologic evidence of new bone formation.

MRI provides a sensitive method of detecting early Legg-Perthes disease without the use of radiation. MRI performed in the coronal and transaxial planes is useful for visualization of the entire femoral head. The loss of normal high signal intensity in the marrow is typical of the early ischemic phase. Infarction is believed to lead to reduction of the lipid content and therefore to loss of the signal. During revascularization, the signal returns to normal in the femoral epiphyseal ossification center. During resorption and reossification, the involved area takes on a speckled appearance of intermixed high- and low-intensity areas as a result of heterogeneous revascularization or recurrent vascular insults. Irregularity of the articular surface, loss of containment to the femoral head, and changes in the

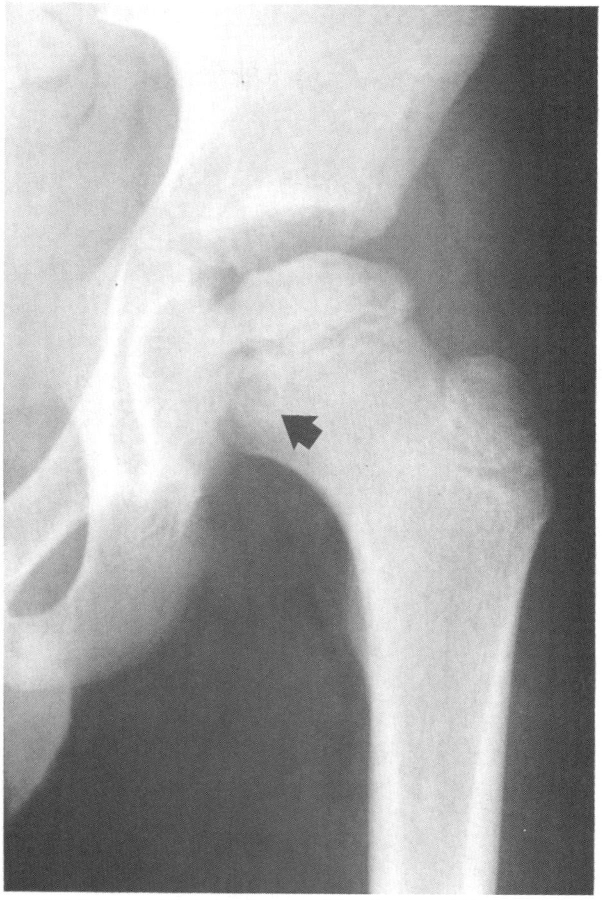

Figure 5-24. Legg-Perthes disease. This 6-year-old boy has had Legg-Perthes disease for approximately 8 months. A radiograph shows flattening of the left femoral head and sclerosis. A small metaphyseal cyst is present below the growth plate (arrow). Slight widening of the joint space is attributable to the associated cartilage hypertrophy.

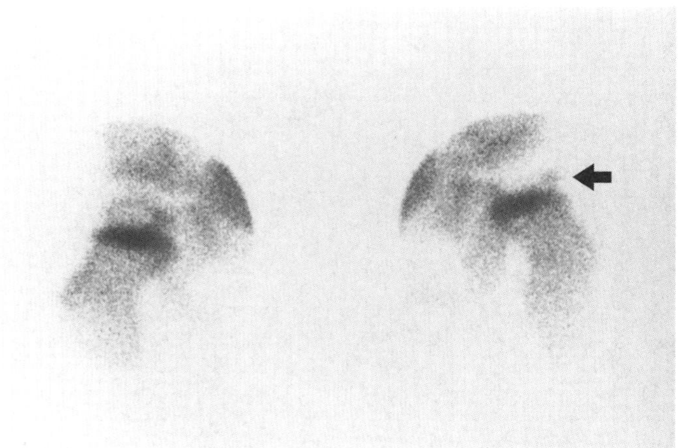

Figure 5-25. Legg-Perthes disease. Tc-99m MDP pinhole images demonstrate changes of Legg-Perthes disease on the left, with the appearance of a lateral column of tracer uptake (arrow) in the otherwise photon-deficient femoral epiphyseal ossification center. This is a result of early revascularization of the femoral head.

femoral epiphyseal ossification center are apparent. Although MRI can evaluate cartilage, it usually is not necessary as a diagnostic examination since radiographs are usually abnormal, establishing the diagnosis and identifying the stage of disease (Figure 5-26).

The goal of treatment is to enable the patient to maintain a normal range of motion and to contain the femoral head within the acetabulum. A necrotic femoral epiphyseal ossification center is vulnerable to mechanical stress, and placement of the femoral head deep within the acetabulum helps to prevent lateral excursion and collapse. The femoral head is contained with bracing or casting. The standard treatment program continues until the dense, sclerotic bone has disappeared and a relatively round, reconstituting femoral head is present. These findings can usually be identified by standard radiographic examination. MRI is not essential for assessing the response to treatment in most patients **(Option (E) is false).**

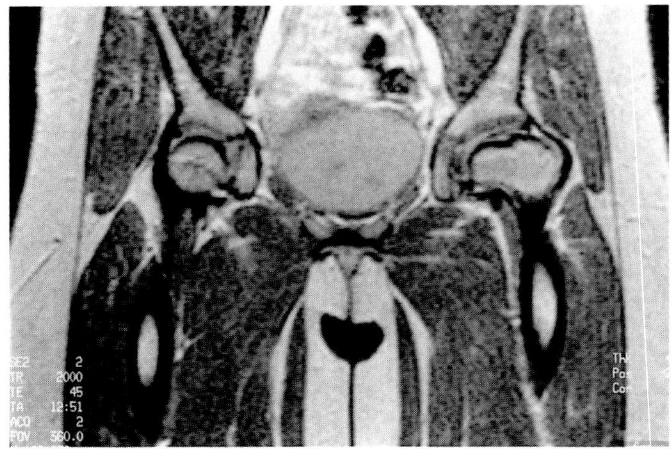

Figure 5-26. Legg-Perthes disease. This 8-year-old boy has a long-standing history of Legg-Perthes disease of the left hip. A coronal MR image shows irregularity of the articular surface and a slight loss of containment of the femoral head. Note the mild cartilage hypertrophy and reossification of the abnormally shaped head.

SUGGESTED READINGS

OSTEOMYELITIS

1. Amundsen TR, Siegel MJ, Siegel BA. Osteomyelitis and infarction in sickle cell hemoglobinopathies: differentiation by combined technetium and gallium scintigraphy. Radiology 1984; 153:807–812
2. Barron BJ, Dhekne RD. Cold osteomyelitis. Radionuclide bone scan findings. Clin Nucl Med 1984; 7:392–393
3. Erdman WA, Tamburro F, Jayson HT, Weatherall PT, Ferry KB, Peshock RM. Osteomyelitis: characteristics and pitfalls of diagnosis with MR imaging. Radiology 1991; 180:533–539
4. Gavilán MG, López JB, Artola BS. Peculiarities of osteo-articular infections in children. Baillieres Best Pract Res Clin Rheumatol 1999; 13:77–94
5. Rosovsky M, Goldfarb CR, Finestone H, Ongseng F. "Cold spots" in pediatric imaging. Semin Nucl Med 1994; 24:184–186
6. Schlesinger AE, Hernandez RJ. Diseases of the musculoskeletal system in children: imaging with CT, sonography, and MR. AJR 1992; 158:729–741
7. Sullivan JA, Vasileff T, Leonard JC. An evaluation of nuclear scanning in orthopaedic infections. J Pediatr Orthop 1981; 1:73–79
8. Treves S, Khettry J, Broker FH, Wilkinson RH, Watts H. Osteomyelitis: early scintigraphic detection in children. Pediatrics 1976; 57:173–186
9. Tuson CE, Hoffman EB, Mann MD. Isotope bone scanning for acute osteomyelitis and septic arthritis in children. J Bone Joint Surg [Br] 1994; 76:306–310

LEUKEMIA

10. Caudle RJ, Crawford AH, Gelfand MJ, Gruppu RA. Childhood acute lymphoblastic leukemia presenting as "cold" lesions on bone scan. A report of two cases. J Pediatr Orthop 1987; 7:93–95
11. Clausen N, Gotze H, Pedersen A, Riis-Petersen J, Tjalve E. Skeletal scintigraphy and radiography at onset of acute lymphocytic leukemia in children. Med Pediatr Oncol 1983; 11:291–296
12. Kuntz DJ, Leonard JC, Nitschke RM, Vanhoutte JJ, Wilson DA, Basmadjian GP. An evaluation of diagnostic techniques utilized in the initial workup of pediatric patients with acute lymphocytic leukemia. Clin Nucl Med 1984; 9:405–408
13. Moore SG, Bisset GS III, Siegel MJ, Donaldson JS. Pediatric musculoskeletal MR imaging. Radiology 1991; 179:345–360
14. Parker BR, Marglin S, Castellino RA. Skeletal manifestations of leukemia, Hodgkin disease, and non-Hodgkin lymphoma. Semin Roentgenol 1980; 15:302–315
15. Rogalsky RJ, Black GB, Reed MH. Orthopaedic manifestations of leukemia in children. J Bone Joint Surg [Am] 1986; 68:94–105
16. Samuda GM, Cheng MY, Yeung CY. Back pain and vertebral compression: an uncommon presentation of childhood acute lymphoblastic leukemia. J Pediatr Orthop 1987; 7:175–178
17. Siegel MJ, Luker GG. Bone marrow imaging in children. Magn Reson Imaging Clin N Am 1996; 4:771–796
18. Troncone L, Rufini V, Turba R, Mastrangelo R, Riccardi R, Donfrancesco F. Nuclear medicine imaging in pediatric oncology. J Nucl Biol Med 1994; 38:76–84
19. Willson JKV. The bone lesions of childhood leukemia. A survey of 140 cases. Radiology 1959; 72:672–681

NEUROBLASTOMA

20. Bonnin F, Lumbroso J, Tenenbaum F, Hartmann O, Parmentier C. Refining interpretation of MIBG scans in children. J Nucl Med 1994; 35: 803–810
21. Cohen MD, Bugaieski EM, Haliloglu M, Faught P, Siddiqui AR. Visual presentation of the staging of pediatric solid tumors. RadioGraphics 1996; 16:523–545
22. Gelfand MJ. Meta-iodobenzylguanidine in children. Semin Nucl Med 1993; 23:231–242
23. Hoefnagel CA, Voute PA, de Kraker J, Marcuse HR. Radionuclide diagnosis and therapy of neural crest tumors using iodine-131 metaiodobenzylguanidine. J Nucl Med 1987; 28:208–214
24. Krenning EP, Kwekkeboom DJ, Bakker WH, et al. Somatostatin receptor scintigraphy with [^{111}In-DTPA-D-Phe^{1}]- and [^{123}I-Tyr^{3}]-octreotide: the Rotterdam experience with more than 1,000 patients. Eur J Nucl Med 1993; 20:716–731
25. Ng YY, Kingston JE. The role of radiology in the staging of neuroblastoma. Clin Radiol 1993; 47:226–235
26. Olsen JO, Pozderac RV, Hinkle G, et al. Somatostatin receptor imaging of neuroendocrine tumors with indium-111 pentetreotide (Octreoscan). Semin Nucl Med 1995; 25:251–261
27. Siegel MJ, Ishwaran H, Fletcher BD, et al. Staging of neuroblastoma by imaging. Report of the Radiology Diagnostic Oncology Group. Radiology 2002; 223:168–175
28. Sisson JC, Shulkin BL. Nuclear medicine imaging of pheochromocytoma and neuroblastoma. Q J Nucl Med 1999; 43:217–223
29. Sty JR, Wells RG. Radiographic imaging in neuroblastoma. In: Pochedly C (ed), Neuroblastoma: tumor biology and therapy. Boca Raton, FL: CRC Press; 1990:147–170
30. Yeh SD, Helson L, Benua RS. Correlation between iodine-131 MIBG imaging and biological markers in advanced neuroblastoma. Clin Nucl Med 1988; 13:46–52

LEGG-PERTHES DISEASE

31. Barker DJ, Hall AJ. The epidemiology of Perthes disease. Clin Orthop 1986; 209:89–94
32. Bos CF, Bloem JL, Bloem RM. Sequential magnetic resonance imaging in Perthes' disease. J Bone Joint Surg [Br] 1991: 73:219–224
33. Caterall A, Roberts GC, Wynne-Davies R. Association of Perthes disease with congenital anomalies of genitourinary tract and inguinal region. Lancet 1971; 1:996–997
34. Connolly LP, Treves ST. Assessing the limping child with skeletal scintigraphy. J Nucl Med 1998; 39:1056–1061
35. Egund N, Wingstrand H. Legg-Calvé-Perthes disease: imaging with MR. Radiology 1991; 179:89–92
36. Fisher RL. An epidemiological study of Legg-Perthes disease. J Bone Joint Surg [Am] 1972; 54:769–778
37. Houston SC. Pelvis and hips. In: Reed MH (ed), Pediatric skeletal radiography. Baltimore: Williams & Wilkins; 1992:326–346
38. Lahdes-Vasama T, Lamminen A, Merikanto J, Marttinen E. The value of MRI in early Perthes' disease: an MRI study with a 2-year follow-up. Pediatr Radiol 1997; 27:517–522
39. MacLeod MA, Houston AS. Functional bone imaging in the detection of ischemic osteopathies. Clin Nucl Med 1997: 22:1–5
40. Mitchell DG, Rao VM, Dalinka MK, et al. Femoral head avascular necrosis: correlation of MR imaging, radiographic staging, radionuclide imaging, and clinical findings. Radiology 1987; 162:709–715
41. Ozonoff MB. Pediatric orthopedic radiology, 2nd ed. Philadelphia: WB Saunders; 1992:244–267
42. Roy DR. Current concepts in Legg-Calvé-Perthes disease. Pediatr Ann 1999; 28:748–752
43. Rush BH, Bramson RT, Ogden JA. Legg-Calvé-Perthes disease: detection of cartilaginous and synovial changes with MR imaging. Radiology 1988; 167:473–476
44. Tsao AK, Dias LS, Conway JJ, Straka P. The prognostic value and significance of serial bone scintigraphy in Legg-Calvé-Perthes disease. J Pediatr Orthop 1997; 17:230–239

TRANSIENT SYNOVITIS OF THE HIP

45. Gershuni DH, Hargens AR, Lee YF, Greenberg EN, Zapf R, Akeson WH. The questionable significance of hip joint tamponade in producing osteonecrosis in Legg-Calvé-Perthes syndrome. J Pediatr Orthop 1983; 3: 280–286
46. Hardinge K. The etiology of transient synovitis of the hip in childhood. J Bone Joint Surg [Br] 1970; 52:100–107
47. Haueisen DC, Weiner DS, Weiner SD. The characterization of "transient synovitis of the hip" in children. J Pediatr Orthop 1986; 6:11–17
48. Kloiber R, Pavlosky W, Portner O, Gartke K. Bone scintigraphy of hip joint effusions in children. AJR 1983; 140:995–999
49. Minikel J, Sty J, Simons G. Sequential radionuclide bone imaging in avascular pediatric hip conditions. Clin Orthop 1983; 175:202–208
50. Miralles M, Gonzalez G, Pulperio JR et al. Sonography of the painful hip in children: 500 consecutive cases. AJR 1989; 152:579–582
51. Nelson JD, Koontz WC. Septic arthritis in infants and children: a review of 117 cases. Pediatrics 1966; 38:966–971
52. Robben SG, Lequin MH, Diepstraten AF, den Hollander JC, Entius CA, Meradji M. Anterior joint capsule of the normal hip and in children with transient synovitis: US study with anatomic and histologic correlation. Radiology 1999; 210:499–507
53. Schaller JG. Arthritis and infections of bone and joints in children. Pediatr Clin North Am 1977; 24:775–790
54 Wilson DJ, Green DJ, McLarnon JC. Arthrosonography of the painful hip. Clin Radiol 1984; 34:17–19

GENERAL

55. Mandell GA, Harcke HT, Kumar SJ. Generalized skeletal and related disorders. Imaging strategies in pediatric orthopedics. Gaithersburg, Md: Aspen; 1990
56. Miller JH, Heisel MA. Leukemia. In: Miller JH (ed), Imaging in pediatric oncology. Baltimore: Williams & Wilkins; 1985:406–408
57. Sty JR, Wells RG, Starshak RJ, Gregg DC. The musculoskeletal system. Diagnostic imaging of infants and children. Gaithersburg, Md: Aspen; 1992

Marilyn J. Siegel, M.D.

Acute Pyelonephritis

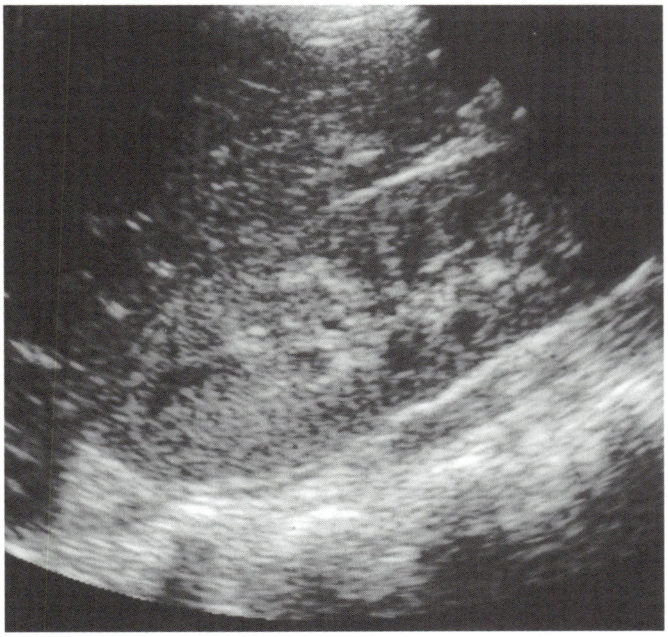

Figure 6-1

Question 30

This 7-year-old boy has low-grade fever and abdominal pain. You are shown gray-scale (Figure 6-1) and color Doppler (Figure 6-2) images.

Which *one* of the following is the MOST likely diagnosis?

(A) Acute pyelonephritis
(B) Reflux nephropathy
(C) Wilms' tumor
(D) Hemolytic uremic syndrome
(E) Infected upper-pole moiety of a duplex system

The longitudinal sonographic image of the right kidney (Figure 6-1) shows a poorly marginated area of increased echogenicity in the upper pole (Figure 6-3). The color Doppler study (Figure 6-2) shows no flow in the right upper pole (Figure 6-4). Normal flow is noted in the remainder of the kidney. The sonographic findings in the test patient are typical of acute pyelonephritis. The patient's clinical findings also support this diagnosis **(Option (A) is correct).**

Acute pyelonephritis is a bacterial infection of the renal parenchyma. Most affected children present with fever and signs or symptoms referable to the kidney, such as flank pain or costovertebral tenderness. Radiologic evaluation is routinely

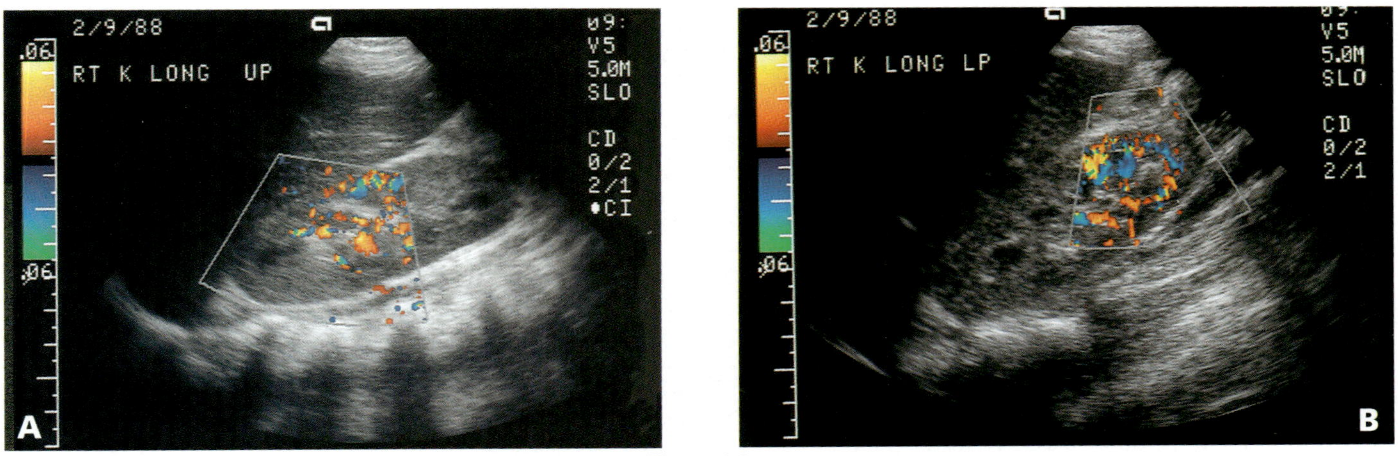

Figure 6-2

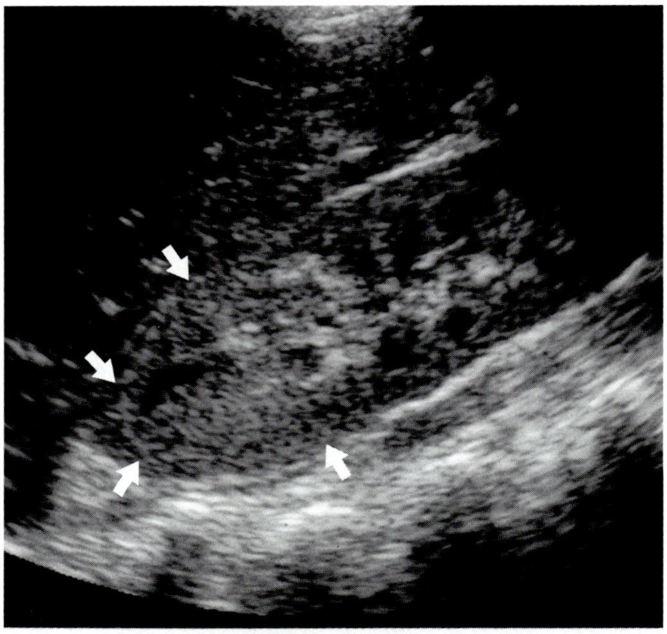

Figure 6-3 (Same as Figure 6-1). Acute pyelonephritis. A longitudinal sonogram through the right flank shows a slightly enlarged kidney. There is diffusely increased echogenicity in the upper portion and midportion of the right kidney (arrows).

performed to evaluate for underlying anomalies predisposing to infection.

Pyelonephritis can produce diffuse or focal renal enlargement. Pyelonephritis with focal involvement has been termed acute focal pyelonephritis. This condition had previously been referred to by a variety of names, including focal bacterial nephritis, acute focal bacterial nephritis, lobar nephronia, and renal cellulitis, all of which refer to severe inflammation without drainable pus. It is now recommended that these terms be replaced by the term "acute focal pyelonephritis." Acute focal pyelonephritis usually produces an ill-defined, oval to round mass within the renal parenchyma. It can be iso-, hypo-, or hyperechoic with respect to the surrounding parenchyma. Variations in echogenicity represent the presence or absence of associated hemorrhage. Duplex sonography and Doppler sonography usually demonstrate diminished or absent flow in the area of involvement.

Reflux nephropathy (Option (B)) is defined as scarring of the renal parenchyma as a result of previous bacterial infection. The scarring begins as a focal area of fibrosis in the medulla that subsequently enlarges and involves the entire thickness of the renal parenchyma. As a result, the renal cortex retracts inward and the renal papilla is pulled outward, destroying the calyx. The scars are typically polar in location. Patients with reflux nephropathy often present with nonspecific signs, such as fever, failure to thrive, growth retardation, and hypertension. Sonographic findings include a small kidney with focal or diffuse loss of parenchyma (Figure 6-5). The most severe changes involve the polar regions. The parenchymal echogenicity can be normal or increased. Although there is little published information regarding Doppler sonography in reflux nephropathy, one would expect flow in a region of scarring to be normal or decreased. The normal-sized kidney in the test patient and the smooth renal margins make reflux nephropathy an unlikely diagnosis.

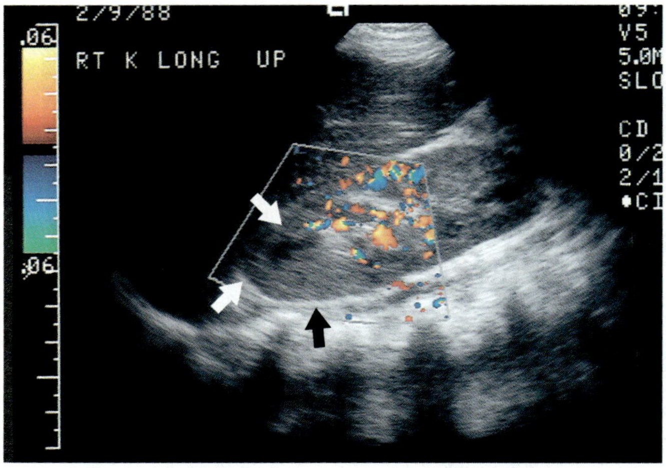

Figure 6-4 (Same as Figure 6-2A). Acute pyelonephritis. A color Doppler image shows decreased flow in the upper half of the right kidney (arrows). Edema and vasoconstriction in the inflamed areas of the kidney are believed to be the cause of the decreased parenchymal blood flow.

Wilms' tumor (Option (C)) is the most common cancer of the kidney in childhood. Most children present between 1 and 5 years of age (mean age, 3 years). An asymptomatic abdominal mass is the most common presenting feature, occurring in more than 90% of patients. Other clinical findings include fever, abdominal pain, microscopic or gross hematuria, and hypertension. On gross examination, Wilms' tumor is a large mass that arises in the cortex and replaces most of the renal parenchyma. It grows exophytically, with a large portion of the tumor protruding from the kidney.

The sonographic findings are those of a large intrarenal or at least partially intrarenal mass. The tumor can be either homogeneously echogenic or heterogeneously echogenic with cystic areas representing hemorrhage, necrosis, or a combination of the two (Figure 6-6). Findings on Doppler sonography include mildly increased vascularity, mass effect with displacement of vessels, and vessel amputation or invasion. Wilms' tumor spreads either by direct extension into the retroperitoneum or by invasion of the renal vein and propagation into the inferior vena cava. The age of the test patient and the sonographic findings, including the hypovascularity and the absence of an exophytic component, make Wilms' tumor an unlikely diagnosis.

Hemolytic uremic syndrome (Option (D)) is a disorder characterized by the classic triad of microangiopathic hemolytic anemia, thrombocytopenia, and renal failure. It is believed to be caused by an antigen-antibody reaction to bacterial toxins. Histologically, obstruction of small arteries and capillaries by thrombi and intimal inflammation, leading to renal impairment and platelet consumption, are seen. Most affected children are younger than 5 years and present with a prodromal phase of diarrhea, which is frequently bloody, followed by the onset of renal failure. Spontaneous recovery generally occurs

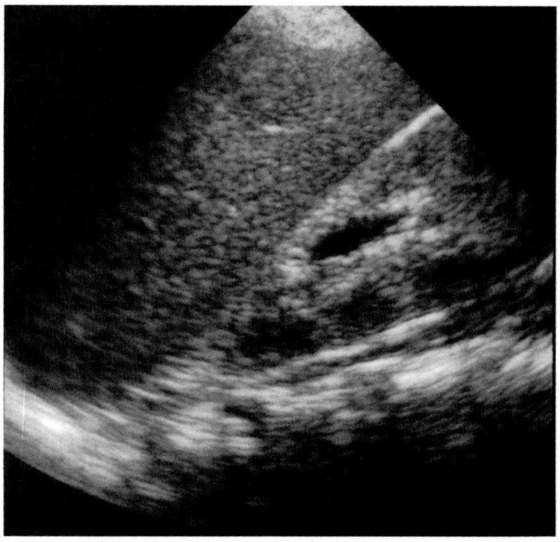

Figure 6-5. Reflux nephropathy. A longitudinal sonogram of the left kidney shows a dilated upper-pole collecting system and the surrounding loss of parenchyma.

within 3 weeks, but during that time the patient usually needs dialysis.

Sonography can be normal in patients with mild disease, whereas in those with severe involvement, there can be increased cortical echogenicity. Duplex Doppler findings also vary with the extent of disease. During the phase of oliguria or anuria, diastolic flow is absent, reversed, or markedly diminished (Figure 6-7). During the recovery phase, with the onset of diuresis, diastolic Doppler shifts return to normal. The absence of a history of bloody diarrhea and the focal renal abnormality on gray-scale sonography in the test patient make hemolytic uremic syndrome an unlikely diagnosis.

Duplication anomalies (Option (E)) can be partial or complete. The spectrum of partial duplication ranges from a bifid renal pelvis to Y-shaped ureters with the two ureters fusing somewhere along their course. A single common distal ureter enters the bladder. With complete ureteral duplication, the kidney has two pelvicalyceal systems and two ureters with separate insertions. The ureter of the upper-pole moiety terminates either ectopically or as a ureterocele. The ectopic ureter usually inserts into the vestibule, vagina, or urethra in girls and into the posterior urethra, epididymis, or seminal vesicles in boys. In both sexes, the ectopic ureters can drain into the bladder neck or into the trigone inferomedial to the normal location. The ureter draining the lower moiety inserts superior and lateral to its normal trigonal position. The upper-pole moiety is typically obstructed, while the lower-pole moiety tends to reflux. The symptoms of duplication are those of infection when the obstructed ureter drains above the external sphincter. When the ureter inserts below the external sphincter, urinary incontinence is a frequent complaint.

The upper-pole system can be hydronephrotic or dysplastic. The sonographic features of a hydronephrotic system include a variable degree of dilatation, parenchymal thinning, and a tortuous and dilated ureter. An infected duplicated system contains echogenic material, sometimes with fluid-debris levels (Figure 6-8). A dysplastic upper pole appears highly echogenic with small cysts. Flow in the dysplastic upper-pole moiety of a duplicated system would be expected to be decreased. However, the normal-sized upper pole and the absence of a separate collecting system in the lower pole in the test images virtually exclude the diagnosis of duplication.

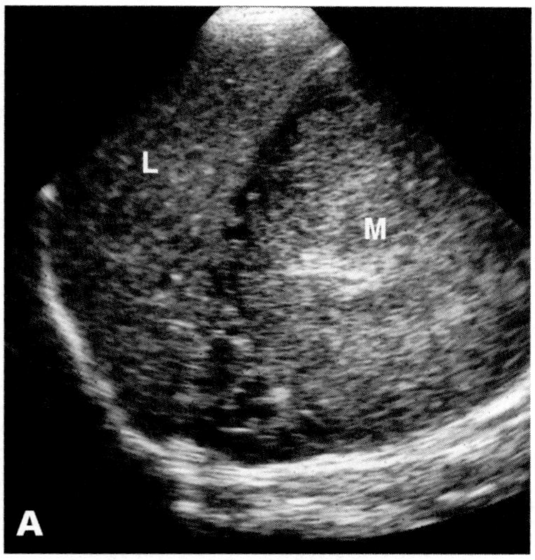

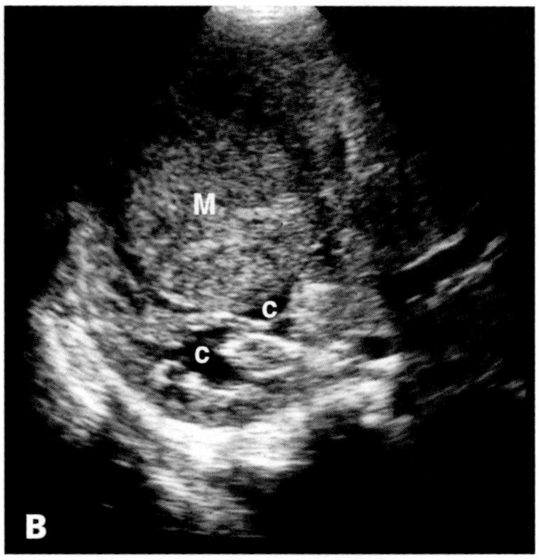

Figure 6-6. Wilms' tumor. Coronal (A) and transverse (B) sonograms of the right kidney show a large, homogeneous echogenic mass (M) arising from the midpole of the kidney and distorting mildly dilated calyces (c). L = liver.

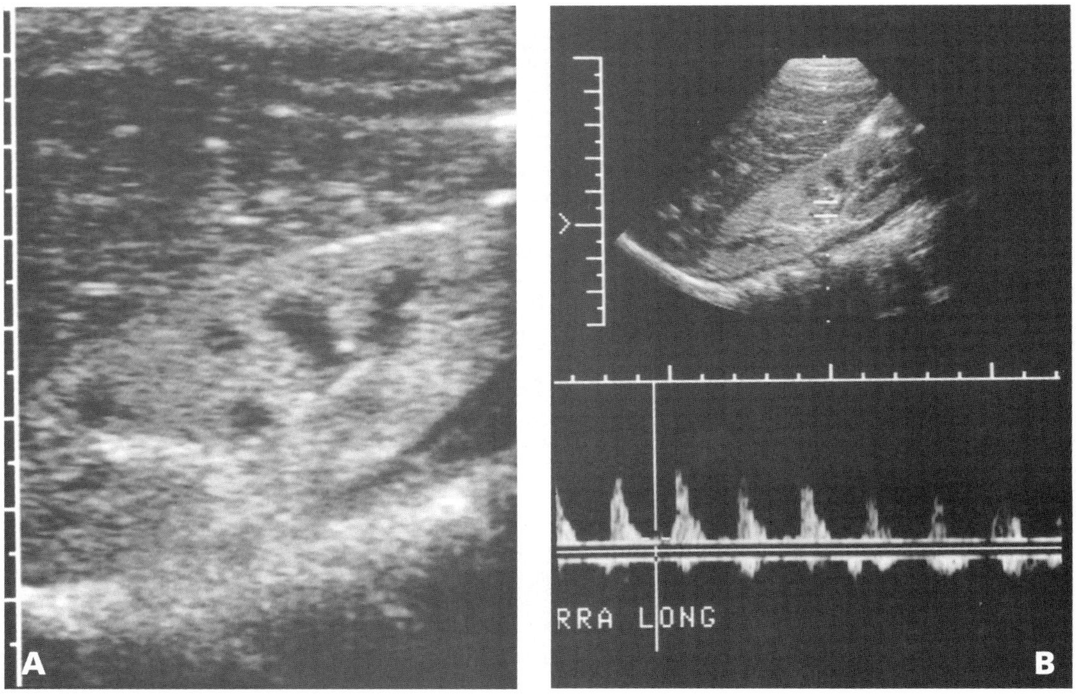

Figure 6-7. Hemolytic uremic syndrome in a 13-year-old girl. (A) A longitudinal sonogram shows diffusely increased renal cortical echogenicity. (B) A duplex Doppler sonogram demonstrates increased intrarenal arterial resistance, with diminished systolic flow and retrograde diastolic flow. At the time of the study, the patient was oliguric.

Question 31

Concerning imaging in children with acute pyelonephritis,

(A) its principal role is to confirm the diagnosis
(B) cystography is routinely performed in children younger than 5 years
(C) the sensitivity of gray-scale sonography for diagnosis is about 80%
(D) the sensitivity of cortical scintigraphy for diagnosis is approximately 90%
(E) striated parenchymal opacification is a typical pattern on CT

Urinary tract infections (UTI) in children can involve the upper urinary tract (kidneys), lower urinary tract (bladder), or both areas. Infections that involve the kidneys are referred to as pyelonephritis, while infections that affect the bladder are referred to as cystitis. Early diagnosis and treatment of UTI, particularly pyelonephritis, is essential to preserve renal function and prevent end-stage renal disease.

Most cases of acute pyelonephritis are attributable to a bacterial infection, and *Escherichia coli* is responsible for more than 90% of the cases in children. The offending *E. coli* organisms often contain typeable capsular polysaccharide antigens (K serotype) or outer membrane antigens (O antigens). Other

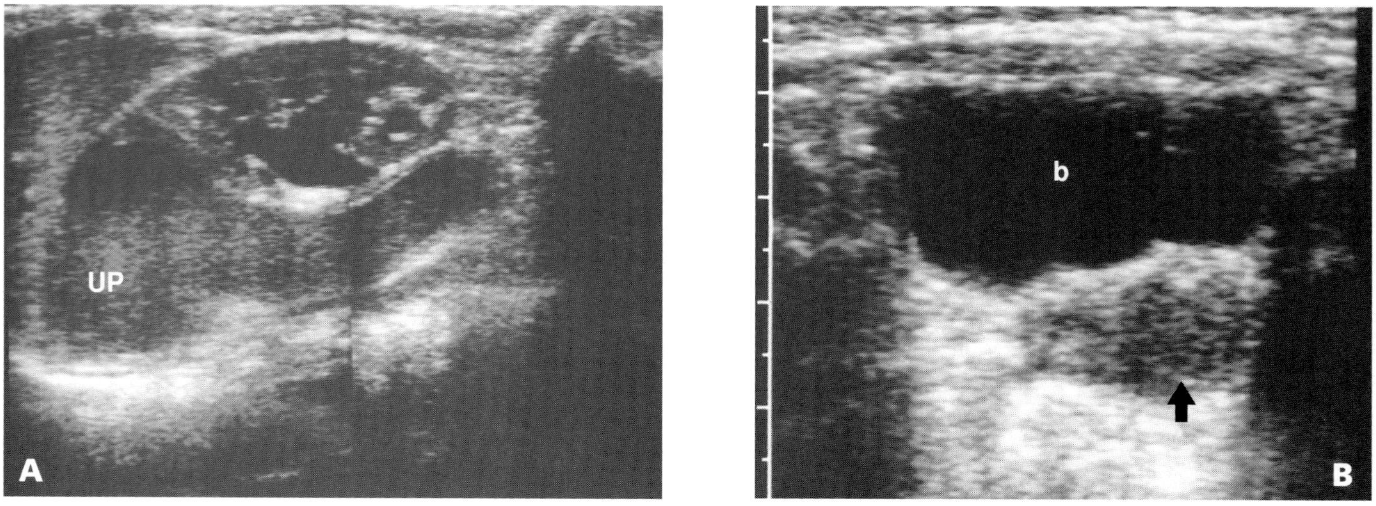

Figure 6-8. Renal duplication with upper-pole obstruction and infection. (A) A coronal sonogram of the left kidney reveals a duplex system with a hydronephrotic upper pole (UP) containing echogenic debris. The collecting system of the lower-pole moiety is dilated as a result of reflux. (B) A transverse sonogram through the pelvis shows a dilated upper-pole ureter (arrow) with internal echoes lying posterior to the urinary bladder (b). Diagnostic needle aspiration of the upper pole confirmed pus within the collecting system, establishing a diagnosis of pyonephrosis.

gram-negative organisms and *Staphylococcus* species are less frequent causes of UTI in childhood. On pathologic examination, acute pyelone-phritis involves both the renal pelvis (uroepithelium) and pa-renchyma. The infection is generally patchy in distribution, but the entire kidney can be involved in patients with severe cases.

The symptoms and signs of acute pyelonephritis vary with patient age. Neonates and infants younger than 2 years usually present with nonspecific systemic manifestations, such as temperature instability or fever, irritability, vomiting, jaundice, poor feeding, and failure to gain weight. Diagnosing UTI, as well as distinguishing lower-tract from upper-tract infection, on the basis of clinical findings can be difficult in this population. Older children and adolescents with acute pyelonephritis generally have signs and symptoms localized to the kidney. Fever, chills, flank pain, costovertebral tenderness, leukocytosis, and leukocyte casts are clinical signs indicative of upper UTI. Frequency, urgency, dysuria, and cloudy or foul-smelling urine are signs suggesting that the patient has lower UTI or cystitis.

The laboratory diagnosis of UTI is based on documentation of bacteriuria. The traditional definition of significant bacteriuria is the growth of more than 100,000 organisms/mL of urine obtained by a clean-catch technique. Counts of less than 100,000 organisms/mL are considered indicative of UTI when the urine is obtained by catheterization or suprapubic aspiration. The likelihood of UTI on the basis of significant bacteriuria in a clean-catch urine specimen is 80% to 85%. The likelihood increases to 95% if significant bacteriuria is found in two consecutive specimens. The reliability of diagnosing bacteriuria on the basis of a bagged urine specimen ranges between 7.5% and 50%. The bagged-urine technique suffers from contamination by perineal bacteria even when the perineum is cleansed. The only time a bagged urine specimen is diagnostic is when there is a negative culture. Other tests used for diagnosis of upper UTI, such as antibody coating of bacteria and C-reactive protein or urinary lactic dehydrogenase analyses, although useful in adults, are unreliable for differentiating pyelonephritis from cystitis in children.

The role of imaging in children with acute pyelonephritis is threefold: (1) to diagnose hydronephrosis or reflux, both of which predispose to infection; (2) to identify complications that require surgical or percutaneous drainage; and (3) to detect pyelonephritic scarring, indicating prior infection. As noted above, the diagnosis of renal infection is based on clinical and laboratory data. Imaging is not needed (or used) to establish or confirm the diagnosis of acute pyelonephritis in most children (**Option (A) is false**).

Most urologists and nephrologists recommend that cystography be performed routinely in all infants and children under 5 years of age with a documented UTI to establish the presence or absence, as well as the grade of, reflux (**Option (B) is true**). Older children and adolescents with infection usually are evaluated by sonography alone because the likelihood of reflux is low. When sonography is normal, further imaging is unnecessary. However, if sonography shows either hydronephrosis or parenchymal scarring, cystography is indicated.

Radiographic voiding cystourethrography (VCUG) is the examination of choice to evaluate for reflux in boys, because it can reliably identify urethral abnormalities that can cause or increase the severity of reflux (Figure 6-9). Because anatomic abnormalities of the bladder and urethra are extremely rare in girls with UTI, radionuclide cystography is increasingly replacing conventional cystography for evaluating the presence and degree of vesicoureteral reflux. Because of its reduced radiation dose, radionuclide cystography has also replaced radiographic cystography in many practices for follow-up evaluation of children who have reflux.

Sonography is performed in all children, regardless of age, to evaluate the upper tract for hydronephrosis or other structural anomalies that can predispose to UTI; this examination

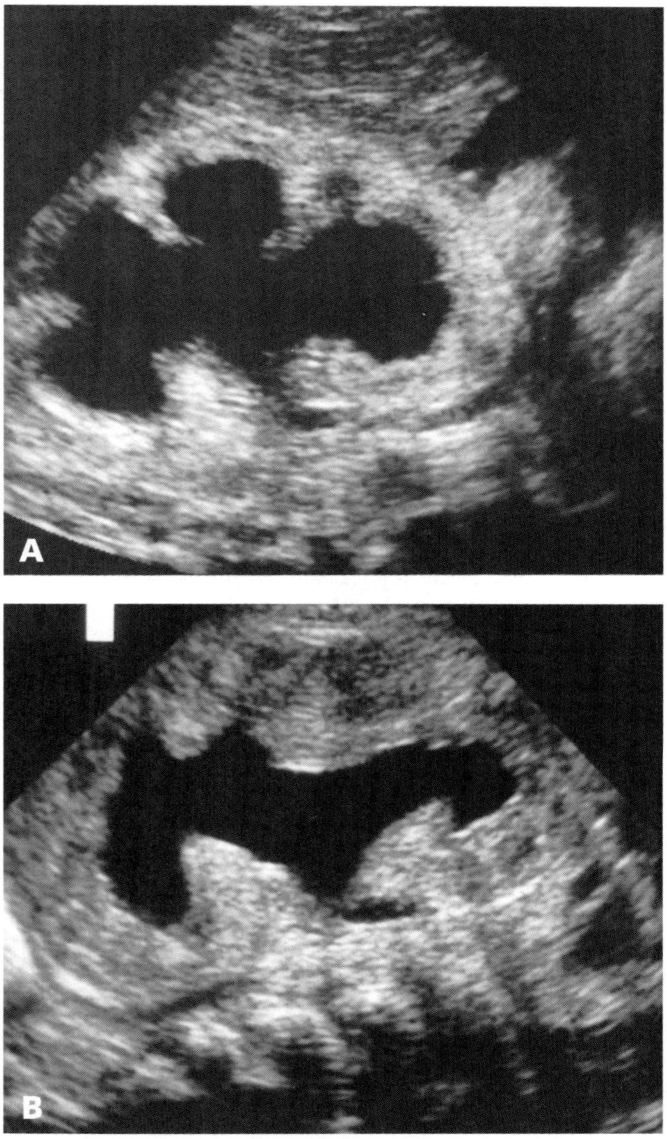

Figure 6-9. Posterior urethral valves. (A and B) Longitudinal sonograms of the right (A) and left (B) kidneys reveal moderate to marked pelvicalyceal dilatation and an echogenic cortex, indicating renal dysplasia.

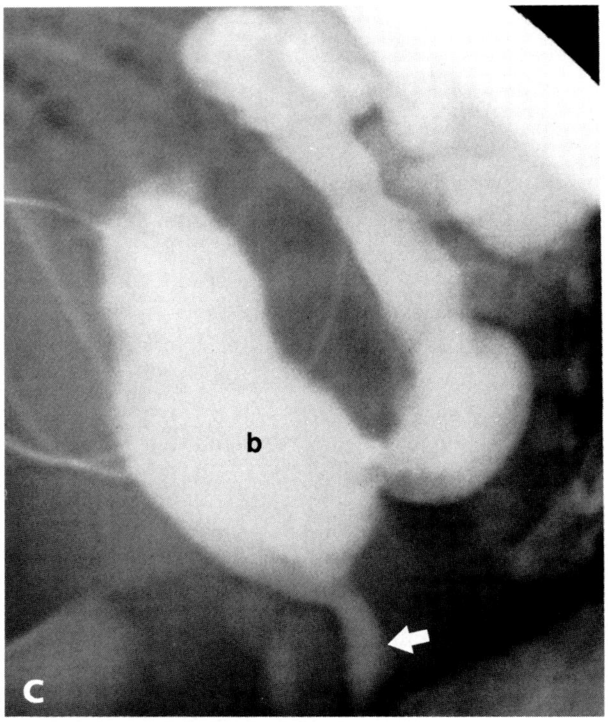

Figure 6-9 (Continued). Posterior urethral valves. (C) A voiding cystourethrogram shows a dilated posterior urethra (arrow), a trabeculated bladder (b), and reflux into a tortuous left ureter.

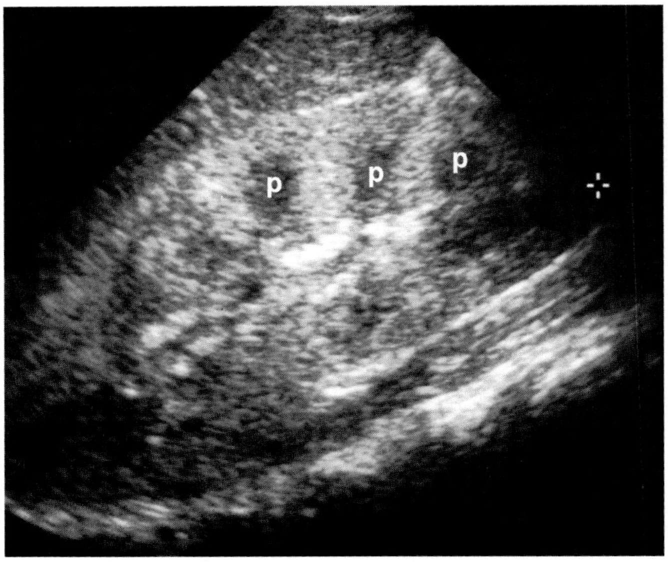

Figure 6-10. Acute pyelonephritis in a 3-year-old girl. Sonography was performed as a screening test to exclude a structural anomaly. A longitudinal sonogram through the right flank shows an enlarged, hyperechoic right kidney, consistent with inflammation. There is no hydronephrosis. Anechoic areas represent pyramids (p).

has replaced the excretory urogram (Figure 6-8). Renal sonography also has been used to detect renal scarring, although it can miss mild damage. If both the VCUG and sonogram are normal, no additional imaging studies are required and the patient is monitored clinically. If the sonogram shows hydronephrosis and evaluation of renal function is desired, scintigraphy is performed.

Most children with acute pyelonephritis have normal gray-scale sonograms. In the studies by Eggli and Eggli and by Björgvinsson et al. of children with acute pyelonephritis, the sensitivity of gray-scale sonography was about 25% to 40% (**Option (C) is false**). Sonographic findings are more likely in patients with severe infection. They include a generalized or focal increase in renal size; abnormal echogenicity of the renal parenchyma, which can be hypo- or hyperechoic relative to normal renal tissue (Figure 6-10); poor definition of the corticomedullary junction; and thickening of the wall of the renal pelvis or ureter.

With the addition of color and power Doppler techniques, the sensitivity of sonography in the diagnosis of renal inflammation increases to 65% and 75%, respectively. Most patients with acute pyelonephritis exhibit diminished or absent color flow in the involved areas, depending on the severity of the associated edema (Figure 6-4).

It has been suggested that measurement of renal volume may be another valuable means for differentiating between upper and lower urinary tract involvement. In a study of 175 children with acute pyelonephritis, Dinkel et al. showed that the kidneys in children with pyelonephritis were markedly enlarged, with a mean average volume 1.75 times that in children with cystitis. The increased renal volume was secondary to parenchymal thickening and not to an enlarged collecting system. The sensitivity and specificity of ultrasonography for diagnosing acute pyelonephritis were 76% and 98%, respectively, when a renal volume of at least 140% normal was used as the diagnostic criterion. When the criterion was a renal volume at least 120% normal, the sensitivity increased to 98% but the specificity decreased to 82%. Renal enlargement was present bilaterally in 50% of children with acute pyelonephritis. Children with cystitis had normal-sized kidneys. These excellent results reported by Dinkel et al. have not been confirmed by most other investigators.

Infection of the renal parenchyma can also be confirmed by cortical imaging studies, with either Tc-99m dimercaptosuccinic acid (DMSA) or Tc-99m glucoheptonate (GH). Tc-99m DMSA binds to the proximal renal tubules and provides excellent images of the parenchyma. Tc-99m GH also binds to tubular epithelial cells, but a large amount is filtered, allowing evaluation of the pelvicalyceal system, ureters, and bladder on early images and of the renal cortex on delayed images. Both agents show cortical involvement well; however, Tc-99m DMSA is preferred over Tc-99m GH because of its lower gonadal dose. Several studies have shown that Tc-99m DMSA scintigraphy, particularly when SPECT is performed, has a sensitivity of about 90% for detecting acute pyelonephritis (**Option (D) is true**). Despite these observations, the role of cortical scintigraphy in patients with acute pyelonephritis has not been clearly defined. There is no consensus about when it should be performed, because there are no convincing data that its increased sensitivity will significantly alter patient management or prognosis. One problem is the 10% false-negative rate, which some nephrologists and urologists believe is too high to allow this test to be used in treatment planning. Second, virtually every pediatric patient with UTI is assumed to be at risk for pyelonephritis and is treated accordingly. Cortical imaging studies can only confirm, but not definitely exclude, pyelone-phritis, and so they are not routinely performed. Cortical imaging is probably best reserved for patients with suspected pyelonephritis in whom the clinical diagnosis or results of other imaging studies are indeterminate.

Findings of acute pyelonephritis on cortical imaging studies include solitary or multiple wedge-shaped or spherical regions of decreased renal activity, most typically in a polar distribution (Figure 6-11). The defects are presumed to result from metabolic alterations in the mechanisms of transport of the radiopharmaceutical across tubular cell membranes or from cortical vasoconstriction attributable to inflammatory cells obstructing paratubular capillaries. The prevalence of cortical defects on scintigraphy in children with febrile UTI is approximately 30% to 70%.

Ga-67 and In-111 leukocyte scintigraphy have also been evaluated for the diagnosis of acute pyelonephritis. Both methods involve relatively high radiation doses and require 24 to 48 hours for imaging. Because of these limitations, they are usually reserved for patients who have unexplained fevers.

CT is not routinely used in the evaluation of children with acute pyelonephritis. Its use is generally reserved for patients who fail to respond to appropriate antibiotic therapy and are suspected of having severe infection or complications, such as a renal or perirenal abscess. It is also valuable for guiding percutaneous catheter drainage of renal or perirenal abscesses. Most patients with mild or uncomplicated pyelonephritis have normal CT scans. In those with severe infection, focal or global renal enlargement and parenchymal perfusion abnormalities can be seen. On postcontrast CT scans, areas of infection appear as wedge-shaped lesions with decreased attenuation, radiating from the renal hilum to the renal capsule (Figure 6-12). These areas do enhance, but to a lesser degree than the normal paren-chyma. They can demonstrate a typical pattern of striated opacification, characterized by bands of alternating increased and decreased densities (Figure 6-13) (**Option (E) is true**). In a series of 16 patients with severe renal infection, Soulen et al. reported a striated pattern in five patients. The abnormal enhancement is thought to represent focal arterial constriction and obstruction of collecting tubules by inflammatory debris and surrounding edema. Early in the course of infection, the parenchymal lesions have well-defined borders, but their borders become indistinct after treatment. Other CT findings in children with acute pyelonephritis include calyceal distortion, thickening of the perinephric fascia, and strands of increased density in the perinephric fat.

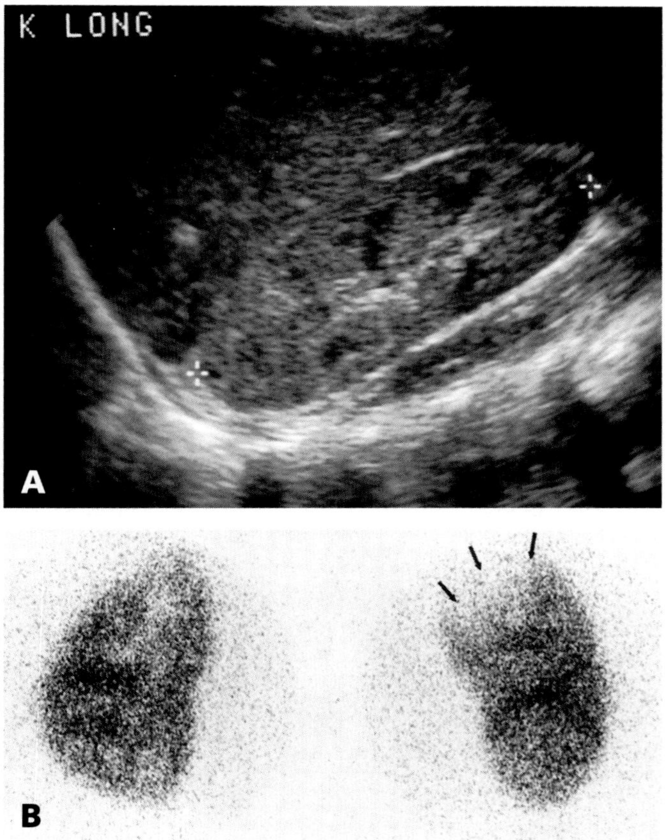

Figure 6-11. Acute pyelonephritis in a 2-year-old girl with recurrent urinary tract infection. (A) A longitudinal sonogram through the right flank shows a slightly echogenic kidney (calipers) of normal size. The cortical echogenicity is equal to that of the liver. In a patient of this age, the echogenicity of the cortex should be lower than that of the liver. (B) Posterior magnification images of the kidneys, obtained with pinhole collimation 3 hours after injection of Tc-99m DMSA, show a large cortical defect (arrows) in the right upper pole. There is no evidence of cortical volume loss that would suggest chronic pyelonephritis.

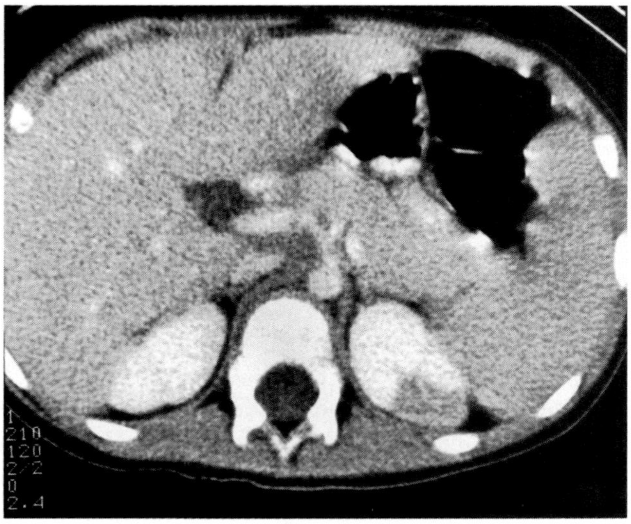

Figure 6-12. Acute pyelonephritis in a 3-year-old girl with prolonged fever and leukocytosis despite appropriate antibiotic therapy. CT was performed to exclude an abscess. A CT scan through the upper abdomen demonstrates a wedge-shaped area of low attenuation in the upper pole of the left kidney, radiating from the area of the medulla to the capsule.

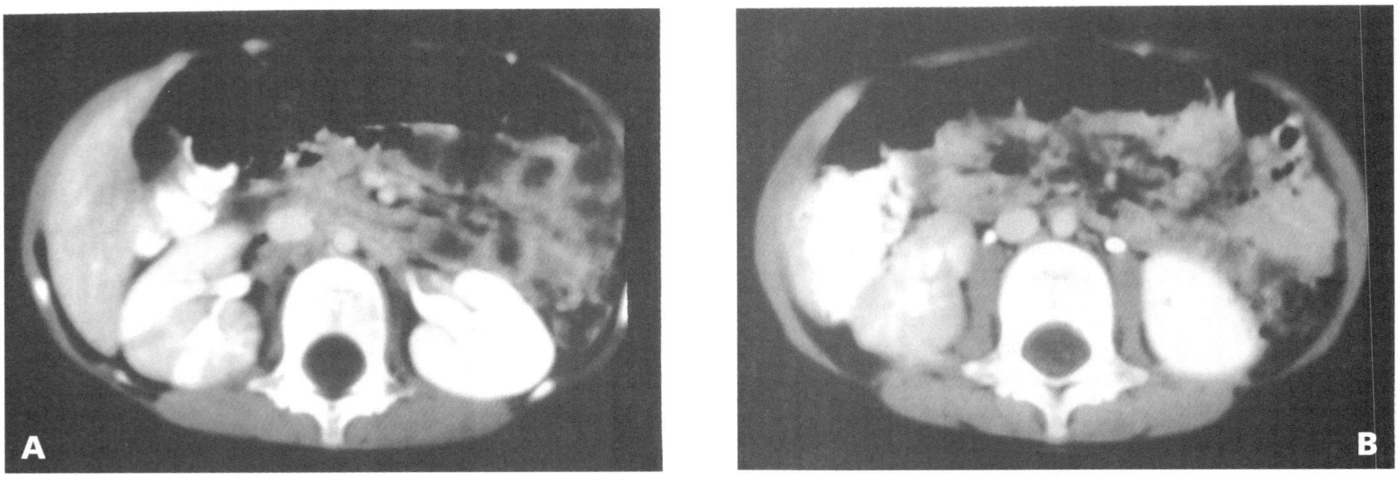

Figure 6-13. Acute pyelonephritis in a 5-year-old girl. CT scans through the middle (A) and lower (B) poles of the kidneys show areas of increased and decreased attenuation in the right kidney, producing a striated appearance.

Question 32

Concerning complications of acute renal infection in children,

(A) a frequent CT feature of renal abscess is thickening of Gerota's fascia
(B) most patients with pyonephrosis have obstruction secondary to ureteral calculi
(C) echogenic material in a dilated collecting system is a specific sign of pyonephrosis
(D) fungal balls are characterized sonographically by nonshadowing echogenic masses

Acute bacterial pyelonephritis is a continuum of changes ranging from mild, uncomplicated infection to more severe pyelonephritis, frank necrosis, and abscess formation. Most complications are detected by sonography. CT, however, is better for defining the extent of disease and for planning therapy, especially interventional procedures. Excretory urography and scintigraphy have limited sensitivity and specificity in the diagnosis of complicated UTI and are rarely, if ever, indicated for diagnosis.

Renal abscess is a sequela of incompletely treated pyelonephritis and is characterized by tissue liquefaction. *E. coli* and *Staphylococcus aureus* are the most common pathogenic organisms. Urinalysis and culture are usually abnormal, although they can give normal results if the patient has received antibiotics or if the abscess has not broken through into the collecting system.

The sonographic findings of renal abscess include a well-defined hypoechoic mass with thick, irregular walls (Figure 6-14). Internal echogenicity, representing necrotic debris or gas, septations, or fluid-debris levels, is sometimes noted. Additional findings include acoustic enhancement, perirenal abscess, and fascial thickening.

The CT appearance of renal abscess is that of a round, low-density mass with thick, irregular walls that usually enhance after intravenous administration of contrast medium (Figure 6-15). Other frequent findings reported by Soulen et al. in a series of 26 patients with renal abscesses included inflammatory changes in the perirenal fat (78% of patients); thickening of Gerota's fascia (42%) (**Option (A) is true**); and extension of disease into the pararenal spaces (27%). Gas has been reported in about 20% of renal abscesses. The chief differential diagnostic consideration is a necrotic Wilms' tumor. The demonstration of gas or perirenal inflammation or fluid supports the diagnosis of abscess rather than a tumor. Imaging with Ga-67 or In-111 leukocytes can also confirm the presence of infection, although this is rarely required if CT is available.

Pyonephrosis is the accumulation of purulent exudate within an obstructed collecting system. In children, the obstruction is most often secondary to a congenital anomaly, such as a ureteropelvic junction obstruction; it is rarely attributable to calculi or stricture (**Option (B) is false**). The diagnosis of pyonephrosis is a urologic emergency and requires urgent percutaneous or surgical drainage. If left untreated, pyonephrosis can

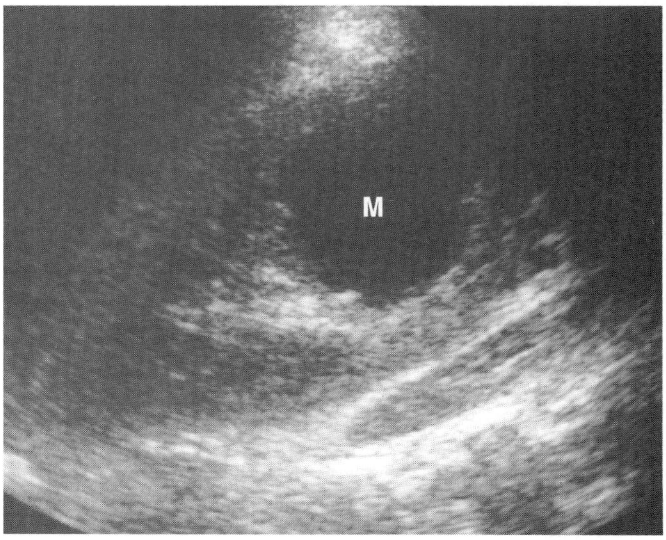

Figure 6-14. Renal abscess in a 16-year-old girl. A longitudinal sonogram of the left kidney shows a large, hypoechoic mass (M) with slightly irregular walls in the lower pole.

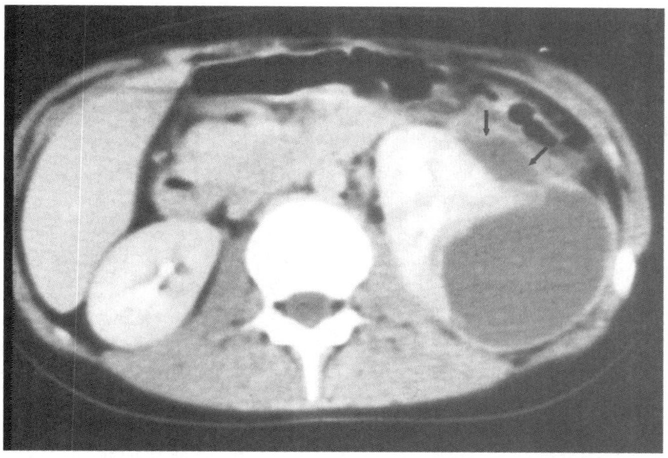

Figure 6-15. Same patient as in Figure 6-14. Renal abscess. A postcontrast CT scan shows an enlarged left kidney containing a low-attenuation mass with enhancing walls. The abscess extends into the perinephric space (arrows). Percutaneous aspiration yielded purulent material.

lead to gram-negative bacteremia, septic shock, and progressive parenchymal destruction with loss of renal function.

The sensitivity of sonography for the diagnosis of pyonephrosis is reported to be between 65% and 90%. The sonographic features of pyonephrosis include a dilated pelvicalyceal system containing low-level echoes or shifting fluid-debris levels (Figure 6-16). The presence of very bright echoes suggests that the infection is due to gas-forming organisms. The demonstration of internal echoes within a dilated system is not specific for pyonephrosis, however (**Option (C) is false**). Hemorrhage or high concentrations of protein also can produce internal echoes and mimic pyonephrosis. On postcontrast CT scans, pyonephrosis appears as a hydronephrotic collecting system with a urine-debris level. Other findings include gas within the dilated pelvicalyceal system and thickening of the perinephric or paranephric soft tissues. Percutaneous aspiration can be accomplished with either CT or sonographic guidance. Cortical imaging studies cannot assess the character of the fluid or the extent

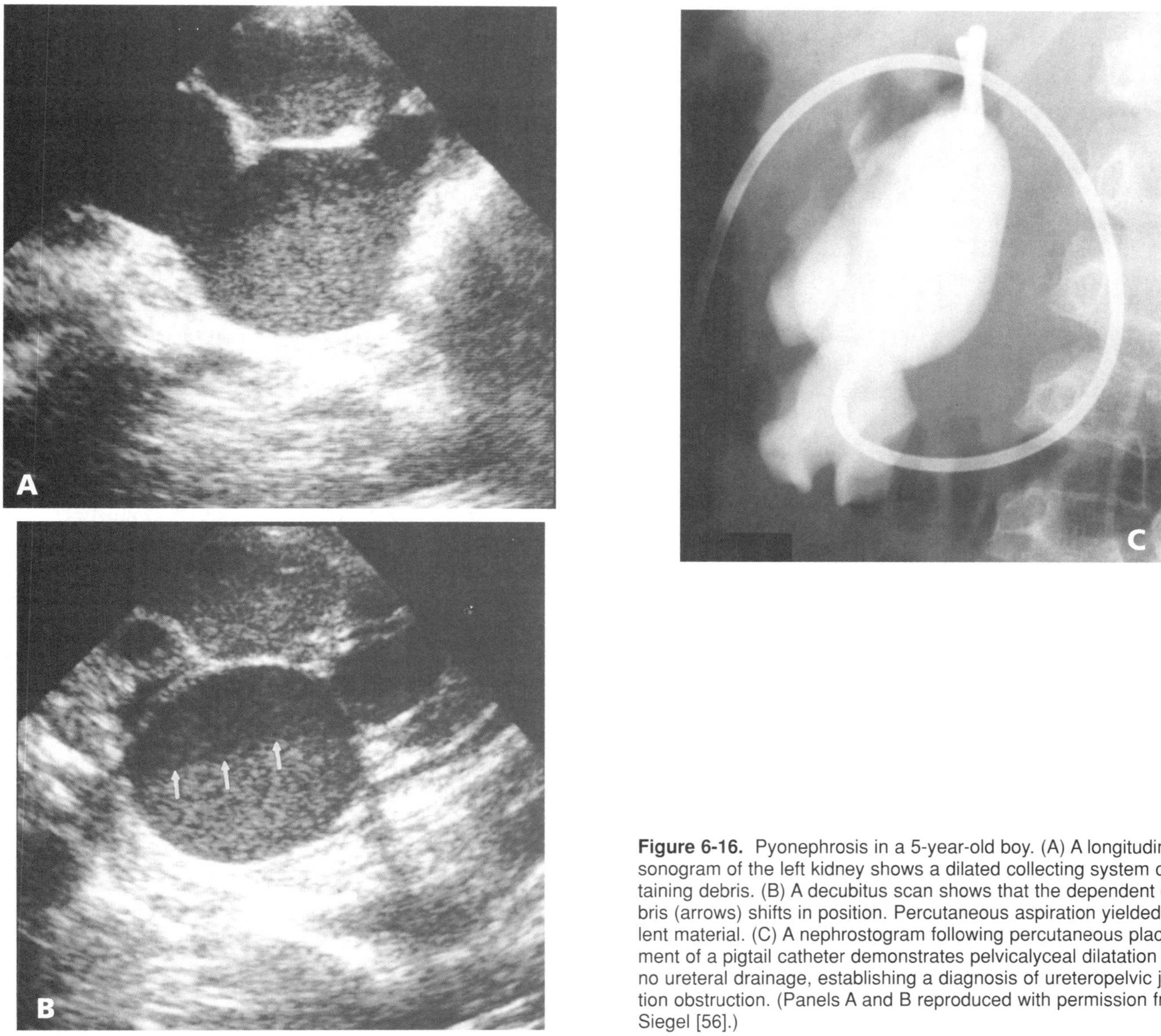

Figure 6-16. Pyonephrosis in a 5-year-old boy. (A) A longitudinal sonogram of the left kidney shows a dilated collecting system containing debris. (B) A decubitus scan shows that the dependent debris (arrows) shifts in position. Percutaneous aspiration yielded purulent material. (C) A nephrostogram following percutaneous placement of a pigtail catheter demonstrates pelvicalyceal dilatation and no ureteral drainage, establishing a diagnosis of ureteropelvic junction obstruction. (Panels A and B reproduced with permission from Siegel [56].)

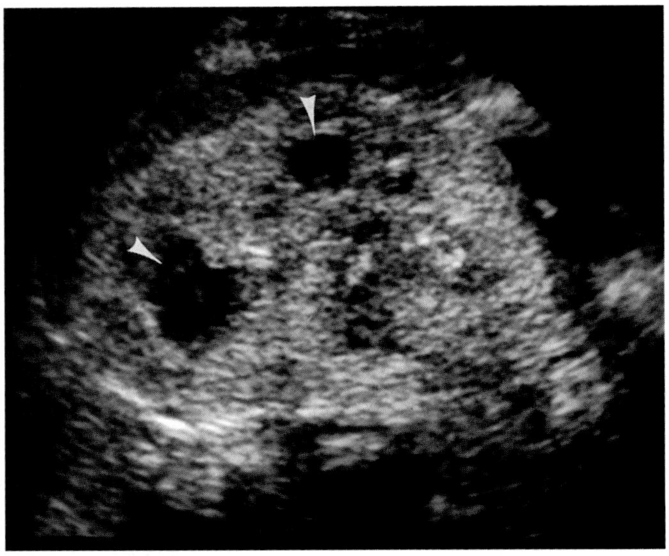

Figure 6-17. Renal candidiasis in a 15-month-old boy. A longitudinal sonogram of the right flank demonstrates an enlarged echogenic kidney with dilated calyces (arrowheads) containing fine echogenic debris. The debris is not masslike and, hence, is not a true fungal ball.

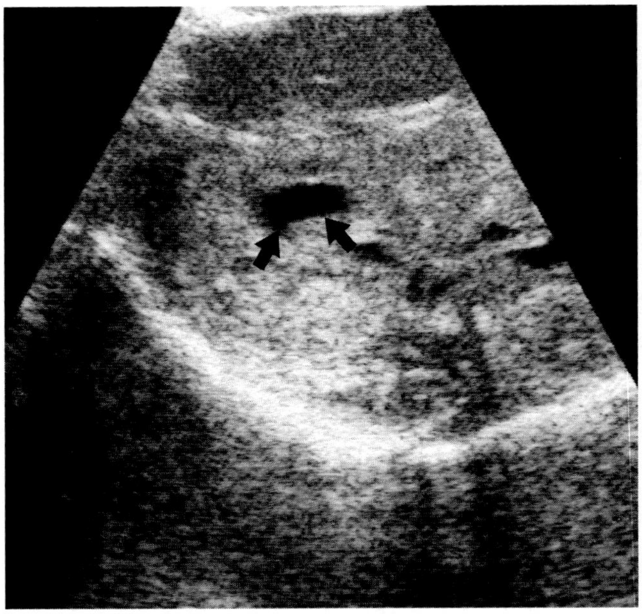

Figure 6-18. Renal candidiasis with fungal balls in a 1-month-old girl with an indwelling catheter for hyperalimentation. A longitudinal sonogram of the left flank with the patient supine demonstrates an echogenic left kidney. The calyx in the upper pole is dilated and contains a nonshadowing echogenic mass (arrows). The mass shifted position with changes in patient position and represents a fungus ball.

of perinephric disease, and for these reasons, they play a limited role in diagnosing pyonephrosis.

Most fungal infections of the kidneys occur in infants and children who have indwelling catheters for hyperalimentation or who are undergoing prolonged antibiotic or immunosuppressive therapy. The most common organism is *Candida albicans,* which usually reaches the kidney as a result of hematogenous spread of systemic disease. This results in acute pyelonephritis, which sometimes progresses to chronic pyelonephritis, characterized by microabscesses and inflammatory infiltrates within the parenchyma, interstitium, and tubules. If the infection remains untreated, the mycelia can clump within the collecting system, resulting in fungal balls and obstructive hydronephrosis.

The sonographic findings of fungal infection are variable and include enlarged hyperechoic kidneys (Figure 6-17), parenchymal abscess, pyonephrosis, and fungal balls. Fungal balls appear as focal, nonshadowing echogenic masses within a dilated collecting system; these can shift position with changes in patient position (Figure 6-18) (**Option (D) is true**). CT is superior to sonography in identifying small abscesses, which appear as bilateral low-density lesions with enhancing rims.

Question 33

Concerning vesicoureteral reflux,

(A) there is a familial tendency
(B) it is usually related to a short intramural ureter
(C) intrarenal reflux predisposes to cortical scarring
(D) associated renal injury is usually diffusely distributed
(E) it cannot be graded reliably by radionuclide cystography
(F) a normal renal sonogram excludes high-grade reflux

Vesicoureteral reflux refers to the retrograde flow of urine from the bladder lumen into the collecting system of the kidney. Urine flows both antegrade through the urethra and retrograde into the ureter and collecting system during micturition. At the end of micturition, the refluxed urine reenters the bladder, where it stagnates until the next episode of voiding, increasing the risk of bacterial colonization. The backflow of urine enables bacteria to have access to the renal parenchyma.

The frequency of reflux in children with asymptomatic UTI (bacteriuria on screening) is approximately 15% to 35%, whereas that in children with symptomatic UTI is 20% to 50%. By comparison, the frequency of vesicoureteral reflux in otherwise healthy children is less than 2%. The natural history of reflux is characterized by diminishing prevalence and severity with increasing patient age. Thus, the younger the child with UTI, the greater the likelihood and severity of reflux.

Vesicoureteral reflux has a higher prevalence in white children than in black children (10:1 ratio) and is familial (**Option**

(A) is true). The chance of a child having reflux is about 66% if a parent had reflux. The chance of a sibling having reflux is 25% to 50% if a child who is the index case has reflux. The risk of reflux in a sibling is even greater if the child who is the index case also has evidence of renal damage. Of additional importance is the fact that 75% of siblings with reflux are asymptomatic.

Vesicoureteral reflux is classified as primary or secondary. Most reflux is primary and the result of an incompetent vesicoureteral junction. In healthy individuals, the submucosal ureter, which lies within the bladder wall, has a relatively long length-to-orifice diameter ratio (normally 4:1 to 5:1). Primary vesicoureteral reflux is thought to be related to an abnormally short intramural ureter (**Option (B) is true**); the ratio of the length to the width has been reported to be as low as 1.4:1. The shape and location of the ureteral orifice also appear to increase the risk of vesicoureteral reflux. Reflux is more common, as well as more severe, when the ureteral orifice has a gaping configuration or is more laterally positioned.

Secondary reflux is attributable to a congenital abnormality, such as posterior urethral valves (Figure 6-9), neurogenic bladder dysfunction, bladder-sphincter dyssynergia, or duplicated system with ectopic ureter or ureterocele (Figure 6-8). These lesions predispose to reflux by increasing the intravesical pressure or by altering the course or length of the ureter.

The significance of vesicoureteral reflux is that it is associated with pyelonephritis and scarring. Although some experimental work has suggested that sterile reflux can cause renal scarring, most clinical and experimental studies have shown that new or progressive renal scarring is dependent on the presence of both vesicoureteral reflux and UTI. It is now believed that intrarenal reflux must be present for renal cortical infection and scarring to occur (**Option (C) is true**). Intrarenal reflux is defined as the retrograde flow of urine from the calyx into the collecting ducts and tubules of the nephrons (Figure 6-19). As a result, bacteria in the collecting system have ready access to the renal parenchyma. Intrarenal reflux is more likely to occur in compound calyces than in simple calyces. Compound calyces have papillary ducts that course perpendicular to the surface of the calyx and hence open easily when there is an increase in intrapelvic pressure, permitting intrarenal reflux. By comparison, simple calyces have obliquely oriented, slitlike duct orifices that are able to close when the intrarenal pressure increases, preventing intrarenal reflux (Figure 6-20). Compound calyces predominate in the polar regions. Hence, renal injury (i.e., scarring) tends to be localized in these areas rather than being diffusely distributed throughout the kidney (**Option (D) is false**).

As mentioned previously, one of the goals of imaging children with UTI is to identify vesicoureteral reflux, since it predisposes to infection and pyelonephritic scarring. Radiographic VCUG with retrograde instillation of iodinated contrast medium into the bladder has been the traditional method used to assess the presence and grade of reflux and to demonstrate the anatomy of the bladder and male urethra. Radiographic VCUG can be performed with fluoroscopic monitoring or hard-copy filming. Images of the bladder, ureters, and kidneys are obtained periodically during bladder filling and voiding. The primary disadvantage of VCUG is a relatively high ovarian radiation dose (1,000 to 1,500 mrem).

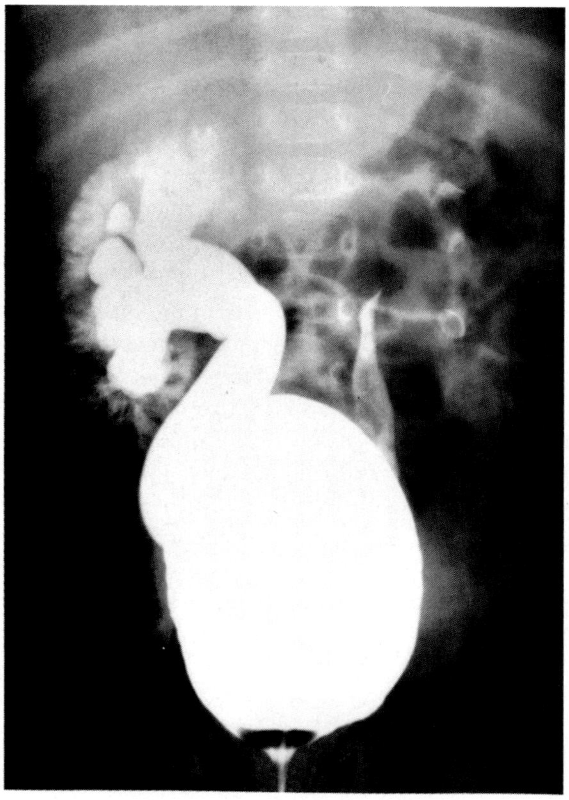

Figure 6-19. Intrarenal reflux. A VCUG shows flow of contrast material into the collecting ducts and the renal parenchyma of the right kidney, consistent with grade V vesicoureteral reflux. Grade II reflux is noted on the left, characterized by reflux into a nondilated collecting system.

The International Reflux Grading System is the system most widely used to grade reflux. This classification recognizes five grades of reflux: grade I, reflux into the ureter only; grade II, reflux into the ureter, renal pelvis, and calyces, without di-

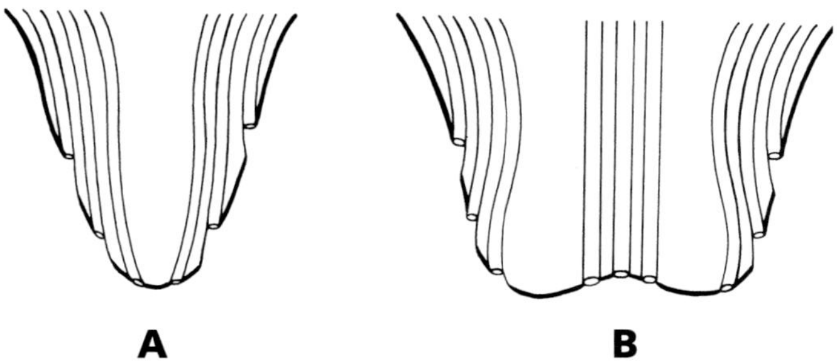

Figure 6-20. Diagrammatic representation of renal papillary anatomy. (A) Simple papillae. Collecting ducts open obliquely into the convex surface of the calyx. (B) Compound papillae. Collecting ducts open at a right angle (perpendicular) to the concave surface. Intrarenal reflux is more likely with this papillary configuration. (Adapted from Ransley [32].)

latation or tortuosity; grade III, mild ureteral and pelvic dilatation with no or mild blunting of the calyceal fornices; grade IV, moderate ureteral and pelvic dilatation with blunting of the calyceal fornices; and grade V, marked ureteral and pelvic dilatation and tortuosity, marked blunting of the calyceal fornices, and lack of papillary impressions in most calyces (Figures 6-21 and 6-22). The grade of reflux directly correlates with the likelihood of renal scarring.

Radionuclide cystography with Tc-99m pertechnetate is replacing the radiographic cystogram in the evaluation of girls with UTI and in the follow-up evaluation of children with known reflux, regardless of gender. Advantages of radionuclide cystography are a lower ovarian radiation dose (10 mrem) and the capability to perform continuous monitoring during bladder filling and voiding, thus increasing the likelihood of detecting transitory reflux. Moreover, the volume of reflux and the bladder capacity at which reflux occurs can be quantified.

Criticisms of the scintigraphic technique are its limited ability to detect grade I reflux, difficulty in grading vesicoureteral reflux, and poor spatial resolution, which is especially important for evaluating bladder and urethral abnormalities. In the series of Strife et al., nuclear cystography showed grade I reflux in only 4% of patients, whereas radiographic cystography showed grade I reflux in 17% to 22% of patients. In another study of 25 children with reflux, Zhang et al. showed that the correlations between radionuclide and radiographic cystography for grading by the International System were 78% for grade II reflux, 100% for grade III reflux, 60% for grade IV reflux, and 100% for grade V reflux. The overall correlation between the two studies was 80%. When only two categories were used (low grade = grades II and III; high grade = grades IV and V), a correlation of 100% was obtained (**Option (E) is false**).

Sonographic cystography is another technique that has been evaluated for the diagnosis of vesicoureteral reflux. Contrast medium or saline is shaken to produce microbubbles and then, following catheterization, the solution is infused into the bladder. The diagnosis of reflux is based on visualization of microbubbles within the ureter or an increased ureteral diameter during bladder filling or voiding. The sensitivity of sonography is 100% for grade III and IV reflux, 60% to 83% for grade II reflux, and 25% to 50% for grade I reflux, with a false-positive rate of 10%.

In some patients, the diagnosis of vesicoureteral reflux is suggested by conventional transabdominal sonography. Findings that suggest reflux include visualization of a dilated distal ureter (Figure 6-23), lateral positioning of the ureteral orifice, changes in ureteral diameter following voiding, and retrograde flow on color-flow Doppler sonography. However, more often than not, sonography is normal in children with reflux. In a study of 177 neonates (132 boys and 45 girls) reported by Tiballs and De Bruyn, approximately 25% of the patients with sonographically normal kidneys had grade III to V reflux on VCUG. In another study of infants and children, Blane et al. found that 74% of 272 kidneys with reflux on cystourethrography were sonographically normal and that 28% of these

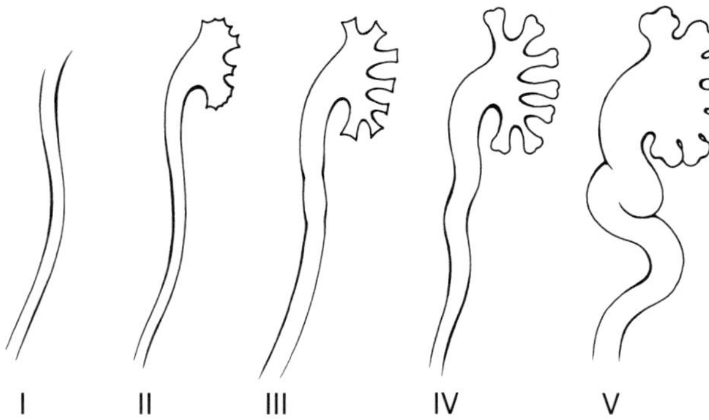

Figure 6-21. International Reflux Grading System. Grade I: reflux into only the ureter. Grade II: reflux into a nondilated renal collecting system; normal calyceal fornices. Grade III: mild ureteral and pelvic distension; slight or no calyceal blunting. Grade IV: moderate ureteral and pelvic distension as well as ureteral tortuosity; mild calyceal blunting. Grade V: marked ureteral and pelvic distension, ureteral tortuosity, and calyceal blunting; loss of papillary impressions. (Adapted from Hoffman and LeRoy [52].)

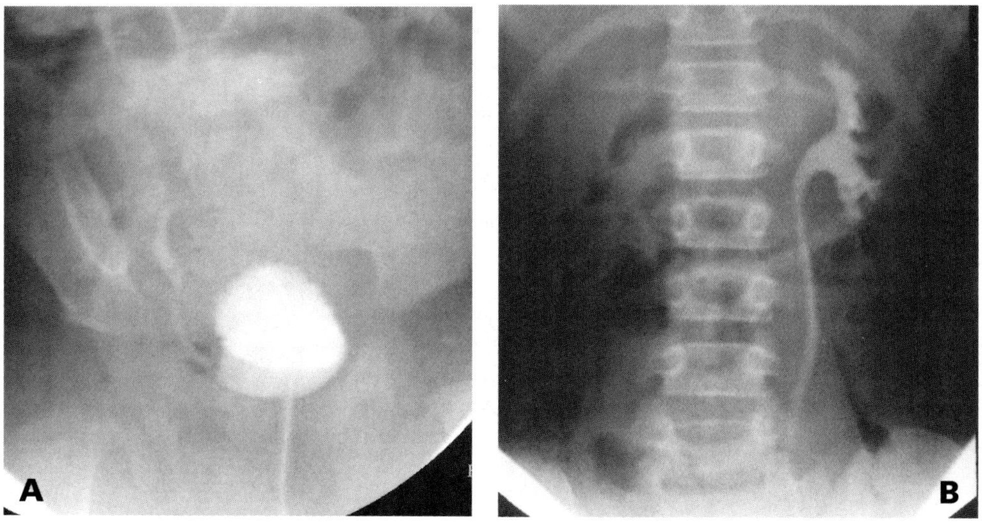

Figure 6-22. Vesicoureteral reflux. Radiographic VCUGs in five different patients. (A) Grade I reflux; (B) Grade II reflux; (C) Grade III reflux; (D) Grade IV reflux; (E) Grade V left reflux and Grade III right reflux.

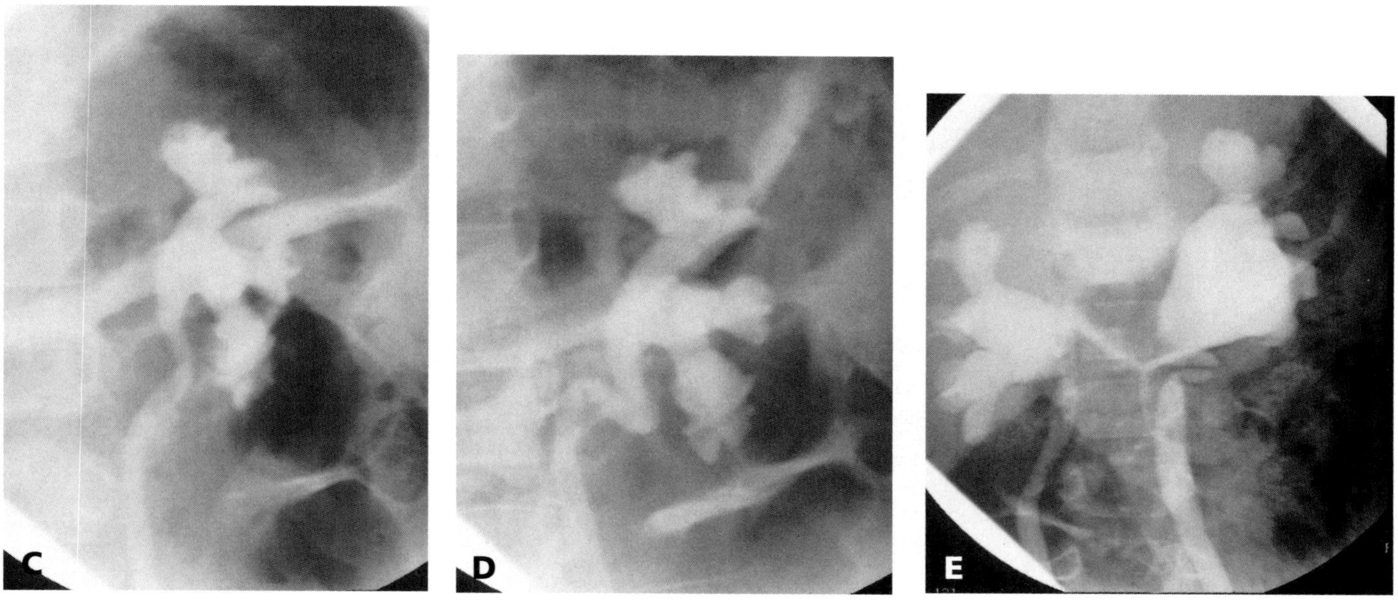

Figure 6-22 (Continued)

sonographically normal kidneys had grade III or higher reflux. Hence, a normal sonogram does not exclude high-grade reflux (**Option (F) is false**).

Most low-grade vesicoureteral reflux is treated medically (low-dose antimicrobial treatment). Medical management is based on the observation that 20% to 35% of cases of reflux spontaneously disappear within 2 years, with a significantly greater likelihood of resolution in patients younger than 12 months at presentation and in those with mild reflux. Surgical reimplantation of the ureter is usually reserved for children who have higher grades of reflux and fail to maintain sterile urine or who develop scars while taking prophylactic antibiotics. The surgical cure rate is greater than 95%. Surgical treatment of vesicoureteral reflux prevents reflux, obviates continuous antibiotic therapy, and significantly reduces the risk of recurrent pyelonephritis, but it may not prevent progression of already established renal scarring.

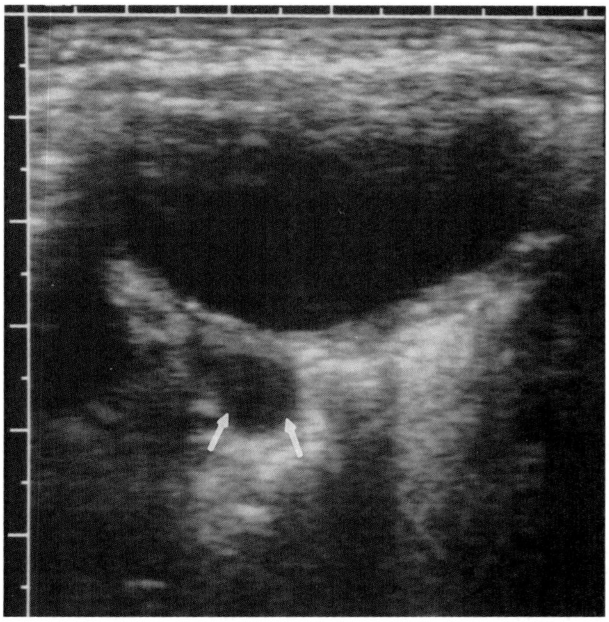

Figure 6-23. Vesicoureteral reflux. A longitudinal sonogram through the bladder demonstrates a dilated distal right ureter (arrows). Grade V reflux was confirmed by VCUG.

The goal of treatment is prevention of cortical damage. Renal scarring secondary to reflux, also referred to as chronic atrophic pyelonephritis, atrophic pyelonephritis, and reflux nephropathy, has been documented in 6% to 10% of children with UTI. The significance of scarring is its association with abnormal renal growth, hypertension, and end-stage renal disease. The frequency of growth retardation is approximately 20%; the frequency of hypertension ranges from 5% to 30%; and the frequency of end-stage renal disease ranges from 10% to 20%. However, for all children with end-stage renal disease, chronic pyelonephritis accounts for less than 2.2% of cases.

The hallmark of renal scarring secondary to vesicoureteral reflux is calyceal clubbing or deformity with overlying parenchymal loss. Cortical scintigraphy is the most reliable method of diagnosing renal scarring. Findings associated with scarring include cortical thinning, a wedge-shaped parenchymal defect, and single or multiple areas of reduced or absent activity (Figure 6-24). Excretory urography and sonography can detect moderate or severe scarring but may miss milder scarring. The urographic findings of chronic pyelonephritis include parenchymal thinning, usually at one of the renal poles, calyceal clubbing or deformity, and decreased renal length and volume (Figure 6-25). Sonographic findings of chronic inflammation are a small echogenic kidney, loss of the normal corticomedullary differentiation, and irregular renal contours.

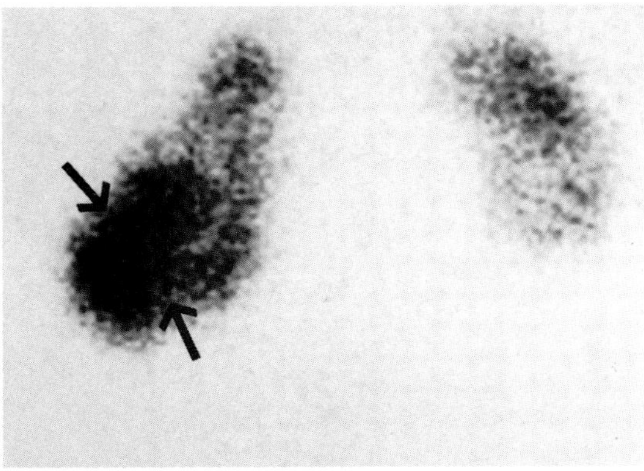

Figure 6-24. Reflux nephropathy. A posterior image of the kidneys obtained 3 hours after administration of Tc-99m DMSA shows that the right kidney is decreased in size, has globally decreased activity by comparison with the left kidney, and contains several focal cortical defects, most notably at both poles. Also noted is atrophy of the left upper pole. The masslike area (arrows) in the left lower pole represents residual functioning tissue.

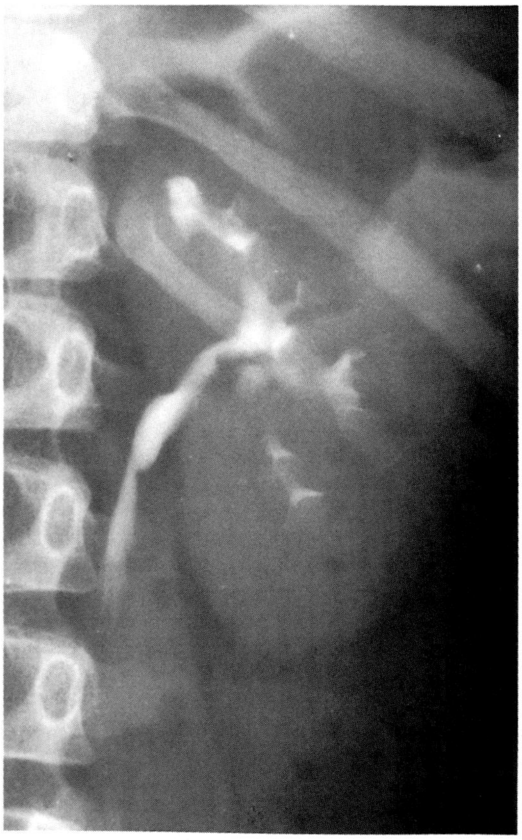

Figure 6-25. Cortical scarring in a 7-year-old girl. An excretory urogram shows calyceal clubbing and adjacent cortical loss in the upper pole of the left kidney, indicative of reflux nephropathy.

Question 34

Concerning hemolytic uremic syndrome,

(A) hemorrhagic colitis usually precedes the development of renal failure when the syndrome is associated with *Escherichia coli* infection
(B) patchy echogenicity of the kidneys is noted on sonography
(C) the resistance in intrarenal arteries is elevated
(D) the prognosis is related more closely to extrarenal than to renal complications

In North America, hemolytic uremic syndrome of childhood has been associated with infection by a variety of organisms, including *Shigella*, *Salmonella*, *Campylobacter*, and *Yersinia* species, as well as enteroviruses. More recently, cases have been reported secondary to infection with toxin-producing *E. coli* O157:H7, most often acquired from a bovine source, either undercooked beef or unpasteurized milk, or from person-to-person contact. *E. coli* O157:H7 produces a verocytotoxin similar to that produced by *Shigella dysenteriae*. This verocytotoxin causes severe damage to human endothelial cells, which is believed to be the inciting event in hemolytic uremic syndrome. The damaged endothelial cells release abnormally large von Willebrand factor multimers, which are capable of aggregating platelets. In addition, the cytotoxin inhibits the production of prostacyclin, which normally regulates platelet aggregation by endothelial cells. These factors work in concert to produce the fibrin microthrombi characteristically seen within small vessels of the kidneys and other organs.

Hemorrhagic colitis develops in 95% of patients with *E. coli* O157:H7-associated hemolytic uremic syndrome and precedes the development of renal failure **(Option (A) is true)**. Radiologic findings of the prodromal colitis include thumbprinting of the bowel wall as a result of submucosal bleeding and edema. Gray-scale sonography and CT demonstrate circumferential thickening of the colonic wall, ascites, and mesenteric edema (Figure 6-26). Although small bowel involvement can occur, it is not as marked or severe as the hemorrhagic colitis. None of these features is distinctive enough to allow a diagnosis of hemolytic uremic syndrome. The differential diagnosis includes neutropenic colitis, acute infectious colitis, and pseudomembranous colitis. Color Doppler sonography appears to be more useful for distinguishing between hemolytic uremic syndrome and other causes of bowel wall thickening. In a series of 37 children with acute colonic diseases, Siegel et al. showed a highly significant relationship between disease type and the presence or absence of color Doppler flow ($P = 0.0013$). The absence of a color Doppler signal in the setting of colonic disease strongly suggested ischemia, either hemolytic uremic syndrome or neutropenic colitis, and virtually excluded inflammation or vasculitis.

The sonographic findings of the renal disease in hemolytic uremic syndrome vary with the stage of disease. In a series of

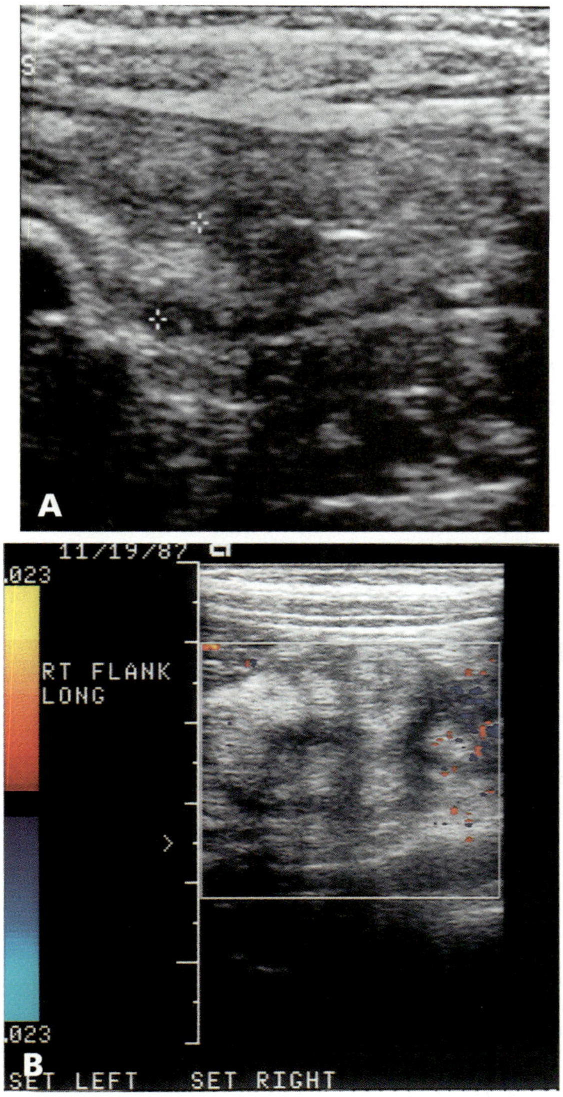

Figure 6-26. Hemolytic uremic syndrome. (A) A longitudinal gray-scale sonogram demonstrates a very thick-walled right colon. The wall of the left colon is approximately 1 cm wide (calipers). (B) A color Doppler sonogram shows no demonstrable blood flow. (Panel B reproduced with permission from Siegel et al. [39].)

17 children with acute renal failure reported by Patriquin et al., the kidneys were normal or slightly enlarged and exhibited diffusely hyperechoic cortex during the stage of oliguria or anuria (**Option (B) is false**). Diastolic flow within intrarenal arteries was absent, greatly reduced, or reversed on duplex Doppler examination, reflecting the reduced arterial lumen and resultant increased resistance (**Option (C) is true**). As the vascular lesions healed, intrarenal resistance decreased and the Doppler flow pattern returned to normal.

The central nervous system is another major site of involvement in patients with hemolytic uremic syndrome. Neuropathologic findings include hemorrhagic or bland infarction in the territories of both large and small vessels, as well as hypoxic changes and cerebral edema. Before the introduction of dialysis, hemolytic uremic syndrome had a very high mortality rate (50% to 75%) as a result of extensive renal damage, including renal cortical necrosis. The mortality has dramatically decreased to 10% to 20%, primarily because of the use of prompt dialysis. Currently, most deaths in patients with hemolytic uremic syndrome are related to extrarenal manifestations, particularly involvement of the central nervous system (**Option (D) is true**).

SUGGESTED READINGS

ACUTE PYELONEPHRITIS

1. Benador D, Benador N, Slosman DO, Nussle D, Mermillod B, Girardin E. Cortical scintigraphy in the evaluation of renal parenchymal changes in children with pyelonephritis. J Pediatr 1994; 124:17–20
2. Berman LH, Stringer DA, St Onge O, Daneman A, Whyte H. An assessment of sonography in the diagnosis and management of neonatal candidiasis. Clin Radiol 1989; 40:577–581
3. Björgvinsson E, Majd M, Eggli KD. Diagnosis of acute pyleonephritis in children: comparison of sonography and ^{99m}Tc-DSMA scintigraphy. AJR 1991; 157:539–543
4. Dacher JN, Boillot B, Eurin D, Marguet C, Mitrofanoff P, LeDosseur P. Rational use of CT in acute pyelonephritis: findings and relationships with reflux. Pediatr Radiol 1993; 23: 281–285
5. Dacher JN, Pfister C, Monroc M, Eurin D, LeDosseur P. Power Doppler sonographic pattern of acute pyelonephritis in children: comparison with CT. AJR 1996; 166:1451–1455
6. Dinkel E, Orth S, Dittrich M, Schulte-Wissermann H. Renal sonography in the differentiation of upper from lower urinary tract infection. AJR 1986; 146:775–780
7. Eggli KD, Eggli D. Color Doppler sonography in pyelonephritis. Pediatr Radiol 1992; 22:422–425
8. Majd M, Rushton HG. Renal cortical scintigraphy in the diagnosis of acute pyelonephritis. Semin Nucl Med 1992; 22:98–111
9. Montgomery P, Kuhn JP, Afshani E. CT evaluation of severe renal inflammatory disease in children. Pediatr Radiol 1987; 17:216–222
10. Papanicolaou N, Pfister RC. Acute renal infections. Radiol Clin North Am 1996; 34:965–995
11. Rosenberg AR, Rossleigh MA, Brydon MP, Bass SJ, Leighton DM, Farnsworth RH. Evaluation of acute urinary tract infection in children by dimercaptosuccinic acid scintigraphy: a prospective study. J Urol 1992; 148:1746–1749
12. Rushton HG, Majd M. Dimercaptosuccinic acid renal scintigraphy for the evaluation of pyelonephritis and scarring: a review of experimental and clinical studies. J Urol 1992; 148:1726–1732
13. Talner LB, Davidson AJ, Lebowitz RL, Dalla Palma L, Goldman SM. Acute pyelonephritis: can we agree on terminology? Radiology 1994; 192: 297–305
14. Traisman ES, Conway JJ, Traisman HS, et al. The localization of urinary tract infection with ^{99m}Tc glucoheptonate scintigraphy. Pediatr Radiol 1986; 16:403–406
15. Winters WD. Power Doppler sonographic evaluation of acute pyelonephritis in children. J Ultrasound Med 1996; 15:91–96

REFLUX AND REFLUX NEPHROPATHY

16. Belman AB. Vesicoureteral reflux. Pediatr Clin North Am 1997; 44: 1171–1190
17. Bisset GS III, Strife JL, Dunbar JS. Urography and voiding cystourethrography: findings in girls with urinary tract infection. AJR 1987; 148: 479–482
18. Blane CE, DiPietro MA, Zerin JM, Sedman AB, Bloom DA. Renal sonography is not a reliable screening examination for vesicoureteral reflux. J Urol 1993; 150:752–755

19. Ditchfield MR, de Campo JF, Cook DJ, et al. Vesicoureteral reflux: an accurate predictor of acute pyelonephritis in childhood urinary tract infection? Radiology 1994; 190:413–415
20. Ditchfield MR, De Campo JF, Nolan TM, et al. Risk factors in the development of early renal cortical defects in children with urinary tract infection. AJR 1994; 162:1393–1397
21. Fettich JJ, Kenda RB. Cyclic direct radionuclide voiding cystography: increasing reliability in detecting vesicoureteral reflux in children. Pediatr Radiol 1992; 22:337–338
22. Hellstrom M, Jacobsson B, Marild S, Jodal U. Voiding cystourethrography as a predictor of reflux nephropathy in children with urinary-tract infection. AJR 1989; 152:801–804
23. Hodson CJ, Maling TMJ, McManamon P, Lewis MG. The pathogenesis of reflux nephropathy (chronic atrophic pyelonephritis). Br J Radiol 1975; 13(suppl):1–26
24. Jequier S, Jequier JC. Reliability of voiding cystourethrography to detect reflux. AJR 1989; 153:807–810
25. Lavocat MP, Granjon D, Allard D, Gay C, Freycon MT, Dubois F. Imaging of pyelonephritis. Pediatr Radiol 1997; 27:159–165
26. Lebowitz RL. The detection of vesicoureteral reflux in the child. Invest Radiol 1986; 21:519–531
27. Lebowitz RL, Olbing H, Parkkulainen KV, Smellie JM, Tamminen-Mobius TE. International system of radiographic grading of vescioureteric reflux. International Reflux Study in Children. Pediatr Radiol 1985; 15: 105–109
28. Lerner GR, Fleischmann LE, Perlmutter AD. Reflux nephropathy. Pediatr Clin North Am 1987; 34:747–770
29. Majd M, Belman AB. Nuclear cystography in infants and children. Urol Clin North Am 1979; 6:395–407
30. Mentzel HJ, Vogt S, Patzer L, et al. Contrast-enhanced sonography of vesicoureterorenal reflux in children: preliminary results. AJR 1999; 173: 737–740
31. Paltiel HJ, Rupich RC, Kiruluta HG. Enhanced detection of vesicoureteral reflux in infants and children with use of cyclic voiding cystourethrography. Radiology 1992; 184:753–755
32. Ransley PG. Opacification of the renal parenchyma in obstruction and reflux. Pediatr Radiol 1976; 4:226–232
33. Rolleston GL, Maling TM, Hodson CJ. Intrarenal reflux and the scarred kidney. Arch Dis Child 1974; 49:531–539
34. Tibballs JM, De Bruyn R. Primary vesicoureteric reflux—how useful is postnatal ultrasound? Arch Dis Child 1996; 75:444–447
35. Willi U, Treves S. Radionuclide voiding cystography. Urol Radiol 1983; 5:161–173

HEMOLYTIC UREMIC SYNDROME

36. Choyke PL, Grant EG, Hoffer FA, Tina L, Korec S. Cortical echogenicity in the hemolytic uremic syndrome: clinical correlation. J Ultrasound Med 1988; 7:439–442
37. Friedland JA, Herman TE, Siegel MJ. *Escherichia coli* O157:H7-associated hemolytic-uremic syndrome: value of colonic color Doppler sonography. Pediatr Radiol 1995; 25:S65–S67
38. Patriquin HB, O'Regan S, Robitaille P, Paltiel H. Hemolytic-uremic syndrome: intrarenal arterial Doppler patterns as a useful guide to therapy. Radiology 1989; 172:625–628
39. Siegel MJ, Friedland JA, Hildebolt CF. Bowel wall thickening in children: differentiation with US. Radiology 1997; 203:631–635

DUPLICATED COLLECTING SYSTEM

40. Bisset GS III, Strife JL. The duplex collecting system in girls with urinary tract infection: prevalence and significance. AJR 1987; 148:497–500
41. Cremin BJ. A review of the ultrasonic appearances of posterior urethral valve and ureteroceles. Pediatr Radiol 1986; 16:357–364
42. Nussbaum AR, Dorst JP, Jeffs RD, Gearhart JP, Sanders RC. Ectopic ureter and ureterocele: their varied sonographic manifestations. Radiology 1986; 159:227–235

PYONEPHROSIS/ABSCESS

43. Jeffrey RB, Laing FC, Wing VW, Hoddick W. Sensitivity of sonography in pyonephrosis: a reevaluation. AJR 1985; 144:71–73
44. Lang EK. Renal, perirenal, and pararenal abscesses: percutaneous drainage. Radiology 1990; 174:109–113
45. Schneider K, Helmig FJ, Eife R, et al. Pyonephrosis in childhood—is ultrasound sufficient for diagnosis? Pediatr Radiol 1989; 19:302–307
46. Soulen MC, Fishman EK, Goldman SM, Gatewood OM. Bacterial renal infection: role of CT. Radiology 1989; 171:703–707

URINARY TRACT INFECTION—GENERAL

47. Conway JJ, Cohn RA. Evolving role of nuclear medicine for the diagnosis and management of urinary tract infection. J Pediatr 1994; 124:87–90
48. Dick PT, Feldman W. Routine diagnostic imaging for childhood urinary tract infections: a systematic overview. J Pediatr 1996; 128:15–22
49. Eggli DF, Tulchinsky M. Scintigraphic evaluation of pediatric urinary tract infection. Semin Nucl Med 1993; 23:199–218
50. Hayden CK Jr, Swischuk LE, Fawcett HD, Rytting JE, McCord G. Urinary tract infections in childhood: a current imaging approach. RadioGraphics 1986; 6:1023–1038
51. Hilton SW. The child with a urinary tract infection. In: Hilton SW, Edwards DK (eds), Practical pediatric radiology. 2nd ed. Philadelphia: WB Saunders; 1994:495–531
52. Hoffman AD, LeRoy AJ. Uroradiology: procedures and anatomy. In: Kelalis PP, King LR, Belman AB (eds), Clinical pediatric urology. 3rd ed. Philadelphia: WB Saunders; 1992:66–116
53. Lebowitz RL, Mandell J. Urinary tract infection in children: putting radiology in its place. Radiology 1987; 165:1–9
54. Rushton HG. Urinary tract infections in children: epidemiology, evaluation, and management. Pediatr Clin North Am 1997; 44:1133–1169
55. Rushton HG. Genitourinary infections. In: Kelalis PP, King LR, Belman AB (eds), Clinical pediatric urology. 3rd ed. Philadelphia: WB Saunders; 1992:286–364
56. Siegel MJ. Urinary tract. In: Siegel MJ (ed), Pediatric sonography. 3rd ed. New York: Lippincott Williams & Wilkins; in press
57. Siegel MJ. Pediatric urinary tract infection. In: Pollack HM, McClennan BL, Dyer RB, Kennedy JP (eds), Clinical urography. Philadelphia: WB Saunders; 2000:1103–1121
58. Siegel MJ. Pediatric body CT. Philadelphia: Lippincott Williams & Wilkins; 1999:226–252
59. Sty JR, Wells RG, Starshak RJ, Schroeder BA. Imaging in acute renal infection in children. AJR 1987; 148:471–477

Lane F. Donnelly, M.D.

Graft-versus-Host Disease

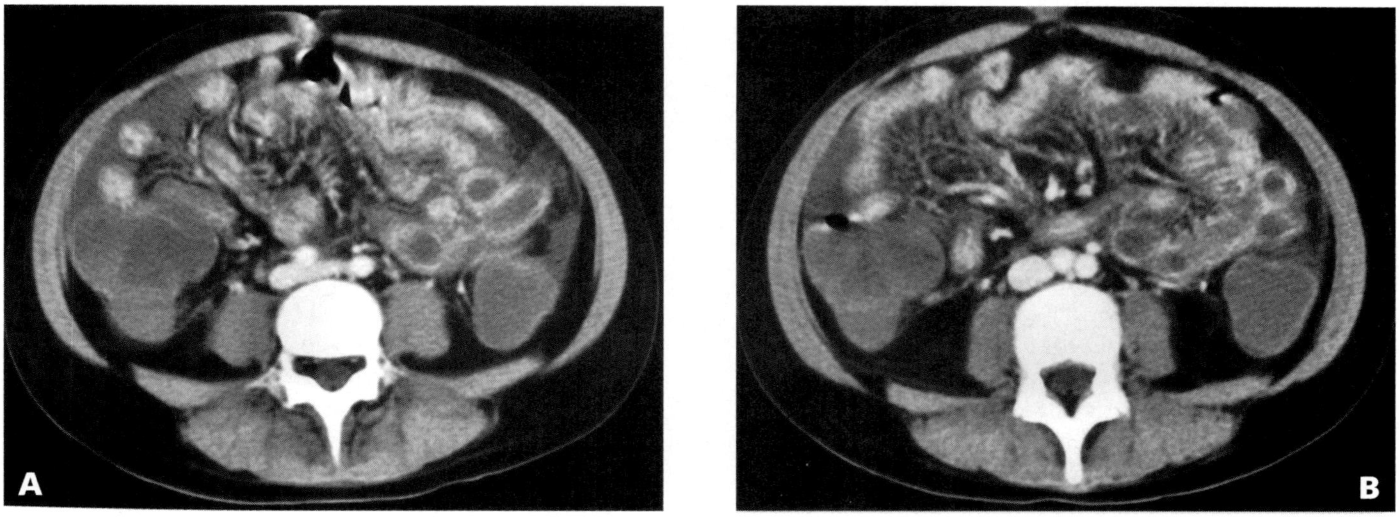

Figure 7-1

Question 35

This 6-year-old boy underwent bone marrow transplantation for acute myelogenous leukemia 1 month ago and now has abdominal pain, nausea and vomiting, diarrhea, and fever. You are shown two postcontrast CT images (Figure 7-1).

Which *one* of the following is the MOST likely diagnosis?

(A) Typhlitis
(B) Lymphoproliferative disorder
(C) Pseudomembranous colitis
(D) Graft-versus-host disease
(E) Radiation enterocolitis

The abdominal CT scan of the test patient (Figure 7-1) demonstrates diffuse bowel abnormality with multiple fluid-filled, mildly to moderately dilated loops of both large and small bowel (Figure 7-2). There is abnormal mucosal enhancement of both large and small bowel, with bowel wall thickening being absent in the colon and mild within several loops of the small bowel. There is associated infiltration of the mesenteric fat (Figure 7-2). In this 6-year-old bone marrow transplant recipient with nonspecific abdominal symptoms, all of the listed choices are possible. However, the CT findings in the test patient are most consistent with gastrointestinal involvement from graft-versus-host disease (GVHD) (**Option (D) is correct**). Moreover, acute GVHD is encountered exclusively in bone marrow transplant recipients.

Typhlitis (neutropenic colitis, necrotizing enteropathy) (Option (A)) is a pathologic process that consists of necrosis and inflammation of the cecum and ascending colon with associated ischemia, secondary bacterial invasion, and resultant sepsis. The term "typhlitis" is derived from the Greek word *typhlon*, meaning cecum. The pathogenesis is poorly understood, but the disease process is related to the presence of neutropenia. The cecum may be predisposed to disease because of relative stasis of bowel contents at this location, leading to overgrowth of bacteria. Typhlitis is most commonly seen in patients with acute leukemia, but can occur in any patient with neutropenia, including neutropenia associated with other hematologic cancers, aplastic anemia, bone marrow transplantation, renal transplantation, and human immunodeficiency virus (HIV) infection. Clinical features include fever, diarrhea, abdominal pain, and occasionally a palpable mass in the right lower quadrant. CT imaging shows bowel wall thickening, pericolonic fluid, and inflammation of the pericolonic fat, usually isolated to the cecum and ascending colon (Figure 7-3).

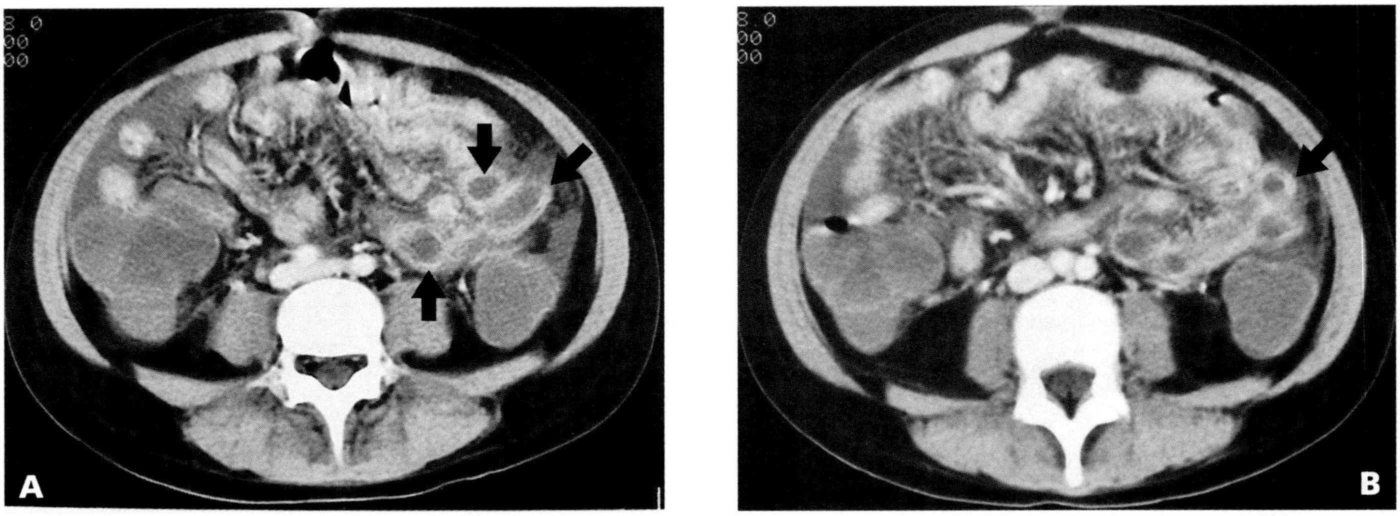

Figure 7-2 (Same as Figure 7-1). Gastrointestinal involvement by graft-versus-host disease. Two CT images show multiple fluid-filled, mildly to moderately dilated loops of both large and small bowels. There is abnormal mucosal enhancement of multiple loops of both large and small bowels. Bowel wall thickening is mild within the small bowel (arrows) and absent in the large bowel. There is infiltration of the mesenteric fat (seen best in panel B). There is a small amount of ascites.

Pneumatosis also can be present (Figure 7-4). The terminal ileum also can be involved, but diffuse involvement of the small and large bowels, as seen in the test images, is not a finding. Rarely, more distal portions of the colon also can be involved. Radiographs are usually nonspecific, but can show ileus, paucity of gas in the right lower quadrant, right-sided colonic wall thickening, cecal pneumatosis, or small bowel obstruction. Sonography also can demonstrate the colonic wall thickening and pericolonic inflammatory changes, but does not reliably demonstrate complications, such as perforation. Historically, barium enema showed cecal wall thickening with thumbprinting, but it is no longer a recommended diagnostic procedure in patients suspected of having typhlitis, because of the risk of perforation. Treatment is usually conservative, with management consisting of fluids and antibiotics. Clinical improvement usually follows a return of adequate numbers of neutrophils. Surgical management is reserved for patients with bowel perforation (Figure 7-5).

Immunocompromised patients are at increased risk for developing lymphoproliferative disorders (Option (B)). Lymphoproliferative disorders consist of a spectrum of diseases ranging from polyclonal B-cell hyperplasia to monoclonal B-cell lym-

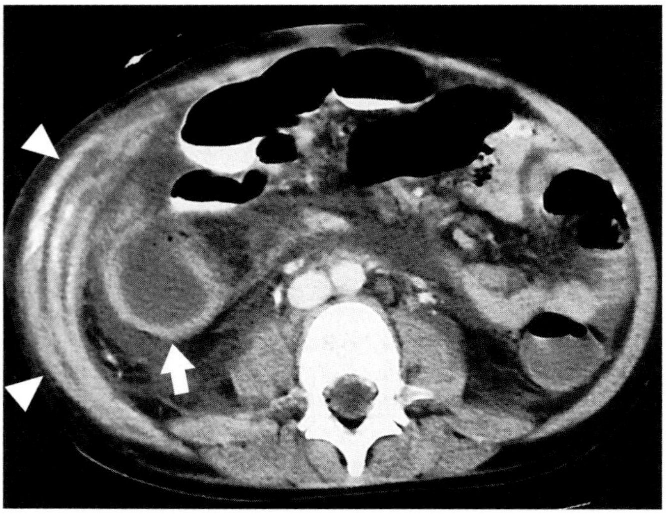

Figure 7-3. Typhlitis in a 6-year-old boy with aplastic anemia. A CT image demonstrates a fluid-filled ascending colon with bowel wall thickening (arrow) and adjacent pericolonic inflammatory changes. The inflammation extends into the adjacent abdominal wall, with asymmetric thickening and heterotopic calcification of the abdominal wall musculature (arrowheads) and soft tissue infiltration of the subcutaneous fat of the abdominal wall musculature. These abdominal wall changes are unusual manifestations of typhlitis.

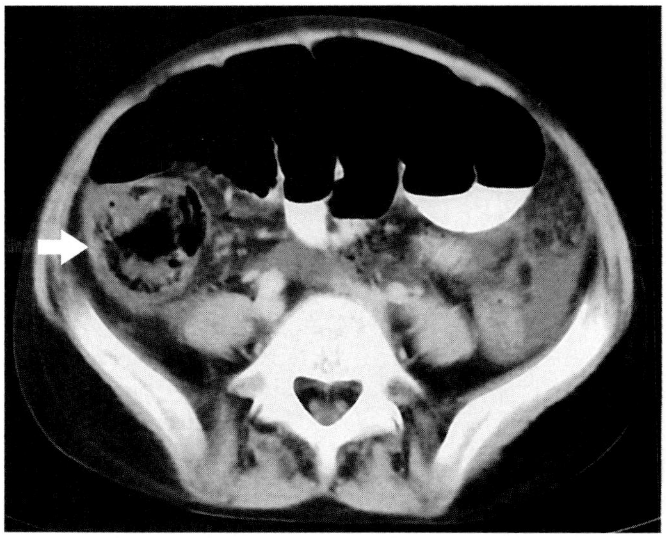

Figure 7-4. Typhlitis with pneumatosis in a 10-year-old boy. A CT image shows bowel wall thickening and pneumatosis (arrow) involving the cecum. Pericolonic inflammatory change is apparent. The small bowel and descending colon do not demonstrate bowel wall thickening.

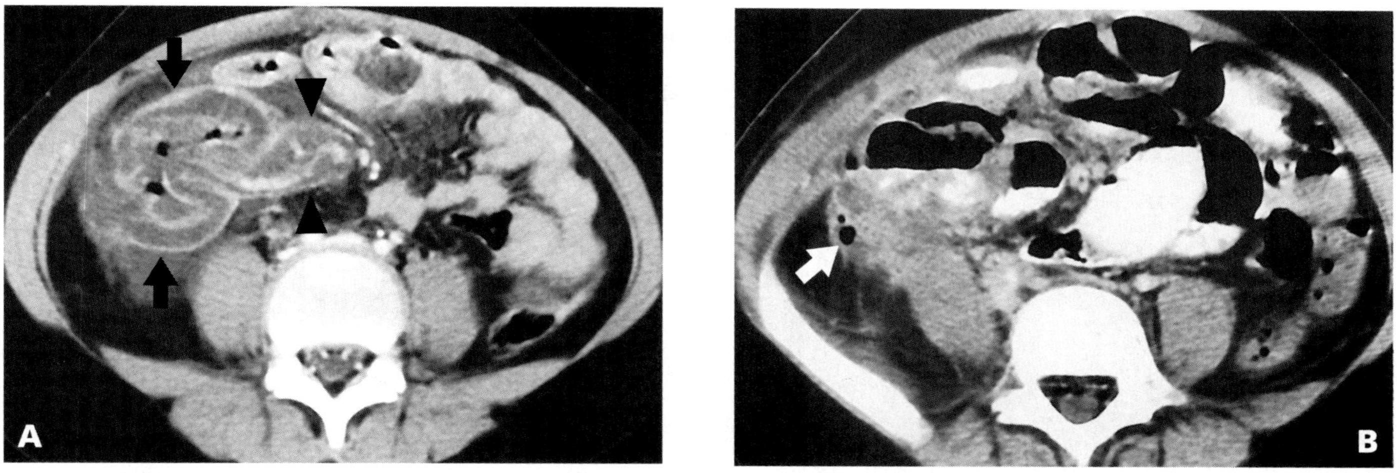

Figure 7-5. Typhlitis with perforation in an 11-year-old girl with a history of acute lymphocytic leukemia and right lower quadrant pain and diarrhea. (A) A CT scan shows marked bowel wall thickening, adventitial enhancement, and pericolonic inflammatory change involving both the cecum (arrows) and terminal ileum (arrowheads). The descending colon and remainder of the small bowel appear normal. (B) A CT scan 2 weeks later shows extraluminal gas (arrow) consistent with interval perforation attributable to progressive transmural necrosis. (Reprinted with permission from Donnelly [25].)

phoma. The process is thought to be related to the loss of normal T-cell control of Epstein-Barr virus-infected B cells. The infected cells proliferate and cause lymphoma-like diseases. The Epstein-Barr virus genome is usually present in DNA extracted from the hyperplastic or malignant cells. Lymphoproliferative disorders often involve the chest and abdomen. In the series of Donnelly et al., the distribution of disease included the abdomen (63%), chest (37%), neck (30%), and brain (4%). Abdominal involvement by lymphoproliferative disorders can appear as a wide spectrum of disease, with almost any abdominal organ being involved. Imaging findings include diffuse lymphadenopathy, focal mass, hepatic disease, and bowel involvement. Hepatic disease is common and can appear as focal liver masses or periportal low attenuation. When the bowel is involved, focal bowel wall thickening is the most common finding. The diffuse distribution of disease and lack of significant bowel wall thickening in the test patient make lymphoproliferative disorder an unlikely diagnosis. Clinical symptoms vary depending on the location of involvement, e.g., liver dysfunction, small bowel obstruction, or palpable mass. Some lymphoproliferative disorders will resolve with reduction of immunosuppressive agents. Other therapeutic options include antiviral or chemotherapeutic agents.

Pseudomembranous colitis (Option (C)) is a consequence of overgrowth by *Clostridium difficile,* which releases a toxin that is the direct cause of the disorder. It is most commonly related to treatment with broad-spectrum antibiotics, which facilitates the bacterial overgrowth. Because immunocompromised children are often on antibiotic therapy for prolonged periods, they are at risk for developing pseudomembranous colitis. On CT, most cases of pseudomembranous colitis show marked bowel wall thickening (average, 15 mm) isolated to the large bowel. These findings are not seen in the test patient.

Radiation enterocolitis (Option (E)) is a less common cause of intra-abdominal crisis in immunocompromised children than are the other listed options. Pathophysiologically, radiation enterocolitis is related to damage to small arterioles and a resultant obliterative endarteritis. This results in both acute and chronic inflammation and eventually fibrosis. A radiation dose in excess of 4,000 to 5,000 rads is necessary to cause significant enterocolitis. Therefore, radiation enterocolitis is usually the result of focal radiation therapy and does not occur as a result of whole-body irradiation, which was administered to the test patient as part of the bone marrow transplantation procedure. It is therefore not the correct diagnosis. Clinical symptoms include crampy abdominal pain, diarrhea, and occult intestinal bleeding. The CT findings include bowel wall thickening, adherence of adjacent bowel loops, and infiltration of the adjacent mesenteric fat. Strictures can develop over a period of years after therapy and can lead to bowel obstruction (Figure 7-6). The diffuse distribution of disease seen in the test patient is not consistent with radiation enterocolitis.

Other considerations in the differential diagnosis of the test patient include infectious causes of enterocolitis. Immunocompromised children are at increased risk for infectious enterocolitis. Potential organisms include cytomegalovirus, coxsackie A and B viruses, *Cryptosporidium, Mycobacterium tuberculosis* or *M. avium-intracellulare,* and HIV. Cytomegalovirus colitis is one of the most common causes of infectious colitis in these children and appears as thickening of the wall of the cecum and terminal ileum on CT studies. It is often difficult to differentiate, both clinically and radiographically, from typhlitis. Children treated with immunosuppressive therapy for cancer can present with acute abdominal symptoms related to recurrent neoplasm, and the presentation can be similar to that of other causes of acute abdomen. Common causes of abdominal pain in immunocompetent children, such as appendicitis and intussusception, also occur in immunocompromised patients and should not be overlooked simply because the child has an altered immune status.

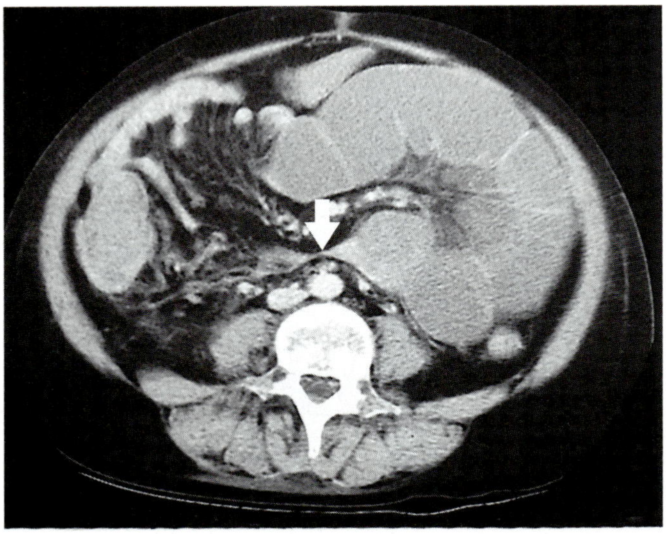

Figure 7-6. Bowel obstruction caused by a radiation-induced stricture in a 13-year-old boy with a history of radiation therapy for neuroblastoma 7 years previously. A CT image shows a beak-like area of narrowing at the level of the stricture (arrow) and resultant dilated, obstructed small bowel proximal to the stricture. (Reprinted with permission from Donnelly [25].)

Question 36

Concerning pseudomembranous colitis,

(A) it is most commonly a pancolitis
(B) colonic wall thickness is usually greater than 10 mm
(C) pericolonic inflammatory changes are usually disproportionately greater than the degree of bowel wall thickening
(D) on CT, the "accordion sign" is seen most often in the transverse colon

Pseudomembranous colitis is a descriptive term for colitis with characteristic pathologic and radiologic appearances. Most cases are related to overgrowth by *C. difficile* and overproduction of its toxin, most often related to antibiotic use. Virtually all antibiotics have been linked to the development of pseudomembranous colitis, with clindamycin being the most strongly implicated. However, the antibiotics most commonly associated with pseudomembranous colitis are most probably cephalosporins and ampicillins because of their widespread use. The onset of pseudomembranous colitis can occur within days of the initiation of antibiotic therapy or can be delayed as long as 6 weeks after the antibiotic therapy has been discontinued.

Direct endothelial damage by the *C. difficile* toxin is the accepted theory for the pathogenesis of pseudomembranous colitis. A disturbance in the balance of the normal bacterial flora of the colon, secondary to antibiotic therapy, is thought to result in a proliferation of *C. difficile*, which then results in overproduction of its toxin. Pseudomembranous colitis is truly a toxin-related disease because *C. difficile* does not invade the gut epithelium.

Gross pathologic evaluation and endoscopy demonstrate the presence of discrete, yellow plaques (pseudomembranes) adherent to the mucosal surface of the colon (Figure 7-7). The pseudomembranes are separated by normal-appearing mucosa. Although small bowel involvement has been described, the vast majority of cases involve only the colon. The colonic disease is usually a pancolitis (**Option (A) is true**) or, less commonly, shows isolated left colonic involvement. Focal epithelial necrosis, formation of exudate, and extensive transmural edema are found microscopically.

Patients usually present with diarrhea, abdominal pain, fever, and lymphocytosis. The diarrhea is typically watery, although it can be hemorrhagic or contain mucus. There is an age-related susceptibility for pseudomembranous colitis, with older adults being most susceptible. Although pseudomembranous colitis is more common in adults than children, it is not an uncommon cause of colitis in children.

The CT findings, although nonspecific, are often highly suggestive of pseudomembranous colitis. There is usually diffuse colonic involvement with marked wall thickening. The degree of colonic wall thickening (average, 15 mm) (**Option (B) is true**) usually exceeds that in patients with other types of colitis (Figures 7-8 and 7-9). The marked colonic wall thickening is believed to be related to the combined thickness of the colonic wall edema and pseudomembranes. Because the inflammatory component of the disease process involves predominantly mucosa and submucosa, the degree of inflammatory change in the pericolonic fat is often disproportionately smaller than would be expected for the degree of wall thickening (**Option (C) is false**). Intraluminal contrast material often insinuates between the pseudomembranes and swollen haustra, form-

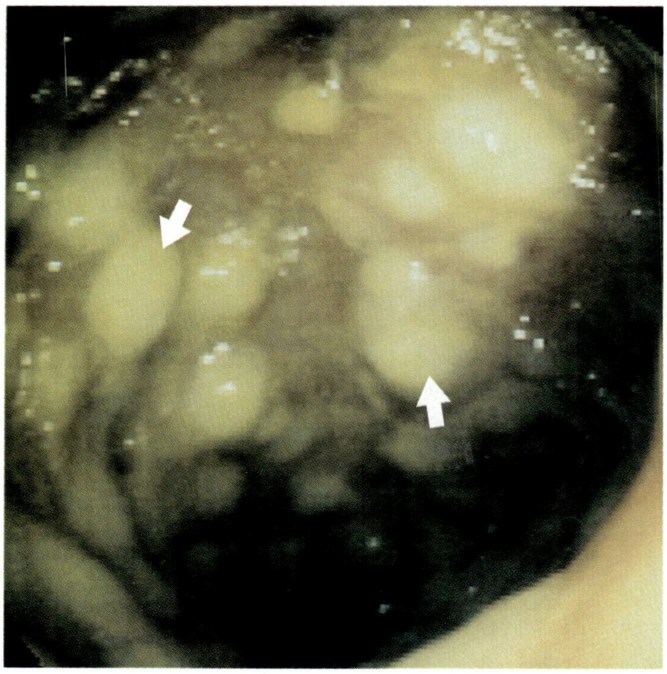

Figure 7-7. Pseudomembranous colitis. Endoscopy demonstrates multiple yellow, discrete plaques (arrows) separated by normal-appearing mucosa. (Reprinted with permission from Donnelly [25].)

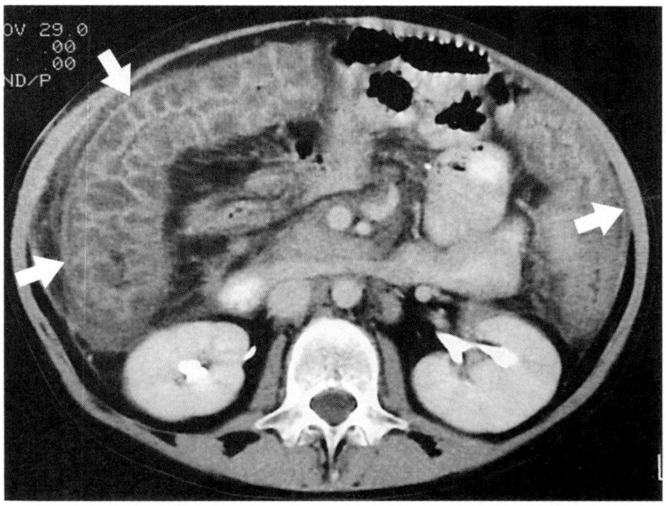

Figure 7-8. Pseudomembranous colitis in a child with a history of liver transplantation. A CT image demonstrates marked bowel wall thickening (16 mm) diffusely throughout the colon (arrows). There is adjacent pericolonic inflammatory change.

ing an "accordion sign," which has been described as highly suggestive of pseudomembranous colitis (Figure 7-10). The accordion sign is seen most often in the transverse colon on CT scans (**Option (D) is true**) because the transverse colon is visualized in the longitudinal plane on axial images, in contrast to the ascending and descending colon, which are seen in cross section on these images. The greater frequency of the accordion sign in the transverse colon is therefore a result of the plane of imaging rather than a propensity for severe disease in this region.

The radiographic findings in patients with severe cases include marked colonic thumbprinting, nodular haustral thickening, and evidence of ascites. Colonic dilatation can be an indication of toxic megacolon complicating pseudomembranous colitis. Barium enema has played a limited role in the diagnosis of pseudomembranous colitis since the advent of cross-sectional imaging, but it can demonstrate thick haustra, confluent plaques, and mucosal irregularity diffusely throughout the colon. Sonography can be helpful in confirming the diagnosis in patients who are too ill to travel from the intensive care unit to the CT facility and demonstrates the marked colonic wall thickening and ascites.

Treatment includes elimination of the offending antibiotic, oral metronidazole therapy, and maintenance of fluid and electrolyte balances. CT is also helpful for monitoring for complications of pseudomembranous colitis that require surgical intervention, such as bowel perforation or abscess formation or both. Although severe cases can lead to progressive sepsis, shock, and death, conservative therapy is successful in treating most patients.

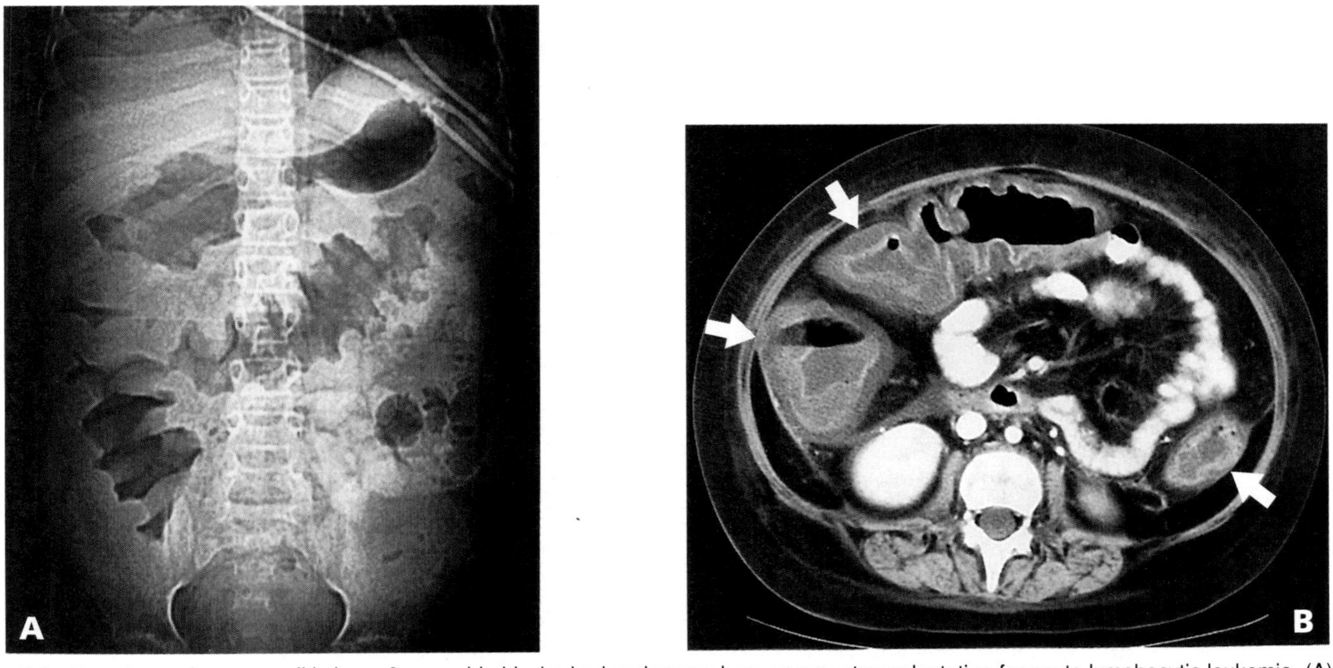

Figure 7-9. Pseudomembranous colitis in an 8-year-old girl who had undergone bone marrow transplantation for acute lymphocytic leukemia. (A) A localization image from an abdominal CT examination shows severe thumbprinting diffusely throughout the colon. (B) A CT image shows marked colonic wall thickening with mucosal enhancement and pericolonic inflammatory change throughout the colon (arrows). Thickening of the small bowel wall is absent.

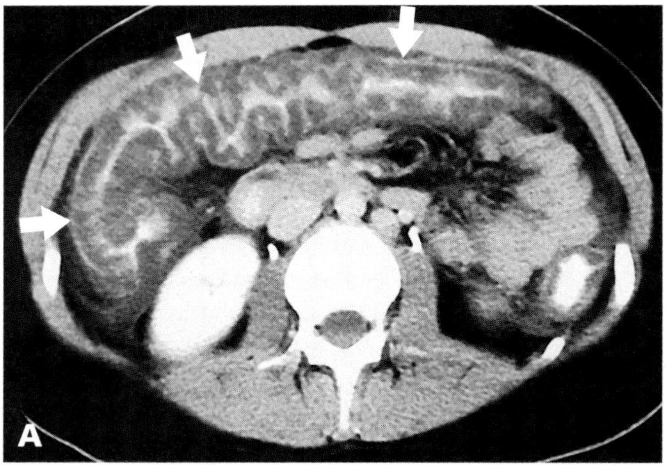

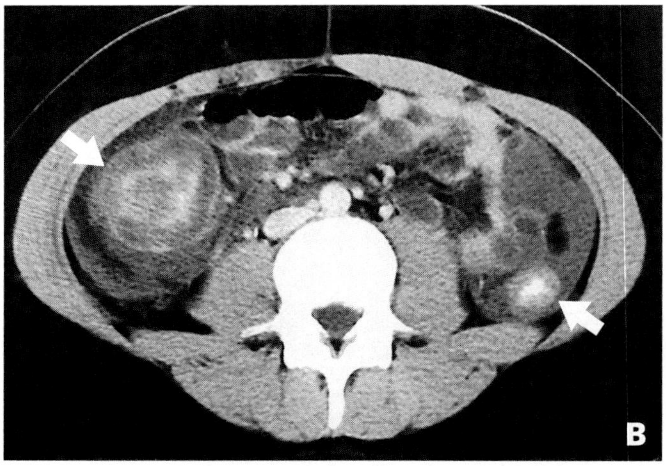

Figure 7-10. Same patient as in Figure 7-7. Pseudomembranous colitis in an 18-year-old woman with abdominal pain, diarrhea, lymphocytosis, and a history of taking antibiotics. CT images at the level of the transverse colon (A) and more inferiorly at the level of the ascending and descending colon (B) show pancolitis characterized by marked bowel wall thickening (arrows). There is inflammatory change within the adjacent fat as well as diffuse ascites. The accordion sign, which is caused by intraluminal contrast material interposed between markedly thickened haustra, is best seen in panel A and is highly suggestive of pseudomembranous colitis. (Reprinted with permission from Donnelly [25].)

Question 37

Concerning graft-versus-host disease,

(A) it is attributable to epithelial damage of recipient target organs by donor T-cell lymphocytes
(B) it occurs in fewer than 20% of matched allogeneic bone marrow transplant recipients
(C) the skin is the most common target organ
(D) patients rarely present with gastrointestinal symptoms

GVHD is a disease process specific to patients who undergo bone marrow transplantation. In this disease, donor T lymphocytes cause selective epithelial damage of the target organs of the recipient (**Option (A) is true**).

GVHD is divided into acute and chronic forms based on whether symptoms occur before or later than 100 days after transplantation. The two forms have different clinical manifestations. Chronic GVHD is less common, occurring in approximately 30% of allogeneic transplant recipients, and typically involves the skin, oral mucosa, gastrointestinal tract, liver, skeletal muscle, hematopoietic system, and lungs. The findings resemble those of a connective tissue disorder; the most common clinically significant complication is long-lasting immunodeficiency. The remainder of this discussion pertains to the more common acute GVHD.

Acute GVHD occurs commonly in bone marrow transplant recipients, with moderate to severe acute GVHD occurring in 30% to 50% of matched allogeneic bone marrow transplant recipients (**Option (B) is false**). The organs most commonly involved include the skin, liver, and gastrointestinal tract. Cutaneous manifestations include a maculopapular rash, which is the most common and often the presenting finding (**Option (C) is true**). Hyperbilirubinemia and hepatic dysfunction occur secondary to damaged biliary epithelium. Involvement of the gastrointestinal tract usually appears after the skin rash and is rarely the presenting or only manifestation (**Option (D) is true**). Intestinal symptoms include abdominal pain, anorexia, fever, nausea and vomiting, diarrhea, and, in severe cases, intestinal hemorrhage. These nonspecific abdominal symptoms often lead to CT evaluation to exclude other sources of abdominal sepsis. The appropriate identification of gastrointestinal GVHD on CT scans has both important prognostic and therapeutic implications and obviates further diagnostic testing to identify the source of sepsis and abdominal symptoms. The prognosis of patients with GVHD is worse when there is definitive gastrointestinal involvement than when the gastrointestinal tract is not involved and correlates with the severity of diarrhea. Gastrointestinal involvement and the resultant electrolyte imbalances and sepsis are the leading cause of death in patients with GVHD.

Treatment of GVHD is aimed at rendering donor T cells ineffective. Glucocorticoids, cyclosporin A, and polyclonal or monoclonal anti-T-cell antibodies have been used to decrease T-cell activity.

Question 38

Concerning the appearance of graft-versus-host disease on abdominal CT scans,

(A) the bowel wall thickness is usually more than 6 mm
(B) mucosal enhancement is a feature
(C) infiltration of the mesenteric fat is common
(D) involvement of both the large and small bowels indicates severe disease

The pathologic process of gastrointestinal involvement by acute GVHD consists of extensive "crypt cell necrosis" and often diffuse mucosal destruction. The destroyed mucosa is replaced by a thin layer of highly vascular granulation tissue (Figure 7-11). The distribution of disease is usually diffuse, with involvement from the duodenum to the rectum. There is no direct correlation between the extent of bowel involvement and the severity of disease **(Option (D) is false).**

CT findings include a diffuse bowel abnormality from the duodenum to the rectum (Figure 7-12). Bowel wall thickening can be mild and isolated to the small bowel or, not uncommonly, is absent (Figure 7-13). Bowel wall thickening is present in the small bowel in 50% of patients and in the large bowel in only 19%; when present, it usually does not exceed 3 to 4 mm **(Option (A) is false).** Characteristically, abnormal enhancement is visualized in the region of the mucosa and corresponds pathologically to the thin layer of vascular granulation tissue that replaces the destroyed mucosa (Figure 7-14) **(Option (B) is true).** Mucosal enhancement is present in nearly all patients. Because of the voluminous diarrhea and ileus associated with GVHD, the small and large bowels are usually diffusely fluid filled and dilated (this finding is nearly always present) (Figures 7-12 and 7-15).

Common extraintestinal abdominal CT findings include infiltration of the mesenteric fat (88% of patients) **(Option (C) is true),** hepatomegaly (44% of patients), decreased hepatic periportal attenuation (31% of patients) (Figure 7-16), and ascites (50% of patients). Ringlike mucosal enhancement, similar in appearance to that within the bowel, can also occur in the gallbladder and urinary bladder walls (Figure 7-17).

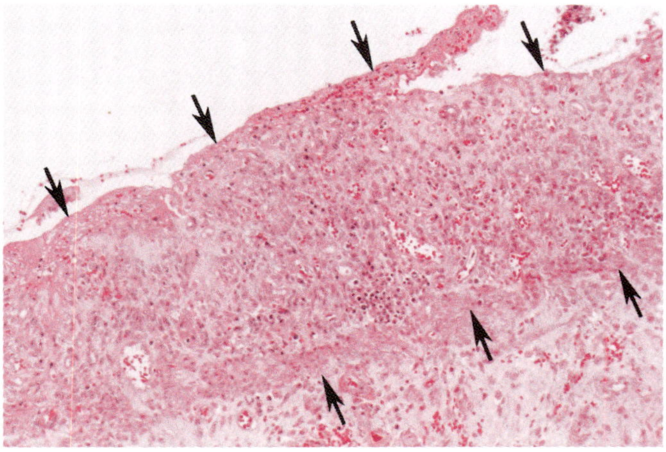

Figure 7-11. Histologic changes of graft-versus-host disease in a specimen obtained at autopsy. The intestinal mucosa has been completely destroyed and replaced by a thin layer of highly vascular granulation tissue (arrows). These findings correlate with the thin, central ring of mucosal enhancement seen on CT scans. Submucosal edema and inflammatory cells are also present. (Reprinted with permission from Donnelly and Morris [3].)

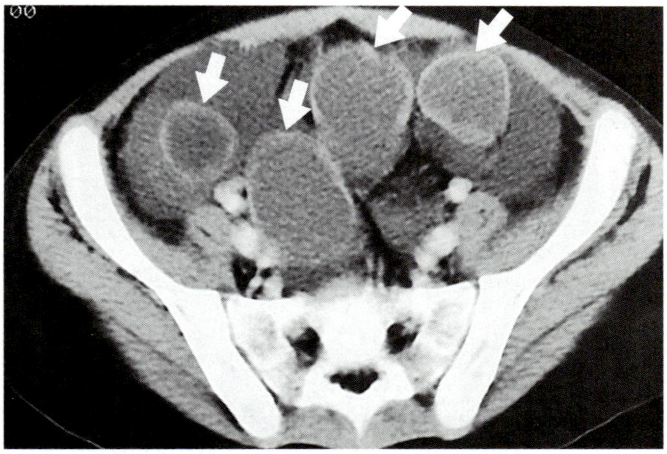

Figure 7-13. Gastrointestinal graft-versus-host disease in a 10-year-old girl who has undergone bone marrow transplantation for Fanconi's anemia. A CT image demonstrates multiple fluid-filled, dilated loops of colon with abnormally enhancing but nonthickened bowel wall (arrows). Ascites is also present. (Reprinted with permission from Donnelly and Morris [3].)

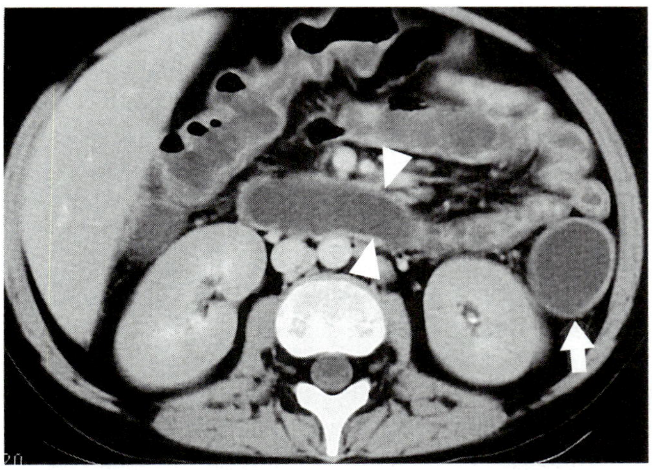

Figure 7-12. Diffuse distribution of graft-versus-host disease. A CT image demonstrates fluid-filled, dilated bowel loops with abnormally enhancing but nonthickened bowel wall extending from the duodenum (arrowheads) to the descending colon (arrow). (Reprinted with permission from Donnelly and Morris [3].)

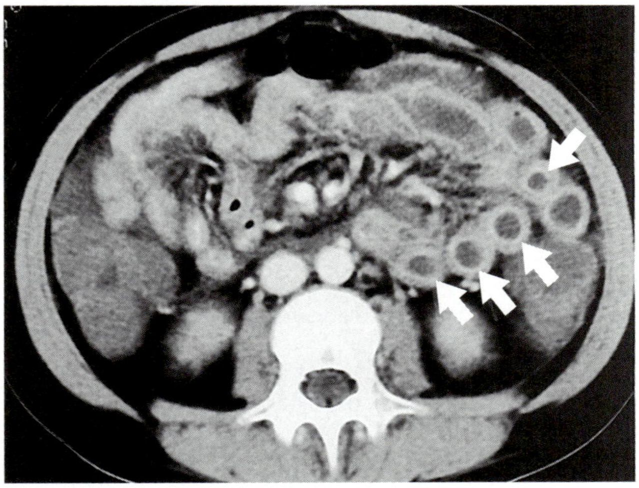

Figure 7-14. Gastrointestinal involvement by graft-versus-host disease. A CT image shows multiple fluid-filled, dilated loops of both large and small bowels. The small bowel wall (arrows) is mildly thickened with central ring enhancement of the mucosal layer. There is soft tissue infiltration of the mesentery. The colon wall is not thickened. (Reprinted with permission from Donnelly and Morris [3].)

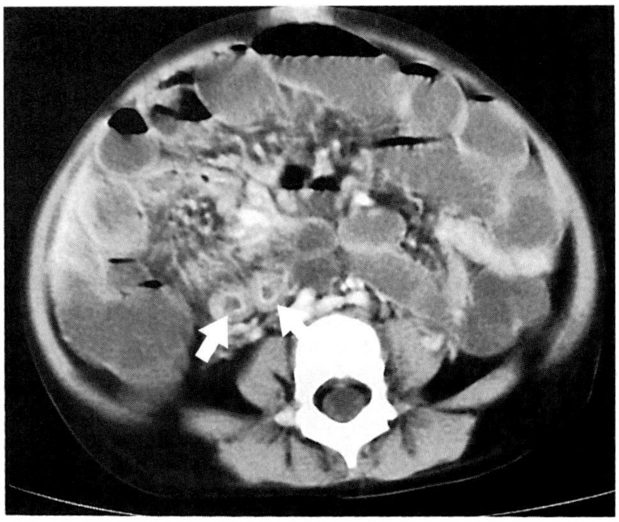

Figure 7-15. Gastrointestinal involvement by graft-versus-host disease. A CT image shows diffusely fluid-filled, dilated small and large bowels. Most of the bowel loops show no bowel wall thickening. One area of small bowel (arrows) shows mild small bowel wall thickening and mucosal enhancement. There is soft tissue infiltration in the mesenteric fat.

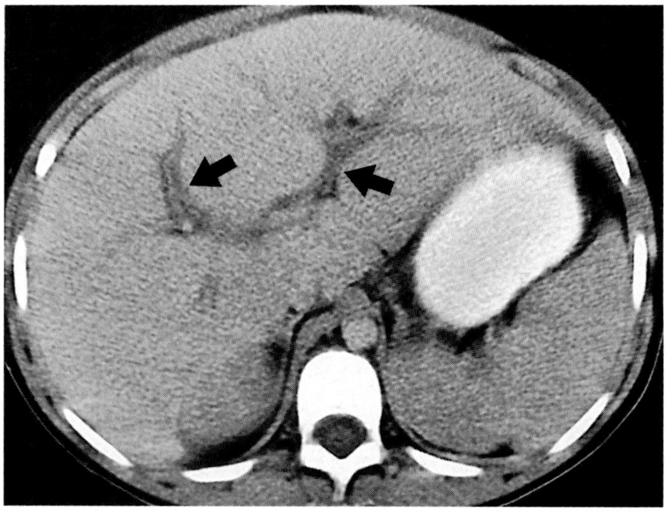

Figure 7-16. Graft-versus-host disease. A CT image demonstrates nonspecific periportal low attenuation (arrows), a common but nonspecific finding in patients with GVHD. (Reprinted with permission from Donnelly and Morris [3].)

Question 39

Concerning acute abdominal disease in immunocompromised children,

(A) abscess is the most common cause of abdominal symptoms
(B) abscess is more often attributable to fungal infection than to bacterial infection
(C) percutaneous drainage of an intraperitoneal abscess is contraindicated
(D) on CT, cecal thickening with surrounding inflammatory changes reliably indicates typhlitis
(E) severe colonic wall thickening is an indication for colostomy

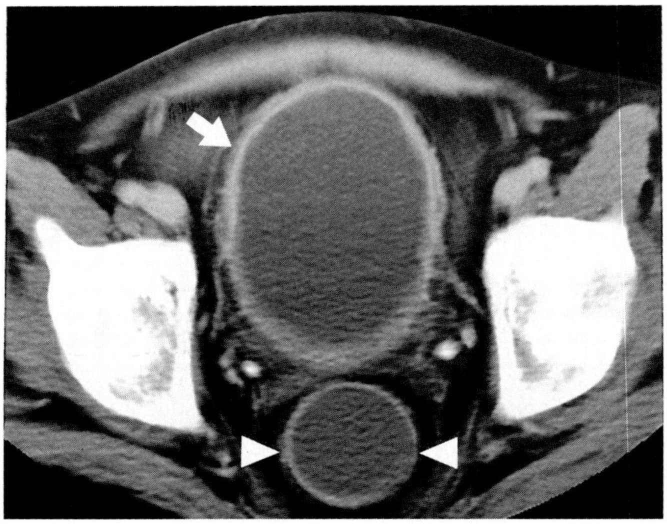

Figure 7-17. Graft-versus-host disease. A CT image shows mucosal enhancement of the urinary bladder (arrow) as well as of a nonthickened rectal wall (arrowheads). (Reprinted with permission from Donnelly and Morris [3].)

The number of immunocompromised children has increased over the past decade because of the increased use of bone marrow transplantation, the increased use of immunosuppressive therapy (for neoplasms, autoimmune disease, and solid organ transplantation), and the spread of HIV infection. Intra-abdominal crises are a common cause of morbidity and mortality in these immunocompromised children. Most of the pathologic causes of acute abdominal processes in immunocompromised children produce similar symptoms at presentation: abdominal pain, diarrhea, nausea and vomiting, fever, and leukocytosis. Because these abdominal symptoms are nonspecific and there is a need for prompt diagnosis in these fragile patients, CT of the abdomen and pelvis is often performed. There is some overlap in the CT appearance of the different entities that cause abdominal symptoms in immunocompromised children, but the findings are frequently specific enough to suggest a diagnosis (Table 7-1). Most often, the distribution of disease is the most helpful finding.

Because the different types of enterocolitis, such as GVHD, pseudomembranous colitis, infectious enterocolitis, and typhlitis, require different types of medical management (see the above discussions), the identification of a specific disease process by CT is helpful. CT is also helpful in excluding the presence of complications of these enterocolitides that require surgical or interventional management, such as bowel perforation or abscess. The degree of colonic wall thickening is not a factor in the decision about whether to perform surgery (**Option (E) is false**). Although immunocompromised children are often referred for abdominal CT imaging to "rule out abscess," abdominal symptoms are more often related to causes of enterocolitis than to abscesses (**Option (A) is false**). Drainable focal intra-abdominal fluid collections, such as those seen in patients with bacterial abscesses, are uncommon. Intra-abdominal abscesses are much more likely to be related to systemic fungal infection by organisms such as *Candida albicans*

Table 7-1: CT findings helpful in differentiating among bowel diseases affecting immunocompromised children[a]

Entity	Typical distribution	Imaging features
Pseudomembranous colitis	Diffuse colonic or less commonly left colonic involvement Rarely, small bowel involvement	Marked bowel wall thickening Disproportionately mild pericolonic inflammation "Accordion sign"
Typhlitis	Cecal and ascending (right) colonic involvement Adjacent terminal ileum involvement	Nonspecific bowel wall thickening and adjacent inflammatory changes
Graft-versus-host disease	Diffuse involvement of small and large bowels	Bowel wall thickening usually mild, isolated to small bowel, or absent Characteristic mucosal enhancement Fluid-filled bowel Infiltration of mesenteric fat, periportal low attenuation, ascites, gallbladder and urinary bladder wall enhancement Hepatomegaly
Cytomegalovirus colitis	Cecal (right colon) and terminal ileum involvement Contiguous involvement of distal colon	Nonspecific bowel wall thickening and adjacent inflammatory changes
Radiation enteriocolitis	Small bowel and/or, less commonly, large bowel	Thickened bowel wall and adherence of adjacent loops Infiltration of adjacent mesenteric and retroperitoneal fat Strictures causing bowel obstruction
Appendicitis	Cecum and, less commonly, terminal ileum	Appendicolith Dilated, thickened appendix Nonspecific cecal wall thickening and adjacent inflammatory changes

[a] Adapted from Donnelly and Morris [3].

or *Aspergillus* species than to infection by bacteria **(Option (B) is true).** Fungal abscesses appear as multiple small, low-attenuation lesions within the liver and spleen rather than as focal intraperitoneal fluid collections (Figure 7-18). The identification of these fungal abscesses is an indication for antifungal therapy. When intra-abdominal abscesses are present in the uncommon form of focal walled-off fluid collections, percutaneous drainage is usually the treatment of choice (Figure 7-19). The patient's immune status does not contraindicate percutaneous drainage **(Option (C) is false).**

The CT findings of bowel wall thickening and surrounding inflammatory changes isolated to the cecum and ascending colon are most often secondary to typhlitis. However, the findings are not specific for the diagnosis of typhlitis and can occur in patients with right lower quadrant inflammation from other causes **(Option (D) is false).** Other common causes of right lower quadrant bowel inflammation in immunocompromised children include infectious enterocolitis, especially that attributable to cytomegalovirus infection, and appendicitis. Com-

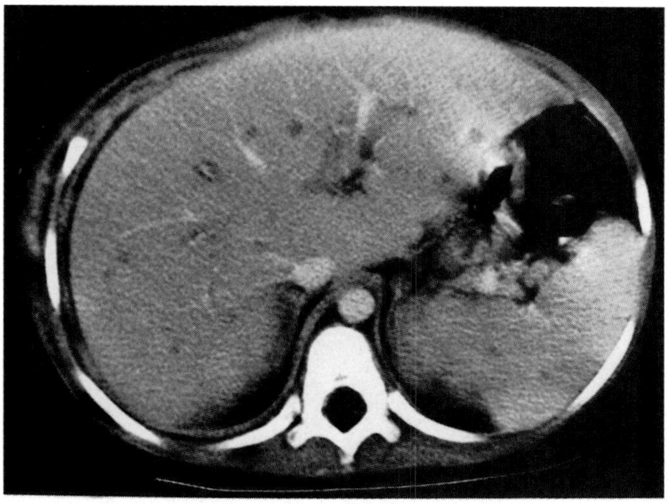

Figure 7-18. Fungal abscesses. A CT image shows multiple small, low-attenuation lesions in the liver and spleen of a 6-year-old boy with aplastic anemia. These are due to *Candida tropicalis* sepsis.

mon childhood diseases such as appendicitis should not be overlooked simply because the affected patient has an altered immune status. In immunocompromised children with CT findings of cecal and right colonic inflammation, specific findings for appendicitis, such as an abnormally thickened or dilated appendix or an appendicolith, should be excluded (Figure 7-20).

SUGGESTED READINGS

GRAFT-VERSUS-HOST DISEASE

1. Benya EC, Sivit CJ, Quinones RR. Abdominal complications after bone marrow transplantation in children: sonographic and CT findings. AJR 1993; 161:1023–1027
2. Day DL, Carpenter BL. Abdominal complications in pediatric bone marrow transplant recipients. RadioGraphics 1993; 13:1101–1112
3. Donnelly LF, Morris CL. Acute graft-versus-host disease in children: abdominal CT findings. Radiology 1996; 199:265–268
4. Ferrara JL, Deeg HJ. Graft-versus-host disease. N Engl J Med 1991; 324:667–674
5. Fisk JD, Shulman HM, Greening RR, McDonald GB, Sale GE, Thomas ED. Gastrointestinal radiographic features of human graft-vs.-host disease. AJR 1981; 136:329–336
6. Jones B, Fishman EK, Kramer SS, et al. Computed tomography of gastrointestinal inflammation after bone marrow transplantation. AJR 1986; 146:691–695
7. Jones B, Kramer SS, Saral R, et al. Gastrointestinal inflammation after bone marrow transplantation: graft-versus-host disease or opportunistic infection? AJR 1988; 150:277–281
8. Maile CW, Frick MP, Crass JR, Snover DC, Weisdorf SA, Kersey JH. The plain abdominal radiograph in acute gastrointestinal graft-vs.-host disease. AJR 1985; 145:289–292
9. Patzic SB, Smith C, Kubicka RA, Kaizer H. Bone marrow transplantation: clinical and radiologic aspects. RadioGraphics 1991; 11:601–610
10. Wick MR, Moore SB, Gastineau DA, Hoagland HC. Immunologic, clinical, and pathologic aspects of human graft-versus-host disease. Mayo Clin Proc 1983; 58:603–612

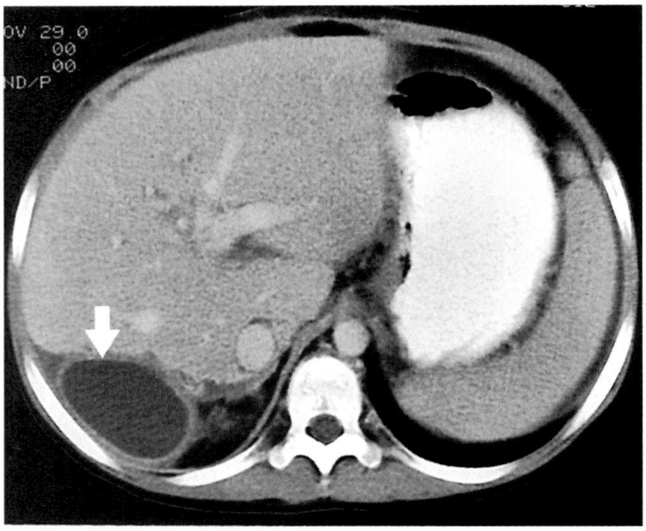

Figure 7-19. Bacterial abscess along the cut edge of a segmental liver transplant. A CT image shows a well-defined fluid collection posterior to the cut edge of the segmental liver transplant (arrow). An immunocompromised state is not a contraindication to percutaneous drainage, which was performed successfully in this patient.

TYPHLITIS (NEUTROPENIC COLITIS)

11. Frick MP, Maile CW, Crass JR, Goldberg ME, Delaney JP. Computed tomography of neutropenic colitis. AJR 1984; 143:763–765
12. Gootenberg JE, Abbondanzo SL. Rapid diagnosis of neutropenic enterocolitis (typhlitis) by ultrasonography. Am J Pediatr Hematol Oncol 1987; 9:222–227
13. Merine DS, Fishman EK, Jones B, Nussbaum AR, Simmons T. Right lower quadrant pain in the immunocompromised patient: CT findings in 10 cases. AJR 1987; 149:1177–1179

LYMPHOPROLIFERATIVE DISORDER

14. Day DL, Shapiro RS, Yueh N, McClain K, Allan BT, Filipovich AH. B-cell lymphoproliferative disorders in children after bone marrow transplantation: radiologic manifestations. Radiology 1987; 162:807–810
15. Donnelly LF, Frush DP, Marshall KW, White KS. Lymphoproliferative disorders: CT findings in immunocompromised children. AJR 1998; 171:725–731
16. Harris KM, Schwartz ML, Slasky BS, Nalesnick M, Makowka L. Post-transplantation cyclosporine-induced lymphoproliferative disorders: clinical and radiologic manifestations. Radiology 1987; 162:697–700

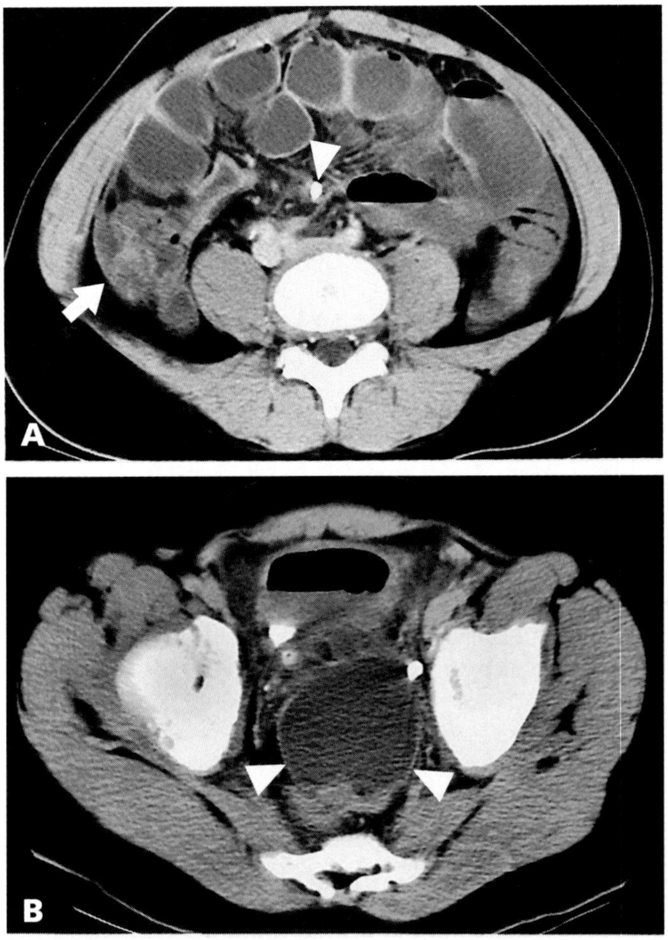

Figure 7-20. Perforated appendicitis in a 5-year-old boy with a history of acute lymphocytic leukemia. (A) A CT image shows bowel wall thickening in the region of the cecum (arrow), multiple dilated loops of small bowel consistent with small bowel obstruction, and a calcified appendicolith (arrowhead) within the midabdomen. (B) A CT image of the inferior pelvis reveals a 5 ˘ 5 cm perirectal fluid collection (arrowheads) consistent with abscess. Immunocompromised children are subject to common diseases, and these diseases should not be overlooked simply because of an altered immune status. (Reprinted with permission from Donnelly [25].)

17. Tubman DE, Frick MP, Hanto DW. Lymphoma after organ transplantation: radiological manifestations in the central nervous system, thorax, and abdomen. Radiology 1983; 149:625–631

PSEUDOMEMBRANOUS COLITIS

18. Blickman JG, Boland GW, Cleveland RH, Bramson RT, Lee MJ. Pseudomembranous colitis: CT findings in children. Pediatr Radiol 1995; 25(Suppl 1):157–159
19. Boland GW, Lee MJ, Cats A, Mueller PR. Pseudomembranous colitis: diagnostic sensitivity of the abdominal plain radiograph. Clin Radiol 1994; 49:473–475
20. Fishman EK, Kavuru M, Jones B, et al. Pseudomembranous colitis: CT evaluation of 26 cases. Radiology 1991; 80:57–60
21. Merine D, Fishman EK, Jones B. Pseudomembranous colitis: CT evaluation. J Comput Assist Tomogr 1987; 11:1017–1020
22. Price AB, Davies DR. Pseudomembranous colitis. J Clin Pathol 1977; 30:1–12
23. Ros PR, Buetow PC, Pantograg-Brown L, Forsmark CE, Sobin LH. Pseudomembranous colitis. Radiology 1996; 198:1–9
24. Stanley RJ, Melson GL, Tedesco FJ. The spectrum of radiographic findings in antibiotic related pseudomembranous colitis. Radiology 1974; 111:519–524

CT IMAGING OF ACUTE ABDOMEN IN IMMUNOCOMPROMISED PATIENTS

25. Donnelly LF. CT imaging of immunocompromised children with acute abdominal symptoms. AJR 1996; 167:909–913
26. Jabra AA, Fishman EK, Taylor GA. CT findings in inflammatory bowel disease in children. AJR 1994; 162:975–979
27. Jones B, Fishman EK. CT of the gut in the immunocompromised host. Radiol Clin North Am 1989; 27:763–771
28. Philpotts LE, Heiken JP, Westcott MA, Gore RM. Colitis: use of CT findings in differential diagnosis. Radiology 1994; 190:445–449
29. Wall SD, Jones B. Gastrointestinal tract in the immunocompromised host: opportunistic infections and other complications. Radiology 1992; 185:327–335
30. Wyatt SH, Fishman EK. The acute abdomen in individuals with AIDS. Radiol Clin North Am 1994; 32:1023–1043

CASE 8

Marilyn J. Siegel, M

Adnexal Masses

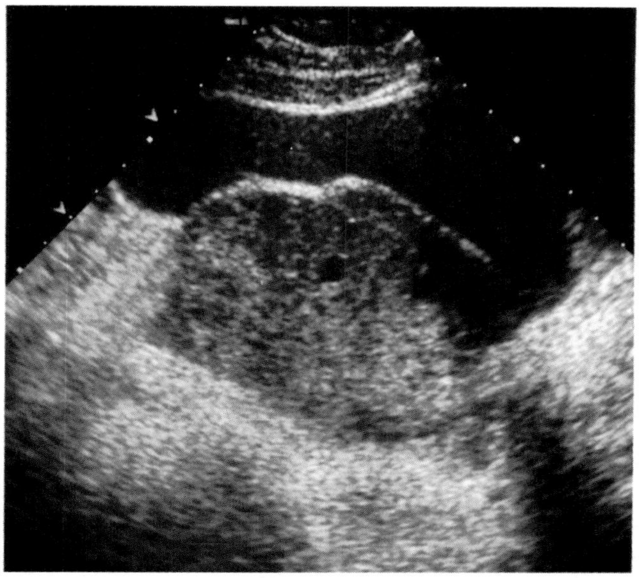

Figure 8-1

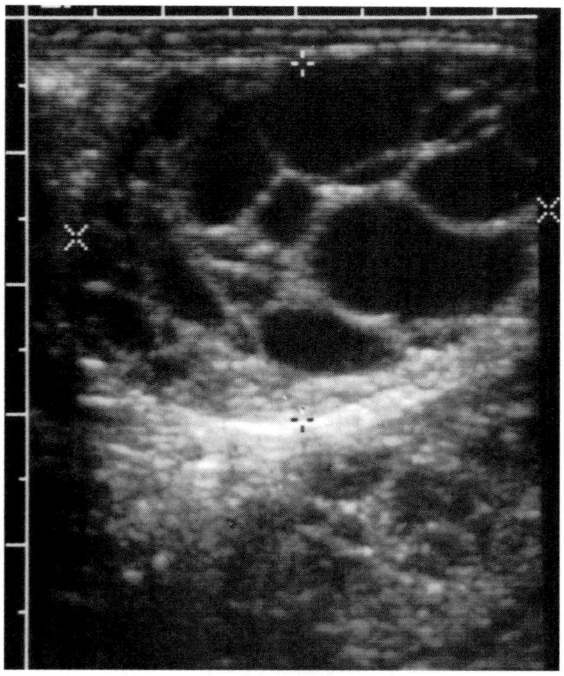

Figure 8-2

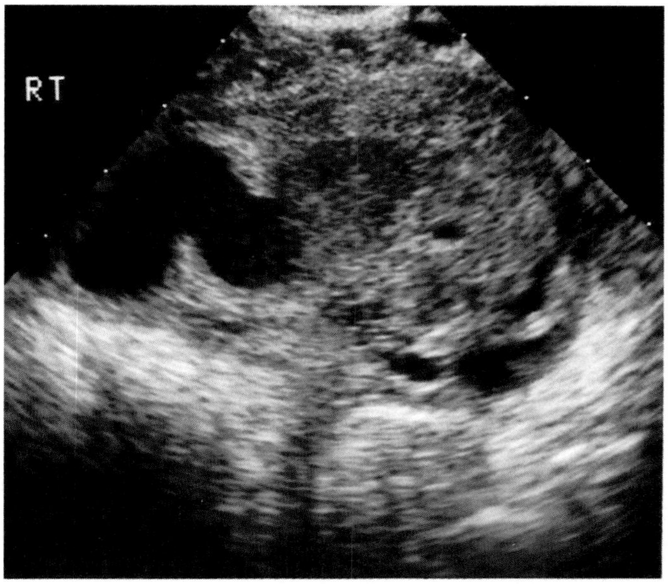

Figure 8-3

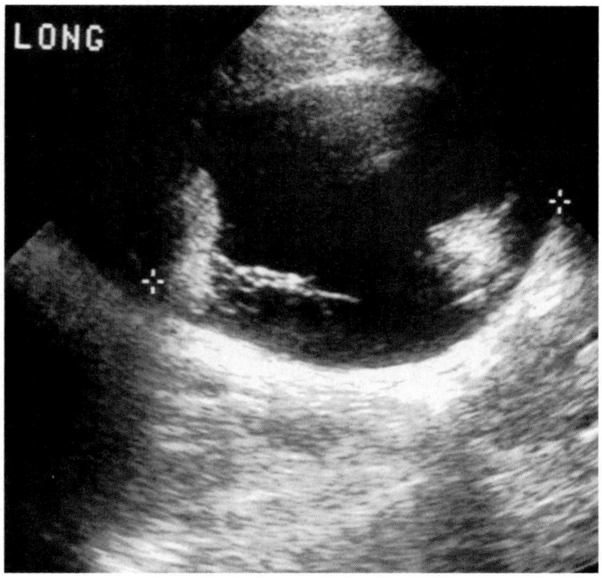

Figure 8-4

through 43

ms of four girls with pelvic pain. For each ...s listed below (Figures 8-1 through 8-4), select the ... diagnosis (A, B, C, D, or E) that is MOST closely associated with it. Each lettered diagnosis may be used once, more than once, or not at all.

40. Figure 8-1
41. Figure 8-2
42. Figure 8-3
43. Figure 8-4

(A) Theca lutein cyst
(B) Pyosalpinx
(C) Torsion
(D) Teratoma
(E) Cystadenoma

Pelvic pain in a young girl can be a diagnostic problem for the examining clinician. Ultrasonography has become the study of choice for the initial evaluation of these patients. Figure 8-1 is a longitudinal sonogram of the pelvis. It shows an ovoid, predominantly solid mass lying behind the bladder. The small hypoechoic areas in the periphery of the mass represent follicles and should suggest that the mass is an enlarged ovary (Figure 8-5). Ovarian torsion is the most likely diagnosis on the basis of the sonographic characteristics (**Option (C) is the correct answer to Question 40**). The absence of large cystic areas excludes both cystadenoma and theca lutein cysts. Benign teratoma is not a consideration, because it should be a complex mass containing a large fluid component and a small amount of solid material. Pyosalpinx is incorrect because it should have a tubular configuration and contain internal echoes.

Figure 8-2 is a longitudinal sonogram of the right ovary. The ovary is enlarged and contains multiple large cysts surrounded by soft tissue. The appearance is most consistent with theca lutein cysts (**Option (A) is the correct answer to Question 41**). None of the remaining options would demonstrate multiple large central and peripheral cysts. A torsed ovary could contain multiple cysts, but they would be peripheral and the ovary would be mostly echogenic with a predominance of soft tissue components. The other lesions are usually solitary, cystic masses.

Theca lutein cysts are nonneoplastic cysts that are thought to represent hyperstimulated follicles. They are found most often in adolescent girls or adult women with gestational trophoblastic disease or who are taking drugs to stimulate ovulation. In contrast to normal follicular and corpus luteum cysts, which are solitary and usually unilateral, theca lutein cysts are multiple and bilateral. The ovaries of affected patients may be larger than 25 cm in diameter.

Figure 8-3, a longitudinal sonogram of the right adnexa, shows a heterogeneous tortuous tubular structure containing debris and lying adjacent to a round, poorly defined solid mass with several peripheral cysts. The tubular component is the dilated fallopian tube, and the round mass is the enlarged ovary (Figure 8-6). The cysts within the ovary represent normal follicles. The planes around the ovary are poorly defined because of inflammation. The appearance should suggest pelvic inflammatory disease and pyosalpinx (**Option (B) is the correct answer to Question 42**). The presence of the dilated fallopian tube containing echogenic debris is characteristic of pyosalpinx and excludes the other diagnoses. The appearance of the ovary could mimic torsion, but torsion is rarely associated with a dilated fallopian tube.

The common causative organisms of pelvic inflammatory

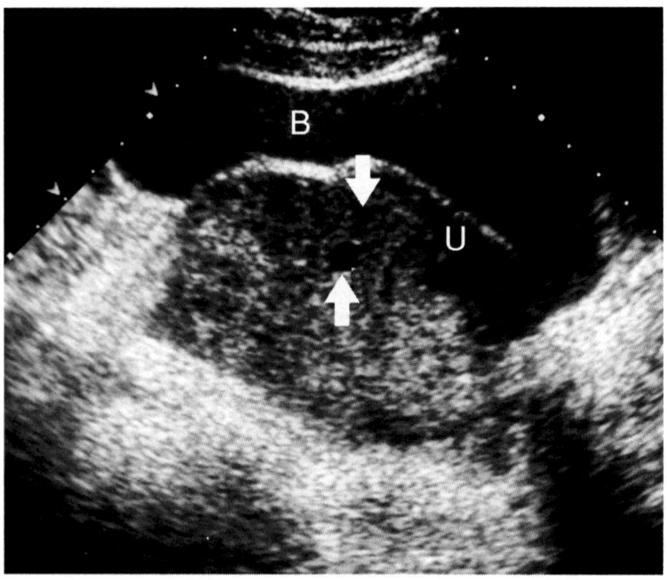

Figure 8-5 (Same as Figure 8-1). Adnexal torsion. A longitudinal sonogram in an 11-year-old girl shows an enlarged right ovary lying behind the bladder (B) and uterus (U). Two small cysts (arrows) are noted in the periphery of the ovary. Laparotomy showed torsion of a normal ovary that contained dilated follicles.

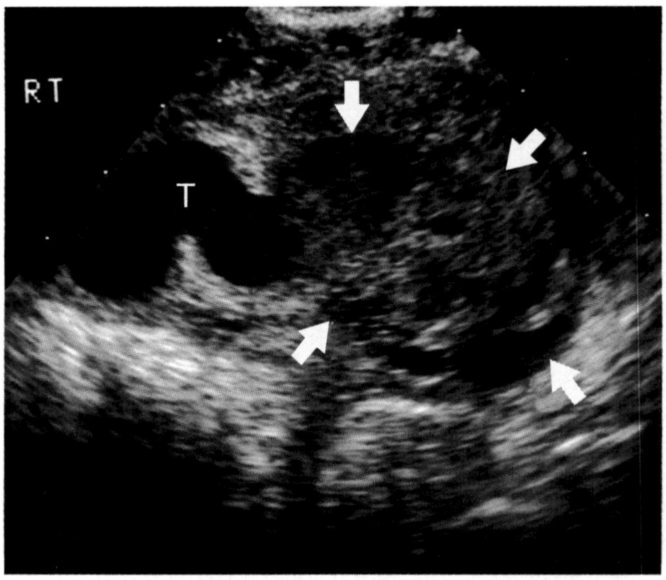

Figure 8-6 (Same as Figure 8-3). Pyosalpinx. A longitudinal sonogram of the right adnexa in a 15-year-old girl shows a tubular structure (T) with echogenic debris, representing an inflamed fallopian tube. The right ovary (arrows) is enlarged and contains several small follicles peripherally.

disease are *Neisseria gonorrhoeae*, *Chlamydia trachomatis*, and endogenous anaerobic organisms. The causative agent first infects the vagina and then ascends to the cervix and uterus. As the infection ascends, the fallopian tubes become filled with purulent exudate, producing a pyosalpinx. Peritoneal spillage of exudate from the tubal fimbrial openings may follow, with subsequent infection of the ovaries and parametria, leading to tubo-ovarian abscess. The frequency of tubo-ovarian abscess in patients with pelvic inflammatory disease is reported to be 7% to 10%.

As expected, the sonographic findings in patients with pelvic inflammatory disease vary with the extent of the inflammatory process. Early in the course of infection, there are minimal or no sonographic findings. Occasionally, the uterine outline is indistinct, a finding known as the indefinite-uterus sign (Figure 8-7). As shown in Figure 8-6, pyosalpinx appears as a tubular structure with internal echoes representing purulent debris. A mature tubo-ovarian abscess appears as a round, unilocular or multilocular cystic mass with irregular, thickened walls and internal debris (Figure 8-8). Fluid-debris levels or septations can be noted in the abscess cavity. Occasionally, the pyosalpinx and tubo-ovarian abscess contain so much debris that they appear echogenic and solid. However, there is usually enhanced through transmission of sound, indicating the cystic nature of the lesion.

Figure 8-4 is a longitudinal sonogram of the right adnexa. It displays a large, round, complex mass that is predominantly cystic, with peripheral echogenic nodules and a septation (Figure 8-9). There is through transmission. Benign teratoma is the most likely diagnosis on the basis of the sonographic characteristics **(Option (D) is the correct answer to Question 43)**. The presence of a solitary, round, cystic mass excludes the other options, except for cystadenoma. For cystadenoma to be a diagnostic possibility, there would have to be a hypoechoic or anechoic mass with thick walls and minimal or no soft tissue contents.

Cystic teratoma is the most common cause of a benign ovarian mass in a child. It is characterized pathologically by the presence of mural nodules, referred to as dermoid plugs or Rokitansky nodules. These plugs contain hair, fat, teeth, bone, or any combination of these elements. On sonography, the dermoid plug is an echogenic focus that protrudes from the inner wall of a chiefly cystic mass. The fluid-filled contents of the cyst represent either sebum or serous fluid. Sebum is liquid and homogeneous at body temperature and hence can mimic fluid on sonography. Benign teratomas are usually unilocular, but they can contain a few thin septa. The wall is typically

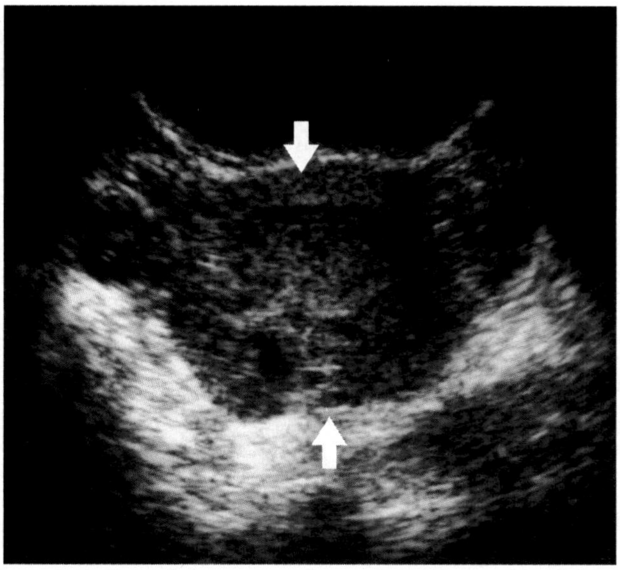

Figure 8-7. Pelvic inflammatory disease in a 16-year-old girl. A transverse sonogram of the pelvis shows an enlarged uterus (arrows). The planes between the uterus and ovaries (arrowheads) are poorly defined (indefinite-uterus sign).

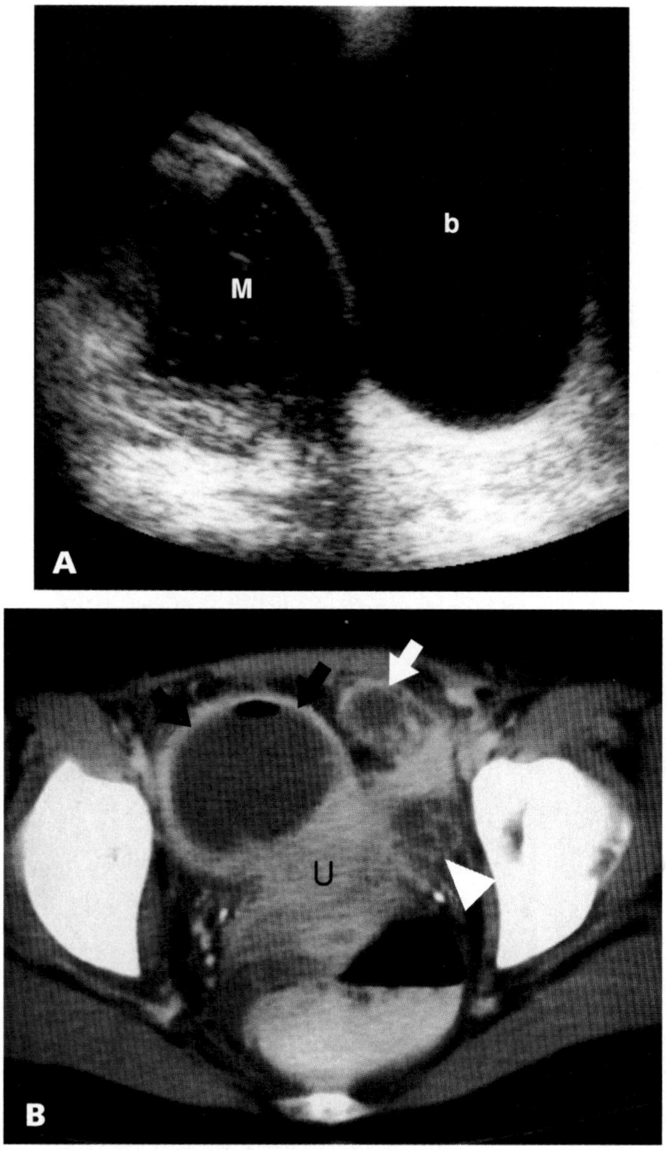

Figure 8-8. Tubo-ovarian abscess in a 12-year-old girl. (A) A longitudinal sonogram of the right ovary shows an anechoic mass (M) containing internal debris and lying behind the bladder (b). (B) A CT scan shows a well-defined fluid collection containing air and surrounded by an enhancing wall (black arrows). This was proven to be a right tubo-ovarian abscess at surgery. A smaller fluid collection (white arrow) is noted anterior to the left ovary (arrowhead). At surgery, this collection was found to be a left pyosalpinx. U = top of uterus.

smooth and between 2 and 5 mm thick.

Cystadenoma (Option (E)) does not correspond to any of the test images. Cystadenomas are rare tumors in children and account for fewer than 10% of benign ovarian neoplasms. The serous type is slightly more frequent than the mucinous type in childhood. Most cystadenomas are large, ranging from 4 to 20 cm in diameter, and present clinically as pelvic masses. On sonography, the tumor typically appears as a thick-walled mass with hypoechoic or anechoic contents (Figure 8-10). Fine echogenicity or septations within the mass are not unusual.

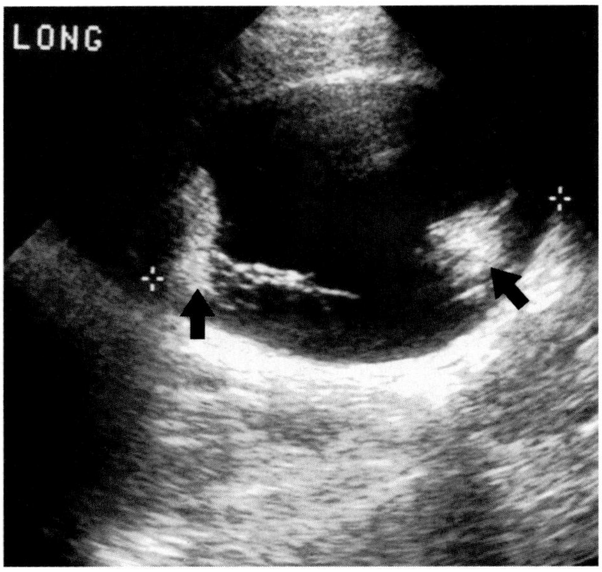

Figure 8-9 (Same as Figure 8-4). Ovarian teratoma. A longitudinal sonogram of the right ovary in a 15-year-old girl shows a cystic mass (between cursors) with peripheral echogenic mural nodules (arrows) and increased through transmission of sound.

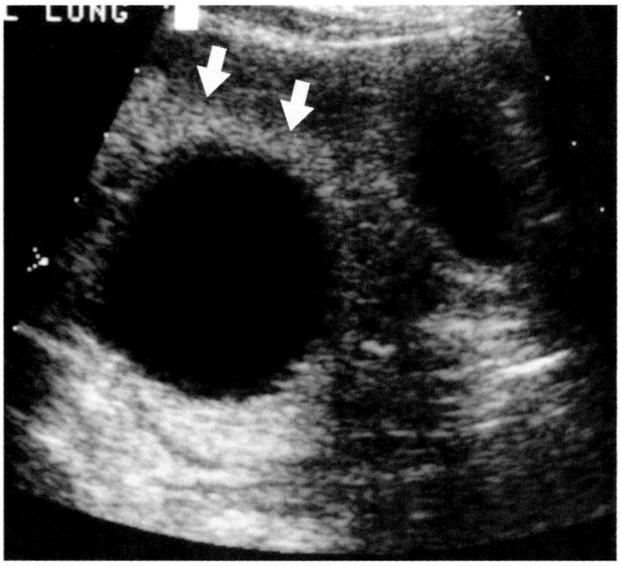

Figure 8-10. Cystadenoma in a 7-year-old girl. A longitudinal sonogram through the right pelvis demonstrates an 8-cm cystic lesion with a thick wall (arrows) and increased through transmission of sound. B = bladder.

Question 44

Concerning ovarian anatomy and development,

(A) the ovaries in neonates are posterolateral to the uterus
(B) the ovaries are infrequently seen in prepubertal girls
(C) multiple follicles are a normal finding in prepubertal girls
(D) most mature follicles are less than 1.5 cm in diameter
(E) the number of immature follicles is increased in patients with polycystic ovary disease
(F) the ovary is supplied by both uterine and ovarian arteries

An understanding of the variations in ovarian position, size, and morphology is important so that they are not mistaken for pathologic findings. The ovaries descend from the upper abdomen into the pelvis during fetal life. At birth, they lie within the superior margin of the broad ligaments. In some neonates, descent is arrested and the ovaries are found anywhere from the inferior edge of the kidneys down to the broad ligaments. Rarely, the ovaries descend below the broad ligaments and lie in the inguinal canal. They do not reach their normal adult position, posterolateral to the uterus, until puberty **(Option (A) is false).**

In the neonatal period, follicle-stimulating hormone (FSH) and estriol levels remain elevated, exerting an end-organ effect for 3 to 4 months. In a sonographic study of 77 infants, 1 day to 24 months of age, Cohen et al. in 1993 showed that mean ovarian volume in the first year of life was approximately 1.0 cm^3. The volume was somewhat lower during the second year of life, averaging 0.67 cm^3. The size of the ovaries during the first 2 years of life is quite variable, however. In the study by Cohen et al., the upper limit of the normal range was 3.6 cm^3 in the first 3 months, 2.7 cm^3 from 4 to 12 months, and 1.7 cm^3 from 12 to 24 months.

In studies of prepubertal girls between 2 and 13 years of age, Salardi et al. and Orsini et al. have reported that the mean ovarian volume ranges from 0.75 to 2.3 cm^3 and from 0.75 to 4.18 cm^3, respectively (Figure 8-11). Of further note, Orsini et al. reported that at least one ovary can be imaged by transabdominal sonography in approximately 80% of children younger than 5 years and in 90% of those older than 5 years. Both ovaries can be seen in approximately 65% and 80% of patients younger and older than 5 years, respectively **(Option (B) is false).**

The ovaries are relatively stable in size until 6 to 7 years of age, when an age-related growth spurt starts. As puberty approaches, the greatest increase in ovarian size occurs. Hall has described normal measurements in postpubertal females as 2.5 to 5.0 cm long, 1.5 to 3.0 cm wide, and 0.6 to 1.5 cm thick. These measurements suggest a volume of between 1.2 and 11.8 cm^3. In a study of ovarian volumes of menstruating women, Cohen et al. showed that the volume ranged from 4.0 to 15.6 cm^3. Ovarian volume peaks in the third decade.

Small cysts representing underdeveloped primordial folli-

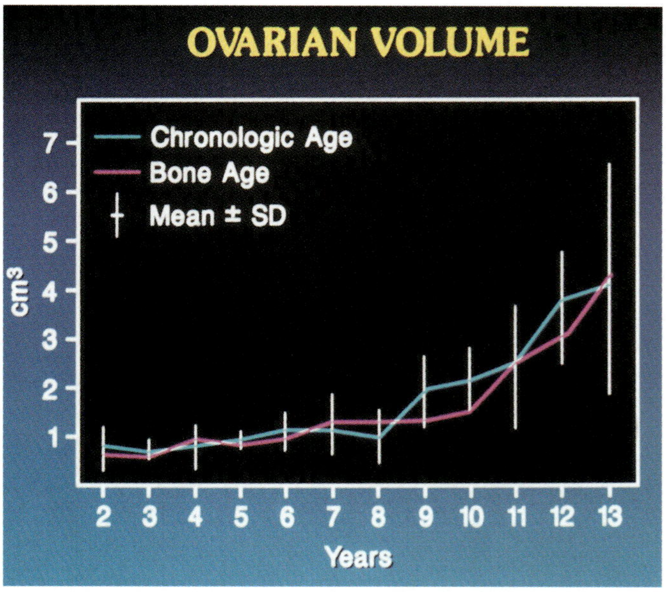

Figure 8-11. Relationship of normal ovarian volumes to both chronological age and bone age. (Adapted from Salardi et al. [34].)

cles are frequent in the ovaries of neonates and infants younger than 24 months. The follicles in premenarchal children are believed to be secondary to pulsatile secretion of low levels of gonadotropin-releasing hormones. Cohen et al. described the appearance of the ovaries sonographically in infants younger than 2 years and in premenarchal girls aged between 2 and 12 years. They detected cysts (i.e., follicles), typically multiple, in 84% of ovaries in infants younger than 2 years and in 68% of ovaries in children aged 2 through 12 years (Figure 8-12) (**Option (C) is true**). In the remaining infants, the ovaries were homogeneous or minimally heterogeneous. The follicular diameter in premenarchal girls younger than 12 years was usually less than 9 mm, with a mean of 6 to 7 mm. Macrocysts greater than 9 mm in diameter were found in 18% of all cystic ovaries in girls younger than 24 months and in 8% of ovaries in girls aged between 2 and 12 years.

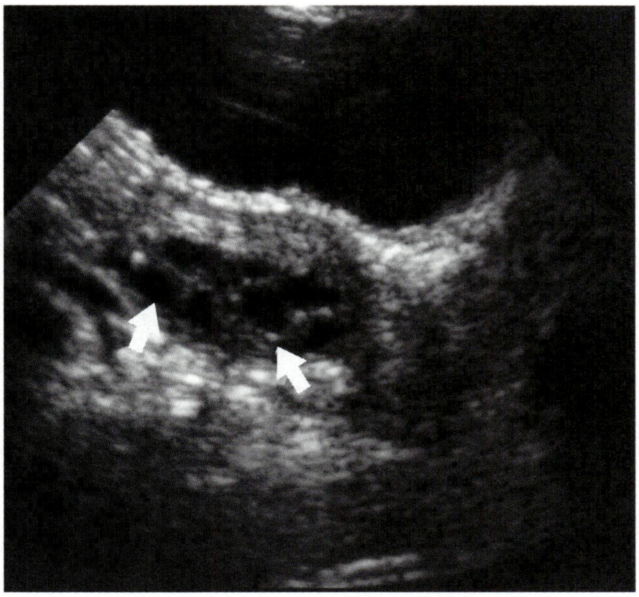

Figure 8-12. Normal prepubertal ovary. A longitudinal sonogram in a 4-year-old girl shows small follicles, measuring less than 9 mm in diameter, in the right ovary (arrows).

The appearance of the pediatric ovary on CT is similar to that reported on sonography. In a series of 125 healthy female children and adolescents, Rigsby and Siegel reported that mean ovarian volume ranged between 0.4 and 3.8 cm^3 in girls aged 2 to 12 years and between 4.3 and 6.9 cm^3 in girls aged 12 years and older. Cysts were seen in about 70% of ovaries, regardless of patient age.

With activation of the hypothalamic-pituitary-ovarian axis at puberty, the ovary becomes more ovoid and descends deeper into the pelvis, ultimately lying posterolateral to the uterus although not necessarily at the same horizontal level. Occasionally, the ovaries fail to descend completely and remain high in the pelvis, lying dorsal or cephalad to the uterus. They can also be found posterior to the uterus if ligamentous attachments are lax.

The appearance of the ovary, as well as its size and position, changes with hormonal stimulation. Grossly, the ovary is composed of two layers: an outer cortical layer and an inner medullary layer. The cortex is larger than the medulla and contains the follicles that undergo maturation. The medulla is composed of fibrous tissue without follicles. Under the influence of pituitary gonadotropins, the ovary goes through three phases during each menstrual cycle: the follicular phase, ovulation, and the luteal phase.

In the follicular phase (days 1 to 14), several previously dormant primordial or immature follicles (composed of an oocyte surrounded by a single layer of epithelium) begin to develop in response to FSH, forming the antral follicles. By day 8 or 9, a dominant follicle, now termed the Graafian follicle, which is destined for ovulation, emerges and continues to mature under the influence of estrogen. The other stimulated follicles, which do not progress to ovulation, will atrophy. By the time of ovulation, the dominant follicle has reached the surface of the ovary. The mature Graafian follicle ruptures in midcycle after the release of luteinizing hormone (LH). With ovulation and extrusion of the ovum, there is a sudden decrease in follicular size. The walls of the follicle collapse inward, and blood accumulates in the lumen. Almost simultaneously with ovulation, a small amount of fluid can be seen in the cul-de-sac. In the luteal phase (days 15 to 28), the granulosa cells remaining in the follicular wall enlarge and accumulate lipid and lutein to form the corpus luteum. The corpus luteum remains for 14 days, after which it rapidly involutes unless the ovum has been fertilized. Eventually, the corpus luteum atrophies and is replaced by collagen-rich cicatricial tissue, forming the corpus albicans.

Developing follicles are between 1 and 2 cm in diameter, and the dominant follicle can reach a diameter of 2.5 cm at maturity. Corpus luteum cysts generally range between 2 and 3 cm in diameter (**Option (D) is false**). Most follicular and corpus luteum cysts can be seen by sonography. Follicular cysts are usually unilocular, anechoic, or hypoechoic structures (Figure

8-13). Corpus luteum cysts may be sonolucent or complex, containing debris or septations as a result of hemorrhage (Figure 8-14).

The differential diagnosis of the normal ovary with multiple follicles includes the spectrum of polycystic ovary disease. This disease is diagnosed on the basis of a combination of clinical, biochemical, and sonographic criteria. It was first described by Stein and Leventhal as a syndrome consisting of amenorrhea, obesity, hirsutism, and sterility in association with bilateral large and cystic ovaries. It is now recognized that polycystic ovary disease represents a spectrum of clinical and pathologic findings and that most patients do not have the full constellation of findings. The consistent clinical feature is chronic anovulation. The endocrine profile of these patients reveals decreased levels of FSH and elevated levels of LH. As a result of the hormonal imbalance, excessive androgen is produced by the ovarian stroma. The ovary continues to produce follicles, but they do not progress to maturation and ovulation.

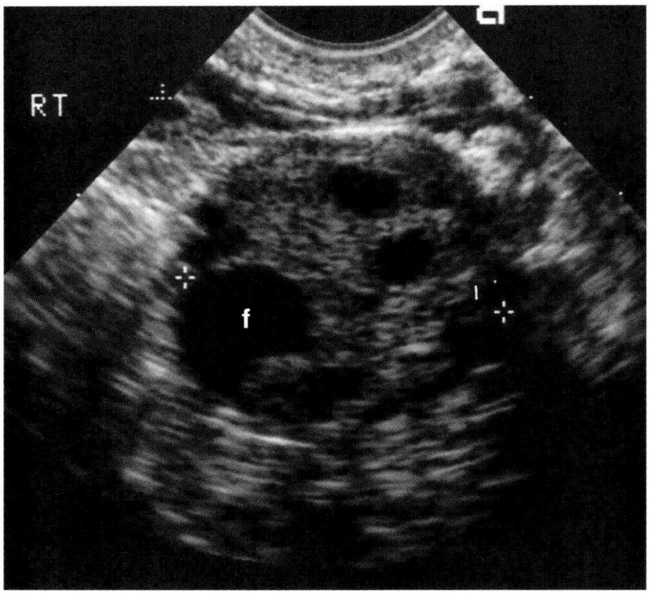

Figure 8-13. Dominant Graafian follicle in a 16-year-old girl. A transverse image from an endovaginal sonogram of the right ovary (calipers) demonstrates a developing follicle (f) measuring 20 × 10 mm. This examination was performed on day 10 of the menstrual cycle.

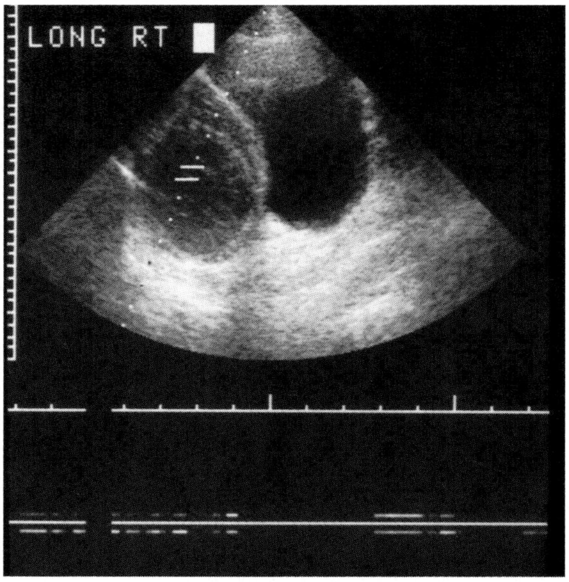

Figure 8-14. Corpus luteum cyst in an 18-year-old girl. A longitudinal Doppler sonogram of the right ovary shows a fluid-filled follicle with scattered internal echoes and increased through transmission of sound. The Doppler cursor is in the center of the lesion, and the absence of Doppler signal confirms the cystic nature of the lesion. The follicle measures 2.5 cm at greatest diameter. The examination was performed on day 22 of the menstrual cycle.

Although Stein and Leventhal originally described bilaterally enlarged ovaries, subsequent studies have made it obvious that there can be normal-sized ovaries and unilateral abnormalities. The two pathologic features of polycystic ovary disease that are consistently identified are hyperstimulated ovarian stroma, caused by the elevated androgen levels, and an increased number of immature and atretic follicles (**Option (E) is true**). The stromal changes range from mild prominence to extensive capsular thickening.

The sonographic features, like the clinical and pathologic findings, are variable. In the studies by Yeh et al. and Hann et al., approximately 70% of patients with polycystic ovary disease had bilaterally enlarged ovaries (mean volume, 14 cm^3). The ovaries were spherical rather than the normal ovoid shape. Normal-sized ovaries were found in 30% of the patients.

Other important sonographic findings in patients with polycystic ovary disease are an increased number of small developing follicles (Figure 8-15) and hyperechoic stroma. Yeh et al. and Parisi et al. found that approximately 75% of ovaries had five or more follicles, ranging between 5 and 8 mm in diameter, in each ovary. By comparison, control subjects had no more than three developing follicles, smaller than 8 mm in diameter, in each ovary. However, Hann et al. reported that only

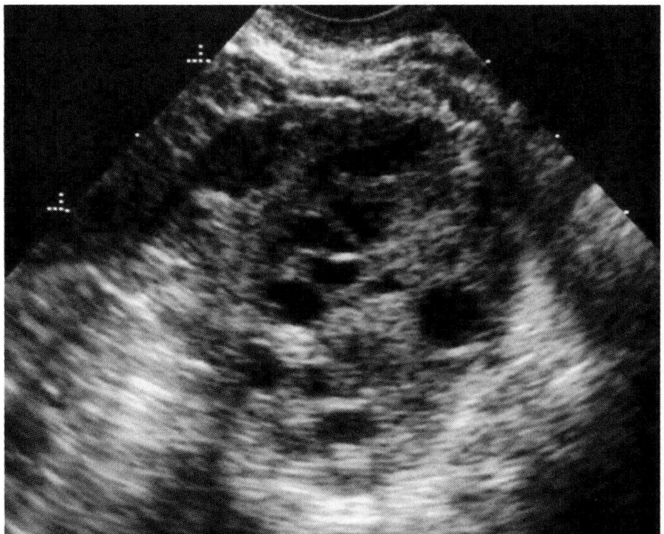

Figure 8-15. Polycystic ovary disease in a 17-year-old girl. A longitudinal sonogram demonstrates an enlarged right ovary containing multiple small follicles (<8 mm in diameter).

39% of patients had small follicles (smaller than 10 mm). The other patients had no discrete follicles. The ovaries were either diffusely hypoechoic or isoechoic relative to the uterus. The discrepancies in the sonographic appearances may reflect differences in technology or the difficulty of detecting the ovaries by transabdominal sonography.

Pache et al. addressed the sonographic appearance of the ovarian stroma. They used transvaginal sonography to study 52 patients, 94% of whom had moderately to markedly increased stromal echogenicity. These investigators found that this feature was the most sensitive (sensitivity, 94%) and specific (specificity, 90%) sonographic sign of polycystic ovary disease. However, they also noted that echogenicity is subjective and therefore may be difficult to use as a diagnostic criterion in clinical practice. They recommended that the combination of ovarian volume and follicular size be used. This combination yielded a sensitivity of 92% and a specificity of 97%.

More recently, there has been more widespread use of Doppler sonography for evaluating ovarian pathologic findings. Therefore, recognition of variations in normal perfusion is important. The ovary receives its blood supply via both the main ovarian artery (arising from the aorta) and the adnexal branches of the uterine artery **(Option (F) is true).** On color flow Doppler sonography, intraovarian arteries appear as short, straight branches. In a series of children and adolescents, Quillin and Siegel found color flow signal in about 80% of prepubertal ovaries and 90% of postpubertal ovaries (Figure 8-16). Duplex Doppler flow varies with the phase of the menstrual cycle. During the early follicular phase (days 0 to 7) and late luteal phase (days 18 to 28), impedance is high and the end-diastolic velocity is low or absent. In the late follicular phase and early luteal phase (days 11 to 17), the end-diastolic flow velocity increases (Figure 8-17), reflecting decreased vascular impedance. Impedance can be quantified by the use of the resistive index (RI). The RI from the late follicular phase to the early luteal phase is approximately 0.5, but it increases during the early and late phases of the cycle to close to 1.0.

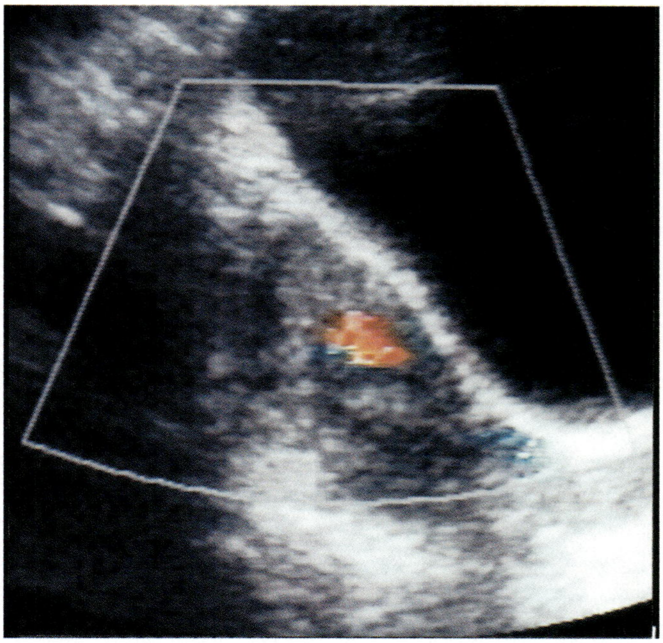

Figure 8-16. Normal ovarian vasculature. A color flow image shows intraovarian arteries in a 12-year-old girl.

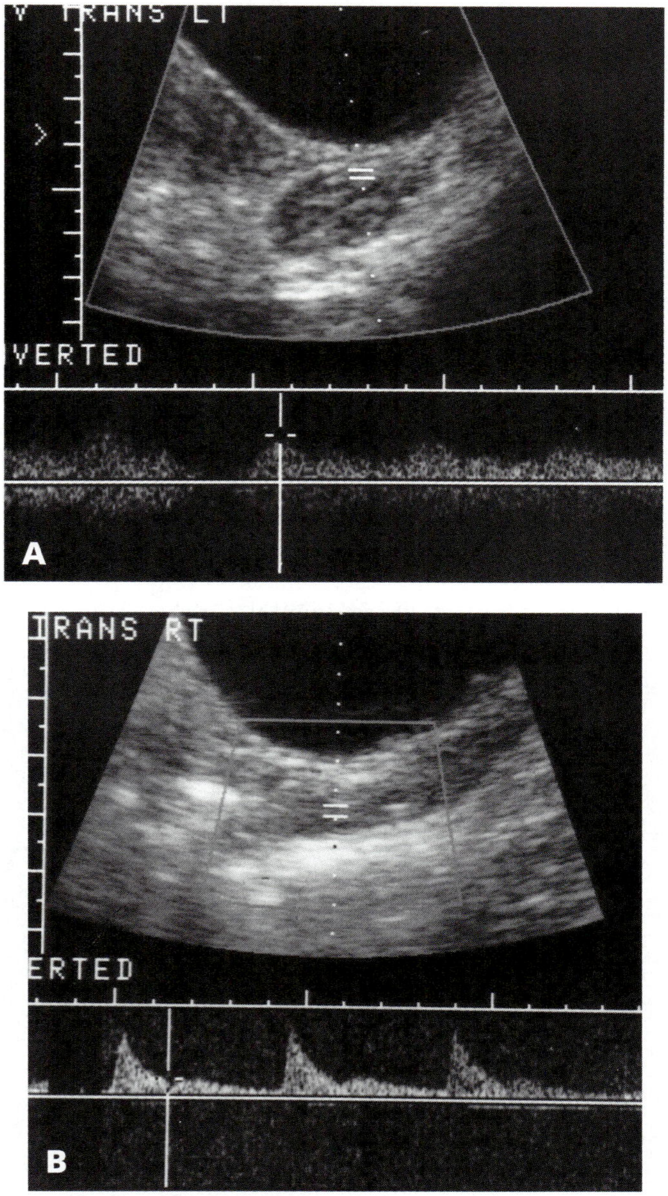

Figure 8-17. Normal ovarian Doppler waveforms. (A) A sonogram of a 14-year-old girl on day 12 of the menstrual cycle shows a low-impedance waveform with high levels of diastolic flow (RI = 0.42). (B) A sonogram of a 16-year-old girl on day 22 of the cycle shows a high-impedance waveform (RI = 0.71).

Question 45

Concerning pathologic ovarian cysts in childhood,

(A) they are a cause of true isosexual precocious puberty
(B) most are 1 to 2 cm in diameter
(C) the typical sonographic appearance of a hemorrhagic cyst is that of a heterogeneous, echogenic mass
(D) acute hemorrhagic cysts have a high signal intensity on both T1- and T2-weighted MR images
(E) short-tau inversion-recovery images are useful in differentiating between hemorrhagic ovarian cyst and teratoma

Cysts account for the majority of ovarian masses. In neonates, ovarian cysts result from exaggeration of normal follicular development secondary to *in utero* stimulation by maternal hormones. In these patients, the cyst can be discovered incidentally on prenatal sonography or can present postnatally as a palpable abdominal or pelvic mass. Large cysts can cause intestinal obstruction or respiratory compromise. Neonatal ovarian cysts can be classified as simple or as complicated by torsion or hemorrhage. A simple cyst is anechoic and has an imperceptible wall. A complicated cyst contains septa, retracting clot, or a fluid-debris level and often has an echogenic wall (Figure 8-18). Neonatal ovarian cysts usually require surgery, but there have been a few cases of spontaneous resolution.

Functional ovarian cysts have been reported in association with precocious puberty. Precocious puberty is defined as the onset of pubertal changes in patients younger than 8 years. This condition can be classified into four groups: (1) true isosexual precocity, characterized by increased serum gonadotropin levels in response to the gonadotropin-releasing factor stimulation test; (2) pseudosexual precocity, characterized by increased estrogen levels but low gonadotropin levels; (3) premature adrenarche, characterized by isolated pubic hair development and increased levels of adrenal androgens; and (4) premature thelarche, characterized by isolated breast development with normal levels of prepubertal hormones. True isosexual precocious puberty is the result of idiopathic activation of the hypothalamic-pituitary-gonadal axis or lesions of the pituitary gland or hypothalamus (**Option (A) is false**). Causes of pseudosexual precocity include functioning ovarian cysts, ovarian neoplasms (granulosa-theca cell tumors, arrhenoblastomas, thecomas, and choriocarcinomas), adrenal adenomas and carcinomas, neurofibromatosis, McCune-Albright syndrome (precocious puberty and polyostotic fibrous dysplasia), and ingestion of estrogen compounds.

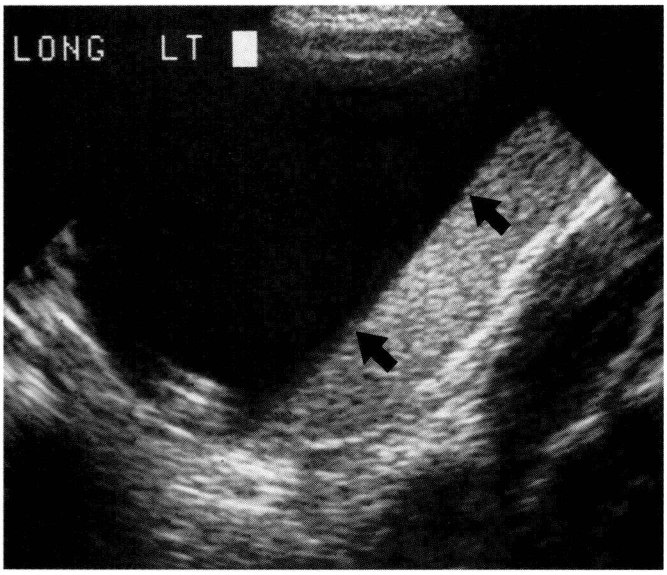

Figure 8-18. Ovarian cyst in a newborn girl. A longitudinal sonogram of the pelvis shows a large cystic mass with increased through transmission of sound and a fluid-debris level (arrows). A torsed hemorrhagic cyst was confirmed at surgery.

The primary role of sonography in patients with precocious puberty is to determine ovarian and uterine sizes and the ratio of corpus length to cervix length. Bilateral ovarian enlargement is indicative of true isosexual precocity (Figure 8-19), whereas unilateral ovarian enlargement is typical of pseudosexual precocity (Figure 8-20). In a sonographic study of 32 girls younger than 8 years with isosexual precocious puberty, King et al. reported mean ovarian volumes of 4.6 cm^3 in those with true isosexual precocity, 4.1 cm^3 in those with pseudosexual precocity, and less than 1 cm^3 in those with premature adrenarche and in a control population. Small follicles (<9 mm) were not a reliable indicator of precocious puberty and were found in slightly more than 50% of both healthy girls and girls with precocious puberty.

In adolescent girls, ovarian cysts result when a Graafian follicle continues to grow after failed ovulation or when a corpus luteum fails to collapse after ovulation. Most cysts are discovered incidentally on pelvic sonograms performed for other reasons. However, a cyst can present as a palpable adnexal mass or cause pain from hemorrhage, rupture, torsion, or pressure.

The sonographic appearance of pathologic ovarian cysts in adolescent girls is variable, depending on the presence or absence of hemorrhage and its age. As discussed above, normal follicles are up to 3 cm in diameter. The definition of a pathologic cyst is arbitrarily accepted as one that is greater than 3 cm in diameter (**Option (B) is false**). Nonhemorrhagic cysts are usually follicular cysts. Most are anechoic, thin-walled, unilocular masses, exhibiting posterior acoustic enhancement (Figure 8-21). Internal septations and debris are seen occasionally. The natural history of simple cysts in adolescent girls is complete involution over time, usually within one or two menstrual cycles.

Hemorrhagic ovarian cysts are usually of luteal origin. There is a wide spectrum of sonographic findings, reflecting the age of the blood. Acute blood is classically anechoic, progressing subacutely to a heterogeneous appearance as clotting and thrombus retraction occur and finally again becoming anechoic with clot lysis. Studies by Baltarowich et al. and Reynolds et al. have shown that approximately 85% of hemorrhagic ovarian cysts exhibit heterogeneous echogenicity (**Option (C) is true**) and are septated, have a fluid-debris level, or contain clotted, retracting blood (Figure 8-22). The remaining cysts are diffusely homogeneous and either hypo- or hyper-

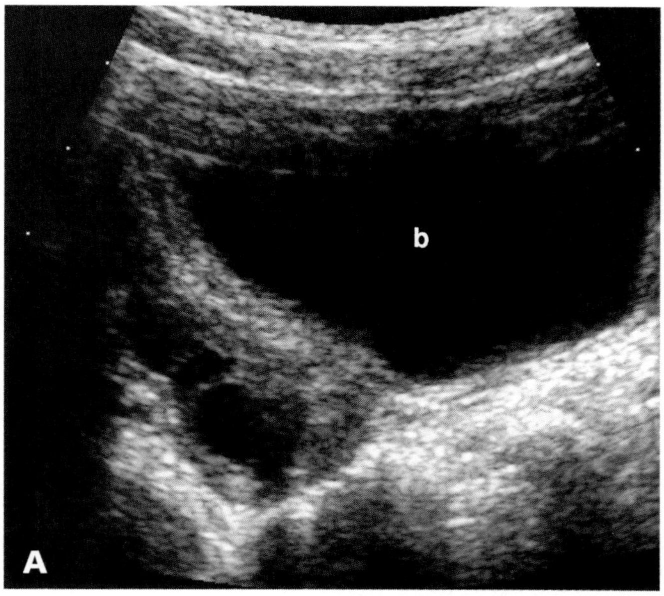

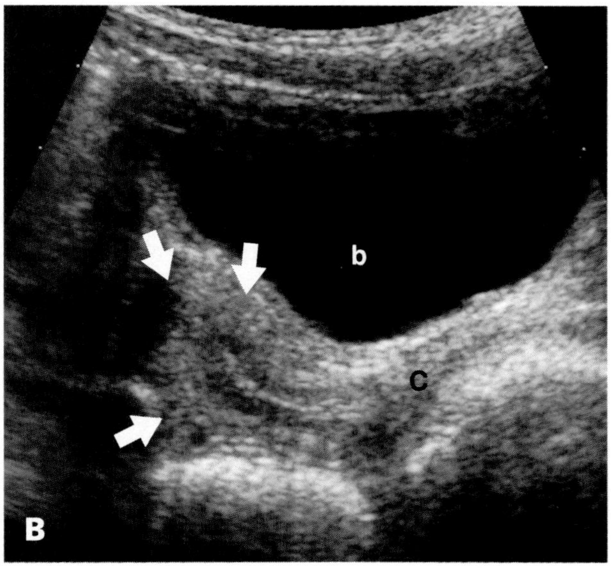

Figure 8-19. True isosexual precocity in a 4-year-old girl. (A) A transverse sonogram shows an enlarged ovary (volume, 4 cm^3) containing small follicles (<9 mm in diameter). (B) A longitudinal sonogram shows an enlarged uterus with a thickened endometrial stripe and an adult configuration, i.e., fundus (arrows) larger than cervix (C). Typically, the prepubertal uterus is tubular and there is no differentiation between the fundus and the cervix. b = bladder.

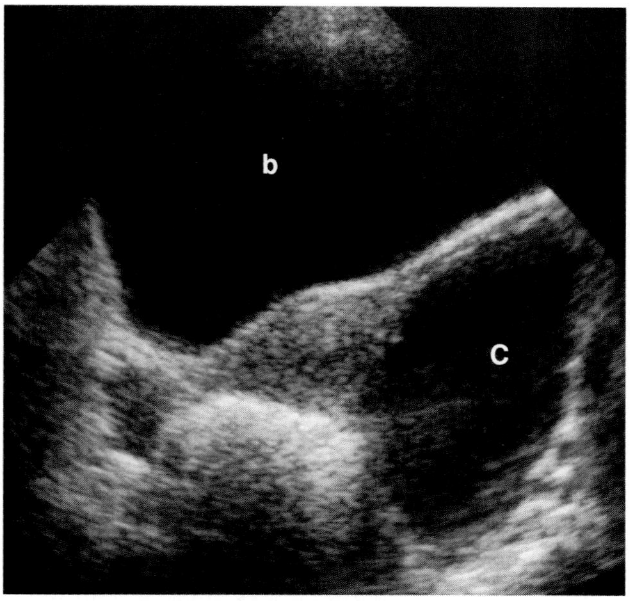

Figure 8-20. Pseudosexual precocity secondary to an autonomous cyst. A longitudinal scan of the pelvis shows a 4-cm cyst (C) in the left ovary. b = bladder.

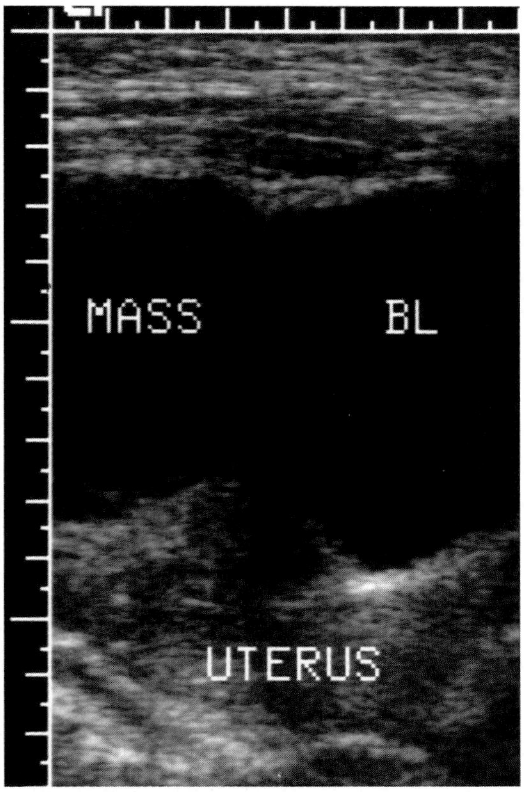

Figure 8-21. Nonhemorrhagic ovarian cyst in an 18-year-old girl. A transverse sonogram of the pelvis shows a 5-cm anechoic mass with imperceptible walls in the expected region of the right ovary. BL = bladder.

echoic relative to surrounding soft tissues. Approximately 90% of lesions have increased through transmission of sound, signifying their fluid content.

The presence of a hyperechoic mass is not pathognomonic of hemorrhagic ovarian cyst. Some teratomas have this sonographic pattern. Differentiation requires identification of calcification or fat, which are features of teratomas, but not of cysts. A complex cystic mass is also nonspecific, and the differential diagnosis includes hemorrhagic cyst, ovarian teratoma, tubo-ovarian or appendiceal abscess, and ectopic pregnancy. Ectopic pregnancy and tubo-ovarian or appendiceal abscess can be diagnosed by clinical and laboratory data. Teratomas and hemorrhagic cysts generally can be distinguished by serial sonography. Hemorrhagic ovarian cysts decrease in size and be-

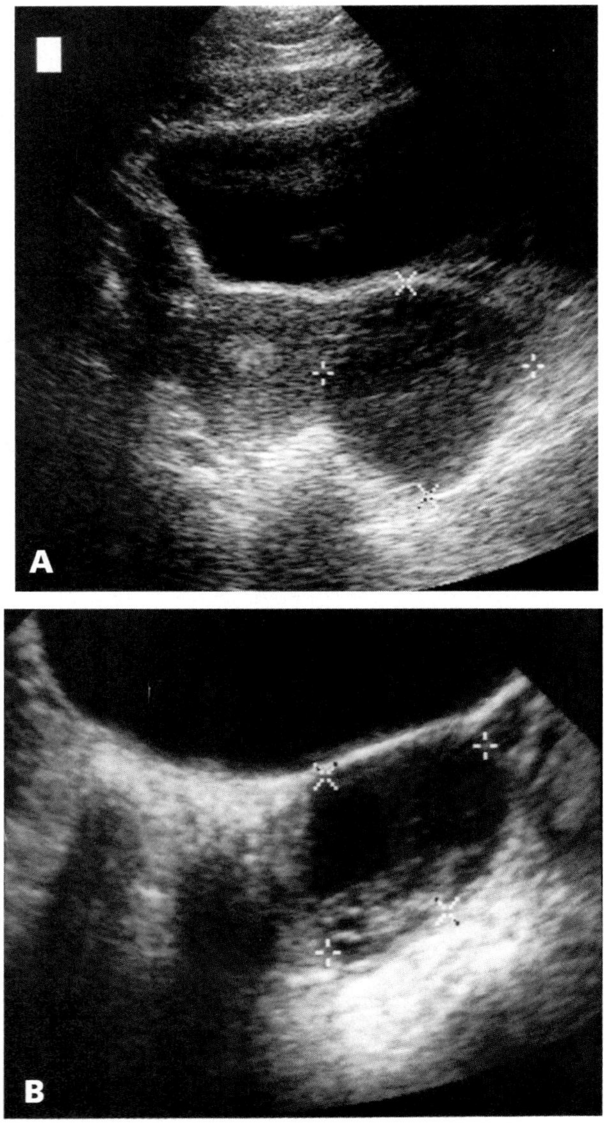

Figure 8-22. Hemorrhagic ovarian cysts. (A) A transverse sonogram in a 14-year-old girl shows a cystic mass (calipers) with internal echoes. There is minimal increased through transmission of sound. (B) A transverse sonogram of the left ovary of a 15-year-old girl demonstrates a cystic mass (calipers) exhibiting increased through transmission of sound and containing a peripheral clot.

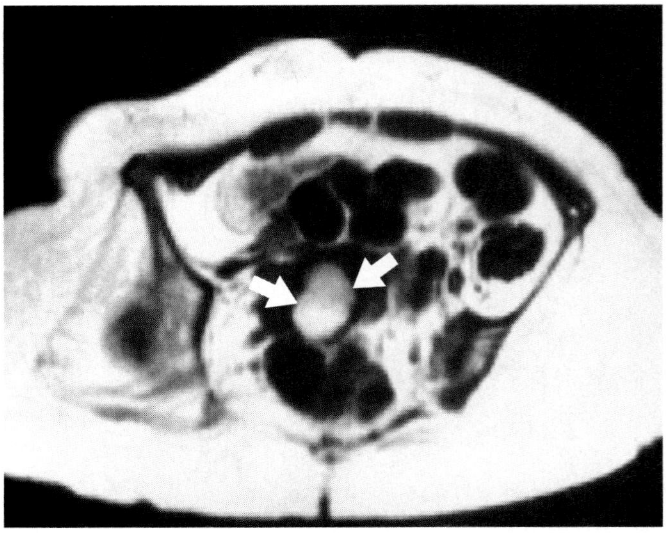

SE 500/17

Figure 8-23. Hemorrhagic ovarian cyst in a 16-year-old girl. A transaxial T1-weighted MR image shows a hyperintense cyst (arrows) in the right ovary. The signal intensity is consistent with subacute blood.

come anechoic over time before involuting completely, whereas cystic neoplasms remain unchanged or increase in size. Similar to simple cysts, involution usually occurs within one or two menstrual cycles. Cystic masses that persist for several cycles should be investigated further by CT, MRI, or percutaneous or surgical aspiration to exclude a cystic neoplasm.

The MRI appearance of blood also varies with the age of the blood. Most acute hematomas (less than 7 days old) exhibit low to intermediate signal intensity on T1-weighted images and low intensity on T2-weighted images (**Option (D) is false**). This appearance relates to the high concentration of deoxyhemoglobin in the erythrocytes. Subacute hematomas (1 week to several months old) appear bright on T1-weighted images because of the formation of methemoglobin. The signal intensity on T2-weighted images is variable (Figure 8-23). In the early subacute stage, when methemoglobin is intracellular, it may be decreased. Following erythrocyte lysis, high intensity on T2-weighted images is seen. Eventually, the methemoglobin breaks down and the central component of the hematoma liquifies. In the chronic stage, the hematoma appears similar to other fluid collections, manifesting low signal intensity on T1-weighted images and high intensity on T2-weighted images.

Fat-suppressed sequences, such as short-tau inversion-recovery, are used to increase the contrast between blood and fat. Signal from fat is nulled on STIR images. Blood is associated with an increased amount of free water, and hence the T1 and T2 relaxation times are usually prolonged; as a result, the blood exhibits a higher signal intensity than does nulled fat, which has a dark signal. Fibrosis and calcification also have low signal intensities on STIR images. Identification of fat or calcification on STIR sequences supports the diagnosis of teratoma rather than a hemorrhagic cyst (**Option (E) is true**).

Question 46

Concerning ovarian teratomas in children and adolescents,

(A) most are malignant
(B) most benign lesions are hypoechoic
(C) hair or fat lies in a dependent position with aqueous fluid on top
(D) hair causes low signal intensity on T1- and T2-weighted MR images
(E) tumors that contain more than 50% soft tissue elements by volume are usually malignant
(F) Doppler sonography shows peripheral flow in benign lesions

Approximately 65% of ovarian tumors in children and adolescents are benign. Cystic teratoma is by far the most common tumor, accounting for more than 90% of all benign ovarian neoplasms. The remaining benign tumors are usually cystadenomas. Approximately 90% of teratomas are benign (**Option (A) is false**).

Cystic teratomas are congenital lesions, arising from pluripotential germinal cells. Although they can occur in pre- and postpubertal girls, the vast majority in the pediatric population (>80%) are found in postpubertal girls. About two thirds of patients present with asymptomatic palpable masses, which can be abdominal because of extension outside of the pelvis. Approximately one third of patients present with acute abdominal or pelvic pain caused by hemorrhage, torsion, or rupture of the tumor.

Ovarian teratomas are usually unilateral, but bilateral tumors have been reported in 10% to 20% of patients. They can vary from 0.5 to 30 cm in maximum dimension, but most measure between 5 and 10 cm in diameter. Benign teratomas occasionally contain a few thin septations, dividing them into two or more compartments. The wall of the teratoma is usually smooth and 2 to 5 mm thick.

Because they arise from all three germ layers, teratomas can have variable sonographic appearances, depending on the relative amounts of sebum, serous fluid, calcium, hair, and fat. The most common sonographic appearance of a benign teratoma is that of a well-circumscribed, predominantly hypoechoic mass (**Option (B) is true**) with echogenic mural nodules. In the study by Sisler and Siegel, 66% of ovarian teratomas had this appearance. The hypoechoic component corresponds to sebum. Pure sebum mimics simple fluid on sonography because it is liquid at body temperature and lacks a significant number of interfaces. The hyperechoic nodules represent dermoid plugs or Rokitansky nodules. These nodules are a classic sign of benign teratoma. They typically protrude from the inner wall of the cystic mass, forming an acute angle with the wall, and they tend to be oval or round. The echogenicity reflects the admixture of tissues, i.e., soft tissue, hair, fat, or calcifications (Figure 8-24).

Acoustic shadowing is another classic sign of cystic teratoma. Sisler and Siegel and Buy et al. reported acoustic shadowing in approximately 50% of ovarian lesions. Acoustic shadowing does not necessarily imply calcified material, such as teeth, but instead can represent a matted mixture of sebum and hair. At times, posterior shadowing from hair or sebum completely obscures visualization of the back wall of the tumor, the "tip of the iceberg" sign. A fat-fluid or hair-fluid level (Figure 8-25) is a unique but less frequent sonographic finding

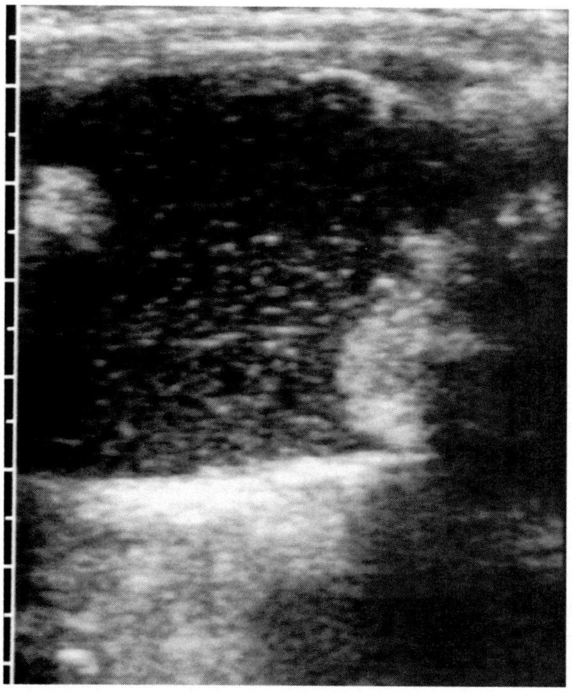

Figure 8-24. Ovarian teratoma in a 2-year-old girl. A longitudinal sonogram of the right adnexa shows a complex mass containing scattered low-level echoes and large echogenic mural nodules. At histopathologic examination, the teratoma contained sebum and the nodules contained hair, fat, and calcification.

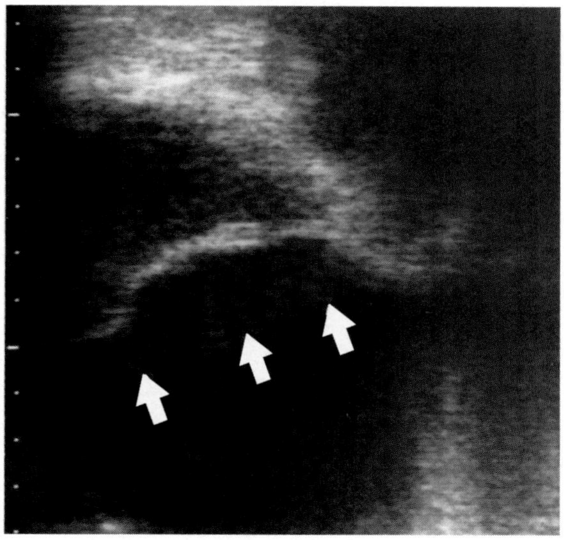

Figure 8-25. Ovarian teratoma. A transverse sonogram of the left ovary shows a complex mass with debris (arrows) floating on fluid. The level shifted when the patient changed position. Surgery demonstrated a benign teratoma containing sebum, fat, and hair.

in ovarian teratomas. In such tumors, fat or hair floats on sebum or serous fluid (**Option (C) is false**). This appearance is different from that seen in hemorrhagic ovarian cysts, in which serous fluid lies on top with proteinaceous debris from old blood in a dependent position.

Although most teratomas are complex on sonography, the spectrum ranges from purely cystic to completely solid. Anechoic or purely cystic teratomas result when the internal contents are made up almost exclusively of serous fluid or sebum. Small mural nodules, usually less than 5 mm in diameter, are seen on pathologic examination, but are too small to be detected by sonography (Figure 8-26). Predominantly solid tumors contain teeth, cartilage, hair, fat, and a sparse amount of fluid or sebaceous material, which results in a very echogenic mass (Figure 8-27).

CT and MRI have improved the ability to characterize the internal morphology of ovarian masses. The diagnosis of benign teratoma is easy on CT when fatty elements or a combination of fat and calcification is identified within a predominantly cystic ovarian mass (Figure 8-28). Other findings in patients with benign cystic teratomas are nodules, fat-fluid levels, and floating debris. In a series of 38 patients with 41 benign cystic teratomas, Buy et al. reported fat in 93%, teeth or calcifications in 56%, mural nodules in 81%, tufts of hair in 65%, and fat-fluid levels in 12%. Benign teratomas have different signal intensities on MRI depending on their tissue composition. Fat appears as an area of high signal intensity on T1-weighted images, whereas serous fluid has low signal intensity. Both fat and serous fluid display high signal intensity on T2-weighted sequences (Figure 8-29). Calcifications, teeth, bone, hair, and fibrous tissue cause low signal intensity on both pulse

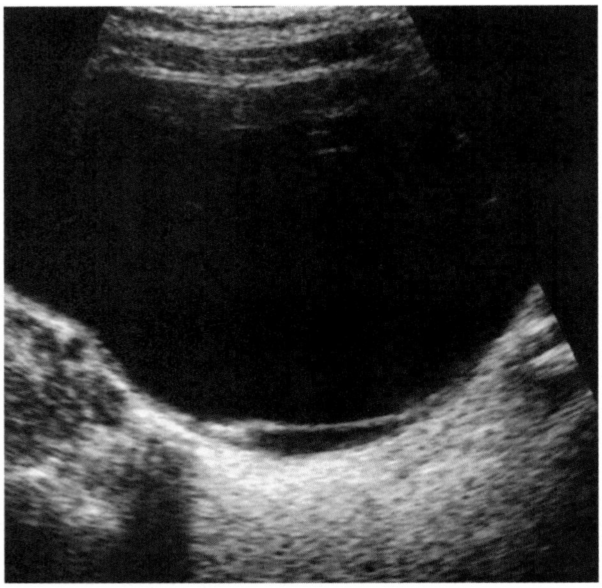

Figure 8-26. Anechoic teratoma mimicking a simple cyst in a 13-year-old girl. A transverse sonogram through the right adnexa shows a large cystic mass with a thin wall. The mass did not involute after several menstrual cycles, and surgery was performed. At pathologic examination, the lesion contained sebum and a 5-mm mural nodule not visible by sonography.

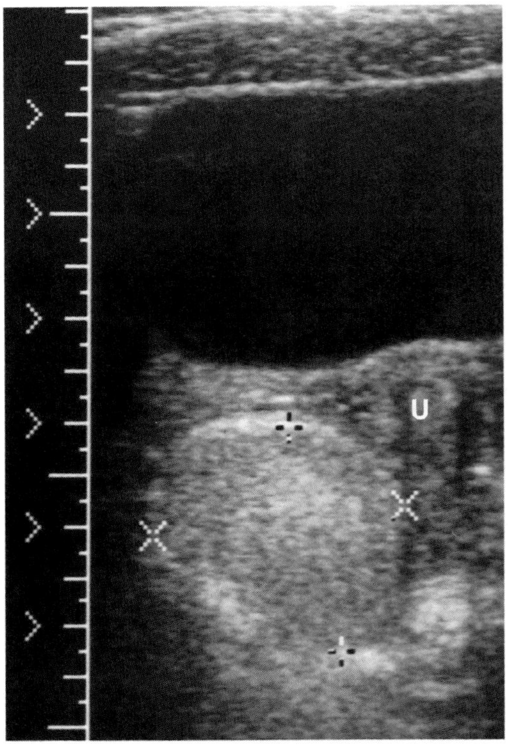

Figure 8-27. Echogenic ovarian teratoma mimicking a malignant neoplasm in a 15-year-old girl. A transverse sonogram shows an echogenic mass (calipers) adjacent to the uterus (U). Surgical exploration confirmed a benign ovarian teratoma containing predominantly fat and calcification.

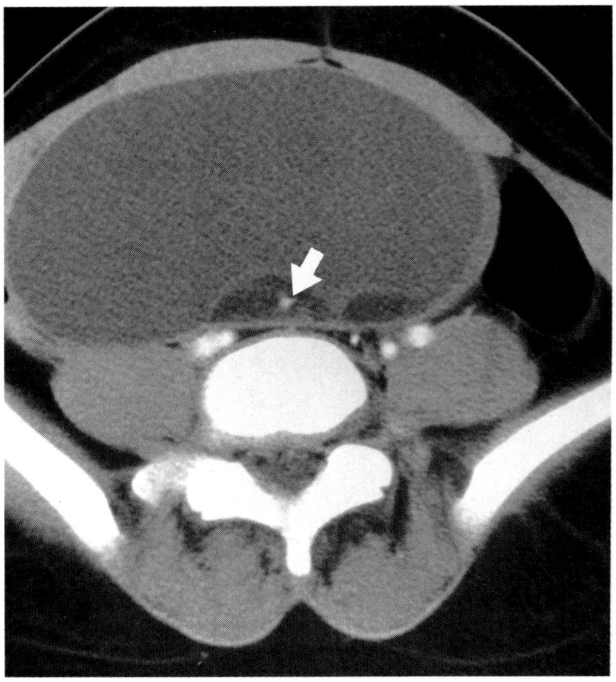

Figure 8-28. Cystic ovarian teratoma in a 13-year-old girl with a complex pelvic mass on sonography. A CT scan through the mid-pelvis shows a large near-water-density mass containing peripheral fat and calcifications (arrow). A mature teratoma was found at surgery.

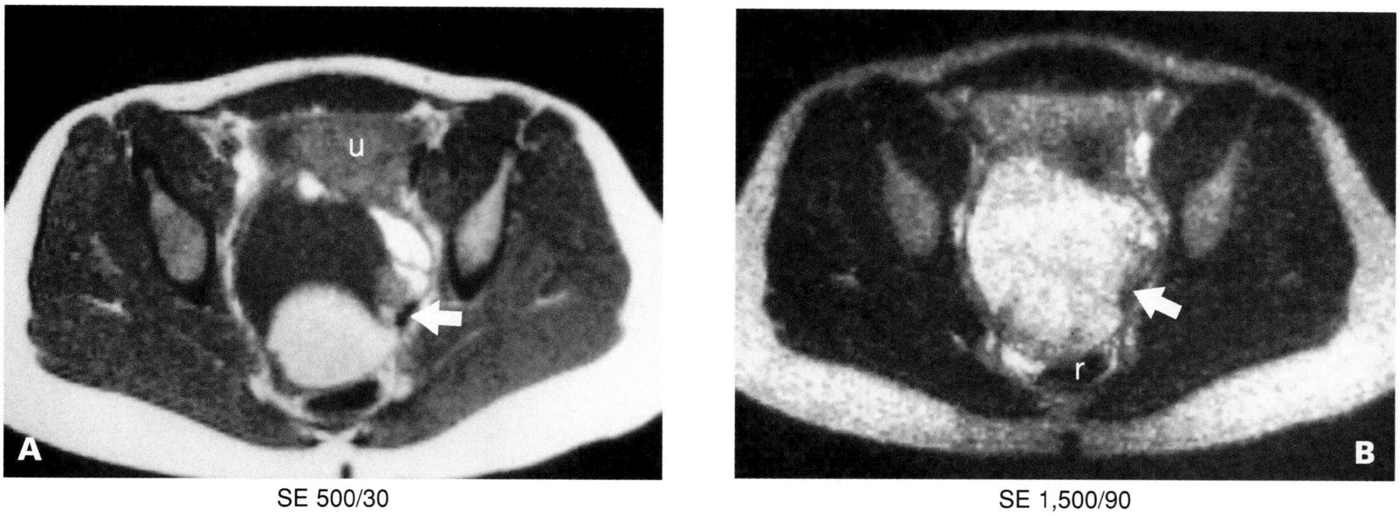

Figure 8-29. Benign cystic teratoma. (A) A transaxial T1-weighted MR image shows a large mixed-intensity mass posterior to the uterus (U). The fluid in the anterior part of the mass has a relatively low signal intensity, while the fat posteriorly and laterally has a high signal intensity. (B) A T2-weighted MR image shows that the signal intensity of the fluid is increased and is equal to that of subcutaneous fat. The focus of low signal intensity laterally (arrow) on both T1- and T2-weighted images corresponded to calcification and hair in the pathologic specimen. r = rectum. (Reprinted with permission from Siegel [45].)

sequences **(Option (D) is true).**

Approximately 10% of ovarian teratomas are malignant. However, teratoma is not the most common malignant ovarian mass in childhood. Of all malignant masses, 60% to 90% are germ cell tumors; 10% to 13% are stromal-sex cord tumors (Sertoli-Leydig, granulosa-theca cell, and undifferentiated), and 5% to 13% are epithelial carcinomas. Of the germ cell tumors, dysgerminoma is the most frequent, followed in order of decreasing frequency by endodermal sinus tumor, malignant teratoma, malignant mixed germ cell tumor, and choriocarcinoma.

Most malignant teratomas are found in peri- or postpubertal girls and present as asymptomatic pelvic or abdominal masses. They are typically larger than 10 cm in diameter at the time of diagnosis. By comparison with benign tumors, which are chiefly cystic, malignant teratomas contain more than 50% soft tissue elements **(Option (E) is true).** Sonographic findings in patients with malignant teratomas are a solid echogenic or complex mass with irregular walls, thick septations, papillary projections, and cul-de-sac fluid (Figure 8-30). Initial reports suggest that Doppler sonography may be able to differentiate between malignant and nonmalignant ovarian masses. In a study of a series of adolescents and adult women, Fleischer et al. reported that malignant ovarian tumors tended to have central, low-resistance arterial Doppler waveforms (pulsatility index of <1.0), whereas benign ovarian masses tended to show peripheral, high-resistance flow (pulsatility index of >1.0). Quillin and Siegel investigated the utility of color Doppler sonography in characterizing benign ovarian lesions in children and adolescents and documented peripheral color flow in approximately 80% of the lesions (Figure 8-31) **(Option (F) is true).** Flow was central in 10% of the remaining lesions and absent in 10%.

The CT and MRI appearance of malignant teratoma is that of a solid or mixed solid-cystic mass with foci or calcification and fat (Figure 8-32). Ascites, lymphadenopathy, and hepatic metastases are signs of intra-abdominal spread. The lungs are also a site of metastatic spread. CT is superior to MRI and sonography in delineating the extent of regional and distant disease, especially lung and small lymph node metastases. Mesenteric or peritoneal implants are not a typical feature of malignant teratomas. Most intraperitoneal seeding is due to epithelial neoplasms rather than to germ cell tumors.

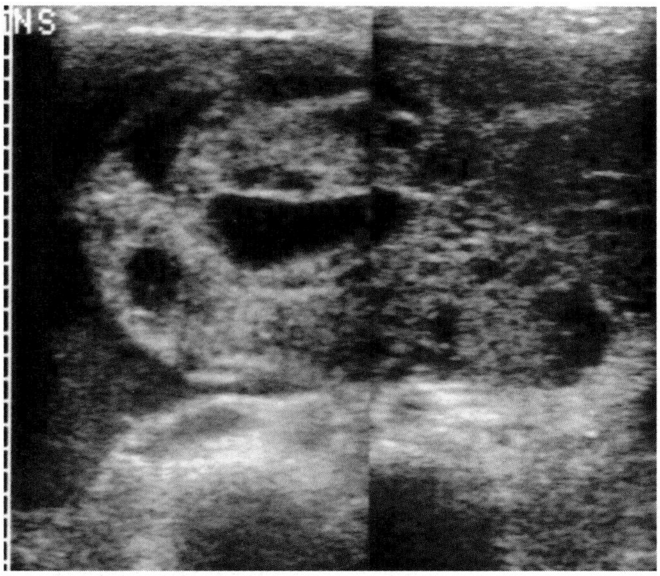

Figure 8-30. Malignant ovarian teratoma. A dual-image transverse sonogram of the right adnexa shows a large, predominantly solid mass. Hypoechoic areas represent necrosis.

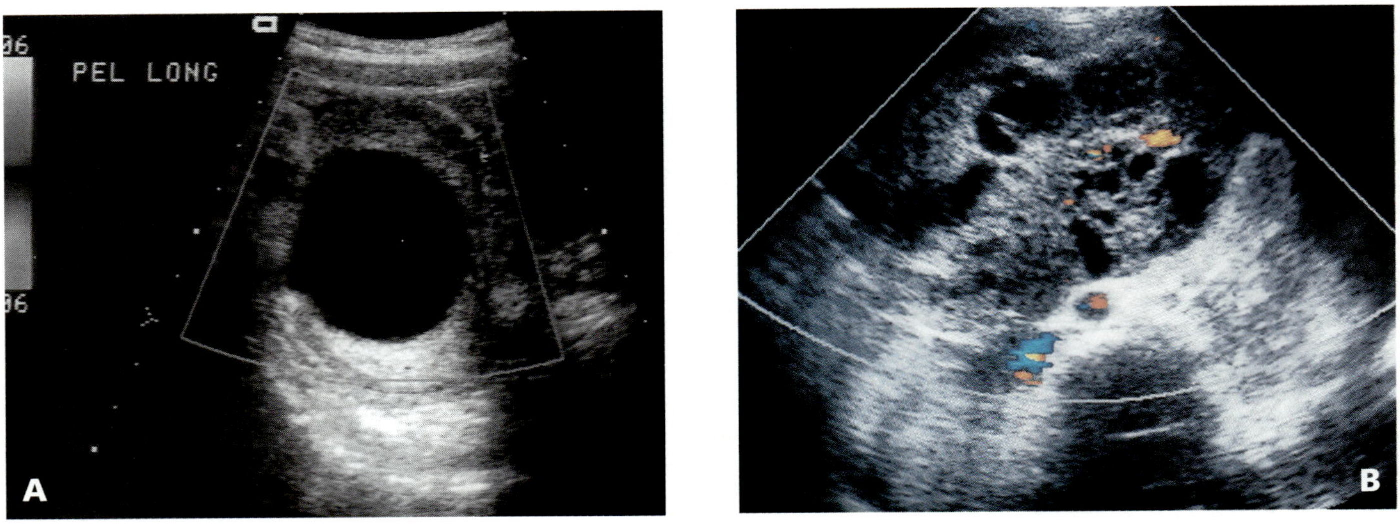

Figure 8-31. Color flow Doppler imaging patterns of ovarian tumors. (A) Same patient as in Figure 8-10. Cystadenoma. A longitudinal image shows peripheral flow in the wall; the cystic area centrally is avascular. (B) Dysgerminoma. Minimal flow is noted within the lesion.

Question 47

Concerning ovarian torsion,

(A) about 50% of patients have a history of recurrent pain
(B) most adolescent girls have a concomitant ovarian mass
(C) in neonates, the typical sonographic appearance is an enlarged ovary with peripheral follicles
(D) an extra-adnexal location in the pelvis is frequent
(E) flow is demonstrated by Doppler sonography in fewer than 5% of patients

Torsion of the ovary and fallopian tube is the result of partial or complete rotation of the ovary on its vascular pedicle. This situation compromises lymphatic, venous, and arterial flow, causing congestion of the ovarian parenchyma and eventually hemorrhagic infarction. Pathologically, the ovarian parenchyma shows a spectrum of findings ranging from massive ovarian edema to ovarian necrosis. The former appearance is more likely to be found in patients with partial obstruction, whereas the latter pattern is usually the result of complete arterial obstruction leading to infarction.

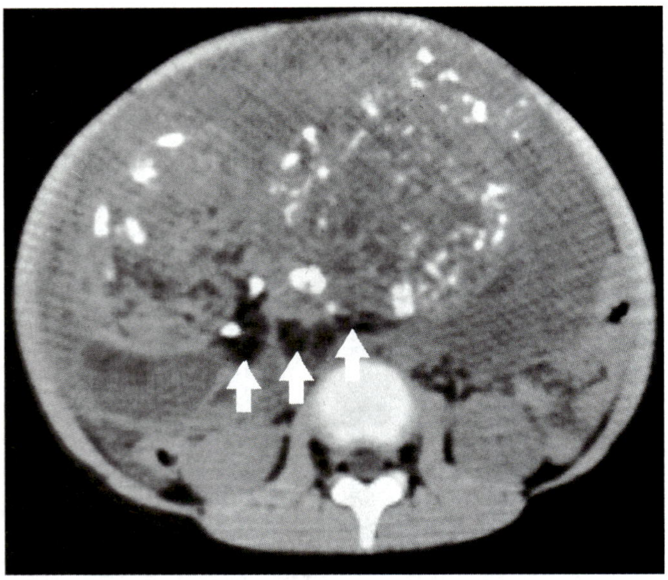

Figure 8-32. Malignant ovarian teratoma. A CT scan shows a predominantly solid mass with areas of fat (arrows) and calcification.

Adnexal torsion has been found in all age groups, but is most common in adolescents and young women. The classic presentation involves acute onset of lower abdominal pain, often associated with nausea or vomiting and leukocytosis. A history of previous episodes of similar pain, presumably reflecting intermittent torsion and detorsion, is found in at least one half of the patients (**Option (A) is true**). A palpable mass is present on physical examination in about 50% of children.

Torsion can occur in a normal adnexa or an abnormal adnexa containing a cyst or tumor. The latter acts as a fulcrum to potentiate torsion of the ovary and fallopian tube. In the series of 20 proven cases of ovarian torsion reported by Stark and Siegel, underlying lesions were more common in neonates and infants than in adolescent girls. Two thirds of the former patients had abnormal ovaries, whereas only 10% of postpubertal girls had pathologic lesions (**Option (B) is false**). The most likely explanation for torsion of a normal adnexa is excessive mobility secondary to lax supporting ligaments. Adnexal torsion is nearly always unilateral. Bilateral torsion is asynchronous.

The torsed ovaries are markedly enlarged, usually at least five to six times larger than the normal ovary. The sonographic appearance is variable and depends on whether the torsion occurs in a normal ovary or one with underlying pathologic changes. The only sonographic appearance considered specific for torsion of a normal ovary is an enlarged ovary with multiple small cysts in the periphery (Figure 8-5). In a series of 11 girls with surgically proven torsion, Graif and Itzchak found that 8 (73%) had enlarged ovaries with multiple enlarged follicles in the periphery. The positive predictive value of multifollicular enlargement was 88%, and the specificity was 93%. The explanation for the cystic changes is transudation of fluid into the follicles secondary to stromal congestion. The remaining patients in the study of Graif and Itzchak had abnormal ovaries with cystic, solid, or mixed cystic and solid masses that were the main sonographic finding. If there is a mass that has potentiated the torsion, the sonogram can have a nonspecific appearance (Figure 8-33). However, the diagnosis of torsion must be considered when the clinical picture is also suspicious for torsion.

Stark and Siegel reported that the sonographic findings of ovarian torsion varied with patient age, reflecting the different frequencies of pathologic masses. Torsed ovaries in neonates virtually always appeared as complex masses with multiple large cysts, septations, and debris. These patients had underlying hemorrhagic cysts at surgery. The multifollicular enlargement considered typical of torsion was infrequently encountered in neonates (**Option (C) is false**). By comparison, 90% of adolescent patients had the typical solid-appearing ovaries with multiple dilated follicles in the periphery.

An extra-adnexal location of the ovary is another classic feature of ovarian torsion. Stark and Siegel noted that approximately 50% of torsed ovaries were located in the lower pelvis or above the bladder. In the study by Helvie and Silver of 26 adolescents and adult women with torsion, approximately 70% of the affected ovaries assumed a midline position, either behind the bladder or cephalad to the uterus (**Option (D) is true**).

Color Doppler imaging can support the diagnosis of torsion by failing to demonstrate color signal in an enlarged ovary (Figure 8-34). However, the absence of color flow is not a reliable criterion of torsion alone, since signal is absent in some normal ovaries. Unfortunately, the presence of an arterial signal does not exclude torsion (Figure 8-35). Stark and Siegel showed flow on color Doppler sonography in approximately 65% of torsed ovaries in children (**Option (E) is false**). Possible explanations for this observation are (1) venous occlusion that produces symptoms before arterial occlusion occurs and (2) persistent arterial flow reflecting the dual ovarian blood supply from the ovarian and uterine arteries. When present, flow can be central or peripheral or can show a combination of the two patterns. Again, other sonographic features should be taken into consideration. If the gray-scale appearance is typical of ovarian torsion, regardless of the color flow pattern, one should be able to suggest a specific diagnosis.

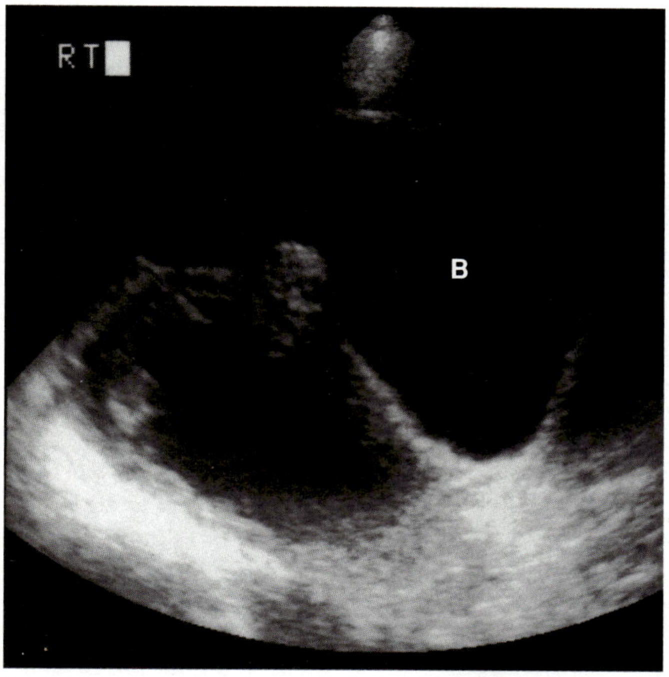

Figure 8-33. Ovarian torsion in a 15-year-old girl. A longitudinal sonogram demonstrates a cystic mass with thick irregular walls in the right adnexa. B = bladder. Surgery revealed a hemorrhagic ovarian cyst with 720° torsion of the fallopian tube. A complex mass, such as the one noted in this patient, is nonspecific, and the differential diagnosis includes torsion as well as a nontorsed hemorrhagic cyst, tubo-ovarian abscess, and ectopic pregnancy. Differentiation requires correlation with clinical and laboratory data and, in some cases, serial sonography.

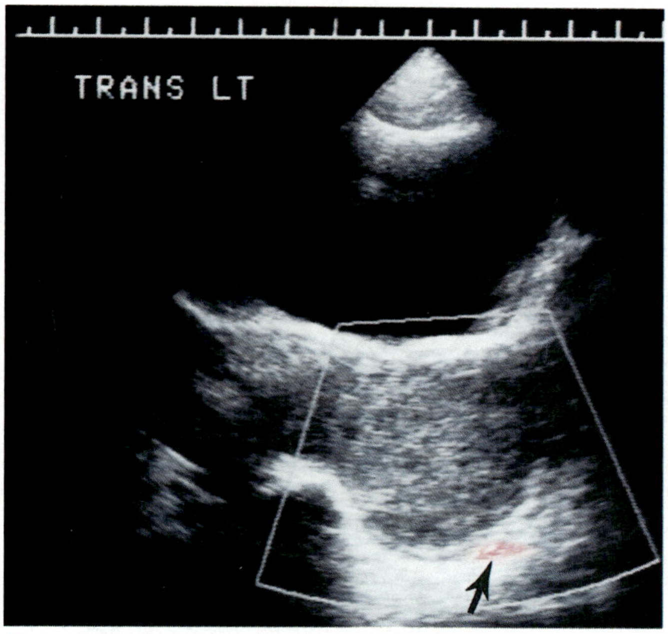

Figure 8-34. Adnexal torsion. A color flow Doppler image shows an enlarged ovary with increased through transmission of sound and no demonstrable flow. The color signal (arrow) adjacent to the ovary is within soft tissues. (Reprinted with permission from Quillin and Siegel [25].)

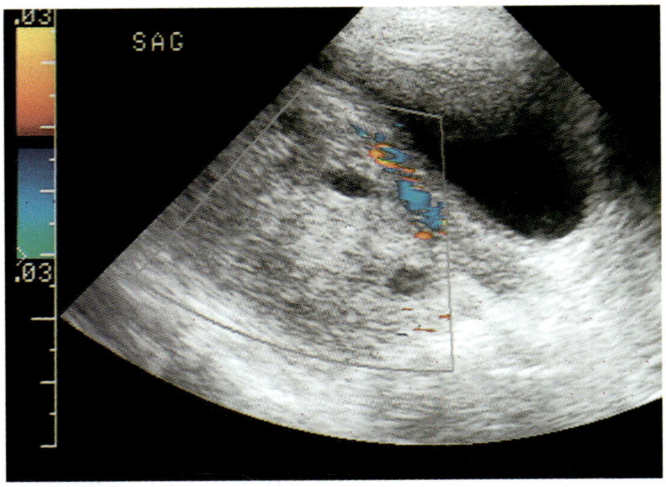

Figure 8-35. Ovarian torsion. A color flow Doppler image shows flow around the periphery of the torsed ovary. The ovary is enlarged and contains several peripheral follicles.

SUGGESTED READINGS

OVARIAN CYSTS

1. Baltarowich OH, Kurtz AB, Pasto ME, Rifkin MD, Needleman L, Goldberg BB. The spectrum of sonographic findings in hemorrhagic ovarian cysts. AJR 1987; 148:901–905
2. Fakhry J, Khoury A, Kotval PS, Noto RA. Sonography of autonomous follicular ovarian cysts in precocious pseudopuberty. J Ultrasound Med 1988; 7:597–603
3. Kier R, Smith RC, McCarthy SM. Value of lipid- and water-suppression MR images in distinguishing between blood and lipid within ovarian masses. AJR 1992; 158:321–325
4. King LR, Siegel MJ, Solomon AL. Usefulness of ovarian volume and cysts in female isosexual precocious puberty. J Ultrasound Med 1993; 12: 577–581
5. Lee HJ, Woo SK, Kim JS, Suh SJ. "Daughter cyst" sign: a sonographic finding of ovarian cyst in neonates, infants, and young children. AJR 2000; 174:1013–1015
6. Neiman HL, Mendelson EB. Ultrasound evaluation of the ovary. In: Callen PW (ed), Ultrasonography in obstetrics and gynecology. Philadelphia: WB Saunders; 1988:423–446
7. Nussbaum AR, Sanders RC, Hartman DS, Dudgeon DL, Parmley TH. Neonatal ovarian cysts: sonographic-pathologic correlation. Radiology 1988; 168:817–821
8. Reynolds T, Hill MC, Glassman LM. Sonography of hemorrhagic ovarian cysts. J Clin Ultrasound 1986; 14:449–453
9. Schmahmann S, Haller JO. Neonatal ovarian cysts: pathogenesis, diagnosis and management. Pediatr Radiol 1997; 27:101–105

PELVIC INFLAMMATORY DISEASES

10. Bulas DI, Ahlstrom PA, Sivit CJ, Blask AR, O'Donnell RM. Pelvic inflammatory disease in the adolescent: comparison of transabdominal and transvaginal sonographic evaluation. Radiology 1992; 183:435–439
11. Golden N, Cohen H, Gennari G, Neuhoff S. The use of pelvic ultrasonography in the evaluation of adolescents with pelvic inflammatory disease. Am J Dis Child 1987; 141:1235–1238
12. Golden N, Neuhoff S, Cohen H. Pelvic inflammatory disease in adolescents. J Pediatr 1989; 114:138–143
13. Shafer MA, Sweet RL. Pelvic inflammatory disease in adolescent females. Epidemiology, pathogenesis, diagnosis, treatment, and sequelae. Pediatr Clin North Am 1989; 36:513–532

TORSION

14. Graif M, Itzchak Y. Sonographic evaluation of ovarian torsion in childhood and adolescence. AJR 1988; 150:647–649
15. Helvie MA, Silver TM. Ovarian torsion: sonographic evaluation. J Clin Ultrasound 1989; 17:327–332
16. Rosado WM Jr, Trambert MA, Gosink BB, Pretorius DH. Adnexal torsion: diagnosis by using Doppler sonography. AJR 1992; 159:1251–1253
17. Stark JE, Siegel MJ. Ovarian torsion in prepubertal and pubertal girls: sonographic findings. AJR 1994; 163:1479–1482

NEOPLASMS

18. Breen JL, Bonamo JF, Maxson WS. Genital tract tumors in children. Pediatr Clin North Am 1981; 28:355–367
19. Buy JN, Ghossain MA, Moss AA, et al. Cystic teratoma of the ovary: CT detection. Radiology 1989; 171:679–701
20. Castleberry RP, Cushing B, Perlman E, Hawkins EP. Germ cell tumors. In: Pizzo PA, Poplack DG (eds), Principles and practice of pediatric oncology. 3rd ed. Philadelphia: Lippincott Raven; 1997:921–945
21. Ehren IM, Mahour GH, Isaacs H Jr. Benign and malignant ovarian tumors in children and adolescents. A review of 63 cases. Am J Surg 1984; 147:339–344
22. Fleischer AC, Rodgers WH, Kepple DM, Williams LL, Jones HW III, Gross PR. Color Doppler sonography of benign and malignant ovarian masses. RadioGraphics 1992; 12:879–885
23. Fried AM, Kenney CM III, Stigers KB, Kacki MH, Buckley SL. Benign pelvic masses: sonographic spectrum. RadioGraphics 1996; 16:321–334
24. Patel MD, Feldstein VA, Lipson SD, Chen DC, Filly RA. Cystic teratomas of the ovary: diagnostic value of sonography. AJR 1998; 171: 1061–1065
25. Quillin SP, Siegel MJ. Transabdominal color Doppler ultrasonography of the painful adolescent ovary. J Ultrasound Med 1994; 13:549–555
26. Sheth S, Fishman EK, Buck JL, Hamper UM, Sanders RC. The variable sonographic appearances of ovarian teratomas: correlation with CT. AJR 1988; 151:331–334
27. Sisler CL, Siegel MJ. Ovarian teratomas: a comparison of the sonographic appearance in prepubertal and postpubertal girls. AJR 1990; 154:139–141

NORMAL OVARY

28. Cohen HL, Eisenberg P, Mandel F, Haller JO. Ovarian cysts are common in premenarchal girls: a sonographic study of 101 children 2–12 years old. AJR 1992; 159:89–91
29. Cohen HL, Shapiro MA, Mandel FS, Shapiro ML. Normal ovaries in neonates and infants: a sonographic study of 77 patients 1 day to 24 months old. AJR 1993; 160:583–586
30. Cohen HL, Tice HM, Mandel FS. Ovarian volumes measured by US: bigger than we think. Radiology 1990; 177:189–192
31. Hall DA. Sonographic appearance of the normal ovary, of polycystic ovary disease, and of functional ovarian cysts. Semin Ultrasound 1983; 4:149–165
32. Orsini LF, Salardi S, Pilu G, Bovicelli L, Cacciari E. Pelvic organs in premenarchal girls: real-time ultrasonography. Radiology 1984; 153:113–116
33. Rigsby CK, Siegel MJ. CT appearance of pediatric ovaries and uterus. J Comput Assist Tomogr 1994; 18:72–76
34. Salardi S, Orsini LF, Cacciari E, Bovicelli L, Tassoni P, Reggiani A. Pelvic ultrasonography in premenarcheal girls: relation to puberty and sex hormone concentrations. Arch Dis Child 1985; 60:120–125

POLYCYSTIC OVARIAN DISEASE

35. Franks S. Polycystic ovary syndrome. N Engl J Med 1995; 333:853–861
36. Hann LE, Hall DA, McArdle CR, Seibel M. Polycystic ovarian disease: sonographic spectrum. Radiology 1984; 150:531–534
37. Pache TD, Wladimiroff JW, Hop WC, Fauser BC. How to discriminate between normal and polycystic ovaries: transvaginal US study. Radiology 1992; 183:421–423
38. Parisi L, Tramonti M, Derchi LE, Casciano S, Zurli A, Rocchi P. Polycystic ovarian disease: ultrasonic evaluation and correlations with clinical and hormonal data. J Clin Ultrasound 1984; 12:21–26
39. Stein IF, Leventhal ML. Amenorrhea associated with bilateral polycystic ovaries. Am J Obstet Gynecol 1935; 29:181–191
40. Yeh HC, Futterweit W, Thornton JC. Polycystic ovarian disease: US features in 104 patients. Radiology 1987; 163:111–116

GENERAL

41. Cohen HL, Haller JO. Pediatric and adolescent genital abnormalities. Clin Diagn Ultrasound 1989; 24:187–215
42. Siegel MJ. Female pelvis. In: Siegel MJ (ed), Pediatric sonography. 3rd ed. Philadelphia: Lippincott Williams & Wilkins; 2001:in press
43. Siegel MJ. Pediatric body CT. Philadelphia: Lippincott Williams & Wilkins; 1999:287–311
44. Siegel MJ. Pediatric gynecologic sonography. Radiology 1991: 179:593–600
45. Siegel MJ. Magnetic resonance imaging of the pediatric pelvis. Semin Ultrasound CT MR 1991; 12:475–505
46. States LJ, Bellah RD. Imaging of the pediatric female pelvis. Semin Roentgenol 1996; 31:312–329
47. Surratt JT, Siegel MJ. Imaging of pediatric ovarian masses. RadioGraphics 1991; 11:533–548

CASE 9

Lane F. Donnelly, M.D.

Giant Cell Tumor of Tendon Sheath

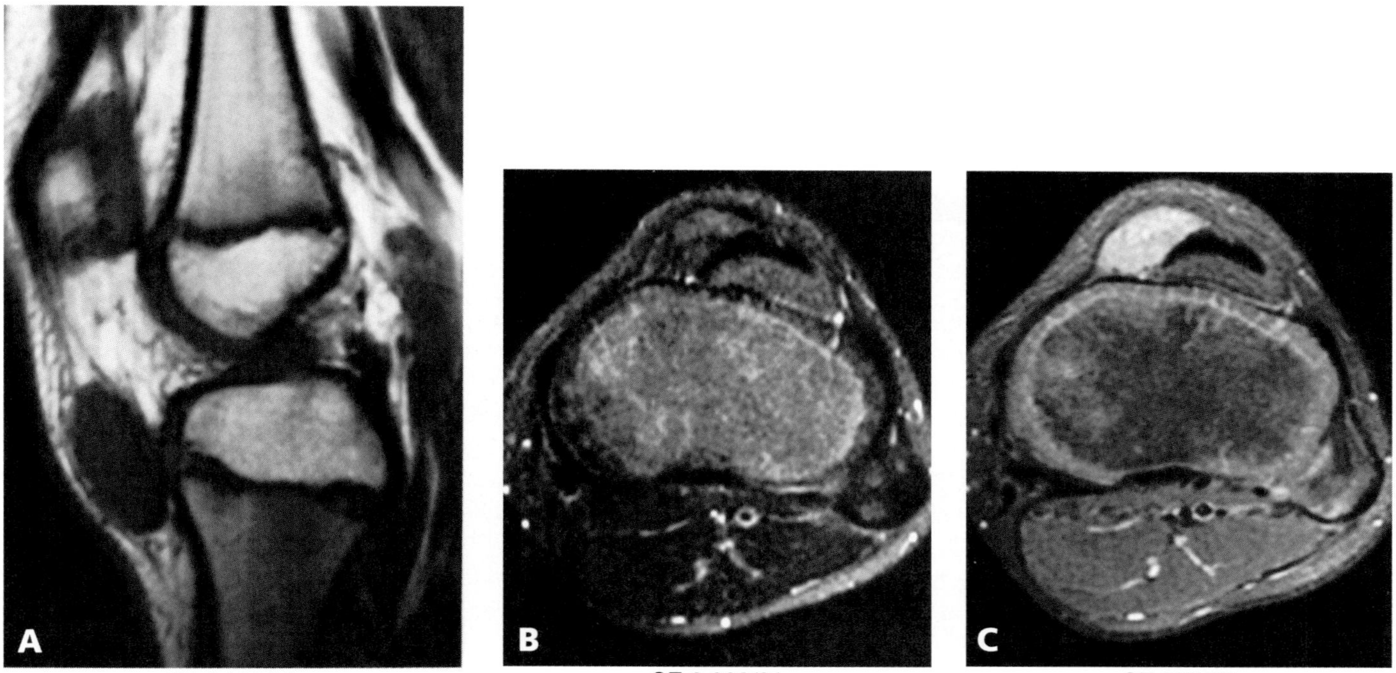

SE 6,100/11   SE 3,000/81   SE 650/20

Figure 9-1

Question 48

This 9-year-old boy has a nontender palpable mass in the infrapatellar region. You are shown sagittal T1-weighted (A), fat-saturated axial T2-weighted (B), and postcontrast T1-weighted (C) MR images (Figure 9-1).

Which *one* of the following is the MOST likely diagnosis?

(A) Hematoma
(B) Pigmented villonodular synovitis
(C) Giant cell tumor of tendon sheath
(D) Aggressive fibromatosis
(E) Synovial sarcoma

The sagittal T1-weighted image through the region of the knee of the test patient (Figure 9-1A) shows a well-defined mass in the infrapatellar region immediately anterior to the patellar tendon (Figure 9-2A). The lesion is hypointense relative to muscle and is homogeneous. The adjacent subcutaneous fat has normal signal intensity without evidence of edema or inflammation. The axial T2-weighted image (Figure 9-1B) again demonstrates the mass, which is located anterior to and abutting the patellar tendon (Figure 9-2B). The mass has a homogeneous, hypointense T2-weighted signal. There is no abnormal signal within the adjacent fat to suggest edema. The borders of the mass are well defined. There is no abnormal signal within the adjacent patellar tendon. The fat-saturated axial T1-weighted image obtained after the intravenous administration of gadolinium chelate (Figure 9-1C) demonstrates diffuse, homogeneous enhancement of the mass (Figure 9-2C). Based on these findings, giant cell tumor of tendon sheath is the most likely diagnosis (**Option (C) is correct**).

Hematomas (Option (A)) are commonly seen in children; minor traumatic injury is almost a "normal" event in the pediatric population. Most minor lacerations and contusions do not require medical management. Most significant hematomas are obviously related to a specific traumatic event, the etiology is

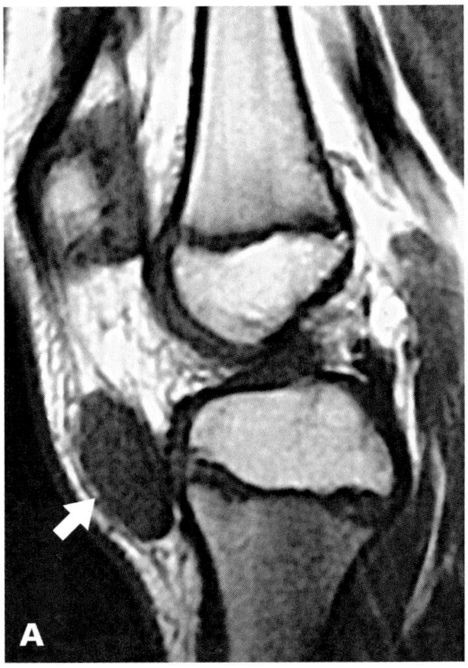

SE 6,100/11

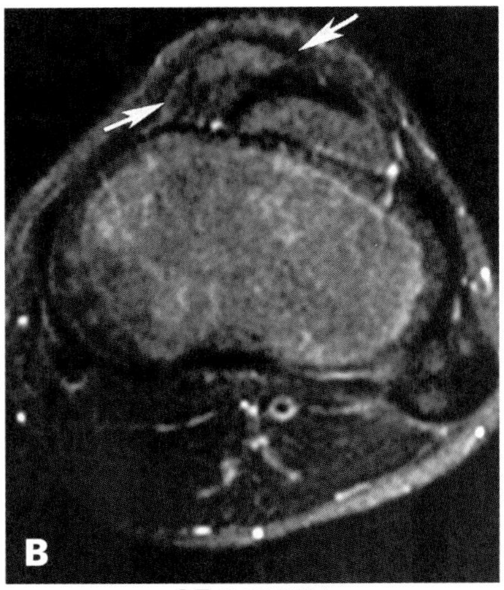

SE 3,000/81

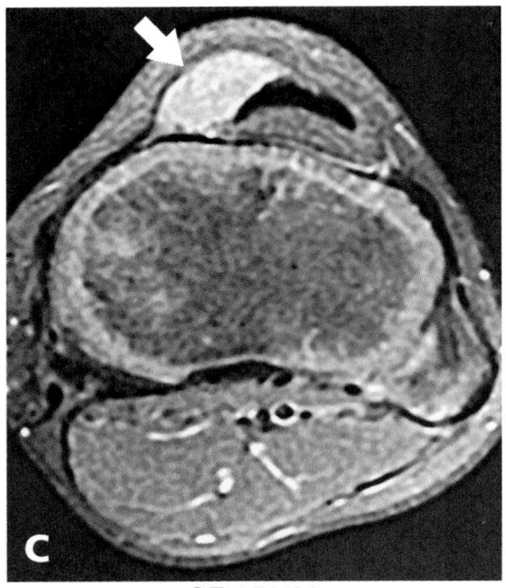

SE 650/20

Figure 9-2 (Same as Figure 9-1). Giant cell tumor of tendon sheath in a 9-year-old boy. (A) A sagittal T1-weighted MR image shows a well-defined, homogeneous, low-intensity mass (arrow) anterior to the proximal tibia. (B) An axial T2-weighted fat-saturated image shows a heterogeneous low-intensity mass (arrows) abutting the patellar tendon. (C) An axial T1-weighted fat-saturated image after intravenous gadolinium chelate administration shows diffuse enhancement of the mass (arrow).

not in question, and imaging is not required. Occasionally, the traumatic history is occult, either unrecognized or trivial, and the child presents with a firm, nonspecific soft tissue mass. In such a presentation, MRI can be performed to exclude neoplasm.

The MRI appearance of hematoma is variable, and the signal intensity depends on the age of the lesion. Hematomas can be categorized into four major phases based on the age of the blood within the lesion: hyperacute, acute, subacute, and chronic. Hyperacute hematomas (1 to 24 hours old) show low signal intensity on T1-weighted images and high signal intensity on T2-weighted images as a result of high concentrations of intracellular oxyhemoglobin. Acute hematomas (1 to 7 days old) show low to intermediate signal intensity on T1-weighted images and low signal intensity on T2-weighted images as a result of the high concentration of intracellular deoxyhemoglobin. Subacute hematomas (1 week to several months old) show high signal intensity on T1-weighted images secondary to the formation of methemoglobin (Figure 9-3A). The signal intensity of subacute hematomas on T2-weighted images depends on whether the methemoglobin is intra- or extracellular. In the early subacute stage, when methemoglobin is intracellular, there is low signal intensity on T2-weighted images. As hemolysis occurs and methemoglobin becomes extracellular, high signal intensity is seen on T2-weighted images (Figure 9-3B). Therefore, the presence of high signal intensity on T1-weighted images and low or high signal intensity on T2-weighted images is characteristic of subacute hematomas. The peripheral portion of the hematoma often becomes hyperintense before the central portion does. Approximately 70% of subacute hematomas also demonstrate a low-intensity rim, which is related to a combination of surrounding hemosiderin-laden macrophages and reactive fibrosis (Figure 9-3). Chronic hematomas have a variable appearance. After the breakdown of methemoglobin, the signal characteristics of chronic hematomas are similar to those of other fluid collections, i.e., low signal intensity on T1-weighted images and high signal intensity on T2-weighted images. Fluid levels also can be present in the center of the hematoma. A variable amount of fibrosis also can be present, generating low signal intensity on T1- or T2-weighted images.

The margins of a hematoma are usually poorly defined. The adjacent subcutaneous fat or muscle often has low signal intensity on T1-weighted images and high signal intensity on T2-weighted images because of posttraumatic edema. In adults, hematomas must be differentiated from the hemorrhagic presentation of a neoplasm. The presence of a nodule or a thick, irregular rim should suggest neoplasm rather than simple hematoma. However, in the pediatric population, hemorrhagic presentation of a malignant neoplasm, mimicking a simple hematoma, is exceedingly rare.

The well-defined border and absence of adjacent edema in the test images and the absence of a history of trauma in the test patient make hematoma unlikely. Although the low signal intensity seen on both T1- and T2-weighted images could be seen in an acute hematoma, the diffuse, homogeneous enhancement of the mass seen on the postcontrast image is inconsistent with hematoma.

Pigmented villonodular synovitis (PVNS) (Option (B)) is a benign proliferative disorder of the synovium of uncertain etiology. The gross pathologic features include a thick, plush synovium with matted masses of villi and synovial folds and sessile or pedunculated nodules. Diffuse involvement of the synovium of a single joint is the most common form, although there is a less common focal nodular variant. Microscopically, synovial cell

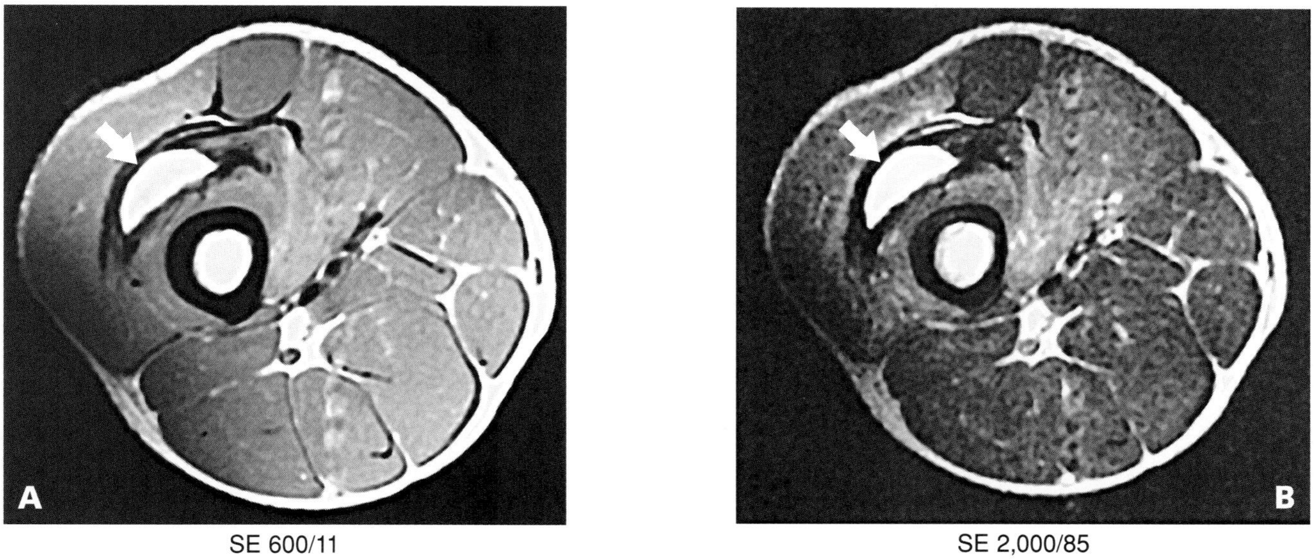

Figure 9-3. Subacute hematoma of the thigh in a 16-year-old boy. (A) An axial T1-weighted MR image shows a mass within the vastus intermedius muscle (arrow). The lesion exhibits central, heterogeneous high signal intensity and has a low-intensity rim. This rim represents hemosiderin-laden macrophages and reactive fibrosis. (B) An axial T2-weighted MR image shows that the mass (arrow) has high signal intensity centrally and a low-intensity rim. The high intensity seen on both T1- and T2-weighted images is consistent with a subacute hematoma.

hyperplasia, multinucleated giant cells, hemosiderin-laden macrophages, and variable amounts of fibrosis are evident. Extracellular and intracellular hemosiderin and aggregates of "foamy" macrophages filled with lipids are important imaging features. PVNS is uncommon, occurring in approximately 1.8 per 10 million individuals. The knee is by far the most frequently affected joint, with less commonly affected joints including the hip, ankle, shoulder, and elbow. Although cases do occur in children, the typical patient presents is in the third or fourth decade. Males and females are equally affected. Classically described findings on radiographs include monoarticular involvement, normal bony mineralization of the affected joint, preservation of the cartilage space, and corticate erosions and cysts on both sides of the joint. The MRI findings reflect the histologic composition of the tumor. Characteristic MRI findings include a lobulated intra-articular synovial mass with predominantly low signal intensity on both T1- and T2-weighted images (Figure 9-4), secondary to the presence of hemosiderin

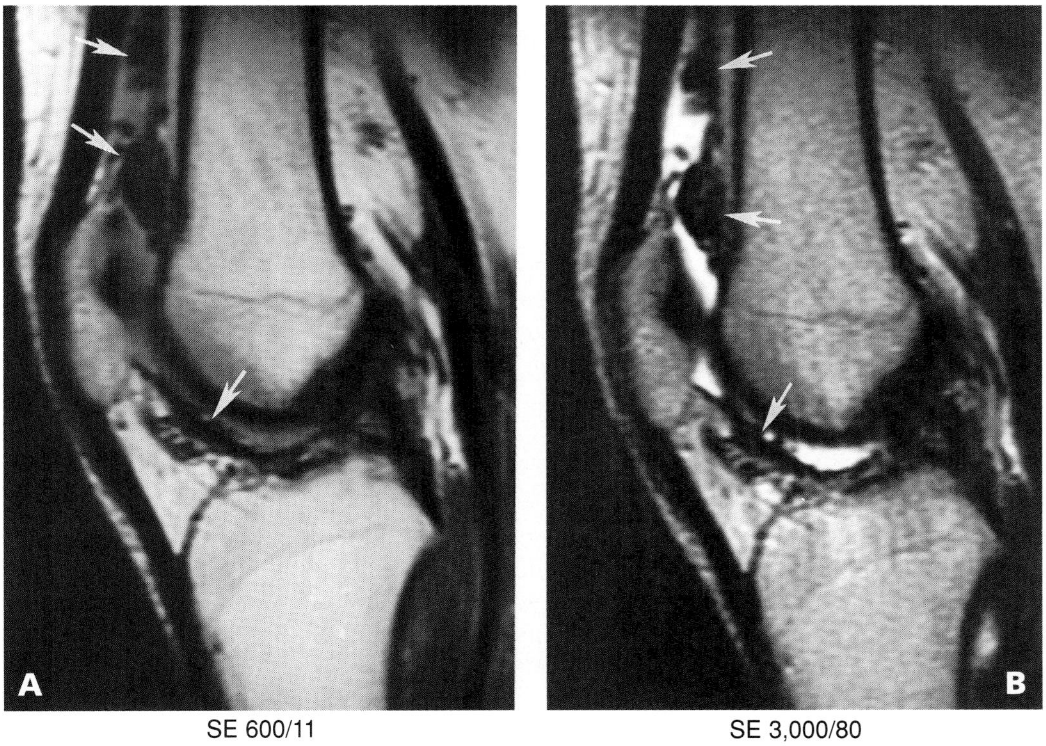

Figure 9-4. Pigmented villonodular synovitis of the knee in a 25-year old woman. Sagittal T1-weighted (A) and T2-weighted (B) MR images show diffuse lobulated synovial masses (arrows) with low signal intensity on both pulse sequences. There is also a joint effusion.

deposition, and thick fibrous tissue. The area of low signal intensity may appear slightly larger and of lower intensity on T2-weighted than on T1-weighted images, secondary to the "blooming" effect of hemosiderin. Other characteristic findings include areas of high "fat" signal intensity within the mass on T1-weighted images as a result of clumps of lipid-laden macrophages and bony erosions. However, the MRI appearance of PVNS varies widely depending on the relative proportions of lipid, hemosiderin, fibrosis, fluid, cyst formation, and cellular elements. Most patients do have a joint effusion. The classic MRI appearance of PVNS is also not specific, since regions of dark synovium also can be observed in patients with rheumatoid arthritis, hemophiliac arthropathy (Figure 9-5), or synovial osteochondromatosis. MRI is helpful in both characterizing the lesion of PVNS and defining the extent of disease for surgical planning. The mass in the test patient is external to the knee joint and is not a synovial process; therefore, PVNS is not a reasonable consideration.

Aggressive fibromatosis (extra-abdominal desmoid) (Option (D)) is a histologically benign disorder that can be locally aggressive. The MRI appearance of these lesions is variable. The signal intensity on T2-weighted images is usually heterogeneous, with high intensity reflecting abundant tumor cellularity (fibroblasts) and intermixed areas of low intensity reflecting areas of fibrosis and hypocellularity (Figure 9-6). The tumor arises in fascial planes of striated muscle, and neurovascular or bone involvement is common. The homogeneous signal intensity and well-defined borders in the test images make aggressive fibromatosis a possible but unlikely diagnosis.

Synovial sarcoma (Option (E)) is a malignant neoplasm of mesenchymal origin. It accounts for approximately 10% of primary soft tissue malignancies, and although most commonly it occurs in the second to fourth decades, it can affect patients of any age from early childhood to late adulthood. The tumor can occur in a variety of locations, including the retroperitoneum, mediastinum, and head and neck, but most synovial sarcomas occur in the extremities, most commonly within the lower extremity. Pathologically, there is a mixture of solid, cystic, fibrous, and hemorrhagic elements. The signal intensity on T2-weighted images is heterogeneous in 82% of patients, reflecting the variable histologic components, but can be homogeneously high, causing the lesions to be mistaken for cystic fluid collections (Figure 9-7). There are often fluid levels and high signal intensity on T1-weighted images, suggestive of hemorrhage. The tumor tends to be found deep in soft tissue, large (85% are greater than 5 cm in diameter), and located with the epicenter of the mass close to a joint. The lesions do not typically arise in the joint space itself, as might be expected with a "synovial" process. Synovial sarcoma has a well-defined margin in approximately 90% of patients. This characteristic makes synovial sarcoma the most common malignant tumor to be mistaken for a benign lesion on MRI (Figure 9-7). Although synovial sarcoma is a consideration in the differential diagnosis of the test patient, the homogeneous low signal intensity on the T1- and T2-weighted images makes it unlikely.

Giant cell tumor of tendon sheath (localized nodular tenosynovitis) is a benign proliferative lesion related to tendon sheaths; the histologic findings are similar to those of PVNS. The characteristic MRI findings are predominantly homogeneous low signal intensity on T1-weighted, proton-density-weighted, and T2-weighted images (Figure 9-2). The low signal intensity is related to fibrosis or hemosiderin deposition. The margins of the lesion tend to be well defined. The location of the characteristic lesion is immediately adjacent to and abutting a tendon sheath. These findings are identical to those seen in the test images.

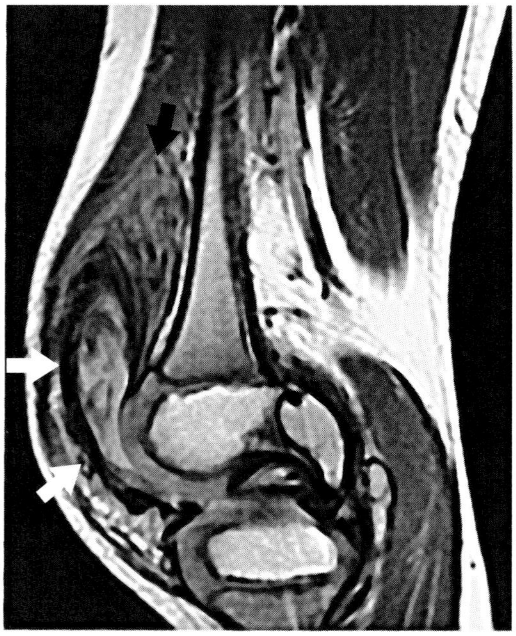

SE 3,000/80

Figure 9-5. Hemophiliac arthropathy in a 6-year-old boy. A sagittal T2-weighted MR image shows complex suprapatellar joint effusion (black arrow) with thickened, low-intensity synovium (white arrows).

Question 49

Concerning giant cell tumor of tendon sheath,

- (A) it most commonly occurs adjacent to small joints
- (B) the most common radiographic pattern is a soft tissue mass with associated osseous pressure erosions
- (C) it most commonly presents during the second decade of life
- (D) it is histologically identical to giant cell tumor of bone

Giant cell tumor of tendon sheath (localized nodular synovitis) is similar histologically to PVNS. Histologically, there is active proliferation of histiocyte-like cells, multinucleated giant

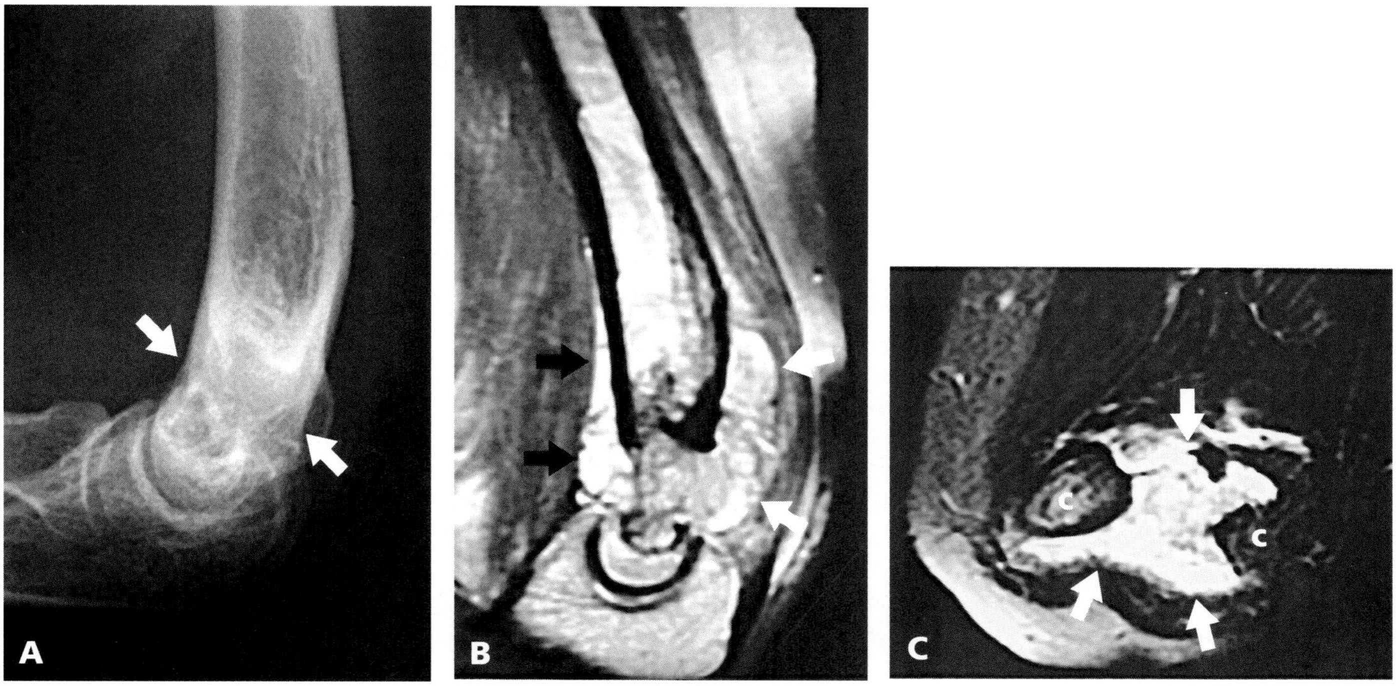

SE 3,000/20 SE 3,000/80

Figure 9-6. Aggressive fibromatosis in a 15-year-old girl. (A) A lateral radiograph of the elbow shows a lytic area (arrows) with surrounding sclerosis in the intracondylar notch. (B) A sagittal proton-density-weighted MR image shows a poorly defined, heterogeneous, aggressive-appearing, high-intensity mass (white arrows) arising in the olecranon fossa and extending through the intracondylar notch of the distal humerus and into soft tissues anteriorly (black arrows). (C) An axial T2-weighted MR image shows the heterogeneous high intensity of the mass (arrows), which extends through the intracondylar notch. c = humeral condyles.

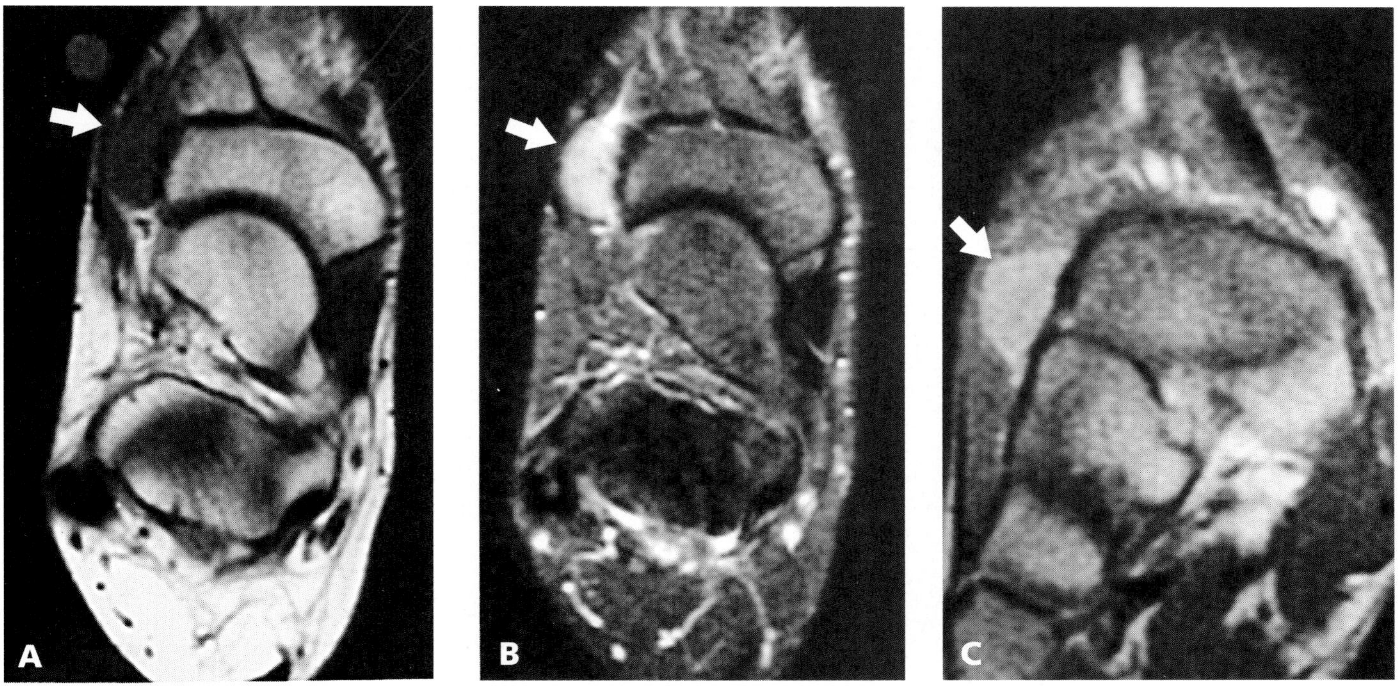

SE 400/11 SE 3,000/85 SE 400/11

Figure 9-7. Synovial sarcoma in a 26-year-old women. (A) An axial (long-axis) T1-weighted MR image shows a homogeneous, well-defined mass (arrow), isointense relative to muscle, adjacent to the lateral aspect of the navicular bone. A vitamin E capsule marks the palpable lesion. (B) An axial (long-axis) T2-weighted MR image shows homogeneous high signal intensity (arrow) and minimal surrounding edema. (C) A coronal (short-axis) T1-weighted MR image obtained after intravenous gadolinium chelate administration, to evaluate whether the lesion was cystic or solid, shows diffuse homogeneous enhancement, consistent with a solid mass (arrow). (Case courtesy of Clyde A. Helms, M.D., Duke University Medical Center, Durham, N.C.)

cells, foam cells, and hemosiderin-laden giant cells. Patients with giant cell tumor of tendon sheath have at least one well-circumscribed discrete soft tissue nodule, usually located along the tendon sheath. In patients with PVNS, there is diffuse proliferation of the synovial membrane with a villous pigmented appearance. There is no histologic relationship between giant cell tumor of tendon sheath and giant cell tumor of hone (**Option (D) is false**). Giant cell tumor of bone (osteoclastoma) consists of fibrostromal elements and variable numbers of giant cells.

Giant cell tumor of tendon sheath most commonly occurs in patients aged 30 to 50 years (**Option (C) is false**), although it can occur at any age. There is a slight female predominance (60% to 67% of cases). Most cases of giant cell tumor of tendon sheath occur in the joints of the fingers and hands (88%), with the index and middle fingers being the most common location (**Option (A) is true**). Less commonly, lesions are affixed to the joint capsules or tendon sheaths of the larger joints, such as the ankle, knee, or hip. In contrast, PVNS more frequently involves larger joints, such as the knee and hip. Giant cell tumor of tendon sheath is the most common solid soft tissue tumor involving the hand and is second only to ganglion as the most common mass lesion of the hand.

Giant cell tumor of tendon sheath grows slowly over a number of years, and patients usually present with an indolent growing mass. The lesions can be stable in size for many years.

The most common radiographic appearance is the presence of a soft tissue mass without bony changes (**Option (B) is false**). Approximately 15% to 20% lesions demonstrate osseous pressure erosions associated with the soft tissue mass. When the lesion involves a small joint, it sometimes causes secondary degenerative or cystic changes and rarely causes an adjacent periosteal reaction. Other digital lesions that can appear similar radiographically include fibroma, enchondroma, synovial chondromatosis, synovial hemangioma, foreign body granuloma, and gout. When the lesions involve larger joints, the differential diagnosis is even more extensive.

The MRI appearance of giant cell tumor of tendon sheath is variable and depends on the proportions of hemosiderin and fibrostromal, cystic, and cellular elements (Figures 9-2 and 9-8). However, the characteristic MRI appearance of giant cell tumor of tendon sheath is a well-defined mass adjacent to a tendon sheath, which demonstrates predominantly homogeneous low signal intensity on T1-weighted, proton-density-weighted, and T2-weighted images (Figure 9-2). The signal characteristics appear to be related to both the fibrotic and hemosiderin components of the tumor. These signal characteristics, however, are not always present (Figure 9-8).

The mass may exhibit nonspecific intermediate signal intensity on T1-weighted images and high signal intensity on T2-weighted images. When local excision, performed to exclude other causes of a mass, demonstrates giant cell tumor of tendon sheath, it is considered curative.

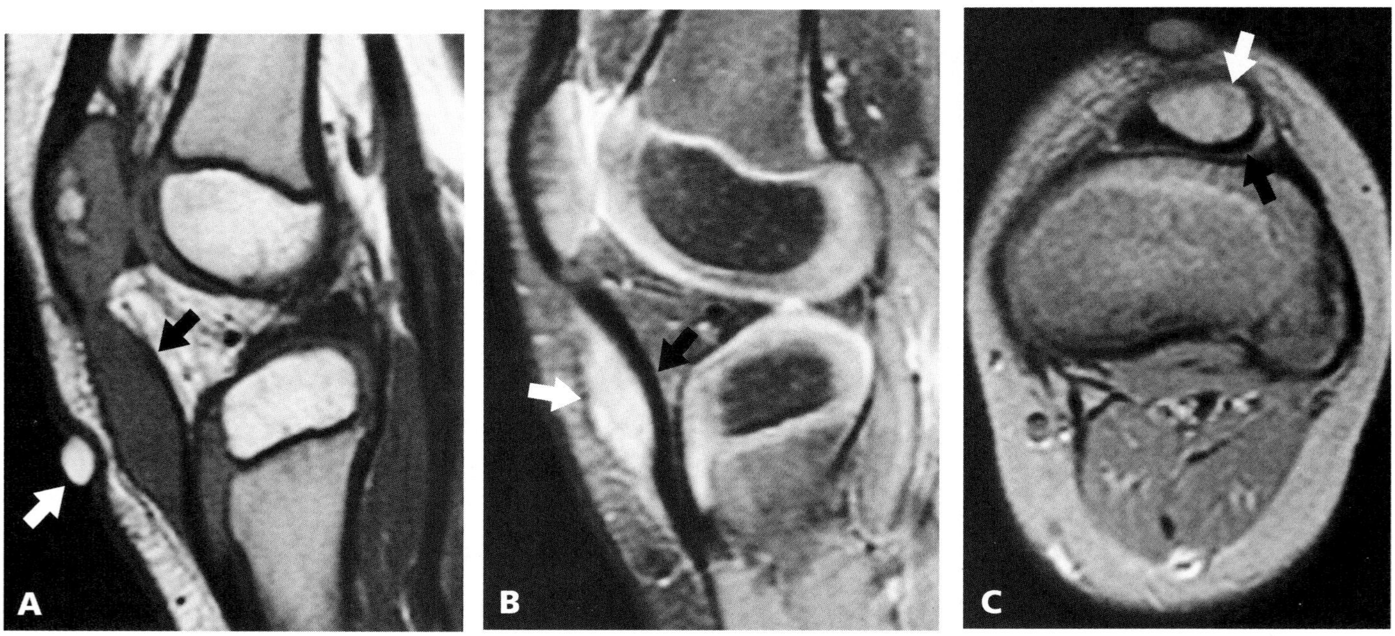

SE 650/11 SE 2,000/11 SE 2,000/80

Figure 9-8. Giant cell tumor of tendon sheath demonstrating variable signal intensity in a 3-year-old girl. (A) A sagittal T1-weighted MR image shows a homogeneous, well-defined mass (black arrow) that is isointense relative to muscle. The lesion is marked by a vitamin E capsule (white arrow). (B) A sagittal proton-density-weighted MR image shows a high-intensity mass (white arrow) abutting the patellar tendon (black arrow). (C) An axial T2- weighted fat-saturated MR image shows that the mass (white arrow) has high signal intensity. The lesion abuts an otherwise normal-appearing patellar tendon (black arrow).

Question 50

Concerning aggressive fibromatosis,

(A) the fibrous nature of the lesion results in low signal intensity on all MRI pulse sequences in most patients
(B) it is a histologically benign lesion
(C) it arises from fascial or musculoaponeurotic coverings
(D) there is a high recurrence rate after surgical resection
(E) there is often a history of previous trauma or surgery

Aggressive fibromatosis (extra-abdominal desmoid) is a neoplasm that arises from fascial or musculoaponeurotic coverings **(Option (C) is true)**. Pathologically, the tumor grossly resembles scar tissue, with variable numbers of well-differentiated fibroblasts in a collagenous, fibrous matrix. Aggressive fibromatosis is a histologically benign lesion with no cytologic features of malignancy and no propensity for distant metastasis **(Option (B) is true)**. Aggressive fibromatosis is a relatively uncommon disorder, with a prevalence of only 2 to 4 cases per 10 million individuals. Although the etiology is unknown, an association with previous trauma or surgery is well documented. However, most reports are small series, and the frequency of anticedent trauma is unknown **(Option (E) is true)**. Other associations include pregnancy, estrogen therapy, and Gardner's syndrome. Aggressive fibromatosis most commonly occurs in the second or third decade of life.

The MRI appearance of aggressive fibromatosis is variable and is often indistinguishable from that of other aggressive soft tissue tumors (Figure 9-6). The epicenter of the tumor is usually in fascial or aponeurotic covering regions of muscle. Neurovascular encasement is present in about 60% of patients, and bone invasion is present in 35%. Approximately 90% of the tumors show poor margination, although they can be well defined. The signal intensity of the lesions is variable and reflects the tumor histology. The tumors do not usually have low intensity on all pulse sequences, as one might expect from their fibrous nature (Figure 9-6) **(Option (A) is false)**. Most lesions have abundant tumor cellularity (fibroblasts), which results in high signal intensity on T2-weighted images and a signal that is iso- or slightly hyperintense relative to that of muscle on T1-weighted images. When a collagenous matrix and hypocellularity predominate, areas of low intensity can be present on all pulse sequences. The signal is heterogeneous in nearly all patients.

The treatment of aggressive fibromatosis is wide surgical resection. The overall mortality rate is low, but local recurrence after surgery is frequent, with recurrence rates reported to be as high as 65% **(Option (D) is true)**.

Question 51

Concerning MRI of focal soft tissue masses in children,

(A) well-defined margins reliably indicate a benign lesion
(B) its primary role is to determine the extent of the disease process
(C) postcontrast T1-weighted images reliably distinguish the margin of a tumor from surrounding edema
(D) a chronic hematoma is often indistinguishable from a hemorrhagic tumor
(E) subcutaneous masses are more likely to be malignant than are masses in muscle

MRI now plays an integral role in the evaluation of soft tissue masses. It establishes the presence of a mass, characterizes the lesion, and accurately depicts the extent of disease. In a patient being imaged for a palpable lesion, MRI has a high negative predictive value and reliably excludes a soft tissue mass. Palpable soft tissue abnormalities are common in children. When the history explains a lesion, such as trauma causing a hematoma, imaging plays a minor role. However, in most patients with palpable soft tissue masses, the clinical history is noncontributory and MRI is critical to the evaluation.

Despite advances in cross-sectional imaging, conventional radiographs are still often the first images obtained in the evaluation of a palpable soft tissue mass. Radiographs may demonstrate that the mass arises from bone, e.g., callus related to a fracture, a benign osteocartilaginous tumor, or a malignant bone tumor, such as Ewing's sarcoma or osteosarcoma. Radiographs can also show specific findings of some benign masses, such as the ossification typical of myositis ossificans or the phleboliths suggestive of hemangioma. When these findings are encountered, further imaging may not be indicated. If the radiographs are nondiagnostic, MRI is the next imaging study of choice. Although sonography is sometimes used to detect and characterize superficial soft tissue lesions, MRI is the primary imaging modality used in the evaluation of soft tissue masses. CT, which can be used to characterize patterns of calcification, also plays only a small supportive role in the evaluation of soft tissue masses. The primary role of MRI is for staging of soft tissue tumors before therapy **(Option (B) is true)**. MRI provides an accurate map of the anatomic regions involved. It accurately demonstrates the extent of the soft tissue tumor, involvement of bone, and involvement of neurovascular structures or joints. This information is important for planning surgical resection or radiation therapy. For malignant lesions, involvement of a large number of fascial planes or muscle groups, neural or vascular structures, or joint space or bone indicates a more difficult surgical dissection and a poorer prognosis. MRI also plays an important role in the follow-up of treatment of malignant soft tissue tumors, identifying both tumor recurrence and other complications.

For the differentiation between benign and malignant lesions and for tissue characterization, the only definitive diagnostic procedure is biopsy. Distinction of benign from malignant soft tissue masses on the basis of MRI criteria is controversial. Certainly, the performance of MRI in tissue characterization has not met initial expectations. Most soft tissue tumors, both benign and malignant, have nonspecific signal intensity characteristics with prolonged T1 and T2 relaxation times. However, a small number of soft tissue tumors have an MRI appearance characteristic of a specific diagnosis. These specific diagnoses are usually related to the presence of fat, vascular structures, subacute blood, or hemosiderin, and they include lipomas (Figure 9-9), hemangiomas, lymphangiomas, hematomas, giant cell tumors of tendon sheath, fibrolipomas of the median nerve (Figure 9-10), cystic hygromas, benign neural tumors, and posttraumatic fat necrosis. When a lesion has the classic appearance of one of these processes, appropriate therapy can be instituted. However, not all cases of these benign lesions demonstrate these characteristic MRI findings, and when there is doubt, biopsy is indicated.

Other parameters that are more often associated with benign than with malignant soft tissue tumors include a diameter of <3 cm, well-defined margins, homogeneous signal intensity on T2-weighted images, absence of neurovascular encasement or bone invasion, absence of adjacent edema, subcutaneous location, and patient age under 20 years. However, unfortunately, studies have shown that these parameters, singly or in combination, cannot reliably differentiate between benign and malignant lesions (**Option (A) is false**). High-grade malignant lesions can be small, well defined, and homogeneous in signal intensity (Figures 9-7 and 9-11), and histologically benign lesions can be large and poorly marginated. Although subcutaneous masses are statistically more likely to be benign than are masses that originate in muscle (**Option (E) is false**), both benign and malignant lesions can involve either the subcutaneous or the muscular planes in children. Aggressive lesions that can involve the subcutaneous space in children include metastatic neuroblastoma and aggressive fibromatosis. The presence of hemorrhage complicating a soft tissue mass also interferes with the differentiation between benign and malignant lesions. Gross hemorrhage complicating soft tissue masses is uncommon in children. A hemorrhagic neoplasm can usually be differentiated from an uncomplicated hematoma by the presence of a nodule or a thick, irregular rim in a neoplasm (**Option (D) is false**).

The technique used for MRI examination of a soft tissue mass is usually tailored to the location and size of the mass and

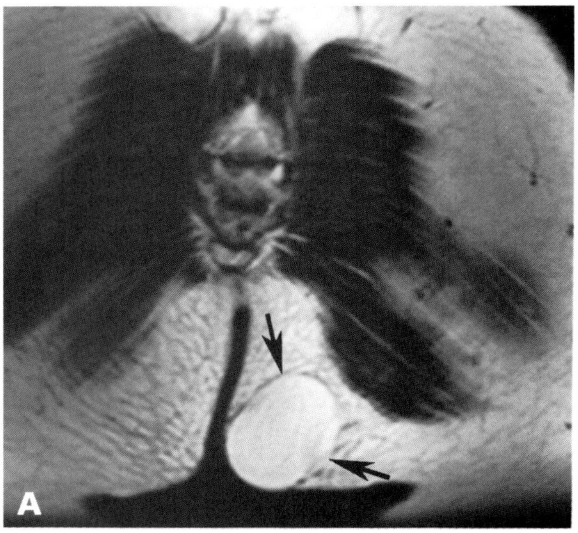

SE 600/11

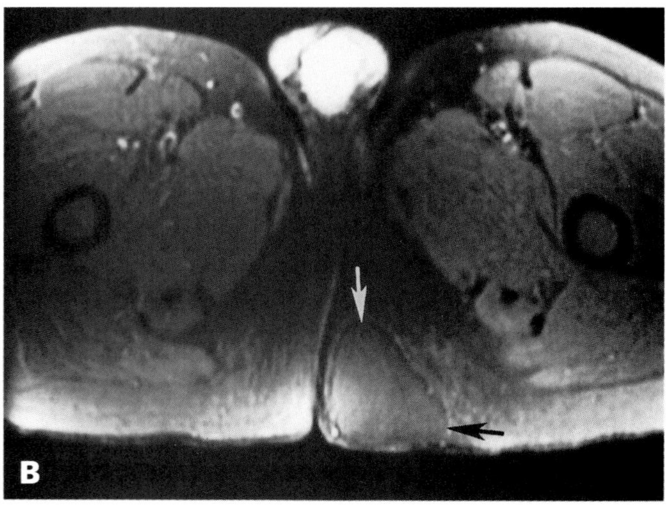

SE 3,000/20

Figure 9-9. Lipoma involving the gluteal subcutaneous tissues of a 16-year-old boy. (A) A coronal T1-weighted MR image shows a well-defined mass (arrows) with a homogeneous signal isointense relative to fat. (B) An axial fat-saturated proton-density-weighted MR image shows low signal intensity within the lesion (arrows), again isointense relative to the ischiorectal fat.

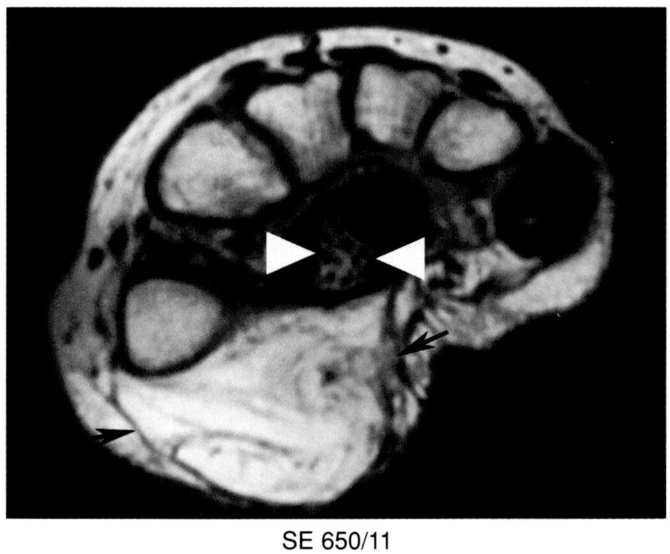

SE 650/11

Figure 9-10. Fibrolipoma of the median nerve in a 15-year-old girl. An axial T1-weighted MR image through the wrist demonstrates masslike enlargement of the median nerve (arrowheads) adjacent to the flexor tendons. The mass has a cablelike appearance, with low-intensity nerve fibers surrounded by high-intensity fatty hamartomatous tissue. The appearance is characteristic of fibrolipoma. The lesion has an exophytic extension into the thenar eminence (arrows). This region of the mass also demonstrates high (fat) signal intensity.

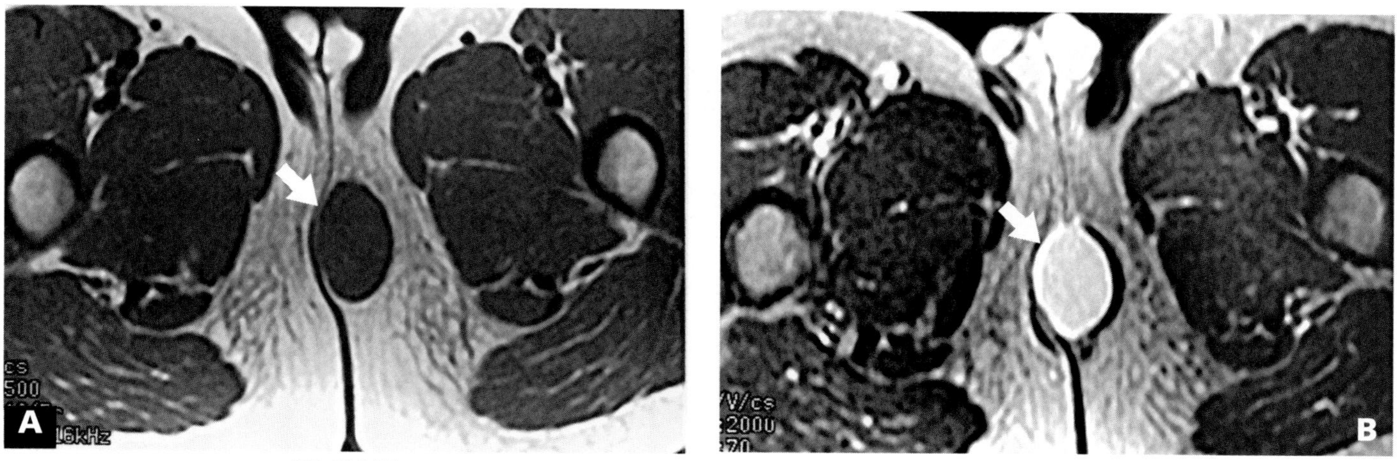

SE 600/11 SE 3,000/85

Figure 9-11. Malignant lesion with "benign" MRI features in a 10-year-old boy. Axial T1-weighted (A) and T2 weighted fat-saturated (B) MR images show a small (3 × 2 cm), well-defined mass (arrow) within the perianal, gluteal subcutaneous fat. The mass demonstrates homogeneous low signal intensity on the T1-weighted image and homogeneous high signal intensity on the T2-weighted image. A biopsy showed this to be an undifferentiated sarcoma.

the size of the patient. The coil choice reflects the size of the body part being examined. In children, choices include head coil, extremity coils, wrap coil, torso array coil, and body coil. Soft tissue tumors are imaged in at least two, and often three, orthogonal planes. Axial images are almost always obtained because of their value in depicting the relationship of the mass to adjacent muscle compartments, neurovascular bundles, and bone. Sagittal or coronal images can then be chosen on the basis of which plane will best demonstrate the mass and its relationship to other adjacent structures. T1-weighted images are usually obtained to evaluate for signal abnormalities that indicate the presence of fat, hemorrhage, or hemosiderin and to help distinguish marrow replacement from normal-appearing fatty marrow. T2-weighted images are also obtained. Some radiologists prefer the use of fat-saturated, fast spin-echo sequences because of the high degree of contrast from the typical high signal intensity of most pathologic lesions and low signal intensity of most normal structures. T2-weighted sequences provide information about the lesion homogeneity, margination, presence of peritumoral edema, and involvement of neurovascular structures and bone. These T2-weighted fat-saturated images are the most helpful images in assessing the extent of a lesion.

The role of contrast enhancement in the evaluation of soft tissue tumors is limited. The use of gadolinium chelate does not increase the sensitivity or specificity. However, there are several specific instances when gadolinium chelate administration is helpful. In the evaluation of a large, partially necrotic soft tissue mass, the administration of gadolinium chelate can be helpful in detecting viable regions of the tissue to identify high-yield biopsy sites. In addition, it can be difficult to differentiate homogeneous soft tissue masses from cystic lesions (Figure 9-7); if the lesion enhances after administration of gadolinium chelate, it is consistent with a solid tumor or inflammatory mass. Postcontrast imaging can also identify enhancing areas when it is necessary to differentiate between hemorrhagic tumors and hematomas. The administration of gadolinium chelate does not reliably distinguish tumor margins from surrounding edema (**Option (C) is false**). Both edema and viable tumor may not enhance with gadolinium chelate. This inability to differentiate tumor invasion from adjacent edema and hemorrhage is a major limitation of MRI.

SUGGESTED READINGS

GIANT CELL TUMOR OF TENDON SHEATH

1. Karasick D, Karasick S. Giant cell tumor of tendon sheath: spectrum of radiologic findings. Skeletal Radiol 1992; 21:219–224
2. Moore JR, Weiland AJ, Curtis RM. Localized nodular tenosynovitis: experience with 115 cases. J Hand Surg [Am] 1984; 9:412–417
3. Sherry CS, Harms SE. MR evaluation of giant cell tumors of tendon sheath. Magn Reson Imaging 1989; 7:195–201
4. Sundaram M, McGuire MH, Fletcher J, Wolverson MK, Heiberg E, Shields JB. Magnetic resonance imaging of lesions of synovial origin. Skeletal Radiol 1986; 15:110–116

HEMATOMA

5. Rubin JI, Gomori JM, Grossman RI, Getter WB, Kressel HY. High-field MR imaging of extracranial hematomas. AJR 1987; 148:813–817
6. Unger EC, Glazer HS, Lee JK, Ling D. MRI of extracranial hematomas: preliminary observations. AJR 1986; 146:403–407

PIGMENTED VILLONODULAR SYNOVITIS

7. Bravo SM, Winalski CS, Weissman BN. Pigmented villonodular synovitis. Radiol Clin North Am 1996; 34:311–326
8. Hughes TH, Sartoris DJ, Schweitzer ME, Resnick DL. Pigmented villonodular synovitis: MRI characteristics. Skeletal Radiol 1995; 24:7–12
9. Jaffe JL, Lichtenstein L, Sutro CJ. Pigmented villonodular synovitis, bursitis, and tenosynovitis. Arch Pathol Lab Med 1941; 31:731–765
10. Jelinek JS, Kransdorf MJ, Utz JA, et al. Imaging of pigmented villonodular synovitis with emphasis on MR imaging. AJR 1989; 152:337–342

AGGRESSIVE FIBROMATOSIS

11. Ackman JB, Whitman GJ, Chew FS. Aggressive fibromatosis. AJR 1994; 63:544
12. Casillas J, Sais GJ, Creve JL, Iparraguirre MC, Morillo G. Imaging of intra- and extra-abdominal desmoid tumors. RadioGraphics 1991; 11: 959–968
13. Hartman TE, Berquist TH, Fetsch JF. MR imaging of extraabdominal desmoids: differentiation from other neoplasms. AJR 1992; 158:581–585.
14. Kransdorf MJ, Jelinek JS, Moser RP Jr, et al. Magnetic resonance appearance of fibromatosis. A report of 14 cases and review of the literature. Skeletal Radiol 1990; 19:495–499
15. Liu P, Thorner P. MRI of fibromatosis: with pathologic correlation. Pediatr Radiol 1992; 22:587–589

SYNOVIAL SARCOMA

16. Cadman NL, Soule EH, Kelly PJ. Synovial sarcoma: an analysis of 134 tumors. Cancer 1965; 18:613–627
17. Jones BC, Sundaram M, Kransdorf MJ. Synovial sarcoma: MR imaging findings in 34 patients. AJR 1993; 161:827–830
18. Ladenstein R, Treuner J, Koscielniak E, et al. Synovial sarcoma of childhood and adolescence. Report of the German CWS-81 study. Cancer 1993; 71:3647–3655
19. Morton MJ, Berquist TH, McLeod RA, Unni KK, Sim FH. MR imaging of synovial sarcoma. AJR 1991; 156:337–340

MRI OF SOFT TISSUE MASSES

20. Berquist TH, Ehman RL, King BF, Hodgman CG, Ilstrup DM. Value of MR imaging in differentiating benign from malignant soft-tissue masses: study of 95 lesions. AJR 1990; 155:1251–1255
21. Bisset GS. MR imaging of soft tissue masses in children. Radiol Clin North Am 1996; 4:697–719
22. Crim JR, Seeger LL, Yau L, Chandnani V, Eckardt JJ. Diagnosis of soft tissue masses with MR imaging: can benign masses be differentiated from malignant ones? Radiology 1992; 185:581–586
23. Kransdorf MJ, Jelinek JS, Moser RP Jr, et al. Soft-tissue masses: diagnosis using MR imaging. AJR 1989; 153:541–547
24. Ma LD, Frassica FJ, Scott WW Jr, Fishman EK, Zerbouni EA. Differentiation of benign and malignant musculoskeletal tumors: potential pitfalls with MR imaging. RadioGraphics 1995; 15:349–366
25. Moulton JS, Blebea JS, Dunco DM, Braley SE, Bisset GS III, Emery KH. MR imaging of soft-tissue masses: diagnostic efficacy and value of distinguishing between benign and malignant lesions. AJR 1995; 164: 1191–1199

CASE 10

Richard B. Towbin, M.D.

Orbital Cellulitis

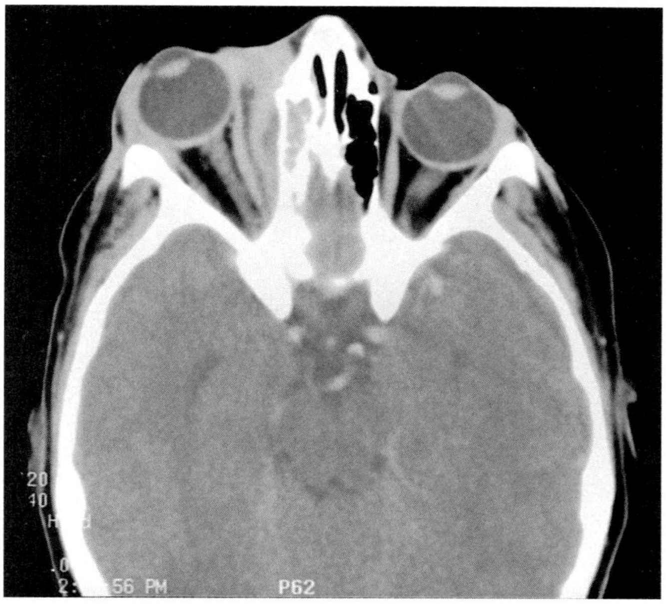

Figure 10-1

Question 52

This 3-year-old girl has periorbital swelling, redness, and slowly progressive proptosis. You are shown an axial postcontrast CT image (Figure 10-1).

Which *one* of the following is the MOST likely diagnosis?

(A) Pseudotumor
(B) Orbital cellulitis
(C) Capillary hemangioma
(D) Rhabdomyosarcoma
(E) Metastatic neuroblastoma

The test image (Figure 10-1) demonstrates a constellation of findings that typifies the features of postseptal orbital cellulitis (**Option (B) is correct**). The medial extraconal space contains a soft tissue mass (Figure 10-2, open arrow) associated with infiltration of the normal fat. This collection is subperiosteal adjacent to the lamina papyracea. The right ethmoid air cells are opacified. The medial rectus muscle (Figure 10-2, solid arrow) is laterally displaced and mildly thickened. The mass effect resulting from the extraconal collection also affects the optic nerve, which is displaced but not enlarged. In this child, the intraconal (retrobulbar) fat is not infiltrated, as is the case in nearly all patients with postseptal cellulitis. The absence of bone destruction helps to exclude a malignant neoplasm.

The child's clinical signs and symptoms resolved rapidly with antibiotic treatment. No intraconal or intracranial complications occurred. An uncomplicated recovery is the usual clinical course in patients with postseptal cellulitis.

Understanding the nomenclature of orbital anatomy is essential for cross-sectional imaging interpretation (Figure 10-3). The term "orbit" is used to identify both the bony skeleton and all the soft tissue components of the eye. The orbit is further classified into the eye proper; the soft tissues surrounding the eye, which include muscles, fat, nerves, and blood vessels;

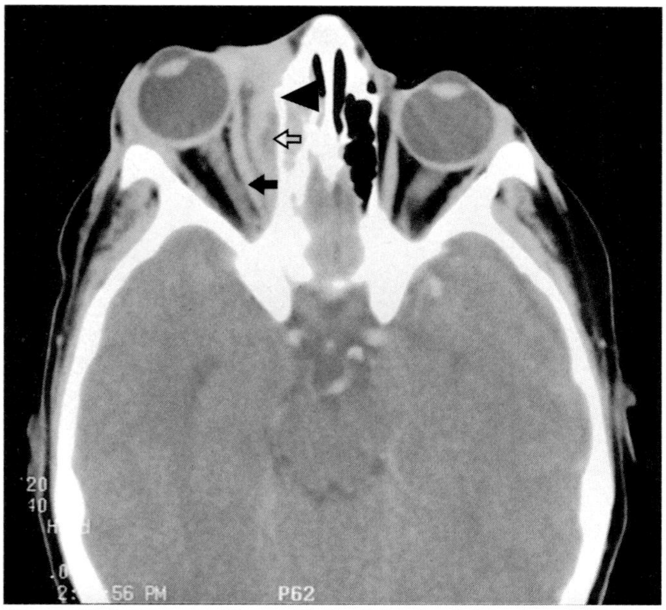

Figure 10-2 (Same as Figure 10-1). Orbital cellulitis. An axial postcontrast CT image demonstrates a normal left eye. On the right there is proptosis of the globe secondary to a postseptal extraconal soft tissue mass (open arrow). This mass is medial to the medial rectus muscle, which is inflamed and enlarged (solid arrow). The intraconal fat is normal, and the optic nerve is uninvolved but slightly displaced by the extraconal mass. The lamina papyracea (arrowhead) is intact, and there is opacification of the ethmoid sinuses.

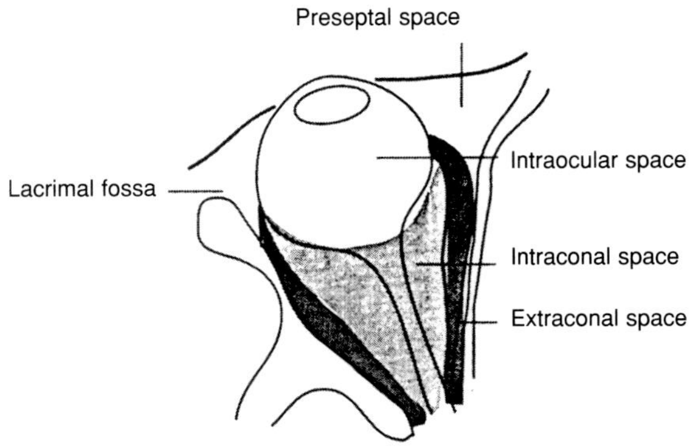

Figure 10-3. Anatomy of orbital spaces. The intraconal space lies inside the rectus muscle pyramid. The extraconal space lies outside the rectus muscle pyramid. The orbital septum represents condensed orbital rim periosteum and attaches to the outer margins of the bony orbit and deep tissues of the lids. It separates all the structures in the orbit from the soft tissues in the face (preseptal vs. postseptal).

and the bony structures. It is useful to classify ophthalmic disease processes as ocular, affecting the eye itself, or orbital, involving the orbital soft tissues or bony orbit. The orbital spaces include the intraconal, extraconal, preseptal, postseptal, and lacrimal fossa spaces. The intraconal space is contained within the rectus muscle pyramid. The extraconal space lies outside the rectus muscle pyramid. The four rectus (superior, inferior, medial, and lateral) muscles and the superior oblique muscle originate in the posterior orbit from the fibrous annulus of Zinn that surrounds the optic canal. The inferior oblique muscle arises from the posterior lacrimal crest. These six muscles form the support structure that surrounds the eye. The muscles are interconnected by fibrous tissues known as the intermuscular septum, which effectively separates the orbit into two compartments, an intraconal space lying within the intermuscular septum and an extraconal space lying between the cone formed by the muscle and the bony orbital wall. The anterior margin of the orbit includes an interconnecting group of fibrous structures. These include the tarsal plates, canthal tendons, and orbital septum. At the margin of the orbital rims, the junction of the external periosteum and the inner periorbita forms the orbital septum which, in conjunction with the tarsal plates, forms a plane of fibrous tissue. The space anterior to the septum is called preseptal, and that posterior to it is called postseptal. The postseptal space consists of the intraconal, extraconal, and subperiorbital compartments.

Orbital pseudotumor (Option (A)) is a nongranulomatous inflammatory disorder of undetermined cause. Histologically, it is represented by reactive lymphoid hyperplasia or an infiltration of the soft tissue structures of the orbit. It is more common in adults than in children and adolescents (with pediatric cases representing about 15% of all cases). About 15% of patients are affected bilaterally. Children with orbital pseudotumor typically have unilateral involvement and usually present with abrupt onset of pain associated with proptosis. In addition, there may be mild lid swelling and redness, chemosis, ophthalmoplegia, and variable loss of vision.

Imaging findings reflect the variable pathologic presentations of pseudotumor of the orbit. The findings can be local, diffuse, or subconjunctival. In the anterior compartment, there can be increased density of the retro-orbital fat. The process can be discrete or poorly defined as an intraconal or extraconal mass. It typically involves muscle and tendon insertions, as opposed to Graves' ophthalmopathy, which has only muscle involvement. Frequently, thickening and enhancement of the sclera near the tendon capsule occur. One or more enlarged muscles close to the insertion in the globe with well-defined margins are identified. The size of the lacrimal gland also can be increased.

The CT features of orbital pseudotumor are variable; however, in most instances there is a relatively localized retrobulbar mass. The retrobulbar findings are manifested as increased attenuation of the retrobulbar fat and lack of definition of the uveal-scleral junction and optic nerve (Figure 10-4). With intravenous administration of contrast material, these structures usually enhance moderately. The extraocular muscles and ten-

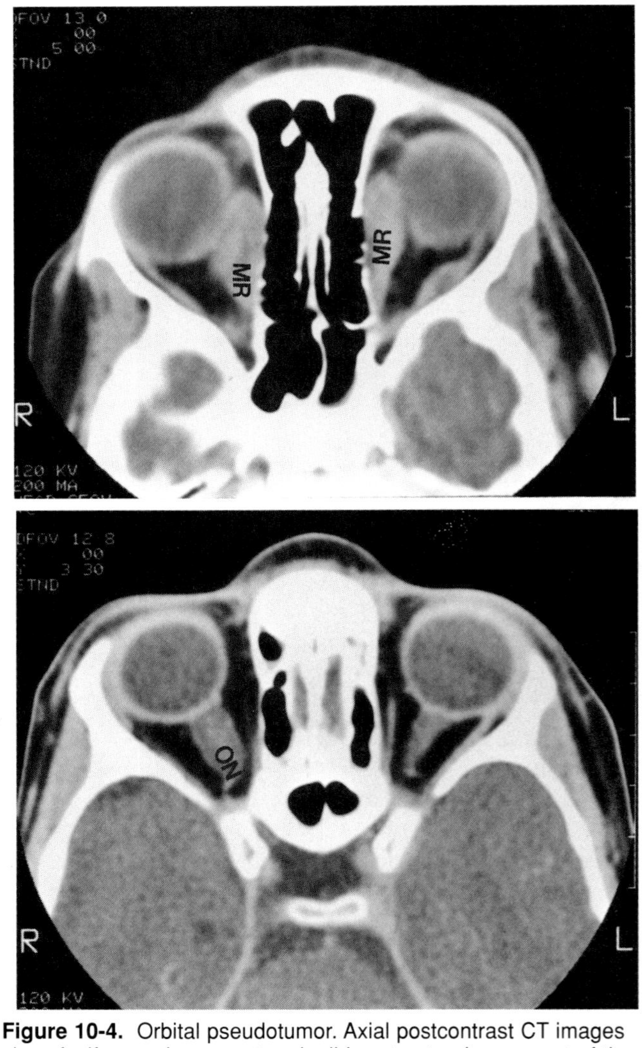

Figure 10-4. Orbital pseudotumor. Axial postcontrast CT images show fusiform enlargement and mild contrast enhancement of the medial rectus (MR) muscles and thickening and poor definition of the interface between the right optic nerve (ON) and adjacent intraconal fat. The child was treated with steroids, and the symptoms resolved.

dons are involved in some patients. Involved muscles appear to have irregular interfaces with the adjacent fat and show enhancement similar to that of the other structures that are infiltrated. Rarely, the entire orbit is involved, leading to proptosis; however, proptosis is not limited to children with involvement of the entire orbit. Occasionally, the lacrimal gland is involved. The CT features of the test patient do not support a diagnosis of pseudotumor because of the absence of intraconal changes and the presence of an extraconal (inflammatory) mass.

Cavernous hemangioma of the orbit is the most common vascular lesion of the orbit, but accounts for only about 2% of pediatric orbital masses. The lesion most often presents in the second to fourth decades of life with progressive proptosis, extraocular motility abnormalities, and impaired visual acuity. These tumors are well-encapsulated retro-ocular masses that tend to enlarge slowly and do not spontaneously involute. They do not invade other orbital structures. On imaging, these lesions most often appear as sharply demarcated oval masses in the superior-temporal portion of the conus. They are capable of expanding the bony orbit, show heterogeneous enhancement, and infrequently contain small calcifications.

In contrast, capillary hemangioma of the orbit (Option (C)) is an invasive, unencapsulated lesion that usually develops within the first weeks of life and presents with rapidly progressive proptosis. The hemangioma is pathologically a benign proliferative capillary malformation and is considered the most common benign mass arising within or adjacent to the orbit in children less than 2 years old. Nearly all cases (95%) are apparent by 6 months of age. About 80% of patients have associated lesions involving the skin of the face or neck or the larynx. The hemangioma is generally rapidly progressive and grows at an unpredictable rate for 2 to 3 years, at which time it regresses spontaneously. Because of this spontaneous regression, most patients are managed conservatively; lesions that do not regress or that cause visual problems are treated with intralesional or systemic steroids, surgery, or embolization. Embolization may be indicated for the treatment of amblyopia, platelet consumption (Kasabach-Merritt syndrome), or local skin ulceration and infection.

CT examination of a child with a capillary hemangioma typically demonstrates both superficial and deep components of the hemangioma (Figure 10-5). In about 90% of patients, an anterior or periorbital component is identified. Conversely, about 75% of lesions with superficial components extend into the postseptal, intraconal space. The imaging features include a variably enhancing mass that involves the superficial, extraconal space and can extend into the retrobulbar region. The degree of enhancement ranges from mild (isodense relative to muscle) to marked. Since most lesions are not encapsulated, they often appear to infiltrate adjacent structures, blurring their margins. Although the tumor is infiltrating, it appears not to destroy the adjacent tissue but, rather, to encase it. The bone adjacent to hemangiomas may become remodeled or thinned; however, true destruction or erosion of bone does not occur. In addition, associated prominent superficial vessels over the bridge of the nose, temporal region, lateral brow, and lateral cheek are present. Phleboliths are often present, as in cavernous hemangiomas and orbital varices. A capillary hemangioma can be excluded as a diagnosis in the test patient by the combination of clinical and imaging features presented. The test patient is older than would be expected for presentation with a capillary hemangioma and does not have an enhancing intraconal mass.

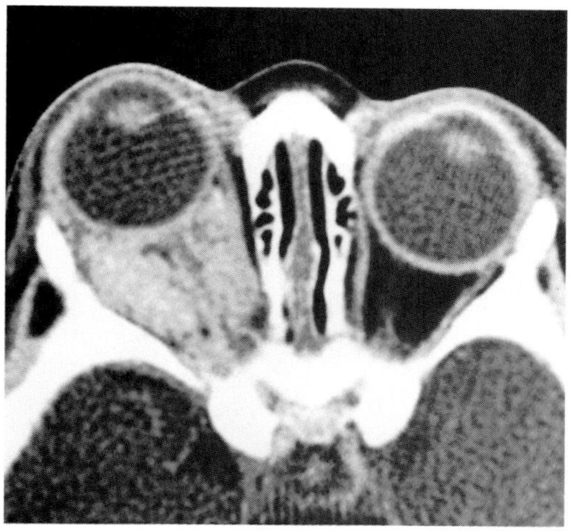

Figure 10-5. Capillary hemangioma. An axial postcontrast CT image shows a large capillary hemangioma in a 3-month-old girl. There is a markedly enhancing, irregularly defined mass in the right retrobulbar (intraconal) region; the hemangioma replaces the normal fat and causes proptosis.

Rhabdomyosarcoma of the orbit (Option (D)) is the most common primary orbital cancer of children. Most children present during the first decade of life with progressive unilateral proptosis; 90% of patients are younger than 16 years at diagnosis, with an average age at presentation of 7 years. Periorbital edema, pain, ophthalmoplegia, and diminished visual acuity also occur. CT demonstrates a noncalcified, soft tissue mass usually arising from an extraocular muscle, with associated proptosis and bone destruction. Preseptal extension is common and is often helpful in differentiating this condition from metastatic neuroblastoma. Bone destruction occurs in most patients (Figure 10-6); this sign strongly suggests cancer but is not specific for rhabdomyosarcoma. Postseptal cellulitis rarely causes gross bone destruction, and in the rare instances when bone destruction occurs, it tends to be subtle and limited to the lamina papyracea. The test images are not compatible with a diagnosis of rhabdomyosarcoma primarily because of the lack of bone destruction or invasion of adjacent structures. Also, orbital rhabdomyosarcoma is generally associated with marked enlargement of an extraocular muscle, which is the site of tumor origin in about 70% of patients.

The MRI appearance of rhabdomyosarcoma of the orbit parallels the findings of rhabdomyosarcoma in other regions of the body. It frequently is isointense relative to normal muscle on T1-weighted images and is isointense or only minimally hyperintense relative to muscle on T2-weighted images. Enhancement occurs to a variable degree on postcontrast T1-weighted images. As with other mass lesions of the orbit, abnormal en-

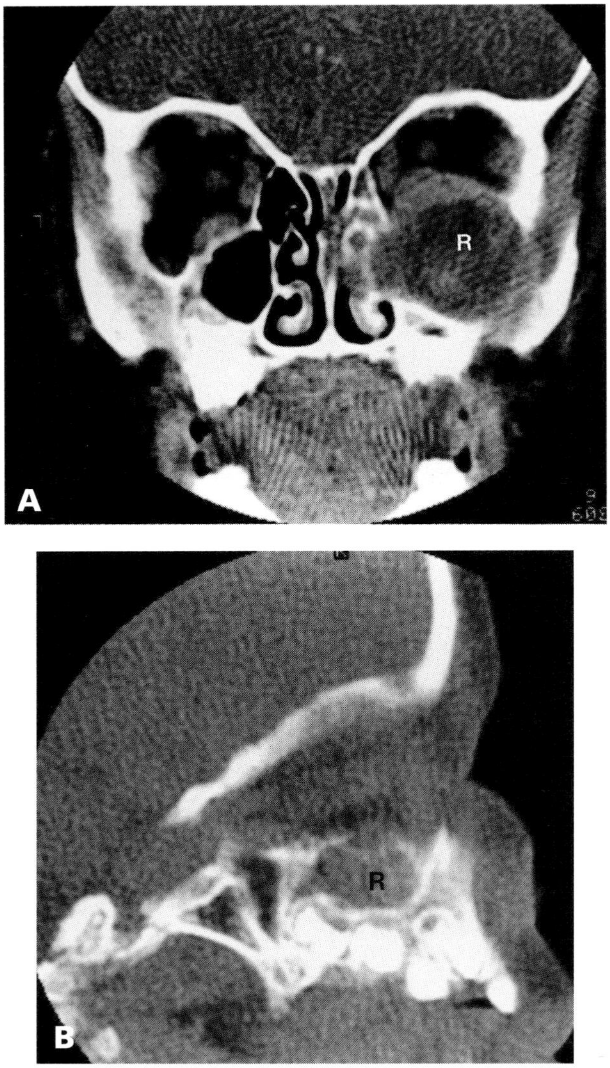

Figure 10-6. Rhabdomyosarcoma. This 2-year-old girl presented with an orbital rhabdomyosarcoma (R), which rapidly enlarged over a 3-month period. Direct coronal (A) and sagittal (B) CT images reveal enlargement of the inferior rectus muscle with adjacent destruction of the orbital floor. The mass extends into the maxillary sinus. Secondary upward displacement of the globe and optic nerve was also present (not shown).

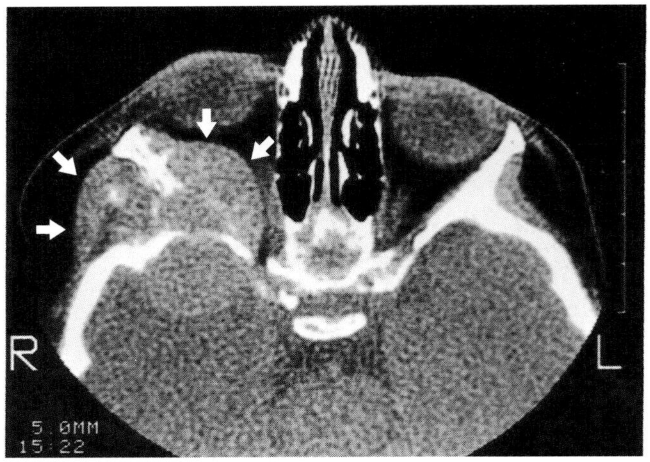

Figure 10-7. Neuroblastoma. This 2-year-old child had proptosis and periorbital discoloration secondary to metastatic neuroblastoma. An axial CT image shows permeative destruction of the lateral orbital wall and sphenoid bone, with a soft tissue mass (arrows) encircling the bone on all three surfaces. This pattern strongly suggests that the lesion has arisen within the bone or bone marrow.

hancement is detected more clearly when fat suppression is used. Intracranial, infratemporal, and lateral extension of orbital rhabdomyosarcomas is evaluated more readily by MRI than by CT.

The most common solid tumors that metastasize to the orbit in children are neuroblastoma (Option (E)) and Ewing's sarcoma. Metastatic neuroblastoma is considerably more common. The lateral orbital wall is a commonly affected site. When this area is involved by hematogenous spread, there is a combination of permeative destruction and a soft tissue mass on all three sides of the bone: temporal, lateral orbit, and epidural (Figure 10-7). The lateral extraconal involvement invariably results in proptosis, and the epidural and temporal components create mass effect, which may or may not produce clinical symptoms. Permeative metastases secondary to neuroblastoma can occur anywhere in the skeleton, including the facial structures. However, when metastases are identified in the facial structures, they are usually a component of widespread disease and indicate a poor prognosis. Orbital neuroblastoma is bilateral in more than 50% of patients. The test images are inconsistent with metastatic neuroblastoma because of the lack of permeative changes or associated soft tissue masses in any of the facial bones, especially the lateral orbital wall.

Question 53

Concerning orbital pseudotumor,

(A) it is more common in children than in adults
(B) it is rarely bilateral
(C) the muscle tendons are spared
(D) CT frequently demonstrates destruction of bone
(E) it is indistinguishable from Graves' ophthalmopathy

Orbital pseudotumor is a nongranulomatous inflammatory disorder of unknown etiology. It may be idiopathic, associated with a systemic disease (sarcoidosis or endocrinopathy), or associated with unrecognized focal infections or a foreign body. The condition is uncommon in childhood; only about 15% of all cases occur in children (**Option (A) is false**). Children present with abrupt onset of orbital pain, which may be associated with proptosis, ophthalmoplegia, lid swelling and erythema, chemosis, decreased vision, or a palpable mass. Approximately 15% to 20% of patients have bilateral involvement (**Option (B) is false**). Several different patterns of orbital involvement have been reported. These consist of (1) a well-defined lesion in the area of the lacrimal gland, (2) a retrobulbar lesion that may or may not involve the sclera, (3) optic neuritis, (4) a poorly defined lesion in the apex of the orbit, (5) myositis, or (6) a diffuse pattern involving several regions. No single pattern predominates in childhood; however, the presence of a well-defined mass in the lacrimal fossa or an ill-defined lesion in the orbital apex is rare in childhood. Optic neuritis, orbital myositis, and the diffuse pattern of pseudotumor are more common in children. Radiologic and laboratory examinations aid in distinguishing orbital pseudotumor from other conditions, including infectious, metabolic, and neoplastic processes. As a result, tissue biopsy is seldom necessary to confirm the diagnosis. When performed, the histopathologic examination reveals a lymphocytic infiltration of the fat, muscles, sclera, or lacrimal gland. This inflammation is often associated with fibrosis and eosinophilia. A clinical trial of steroids generally produces striking resolution of signs and symptoms within 48 hours. Imaging findings similar to those associated with orbital pseudotumor can be seen in children with true orbital infectious processes, sarcoidosis, and Wegener's granulomatosis.

Although the CT features of the disease vary, there is usually a localized infiltration of the retrobulbar region. This cellular infiltration results in a change of the retrobulbar fat to water density. In addition, irregular thickening and increased attenuation of the uveal-scleral interface (Figure 10-8) and the optic nerve are found. After intravenous administration of contrast agent, these areas generally enhance markedly. The extraocular muscles also can be involved and will appear enlarged because of the associated myositis. Again, enhancement usually occurs. The result of this retrobulbar involvement is usually some degree of proptosis. When the muscles are involved there is usually associated thickening of the muscle tendons (**Option (C) is false**), which is one of several features that may help distinguish this condition from Graves' ophthalmopathy (Table 10-1) (**Option (E) is false**). In some patients, there is isolated

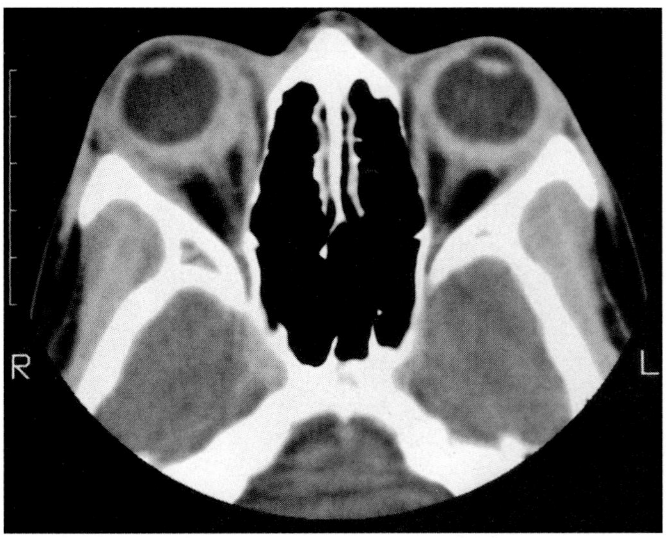

Figure 10-8. Orbital pseudotumor. An axial postcontrast CT image demonstrates uveal-scleral thickening bilaterally. On other axial images, the optic nerve and extraocular muscle were enlarged.

Table 10-1: Features of thyroid ophthalmopathy and orbital pseudotumor[a]

involvement of one or more extraocular muscles, with diffuse

	involvement	Normal
Feature	Thyroid Ophthalmopathy	Orbital
Distribution		Pseudotumor
Muscle enlargement	85% Bilateral	
Tendon involvement	I>M>S>L	85% Unilateral
Fat involvement	Normal	All enlarged
Lacrimal gland	Fat quantity increased	Involved

[a]I = inferior rectus; M = medial rectus; S = superior rectus; L = lateral rectus.

enlargement on CT or MRI. This variation is termed myositic pseudotumor. Isolated involvement of the lacrimal gland is also identified in some children, whereas the entire orbit is involved in others. Bone destruction is not associated with this condition (**Option (D) is false**). The lack of bone destruction is helpful in the differential diagnosis. Bone destruction is more often identified in children with malignant neoplasms, such as orbital rhabdomyosarcoma, esthesioneuroblastoma and metastases, and aggressive inflammatory lesions, such as Wegener's granulomatosis and lethal midline granuloma.

MRI findings are similar to those noted by CT. Again, uveal-scleral thickening, enlargement of the extraocular muscles, and irregular muscle insertions may be seen. The involved areas are generally isointense relative to the extraocular muscles and hypointense relative to fat on T1-weighted images and isointense relative to fat on T2-weighted images.

As a result of cellular infiltration, the fat in the involved orbit usually has decreased signal intensity. Other benign inflammatory conditions often tend to produce a more marked increase in signal intensity on T2-weighted images. As a well-defined mass in the outer aspect of the orbit (lacrimal space), pseudotumor has an appearance very similar to that of leukemia or infiltration of the lacrimal gland by lymphoma. Also, scleral and retrobulbar pseudotumor may have an appearance similar to the pattern found in acute lymphocytic leukemia. The clinical presentation of a sudden onset of painful proptosis helps differentiate orbital pseudotumor from the more insidious and painless onset of leukemia. Characteristic of a local pseudotumor is its rapid and often complete response following steroid therapy. At times, a biopsy may be necessary to distinguish orbital pseudotumor from infiltrative malignancy.

Question 54

Concerning orbital cellulitis,

(A) preseptal cellulitis usually cannot be distinguished from postseptal cellulitis on physical examination
(B) preseptal cellulitis is confined to the eyelid
(C) postseptal cellulitis usually involves the intraconal space
(D) CT reliably differentiates subperiosteal abscess from phlegmon
(E) intracranial complications occur in fewer than 5% of children with postseptal cellulitis

Pneumatization of the paranasal sinuses during childhood follows a predictable sequence; however, the exact age at which each sinus pneumatizes varies. In general, the maxillary and ethmoid sinuses are pneumatized at birth, although they are tiny. The sphenoid sinus develops from anterior to posterior and is usually pneumatized by 4 to 6 years of age. The frontal sinuses are the last to develop and arise as outgrowths from the anterior ethmoid cells. Pneumatization is usually identified at about 10 years of age, and the sinuses continue to enlarge over the next few years. People with persistent metopic sutures may not develop frontal sinuses.

Acute orbital inflammatory disease is defined as suppurative inflammation of the soft tissues of the orbit (orbital cellulitis) or surrounding the orbit (periorbital cellulitis). Acute or chronic ethmoid sinusitis is the most common cause of periorbital cellulitis and orbital cellulitis in children. Transvenous migration represents the most common route by which infection spreads from the ethmoid sinuses to the orbital soft tissues. Hematogenous spread also can occur secondary to periodontal injury, a foreign body, skin infection, or middle ear disease.

Sinonasal orbital inflammation progresses in a predictable manner. Chandler et al. categorized this progression into five stages. In stage 1, preseptal swelling occurs initially in the eyelid and later in the adjacent soft tissues (Figure 10-9). Then, in stage 2, the inflammation extends through the orbital septum to involve the postseptal extraconal space. When this region is involved, the child presents with pain, proptosis, and chemosis (Figure 10-10). Depending on the severity of the infection, there may be associated reduction of extraocular movements as a result of inflammation of the muscle(s). If the infection is untreated, it may progress to stage 3, which involves an extraconal subperiosteal abscess. In addition to the signs and symptoms characteristic of stage 2, the globe is displaced inferolaterally by the mass of the fluid collection. If further progression (i.e., stage 4) occurs, a true orbital abscess develops and involves the postseptal intraconal space. This development is generally associated with severe proptosis, chemosis, ophthalmoplegia, and loss of visual acuity. If septic thrombophlebitis occurs with retrograde extension via the valveless ophthalmic veins (i.e., stage 5), cavernous sinus thrombosis can occur. When this stage is reached, in addition to the signs and symptoms described for stage 4 disease, there is rapidly progressive bilateral ophthalmoplegia.

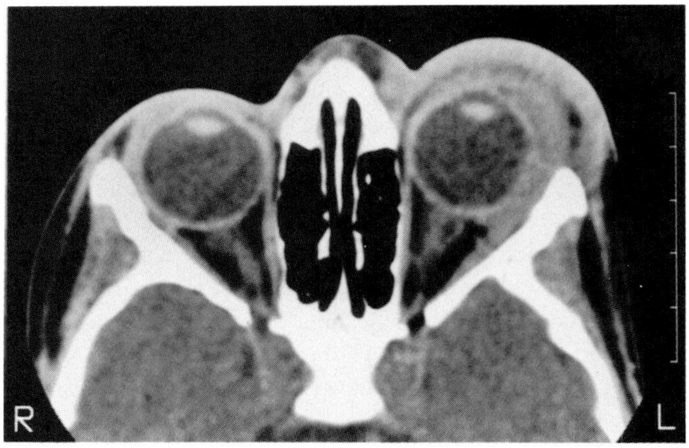

Figure 10-9. Orbital cellulitis. An axial noncontrast CT image shows a swollen left eyelid and adjacent soft tissues in a 3-year-old boy. All swelling is anterior to the orbital septum. This pattern of involvement is characteristic of preseptal cellulitis, in contrast to postseptal cellulitis, which is deep to the lid.

As already noted, periorbital cellulitis is a common condition in childhood and is often but not always a complication of ethmoid sinusitis. In children, the bony septa of the sinus walls are thinner, the vascular foramina are larger, the bones are more porous, and the sutures are still open. These features seem to be especially significant for facilitating the spread of infection. In older children, frontal sinusitis and, rarely, sphenoid sinusitis can cause this condition. CT scans of children with periorbital cellulitis show that more than one sinus is usually involved. In some patients, the sinuses are completely normal and the orbital infection appears to spread by direct extension from an adjacent site such as infected teeth or adjacent soft tissue infection of the face. In rare instances, the periorbital inflammation results from hematogenous spread. The organisms most often isolated include *Staphylococcus* and *Strepto-*

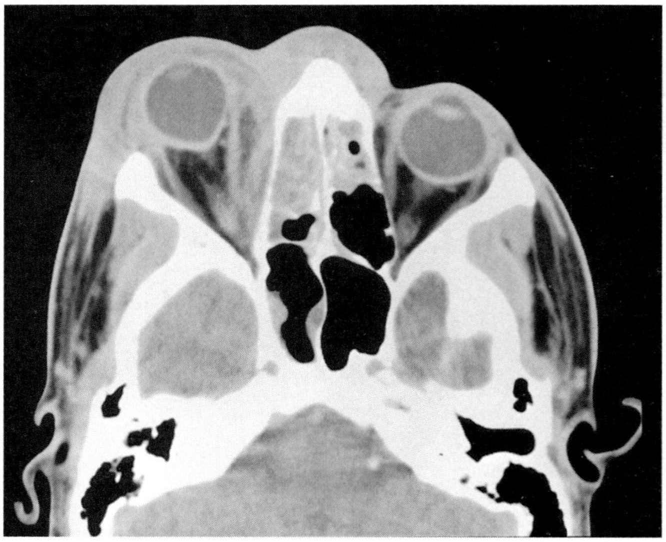

Figure 10-10. Orbital cellulitis. A postcontrast axial CT image shows partial opacification of the ethmoid sinuses. There is preseptal soft tissue thickening attributable to inflammation as well as edema and inflammation in the extraconal fat. Proptosis is present.

coccus species. Infants and toddlers can have *Haemophilus influenzae* infections. These children may have a bluish or purplish hue to the skin overlying the involved sinus.

As noted previously, the orbital contents are divided anteriorly and posteriorly by the orbital septum. The bony orbit is lined by periosteum (periorbita), which reflects anteriorly onto the tarsal plate of the eyelid. This tissue reflection is known as the orbital septum. The tissue anterior to the septum is preseptal, whereas the larger, posterior space is postseptal. The postseptal space is further subdivided into the intraconal and extraconal compartments by the extraocular muscles. The intraconal space contains the globe, retrobulbar fat, and optic nerve.

Preseptal cellulitis typically involves both the eyelid and the facial soft tissues (**Option (B) is false**). Typically, edema and erythema are seen in the lid, and in time they can spread to the adjacent facial soft tissues. Features of preseptal cellulitis that distinguish it from postseptal disease include chemosis, proptosis, lack of visual abnormalities, and a normal range of extraocular motion. Differentiation between these conditions on the basis of these clinical characteristics is therefore generally straightforward (**Option (A) is false**). Most cases of postseptal cellulitis involve the postseptal, extraconal space. Although a range of symptoms can be identified at presentation, pain, chemosis, and proptosis are usually noted. It should be noted that virtually all patients with postseptal cellulitis also have preseptal disease. In addition, conjunctivitis, diminished extraocular motion, and intracranial extension can be seen. Intracranial extension of the infection is uncommon, occurring in fewer than 1% of patients (**Option (E) is true**). Central nervous system involvement is usually the result of hematogenous spread via the small bridging veins that travel through the walls of the sinuses, orbits, and calvaria. Intracranial complications include epidural abscess, subdural abscess, meningitis, brain abscess, and cavernous sinus thrombosis.

Not all patients with periorbital or orbital inflammatory disease require CT evaluation. However, when there is diplopia or loss of visual acuity, CT is indicated as an emergency procedure, because surgical decompression is necessary. Also, if there are questions of central nervous system complications or the diagnosis is not certain, CT is indicated. In the absence of these findings, the patient is first managed medically with intravenous antibiotics. This action will generally result in decreasing clinical symptoms within 24 hours, and imaging is unnecessary. However, if there is lack of improvement or worsening of the clinical condition, orbital CT is indicated.

The approach to diagnostic imaging varies among institutions. CT is generally considered the modality of choice; however, the imaging protocol used may vary. A diagnosis can readily be made with contiguous 5-mm-thick axial, precontrast images, postcontrast images only, or both sequences. The main difference between precontrast and postcontrast images is that the latter show subperiosteal inflammatory masses (phlegmon or abscess) more conspicuously and also demonstrate mild medial rectus muscle involvement more readily because of the enhancement attributable to the associated myositis. When an intracranial complication is suspected, contrast agent administration is required, and both axial and coronal images should be obtained to optimally visualize the brain and extra-axial spaces, with special attention to those adjacent to the orbital roof and planum sphenoidale. Extension of the inflammatory process into the intraconal space rarely occurs today, probably because of the widespread use of antibiotics (**Option (C) is false**).

Although it is usually not difficult to diagnose a postseptal, extraconal inflammatory mass, differentiating between a phlegmon (predominantly solid inflammatory mass) and a mature subperiosteal abscess (central liquefaction) is generally difficult. Differentiation of these two stages of the inflammatory process is important for determining the approach to therapy. If a phlegmon is present, hospitalization and treatment with intravenous antibiotics will usually obviate surgery. However, if a mature abscess with central liquefaction is present, surgery may be necessary. CT is not able to differentiate a phlegmon from an abscess unless a gas-fluid level or an enhancing rim is present (**Option (D) is false**). Low attenuation within the medial or lateral extraconal mass can be seen with cellulitis, as well as with an abscess.

Question 55

Concerning capillary hemangioma of the orbit,

(A) it is usually diagnosed in infancy
(B) it is associated with cutaneous hemangiomas
(C) it often presents with proptosis
(D) it is often associated with spontaneous bleeding
(E) CT often shows bone destruction
(F) it is an extraconal lesion

Capillary hemangioma has two overlapping anatomic patterns. Superficial hemangiomas of the lid are the most common. Frequently they are confined to the preseptal space and usually are located in the upper lid. A second and more aggressive form can occupy the entire bony orbit and result in expansion and remodeling.

Capillary hemangioma of the orbit is a benign neoplasm that usually presents within the first weeks of life (**Option (A) is true**); most cases are diagnosed by 6 months of age. The lesion accounts for about 5% to 15% of all orbital masses in children and more commonly affects girls (3:1 ratio of girls to boys). The capillary hemangioma is invasive and unencapsulated and tends to infiltrate the orbital components without regard to anatomic planes. The most common location is the superior nasal quadrant of the orbit. In rare instances, the capillary hemangioma extends intracranially by direct extension via the superior orbital fissure, orbital roof, or optic canal. Capillary hemangiomas often grow until 2 to 3 years of age, at which time they begin to spontaneously involute. Spontaneous bleeding is rare and occurs more often in patients with orbital lymphangiomas (**Option (D) is false**).

Superficial lesions present with skin discoloration and mass effect, whereas deep lesions usually are initially identified as a result of rapidly progressive proptosis (**Option (C) is true**). Clinically, a capillary hemangioma can enlarge during crying or other maneuvers producing a Valsalva effect, with discoloration of the skin about the orbit or with proptosis. The lesion is associated with cutaneous strawberry hemangiomas of the face or neck or with similar hemangiomas in the larynx or elsewhere in the body in 80% of patients (**Option (B) is true**).

Capillary hemangiomas of the orbit involve the postseptal, intraconal space (**Option (F) is false**). CT and MRI are diagnostic. Approximately 90% of the lesions have an anterior component. Conversely, 75% of superficial lesions extend into the orbit. CT demonstrates a poorly marginated intraconal mass that is isodense relative to muscle on precontrast images and enhances markedly on postcontrast images. The lesion causes mass effect, usually with significant proptosis. In general, the mass encases, but does not invade, the optic nerve and extraocular muscles, making differentiation of these structures from the mass impossible. Capillary hemangiomas do not destroy bone (**Option (E) is false**), but can cause remodeling with associated enlargement of the bony orbit. The identification of bony changes of the orbit depends on the age at the time of imaging. In children in whom the mass has been present for many months, unilateral orbital enlargement without destruction can be seen.

The findings on MRI are similar to those on CT, with the lesion being isointense relative to muscle on T1-weighted images and hyperintense on T2-weighted images. Injection of gadolinium chelate results in obvious enhancement of the mass.

The more aggressive capillary hemangioma is primarily postseptal. This type of lesion eventually can occupy the entire bony orbit, which will become expanded (Figure 10-11). This expansion will result in deviation of the eye. Postseptal involvement can be intraconal, extraconal, or both. Just as with the smaller, superficial hemangiomas, calcification is rare. Despite its size, this variety often remains reasonably well defined and appears homogeneous and hyperintense following contrast enhancement. This type of lesion can extend out of the orbit, through the inferior or superior orbital fissures into the pterygomaxillary fossa or intracranially. A not uncommon exit of venous drainage is intracranially through the cavernous sinus system into the middle cranial fossa.

Cavernous hemangiomas differ from capillary hemangiomas in many ways. Individuals with cavernous hemangiomas usually present between the second and fourth decades, and this condition accounts for only 2% of pediatric orbital masses. A cavernous hemangioma is a well-encapsulated mass that can involve any portion of the orbit. However, it typically involves the intraconal space, usually in the retrobulbar region. Unlike capillary hemangiomas, cavernous hemangiomas usually enlarge slowly and do not involute at any age. Because cavernous hemangiomas are surrounded by a pseudocapsule, they do not invade and encase structures. Instead, they exert mass effect and displace adjacent structures while remaining confined by anatomic planes. As a result of these pathologic features, patients usually present with slowly progressive proptosis, difficulties with extraocular movements, and impaired vision.

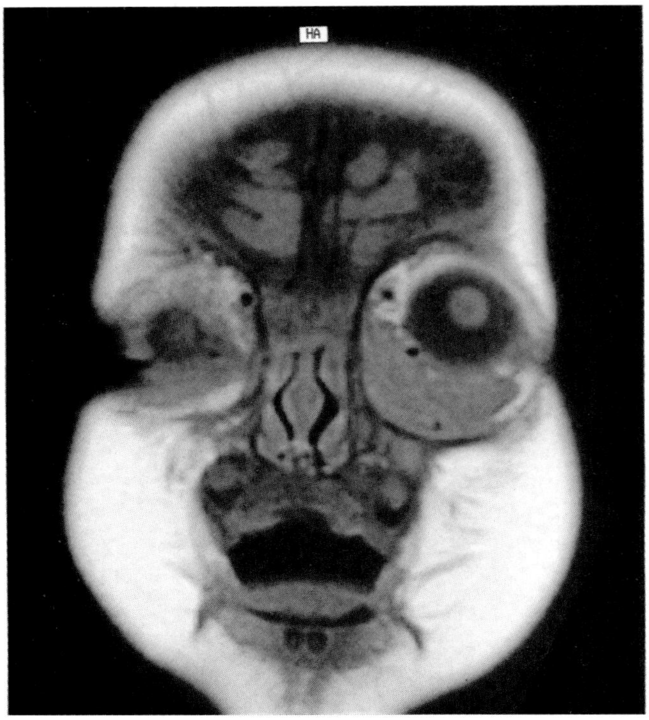

SE 500/13

Figure 10-11. Capillary hemangioma. A coronal T1-weighted MR image shows proptosis and elevation of the left globe. Note the marked expansion of the bony left orbit.

On CT, a cavernous hemangioma appears as a rounded, well-defined, high-attenuation mass with variable contrast enhancement. Depending on the size and location of the mass, there is variable mass effect with resultant displacement of adjacent structures, but without invasion or blurring of adjacent anatomic planes. The appearance of a cavernous hemangioma on MRI is nonspecific. On T1-weighted images, the lesion is usually isointense relative to the extraocular muscles. On T2-weighted sequences, the lesion appears hyperintense. Injection of gadolinium chelate results in a variable degree of enhancement.

Question 56

Concerning orbital rhabdomyosarcoma,

(A) it is the most common primary malignant orbital tumor in children
(B) the embryonal type is the most common histologic form
(C) CT often shows bone destruction
(D) it invades the optic nerve

Neoplasms involving the pediatric orbit can be of primary orbital origin, extend into the orbit from adjacent structures, or be metastatic. The most common primary tumors are optic glioma, rhabdomyosarcoma, neurofibroma, and retinoblastoma. Rarely, lesions such as Langerhans cell histiocytosis, chondrosarcoma, fibrosarcoma, and osteogenic sarcoma arise from the bony orbit. Bony metastases are common in childhood tumors. The most frequently identified metastases in the orbital region are secondary to neuroblastoma and Ewing's sarcoma.

Rhabdomyosarcoma is the most common primary malignant tumor of the orbit in childhood (**Option (A) is true**). The lesion is more common in Caucasians, and 90% of affected children are 16 years of age or younger. Orbital rhabdomyosarcoma accounts for approximately 4% of all orbital masses in childhood. Although rhabdomyosarcoma occurs randomly in the population, a rare association with neurofibromatosis has been reported. There are three histologic types of tumor: embryonal, alveolar, and undifferentiated. The embryonal type is the most common, accounting for about 75% of cases (**Option (B) is true**). The alveolar type is diagnosed in approximately 15% of patients, whereas undifferentiated tumors account for 10% of cases. Most rhabdomyosarcomas of the eye involve the orbit proper (about 70% of cases) (Figure 10-12); the remainder involve the eyelid and the conjunctiva.

Rhabdomyosarcomas can arise anywhere from within or around the orbit. However, they typically originate from mesenchymal tissue other than the extraocular muscles. A preseptal origin in the upper lid or the medial epicanthal region is not uncommon. However, any region of the orbit can be affected. Intraorbital tumors can be intraconal or extraconal or rapidly involve both spaces.

The most common clinical finding with rhabdomyosarcoma of the orbit is rapidly progressive proptosis; however, ptosis, eyelid or conjunctival edema, nasal obstruction, epistaxis, abnormal extraocular movements, pain, and loss of vision also can be found. On average, children present at approximately 7 years of age. The most common sites of presentation are in the supranasal quadrant of the orbit and behind the globe. Once a diagnosis is established, treatment consists of radiation and chemotherapy. Radical surgery is reserved for disease that extends out of the orbit. The prognosis for rhabdomyosarcoma localized to the orbit is better than that for rhabdomyosarcoma in other head and neck sites, with about a 90% 3-year survival rate.

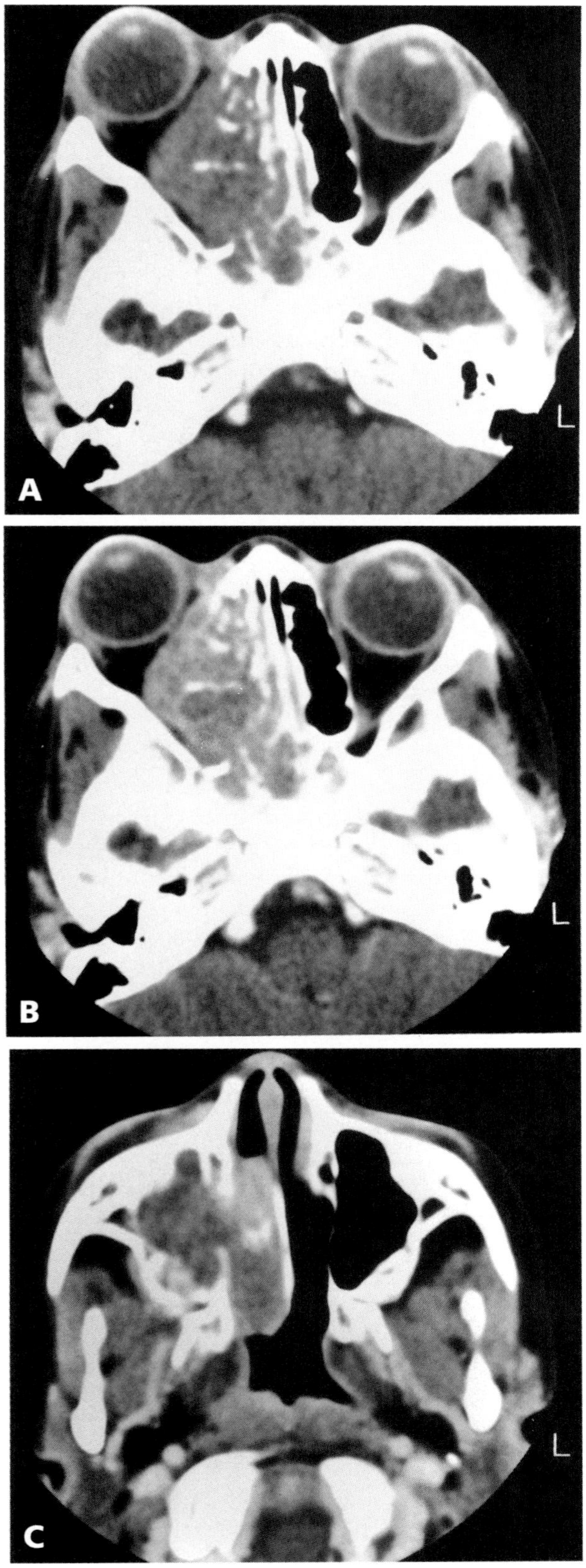

Figure 10-12. Rhabdomyosarcoma. (A and B) Precontrast (A) and postcontrast (B) axial CT images of a 4-year-old girl show that the mass involves the medial rectus muscle, enhances mildly, and destroys the adjacent lamina papyracea, sphenoid bone, and maxilla. (C) A postcontrast axial CT image at a lower level shows that the large soft tissue mass extends into the maxillary sinus and nasal fossa. Numerous flecks of destroyed bone can be seen within the mass.

On CT, rhabdomyosarcoma presents as a variably sized mass that is almost always associated with destruction of adjacent bone (**Option (C) is true**). Small rhabdomyosarcomas that are detected early are typically homogeneous on CT, with attenuation values very similar to those of normal muscle. In addition, tumors smaller than 2 cm can show an irregular contour, but often remain well defined and noninvasive. Tumors larger than 2 cm often contain areas of decreased or heterogeneous attenuation from tumor necrosis. With contrast agent administration, moderate enhancement is common and may be indistinguishable from the enhancement pattern found with other soft tissue malignancies. Tumor extension into an adjacent sinus, nasal cavity, or the skull base occurs. Direct extension into the optic nerve does not seem to occur (**Option (D) is false**). Because of the potential for lesions extending into the skull base to spread into the intracranial, extra-axial space by direct extension via normal fissures and foramina or via bone destruction, it is important to include postcontrast direct coronal images, since axial images alone can miss early disease. In addition, reconstruction with bone algorithms is helpful for differential diagnosis and detection of bone destruction. Although both CT and MRI can be diagnostic for a malignancy, MRI has become the modality of choice in most cases.

The MRI appearance of orbital rhabdomyosarcoma is similar to that of rhabdomyosarcoma elsewhere in the body. On T1-weighted MR images, rhabdomyosarcoma is hypointense relative to fat and isointense relative to muscle. On T2-weighted images, the lesion appears hyperintenserelative to fat and muscle and enhances heterogeneously with injection of gadolinium chelate. As with other masses, abnormal enhancement is detected more readily when a preexcitation radiofrequency pulse is used to suppress fat signal. As with CT, invasion into the paranasal sinuses or pharynx can be identified by MRI.

A specific histologic diagnosis of malignant neoplasia within the orbit is not possible with cross-sectional imaging alone (Figure 10-13). However, the aggressive appearance of such lesions as a whole is indicated by the presence of infiltration, a poorly marginated tumor, surrounding bone destruction, and variable enhancement with CT and MRI as a result of tissue necrosis.

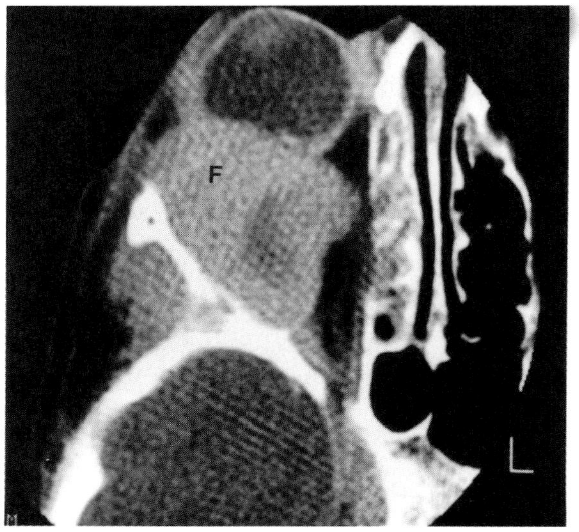

Figure 10-13. Fibrosarcoma. A CT image shows the fibrosarcoma (F), a primary bone tumor, arising from the lateral orbital wall. This neoplasm mimics the features of neuroblastoma and other primary bone tumors and marrow abnormalities that may involve the sphenoid wing and lateral orbital wall.

SUGGESTED READINGS

ORBITAL CELLULITIS

1. Barnes PD, Robson CD, Robertson RL, Poussaint TY. Pediatric orbital and visual pathway lesions. Neuroimaging Clin North Am 1996; 6:179–198
2. Chandler JR, Langenbrunner DJ, Stevens ER. The pathogenesis of orbital complications in acute sinusitis. Laryngoscope 1970; 80:1414–1428
3. Dresner SC, Rothfus WE, Slamovits TG, Kennerdell JS, Curtin HD. Computed tomography of orbital myositis. AJR 1984; 143:671–674
4. Hornblass A, Herschorn BJ, Stern K, Grimes C. Orbital abscess. Surv Ophthalmol 1984; 29:169–178
5. Moloney JR, Badham NJ, McRae A. The acute orbit. Preseptal (periorbital) cellulitis, subperiosteal abscess and orbital cellulitis due to sinusitis. J Laryngol Otol Suppl 1987; 12:1–8
6. Shapiro ED, Wald ER, Brozanski BA. Periorbital cellulitis and paranasal sinusitis: a reappraisal. Pediatr Infect Dis 1982; 1:91–94

PSEUDOTUMOR

7. Atlas SW, Grossman RI, Sovino PJ, et al. Surface-coil MR of orbital pseudotumor. AJR 1987; 148:803–808
8. Berger JW, Rubin PA, Jakobiec FA. Pediatric orbital pseudotumor: case report and review of the literature. Int Ophthalmol Clin 1996; 36:161–177
9. Berrocal T, de Orbe A, Prieto C, et al. US and color Doppler imaging of ocular and orbital disease in the pediatric age group. RadioGraphics 1996; 16:251–272
10. Khan JA, Hoover DL, Giangiacomo J, Singsen BH. Orbital and childhood sarcoidosis. J Pediatr Ophthalmol Strabismus 1986; 23:190–194
11. Mottow LS, Jakobiec FA. Idiopathic inflammatory orbital pseudotumor in childhood. I. Clinical characteristics. Arch Ophthalmol 1978; 96: 1410–1417
12. Nugent RA, Rootman J, Robertson WD, Lapointe JS, Harrison PB. Acute orbital pseudotumors: classification and CT features. AJR 1981; 137:957–962
13. Parelholff ES, Chavis RM, Friendly DS. Wegener's granulomatosis presenting as orbital pseudotumor in children. J Pediatr Ophthalmol Strabismus 1985; 22:100–104

HEMANGIOMA

14. Davis KR, Hesselink JR, Dallow RL, Grove AS Jr. CT and ultrasound in the diagnosis of cavernous hemangioma and lymphangioma of the orbit. J Comput Tomogr 1980; 4:98–104
15. Dyer J, Atkinson L. Cavernous hemangioma of the orbit. Aust NZ J Surg 1985; 55:269–273
16. Flanagan JC. Vascular problems of the orbit. Ophthalmology 1979; 86: 896–913
17. Haik BG, Jakobiec FA, Ellsworth RM, Jones IS. Capillary hemangioma of the lids and orbit: an analysis of the clinical features and therapeutic results in 101 cases. Ophthalmology 1979; 86:760–792
18. Savoiardo M, Strada L, Passerini A. Cavernous hemangioma of the orbit: value of CT, angiography, and phlebography. AJNR 1983; 4:741–744

RHABDOMYOSARCOMA

19. Lallemand DP, Brasch RC, Char DH, Norman D. Orbital tumors in children. Characterization by computed tomography. Radiology 1984;

151:85–88
20. Nicholson DH, Green WR. Tumors of the eye, lids and orbit in children. In: Harley RD (ed), Pediatric ophthalmology. Philadelphia: WB Saunders; 1983:1223–1271
21. Porterfield JF. Orbital tumors in children: a report on 214 cases. Int Ophthalmol Clin 1962; 2:319–335
22. Stefanyszyn MA, Handler SD, Wright JE. Pediatric orbital tumors. Otolaryngol Clin North Am 1988; 21:103–118
23. Vade A, Armstrong MB. Orbital rhabdomyosarcoma in childhood. Radiol Clin North Am 1987; 25:701–714
24. Wharam M, Beltangady M, Hays D, et al. Localized orbital rhabdomyosarcoma. An interim report of the Intergroup Rhabdomyosarcoma Study Committee. Ophthalmology 1987; 94:251–254
25. Yang WT, Kwan WH, Li CK, Metreweli C. Imaging of pediatric head and neck rhabdomyosarcomas with emphasis on magnetic resonance imaging and a review of the literature. Pediatr Hematol Oncol 1997; 14: 243–257

GENERAL

26. Ball WS, Kulwin DR. The eye and orbit. In: Ball WS (ed), Pediatric neuroradiology. Philadelphia: Lippincott-Raven; 1997:565–606
27. Herrick RC, Hayman LA, Taber KH, Diaz-Marchan PJ, Kuo MD. Artifacts and pitfalls in MR imaging of the orbit: a clinical review. RadioGraphics 1997; 17:707–724
28. Starshak RJ, Wells RG, Sty JR, Gregg DC. Extracranial head and neck. In: Sty JR (ed), Diagnostic imaging of infants and children, vol. 2. Gaithersburg, MD: Aspen; 1992:255–341

CASE 11

Lane F. Donnelly, M.D.

Dermatomyositis

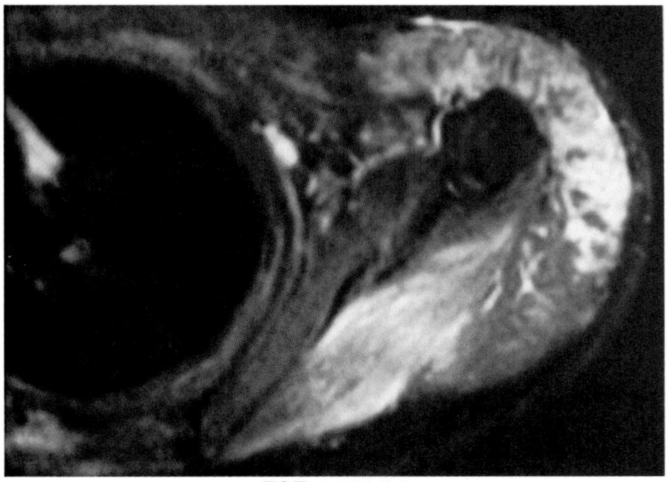

FSE 3,000/80

Figure 11-1

Question 57

This 15-year-old boy has left shoulder pain, swelling, and weakness. You are shown an axial fast spin-echo, T2-weighted image with fat saturation (Figure 11-1).

Which *one* of the following is the MOST likely diagnosis?

(A) Fascioscapulohumeral muscular dystrophy
(B) Dermatomyositis
(C) Plexiform neurofibroma
(D) Hemangioma
(E) Fibrosarcoma

The axial fast spin-echo, T2-weighted MR image of the test patient (Figure 11-1) demonstrates abnormal enlargement and heterogeneously increased signal intensity involving multiple muscles of the left shoulder girdle, including the deltoid, subscapularis, and supraspinatus (Figure 11-2). There is also abnormal increased signal within the adjacent musculofascial planes and subcutaneous tissues. There are no discrete focal masses within either the muscles or the subcutaneous tissues. The bony structures appear normal. Of the options listed, dermatomyositis is the most likely diagnosis based on these MRI findings (**Option (B) is correct**).

Muscular dystrophy is a heterogeneous group of relentlessly progressive muscle diseases. The most common type is Duchenne muscular dystrophy, which is an X-linked recessive disorder. The typical clinical scenario is that of a boy younger than 5 years of age presenting with proximal muscular weakness and a serum creatinine kinase level greater than 50 times the upper limit of normal. A combination of myopathic and neuropathic changes is seen on electromyography. Characteristic findings are short, low-amplitude polyphasic motor unit action potentials and fibrillations. A muscle biopsy shows characteristic findings of a necrotizing vasculitis with perivascular inflammation and small-vessel thrombosis, combined with inflammation, necrosis, and cellular loss of scattered myocytes. Other clinical manifestations include progressive cardiomyopathy, scoliosis, and kyphosis.

The diagnosis is usually made by muscle biopsy, and MRI has not played a significant diagnostic role. However, some reports have advocated the use of MR spectroscopy in the diagnosis, and others have advocated the use of MRI in monitoring

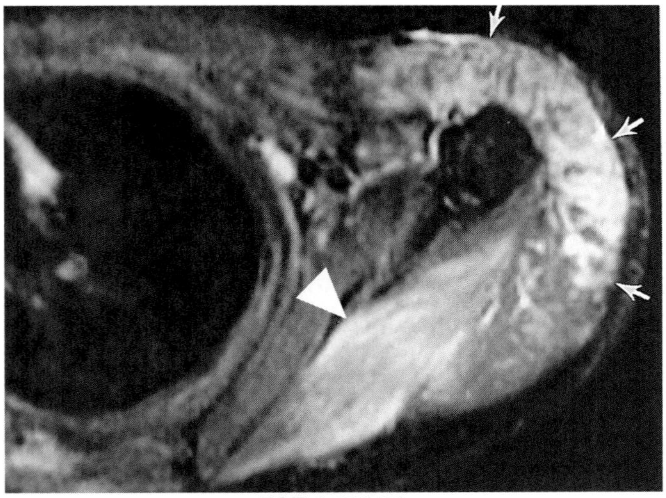

FSE 3,000/80

Figure 11-2 (Same as Figure 11-1). Dermatomyositis. An axial fast spin-echo, T2-weighted MR image with fat saturation shows enlargement and heterogeneously increased signal intensity involving multiple muscles of the shoulder girdle, including the deltoid (arrows) and supraspinatus (arrowhead). There is also abnormal signal within the adjacent musculofascial planes and subcutaneous tissues.

changes related to disease progression. MRI can play an important role in this respect because muscular dystrophy is a relentlessly progressive disease, therapeutic trial is continuous, and repeated biopsy is an unacceptable procedure for monitoring the disease.

The MRI findings are related to muscle atrophy and fatty replacement. T1-weighted images demonstrate heterogeneously increased signal within affected muscles secondary to the fatty replacement (Figure 11-3). In addition, there is an increase in the amount of subcutaneous fat adjacent to affected muscle groups. This is responsible for the "pseudohypertrophic" enlargement of the calves described in affected patients. The proximal muscle groups of the shoulders, thighs, and pelvis are most commonly affected. The most commonly spared muscles include the gracilis, sartorius, semimembranosus, and semitendinosus.

Radiographic findings include widening of the fibular head on frontal radiographs, osteoporosis, and, occasionally, changes that may mimic juvenile rheumatoid arthritis (joint space narrowing, periarticular osteoporosis, apparent overgrowth of epiphyses, and premature epiphyseal closure). Sonography demonstrates increased echogenicity of affected muscles, and CT demonstrates decreased attenuation; both of these are related to the fatty deposition in the atrophic muscles.

Fascioscapulohumeral muscular dystrophy (Option (A)) is a specific type of muscular dystrophy with a propensity to affect the muscles of the shoulder. It has an autosomal dominant inheritance pattern and affects both men and women. Affected patients, in contrast to those with Duchenne muscular dystrophy, present in adolescence rather than before 5 years of age with a characteristic weakness of the shoulder musculature. The scapulae are abnormally positioned in a "winged" configuration. Progression is slow, and the muscles of the trunk, pelvis, legs, and face eventually can become involved. Muscle enzyme levels in serum are usually normal or only slightly increased.

The test image (Figure 11-1) shows enlargement and increased signal intensity of the affected muscles. These features

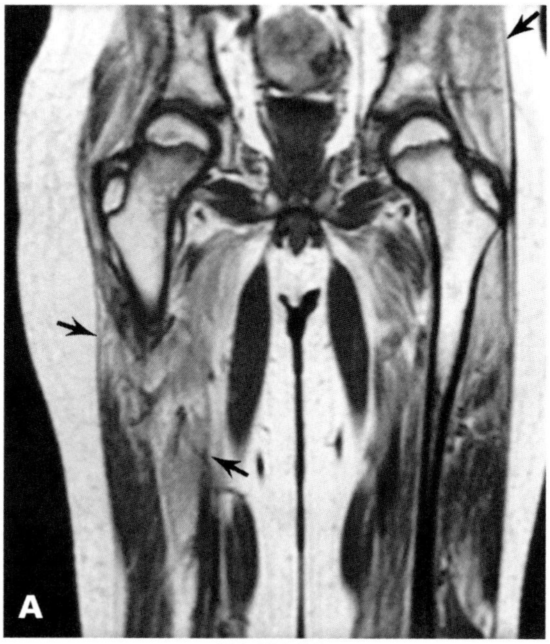

SE 400/11

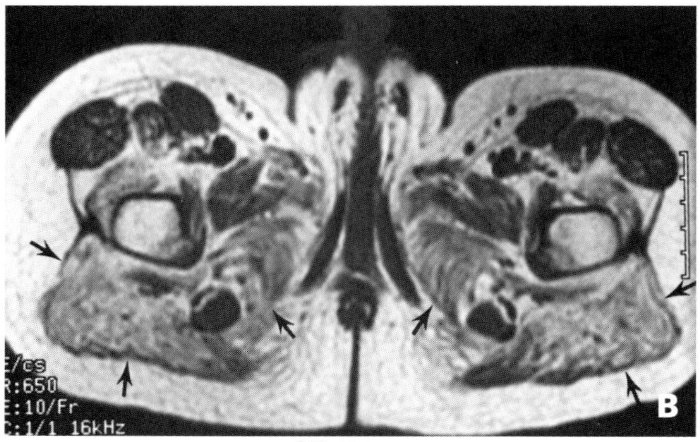

SE 400/11

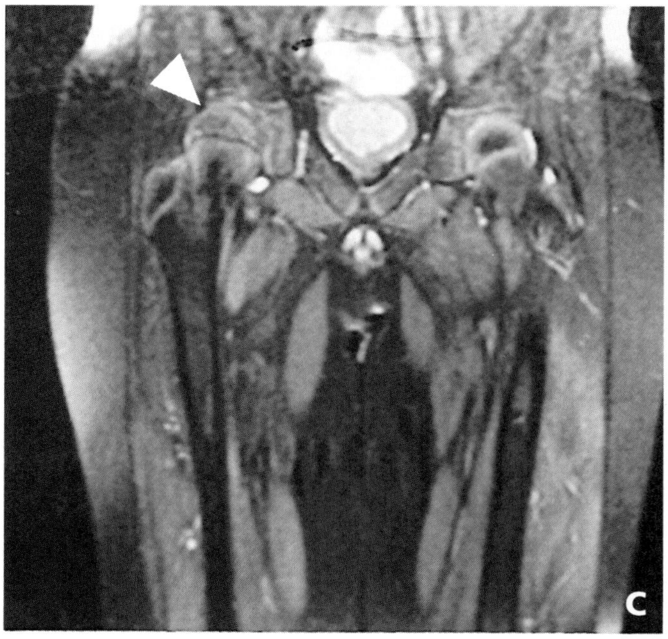

FSE 3,000/85

Figure 11-3. Duchenne muscular dystrophy in a 10-year-old boy with right hip pain. Coronal (A) and axial (B) T1-weighted images of the proximal lower extremities show decreased mass and fatty replacement of muscles. The muscles demonstrate high "fatty" signal (arrows). There is an increase in the thickness of the subcutaneous fat adjacent to the affected muscle groups. (C) A coronal T2-weighted image shows, in contrast to dermatomyositis, no abnormal increased signal in the affected muscles. The muscles have the same signal intensity as subcutaneous fat. There is abnormal high signal intensity in the right femoral head (arrowhead), consistent with avascular necrosis, related to steroid therapy. This explains the right hip pain.

are not consistent with muscular dystrophy, in which there would be muscle atrophy rather than swelling and increased signal intensity on T1-weighted rather than T2-weighted images.

Plexiform neurofibroma (Option (C)) is nearly pathognomonic for neurofibromatosis type 1 (NF1). It can occur in a variety of locations, including the subcutaneous tissues, extremities, head and neck, paraspinal muscles, mediastinum, retroperitoneum, and mesentery. The lesion consists of a network of finger-like extensions of tumor along a nerve and its branches. When it involves the extremities, it can extend from the subcutaneous tissues into adjacent muscles in a contiguous fashion. On T2-weighted MR images, the lesion appears as a large, multilobulated mass with heterogeneous high and low signal intensities (Figure 11-4). Similar to neurofibromas, the appearance of a target sign, consisting of peripheral high signal intensity with central low signal intensity, on T2-weighted images is characteristic (Figure 11-4). One plexiform neurofibroma can exhibit multiple target signs. The involvement of multiple muscles in the test patient does not have the appearance of a contiguous mass because the anatomy of the fascial planes is maintained. No target lesions are identified. These findings make plexiform neurofibroma an unlikely diagnosis.

Hemangiomas (Option (D)) are relatively common tumors and are the most common tumor of soft tissue in children. However, fewer than 5% of these lesions are intramuscular. Hemangiomas can be small and confined to a single tissue or large and involve multiple tissue planes, including subcutaneous tissue, muscle, and bone. The involvement usually occurs in a contiguous fashion. Characteristic MRI findings of hemangiomas include areas of low signal intensity on T1-weighted images and high signal intensity on T2-weighted images (Figure 11-5). They enhance diffusely after administration of gadolinium chelate. The signal voids often exhibit a serpentine configuration. There can be associated muscle atrophy, and the lesions are often oriented along the long axis of the affected muscle. Lymphaatic malformations can have more focal cystic areas of abnormal high signal intensity on T2-weighted images.

The test image shows abnormal increased signal intensity involving multiple muscle groups without a contiguous mass being present. The pattern of signal abnormality is not serpentine, and there is no evidence of flow void to suggest vessels. Hence, hemangioma is an unlikely diagnosis.

Fibrosarcoma (Option (E)) is exceedingly uncommon in children; it most commonly involves the extremities and typically occurs in the second decade of life. As with other soft tissue sarcomas, its MRI appearance is usually nonspecific. Most lesions demonstrate relatively low signal intensity on T1-weighted images and high signal intensity on T2-weighted images. However, there can be low signal intensity on T2-weighted images as a result of a high fibrous tissue content (Figure 11-6). The margins tend to be irregular, the signal intensity is heterogeneous, and invasion of adjacent neurovascular structures and bone is common. There is often peritumoral edema. A specific diagnosis requires biopsy. The involvement of multiple muscle groups without the appearance of a mass in the test image makes fibrosarcoma an unlikely diagnosis.

Dermatomyositis is one of several idiopathic inflammatory myopathies that occur in children. Its etiology is unknown, but it is related to the presence of autoantibodies against muscle. It is a multisystemic disease, characterized by a diffuse, nonsuppurative inflammation involving both striated muscle and skin. Clinical manifestations include progressive proximal muscle weakness, which is sometimes painful, a characteristic

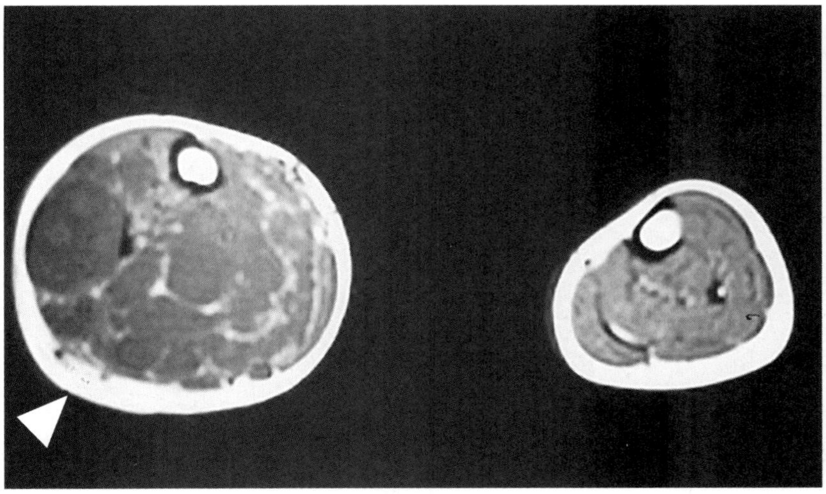

A

SE 400/11

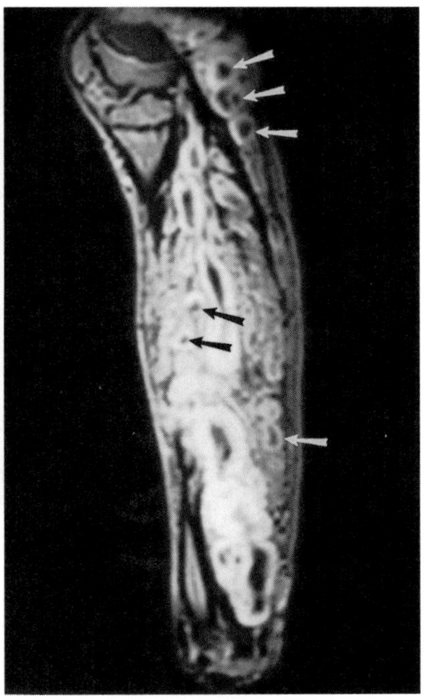

B

FSE 3,000/80

Figure 11-4. Plexiform neurofibroma in an 11-year-old girl with neurofibromatosis. (A) An axial T1-weighted MR image shows a diffuse multilobulated mass, isointense relative to muscle, enlarging the right calf (arrowhead). (B) A sagittal T2-weighted MR image shows a mixed (predominantly high)-signal-intensity lobulated mass with multiple low-signal-intensity target signs (arrows).

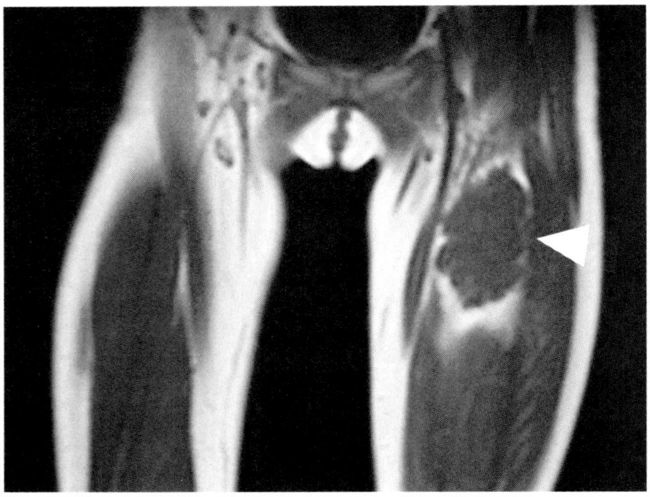

A

SE 600/20

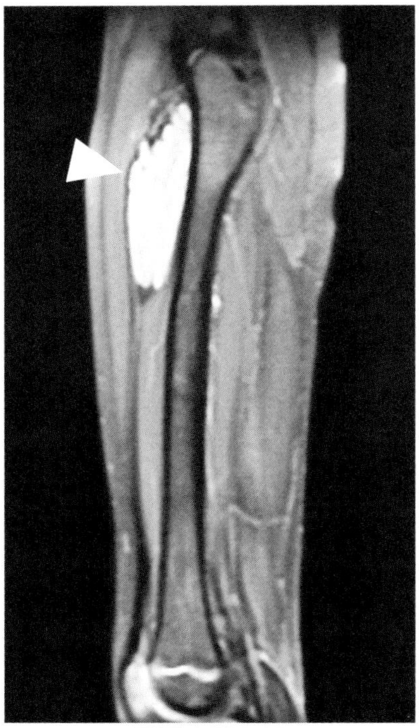

B

FSE 2,500/80

Figure 11-5. Hemangioma in a 5-year-old girl with a palpable mass. (A) A coronal T1-weighted MR image through the thighs shows a well-defined, lobulated mass (arrowhead) with homogeneous signal isointense relative to normal muscle. (B) A sagittal T2-weighted, fat-saturated MR image shows a well-defined mass (arowhead) with heterogeneous high signal intensity. The lesion involves the vastus intermedius muscle.

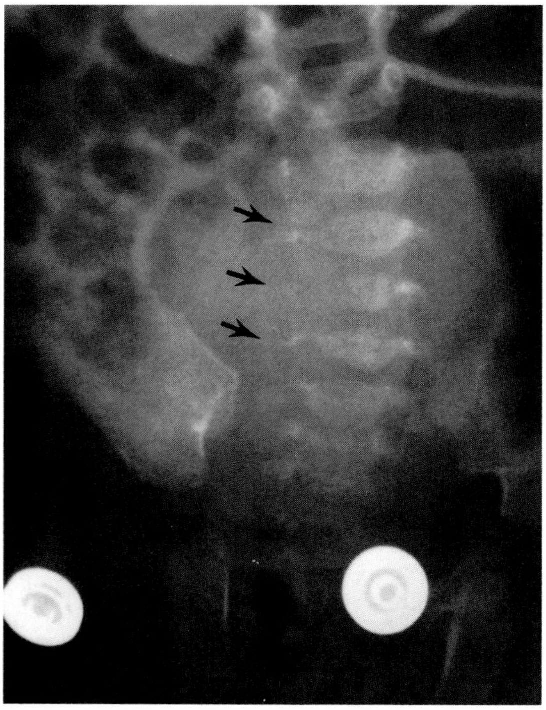

A

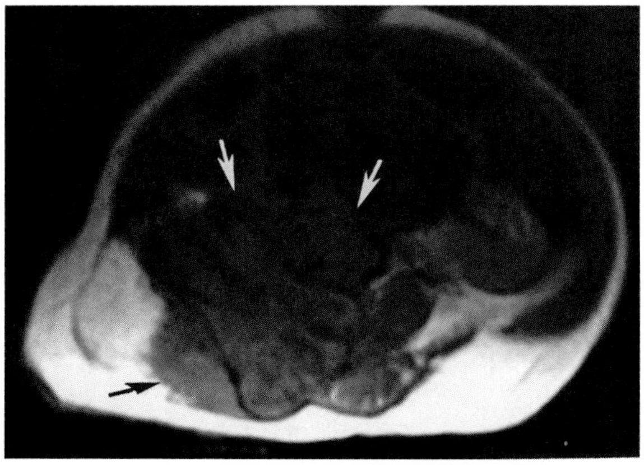

B

SE 400/15

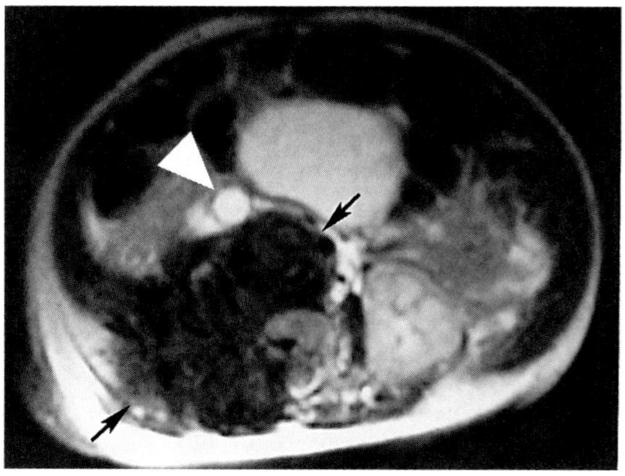

C

FSE 3,000/85

Figure 11-6. Infantile fibrosarcoma in an 8-week-old girl with right lower extremity weakness and decreased range of motion of the right hip. (A) A frontal radiograph of the lumbar spine shows deformity, sclerosis, and loss of height on the right side of the third, fourth, and fifth lumbar and first sacral vertebral bodies (arrows). There is also widening of the right sacroiliac joint. (B and C) Axial T1-weighted and T2-weighted, fat suppressed MR images show a large, poorly defined mass (arrows) involving the right side of the lumbar spine and sacrum and extending into the adjacent soft tissues. There is right hydroureter (arrowhead) secondary to obstruction. The mass is slightly hyperintense relative to muscle on the T1-weighted images and hypointense on the T2-weighted image, because of the prevalence of extracellular fibrous tissue.

skin rash, and other constitutional signs and symptoms. The diagnosis is usually suspected on the basis of clinical findings and elevated serum creatinine kinase levels. A definitive diagnosis can be made by electromyography or muscle biopsy. However, because of the invasive nature of these tests, MRI has been advocated as a means of confirming the diagnosis, directing the biopsy to an area of inflammation, and evaluating the response to therapy.

As noted in the test patient (Figure 11-1), MRI findings of dermatomyositis include increased signal intensity of affected muscles on T2-weighted images; the presence of perimuscular edema, which appears as increased intensity with a myofascial distribution on T2-weighted images; and increased intensity in a reticular pattern within the subcutaneous fat on T2-weighted images.

Question 58

Concerning dermatomyositis,

(A) gadolinium-enhanced imaging is the most sensitive MRI technique for its detection
(B) the presence of subcutaneous edema helps differentiate it from infectious myositis
(C) after treatment, abnormalities on MR images persist long after the clinical symptoms have resolved
(D) patients with clinically active disease rarely have normal MRI studies
(E) MRI is useful for directing biopsy

Dermatomyositis is one of several types of idiopathic inflammatory myopathies that can affect children. Other types include polymyositis and inclusion body myositis. The presence of an inflammatory myopathy is usually suggested by the onset of proximal muscle weakness, often accompanied by muscle tenderness. Constitutional symptoms such as fever or fatigue are often also present. Other medical problems associated with dermatomyositis include arthritis, Raynaud's phenomenon, interstitial lung disease, and a spectrum of rashes. Common rashes include a "V-shaped" chest rash and a "shawl" distribution rash. Disease-specific rashes include erythema of the eyelids (heliotrope rash) and erythematous papules of the knuckles (Gottron's sign). Laboratory abnormalities include a marked elevation of serum creatinine kinase levels. Any number of myositis-specific antimuscle antibodies also can be present, supporting the diagnosis.

In patients in whom there is a clinical suspicion of dermatomyositis, the diagnosis is often confirmed by either muscle biopsy or electromyography. However, both of these procedures have limitations. Electromyography is painful and time-consuming, and the needles utilized in the procedures can actually induce inflammation, which interferes with subsequent biopsy results. The length of time and pain associated with the procedure make it suboptimal for use in children, especially on a sequential basis. Also, because of the patchy distribution of inflammation in cases of dermatomyositis, 10% to 15% of nondirected biopsies are normal in the presence of active myositis. Because of these limitations, MRI has replaced electromyography and limited the use of biopsy in diagnosing and monitoring patients with dermatomyositis at many medical centers. MRI can be useful in confirming the presence of myositis in equivocal cases, directing biopsies to an area of inflammation in order to increase biopsy yield (**Option (E) is true**), so that appropriate treatment can be initiated. Also, in the absence of abnormal MR signal intensity within the muscle, clinical investigations can be directed elsewhere. MRI is also helpful in monitoring the response to therapy. Abnormalities on MRI correlate better with active disease than do creatinine kinase levels in serum. There are also cost savings associated with performing MRI in place of electromyography or muscle biopsy. In a survey of several medical centers, MRI examinations performed better and were five times less expensive than muscle biopsy.

The MRI examination for the evaluation of dermatomyositis should include both T1-weighted and fat-saturated T2-weighted images. The choice of coil depends on the body part being imaged. Most commonly, the lower pelvis and thighs are imaged with a torso array coil. The imaging protocol consists of coronal T1-weighted images, axial fast spin-echo proton-density-weighted and T2-weighted images with fat saturation, and a coronal short-tau inversion-recovery image. Although areas of myositis do enhance on T1-weighted images after gadolinium chelate administration, postcontrast imaging is not more sensitive than T2-weighted imaging (**Option (A) is false**). Therefore, postcontrast images are not typically obtained.

The MRI findings of dermatomyositis include increased signal intensity of involved muscles on T2-weighted images (Figure 11-2 and Figure 11-7). Commonly involved muscles include the gluteus muscles, abductors, quadriceps, hamstring muscles of the thigh, calf muscles, and shoulder muscles. Increased signal intensity surrounding involved muscles is often visible in a myofascial distribution on T2-weighted images (Figure 11-7). This halo of edema can be present even in the absence of abnormal signal intensity in the muscle. There is also often increased signal intensity with a reticular pattern in the subcutaneous fat on T2-weighted images (Figure 11-7). The above findings tend to be bilaterally symmetric; however, the disease can have a very patchy distribution.

Patients with chronic longstanding dermatomyositis can develop muscle calcification (Figure 11-8), which appears as hypointense areas on all pulse sequences. Muscle atrophy and fatty infiltration also can be present in chronically affected patients. In patients with longstanding disease, muscle weakness may be secondary to a combination of active inflammation, muscular atrophy and fatty replacement, and steroid-induced myopathy. The MRI findings help define the contribution of each of these problems to the patient's total weakness and hence aid the thera-

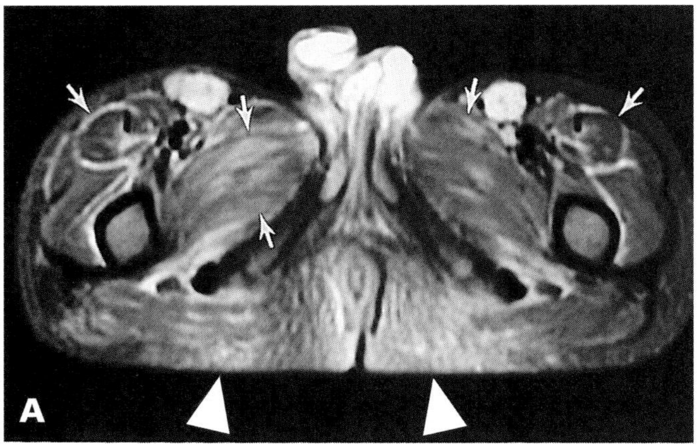

FSE 3,000/80

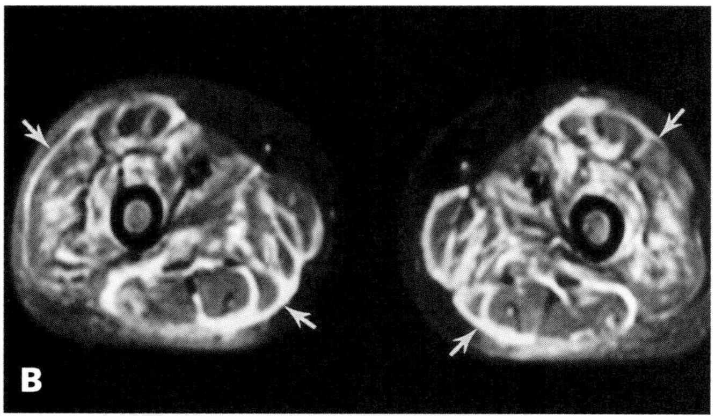

FSE 3,000/80

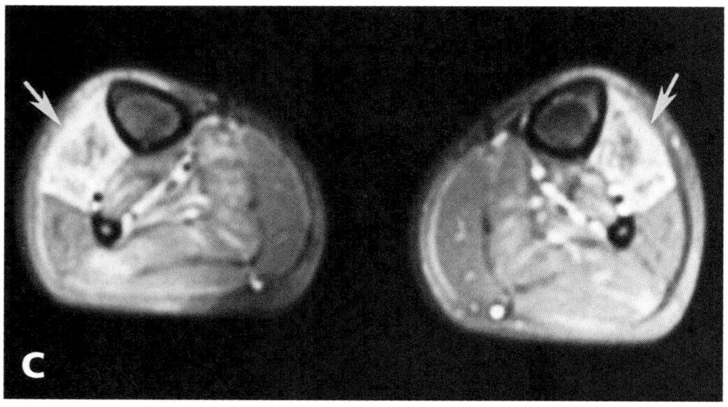

FSE 3,000/80

Figure 11-7. Dermatomyositis in a 4-year-old girl with lower extremity weakness and pain. (A and B) Axial T2-weighted, fat-saturated MR images through the upper thighs (A) and middle thighs (B) show symmetric, increased signal intensity in multiple muscle groups (arrows), including the adductors, gluteus maximus, sartorius, rectus femoris, and vastus lateralis. There are increased signal intensity surrounding the affected muscle groups in a myofascial distribution and increased signal intensity with a reticular pattern in the subcutaneous tissues (arrowheads). (C) An axial T2-weighted, fat-saturated MR image through the calves shows symmetric involvement of the tibialis anterior muscles (arrows).

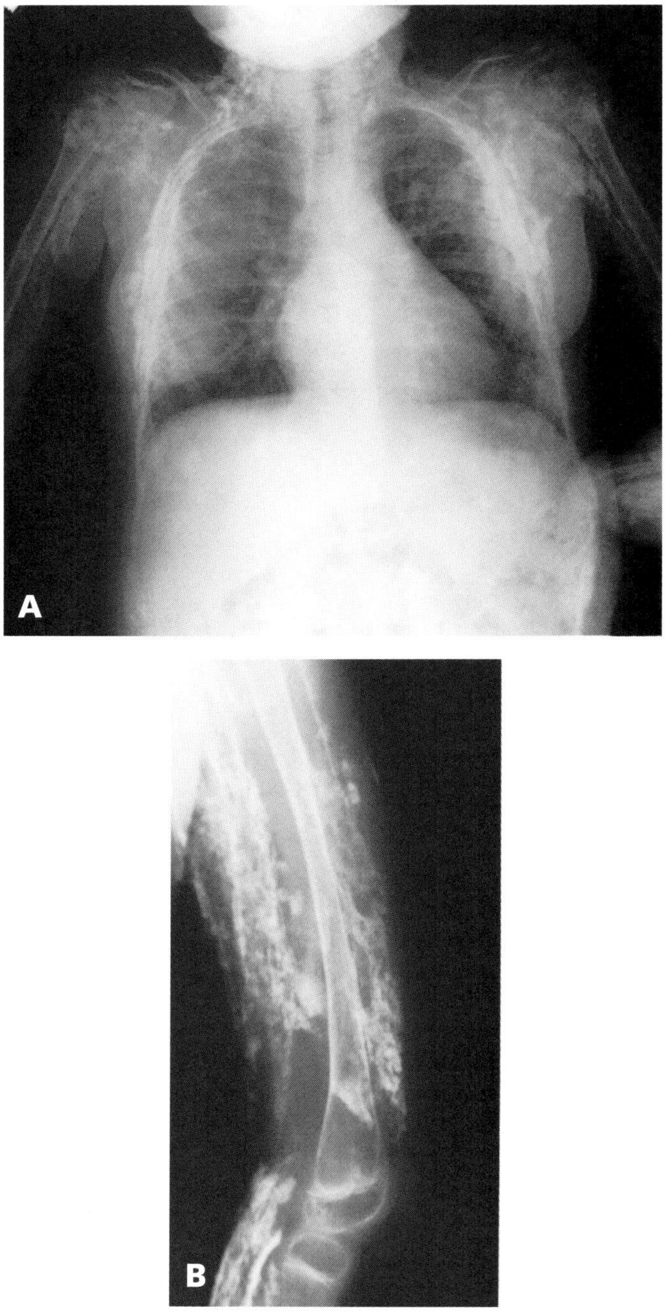

Figure 11-8. Dermatomyositis with extensive calcifications in an 8-year-old girl. Radiographs of the chest (A) and thigh (B) show extensive muscular calcifications.

peutic decisions. The MRI findings are highly sensitive to changes of dermatomyositis. Patients with clinically active disease almost always have abnormal MRI studies (**Option (D) is true**). When patients respond to therapy, there is rapid resolution of the abnormally increased signal intensity of affected muscles on T2-weighted images (**Option (C) is false**).

Pathologically, the increased signal intensity is related to increased water content secondary to intramuscular, fascial, and perivascular inflammation. Muscle necrosis and phagocytosis also can contribute to the increased signal intensity.

The MRI findings of dermatomyositis are not specific. Similar findings can be seen in patients with other types of connective tissue disorders (Figure 11-9) and with infectious myositis (**Option (B) is false**). The differential diagnosis includes other noninfectious causes of myositis, such as polymyositis, infectious myositis (Figure 11-10), subacute denervation related to trauma, and rhabdomyolysis.

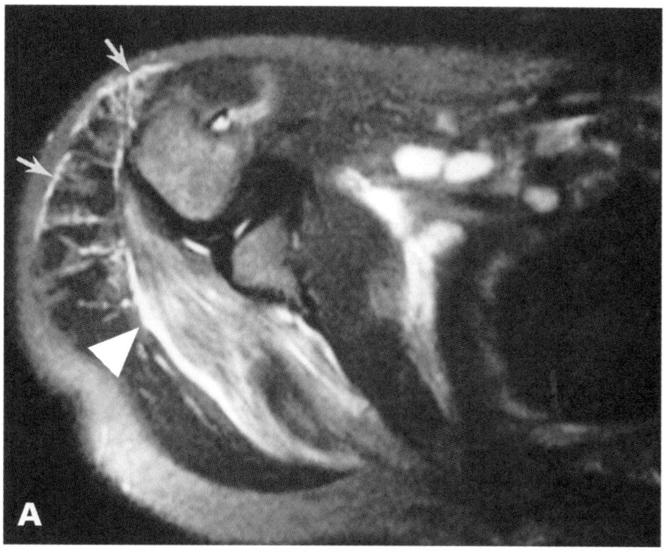

FSE 3,000/85

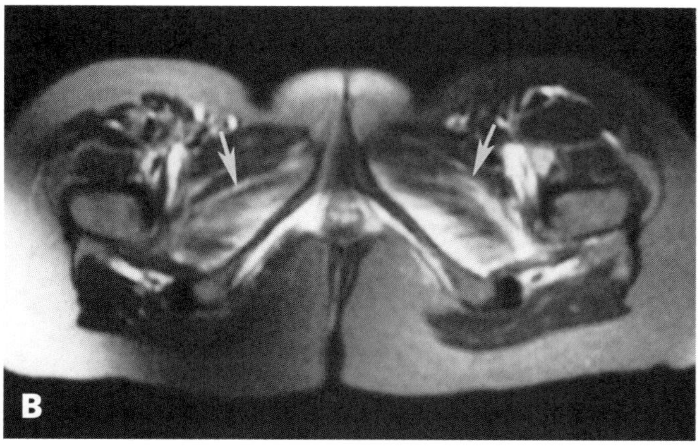

FSE 3,000/85

Figure 11-9. Lupus-related myositis exhibiting MRI findings similar to those of dermatomyositis in a 15-year-old girl with laboratory and clinical findings of systemic lupus erythematosus. (A) An axial T2-weighted, fat-saturated MR image through the shoulder shows abnormal enlargement and heterogeneously increased signal involving the deltoid (small arrows) and subscapularis (arrowhead) muscles. The appearance is very similar to that seen in Figure 11-1. (B) An axial T2-weighted, fat-saturated MR image through the upper thighs shows symmetrically increased signal intensity in the adductor muscles (arrows) with surrounding increased myofascial signal intensity.

Question 59

Concerning plexiform neurofibromas,

(A) they are virtually pathognomonic of neurofibromatosis type 1
(B) histologically, neoplastic Schwann cells and matrix displace rather than infiltrate neuronal axons
(C) retroperitoneal lesions are usually bilateral
(D) their smooth, noninfiltrating margins help to differentiate them from malignant nerve sheath tumors
(E) on T2-weighted MR images, they typically have one or multiple "targets," with a low-intensity center and and a high-intensity rim

NF1 (von Recklinghausen's neurofibromatosis) is a relatively common autosomal dominant disorder, affecting 1 in 2,000 to 1 in 4,000 people. In patients with NF1, the peripheral nerves can be involved with neurofibromas, plexiform neurofibromas, or malignant peripheral nerve sheath tumors. Plexiform neurofibromas are nearly pathognomonic for NF1 (**Option (A) is true**). The presence of a plexiform neurofibroma fulfills one of the two criteria required for the diagnosis of NF1.

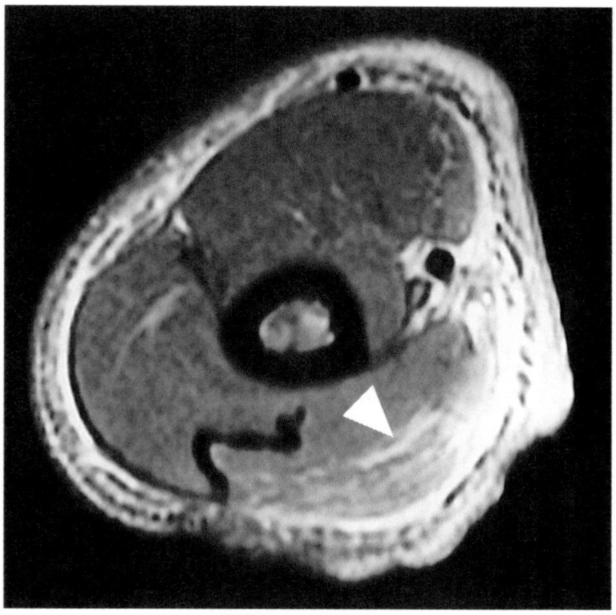

FSE 2,500/80

Figure 11-10. Necrosing fasciitis and pyomyositis complicating chicken pox in a 7-year-old boy. An axial T2-weighted, fat-saturated MR image through the midhumerus shows circumferential increased signal intensity and thickening of the subcutaneous fat and abnormal signal intensity in the long head of the triceps muscle (arrowhead).

Plexiform neurofibromas can occur in a variety of locations. They most commonly involve the skin and subcutaneous tissue, extremities, the head and neck, paraspinous structures, mediatinum, mesentery, and retroperitoneum.

Pathologically, plexiform neurofibromas consist of an interdigitating network of fronds of tumor that arise from and surround a nerve and its branches. Microscopically, there is a disorganized array of wavy Schwann cell bundles dispersed in a collagen matrix. The neuronal axons are surrounded and separated from one another by this engulfing tangle of neoplastic Schwann cells and matrix. It is this histologic feature which allows plexiform neurofibromas to be differentiated from schwannomas and neurofibromas, which displace bundles of neuronal axons rather than infiltrating and separating them **(Option (B) is false).**

Malignant peripheral nerve sheath tumors are the leading cause of cancer death in patients with NF1. The treatment of malignant peripheral nerve sheath tumors is surgical resection. Because functioning neuronal axons are interspersed within the tumor in a plexiform neurofibroma, biopsy or surgical resection can result in sensorimotor nerve deficits. It is clinically difficult to distinguish benign from malignant neuronal tumors in patients with NF1. Because the lesions in these patients can be numerous or deeply situated, repeated multiple biopsies are not an optimal way to monitor for malignant tumors. Large, complex lesions are also subject to sampling errors when blind biopsies are performed. Therefore, an imaging feature that could differentiate between these lesions would be helpful.

MRI is the modality of choice for characterizing and evaluating the extent of nerve sheath tumors. Plexiform neurofibromas appear as large masses that exhibit heterogeneous signal intensity and often extend along the distribution of a peripheral nerve. The lesions can involve skin, subcutaneous tissue, and muscle and can extend into bone (Figure 11-11). Often, more than one anatomic region is involved, but the lesions are usually contiguous. The margins vary from poorly to well defined. Retroperitoneal lesions tend to be bilateral symmetric psoas masses or presacral lesions (Figure 11-12) **(Option (C) is true).** If a psoas lesion is unilateral or asymmetric in size, a malignant lesion should be suspected.

Unfortunately, there is overlap between the MRI features of benign and malignant peripheral nerve tumors, including size, signal heterogeneity, contrast enhancement, peripheral edema, and margination **(Option (D) is false).** It has been suggested that the most helpful differentiating MRI feature is the presence of the target sign on T2-weighted images. Benign neurofibromas have this sign, with a rim of high signal intensity and a central area of low intensity. Histologically, the rim represents myxoid tissue encircling a central zone of collagen and cellular matrix (Figure 11-13). In a complex lesion, the presence of one or multiple target lesions favors a benign plexiform neurofibroma **(Option (E) is true).** These target lesions are reportedly absent in malignant nerve sheath tumors.

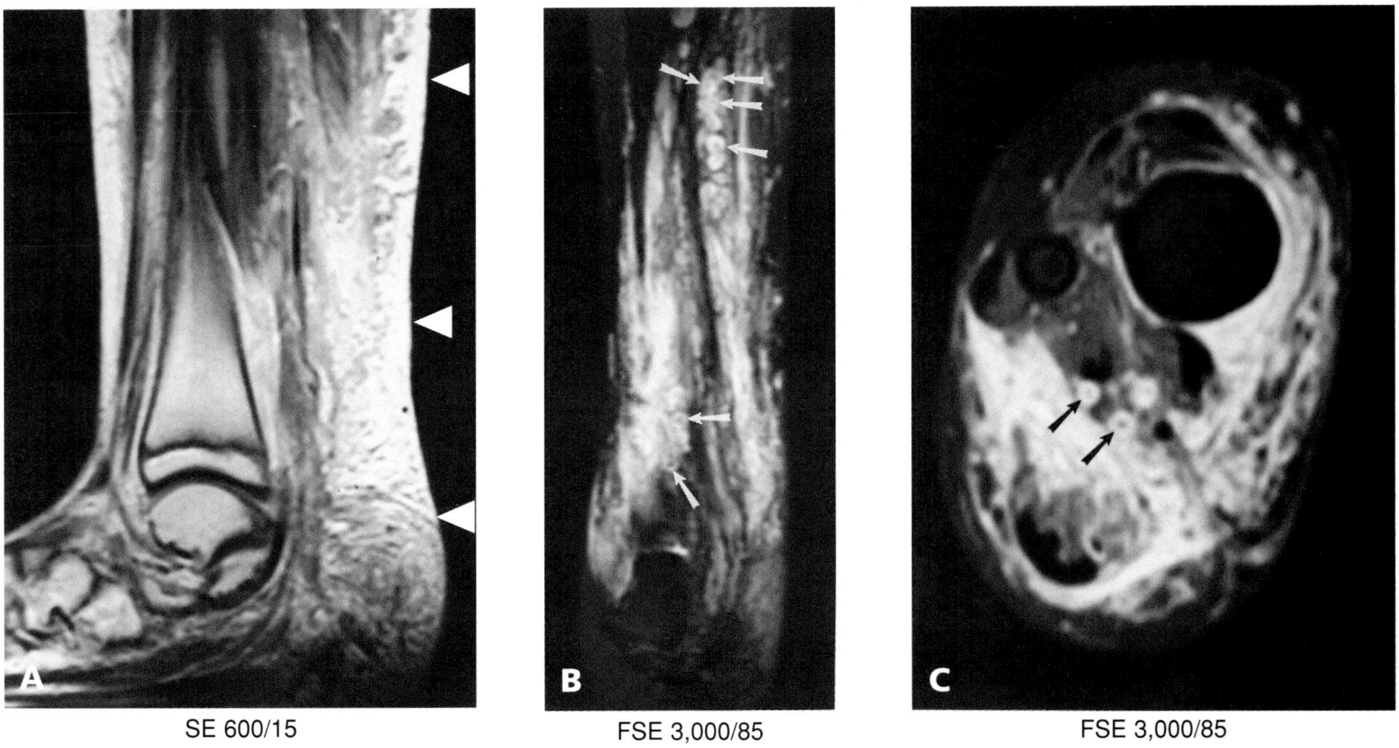

SE 600/15 FSE 3,000/85 FSE 3,000/85

Figure 11-11. Plexiform neurofibroma in an 8-year-old girl with neurofibromatosis. (A) A sagittal T1-weighted image shows a diffuse heterogeneous mass (arrowheads) with poorly defined margins involving the skin, subcutaneous tissues, muscle, and tendons of the posterior lower leg and foot. (B and C) Coronal (B) and axial (C) T2-weighted, fat-suppressed MR images show a mixed heterogeneous, but predominantly high-intensity, mass. There are multiple low-intensity targets (arrows) within the lesion.

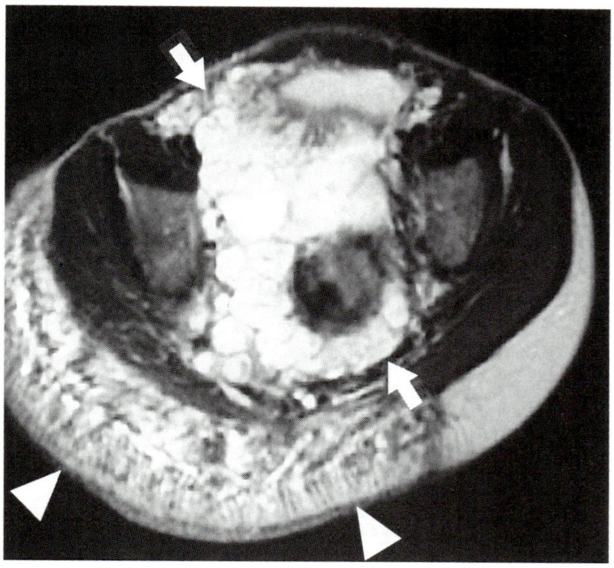

FSE 2,500/80

Figure 11-12. Plexiform neurofibroma in a 7-year-old boy with neurofibromatosis. An axial T2-weighted, fat-suppressed MR image show a heterogeneous, but predominantly high-intensity, mass (arrows) surrounding the rectum and involving the retroperitoneum and the right posterior subcutaneous tissues and skin (arrowheads). There are multiple low-intensity targets within the lesion.

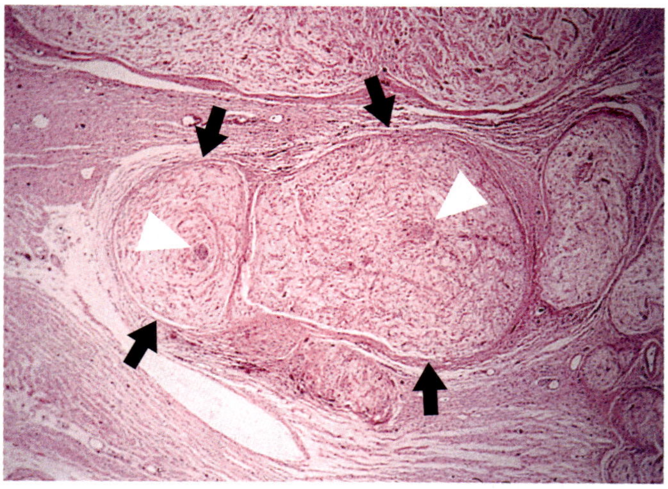

Figure 11-13. Histology of the target sign in a patient with plexiform neurofibroma. The high-intensity rim as seen in T2-weighted MR images represents myxoid tissue (arrows). The low-intensity central zone represents collagen matrix (arrowheads).

Question 60

Concerning soft tissue hemangiomas of childhood,

(A) they are the most common tumors of infancy and childhood
(B) the MRI findings are usually nonspecific
(C) embolization or surgical management is necessary in most patients
(D) most arise in striated muscle
(E) surrounding soft tissue edema is an uncommon finding

Musculoskeletal vascular malformations of childhood include hemangiomas, lymphatic malformations, venous malformations, and high-flow arteriovenous malformations. Hemangiomas are among the most common soft tissue tumors, representing 7% of all benign tumors. Hemangioma is the most frequent tumor of childhood (**Option (A) is true**).

Hemangiomas can be superficial or deep. The superficial lesions have a classic appearance on physical examination and usually do not require imaging for diagnosis. The deep lesions are usually present a more difficult diagnostic challenge and require imaging for diagnosis. Hemangiomas can be small and confined to one tissue or can be large and involve multiple tissues in a contiguous fashion. Most commonly, hemangiomas arise in the subcutaneous tissues but they also can arise from bone, synovium, or skeletal muscle. Fewer than 5% of lesions arise intramuscularly (**Option (D) is false**). Clinically, the superficial lesions can demonstrate a bluish discoloration and sometimes an associated bruit. The deep lesions appear as nonspecific palpable masses.

Hemangiomas represent a cellular proliferation of endothelial cells and are true neoplasms. They most commonly present in infants. Hemangiomas are typically small, at times are not recognized at birth, and then rapidly increase in size over the first 6 months of life. Involution of the mass typically begins at about 10 months of age, and approximately one half of the lesions are resolved by 5 years of age. Most are asymptomatic and do not require medical attention. Hemangiomas can be complicated by the Kasabach-Merritt syndrome (consumptive coagulopathy), compression of adjacent vital structures (such as the airway or orbit), and formation of fissures, ulcerations, or bleeding. They also can cause psychological problems when located on the face, particularly the nose.

Treatment is unnecessary for most hemangiomas unless complications develop (**Option (C) is false**). Therapeutic options include systemic steroid therapy, interferon alfa-1 therapy, surgery, or embolization. Steroid administration is typically the initial therapy of choice.

MRI is the imaging method of choice for evaluating suspected hemangiomas. It has been shown to be valuable in confirming the diagnosis, monitoring the response to therapy, and defining the anatomic extent of hemangiomas. MRI findings are often either specific or highly suggestive of the diagnosis (**Option (B) is false**). An accurate diagnosis can be made for at least 70% of lesions. On MRI, hemangiomas typically appear as well-defined, discrete masses that are hyperintense relative to muscle on T2-weighted images (Fig. 11-14) and isointense relative to muscle on T1-weighted images. The mass enhances diffusely on images obtained after injection of gadolinium chelate. Prominent draining veins can be seen as both central and peripheral vascular structures. These appear as flow voids on standard MRI sequences. An involuting hemangioma can demonstrate fatty signal intensity within the mass. Edema in the surrounding soft tissues is not a common finding (**Option (E) is true**). On sonography, hemangiomas appear as lobulated masses with prominent flow on color flow Doppler images. Al-

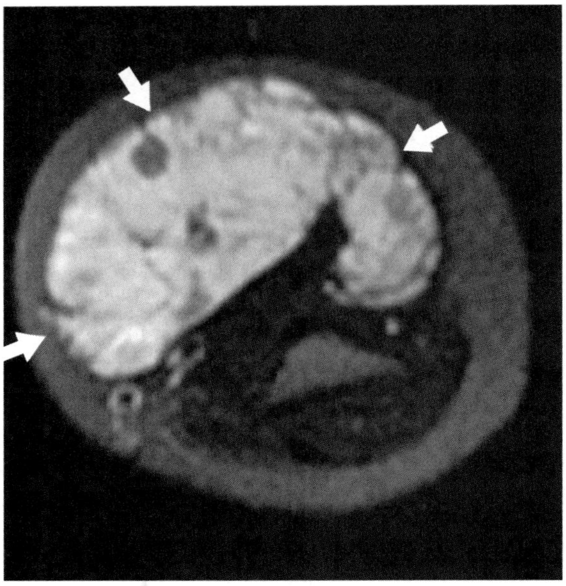

FSE 3,000/85

Figure 11-14. Hemangioma in a 4-year-old boy. A T2-weighted MR image shows a lobulated, well-defined mass (arrows) in the region of the anterior proximal arm. The lesion shows a predominantly high signal intensity and contains several prominent flow voids consistent with draining veins.

though CT typically is not used to make the diagnosis, when seen on CT scans, hemangiomas appear as well-defined, diffusely enhancing masses.

Venous malformations appear on MRI as areas of multiple serpentine channels with a high signal intensity on T2-weighted images (Fig. 11-15). The serpentine channels tend to show enhancement after injection of gadolinium chelate. Phleboliths can be present. Lymphatic malformations appear as multiple cystic masses of various sizes. The cystic areas show a high signal intensity on T2-weighted images (Figure 11-16) and can demonstrate septal but not diffuse enhancement. CT and ultrasonography may also be used to evaluate lymphatic malformations. The lesions appear cystic on both imaging modalities. Arteriovenous malformations appear as tangles of vessels that demonstrate high flow on gradient-echo images (Fig. 11-17). It is important to determine whether a vascular malformation has a component of high arterial flow as these lesions are treated with transarterial embolization rather than direct pericutaneous sclerosis.

Soft tissue sarcomas, such as fibrosarcoma and rhabdomyosarcoma, must be considered in the differential diagnosis of a soft tissue mass presenting in an infant. If the mass does have the typical growth pattern or the characteristic MRI appearance of a vascular malformation, sarcoma should be considered and a biopsy should be performed.

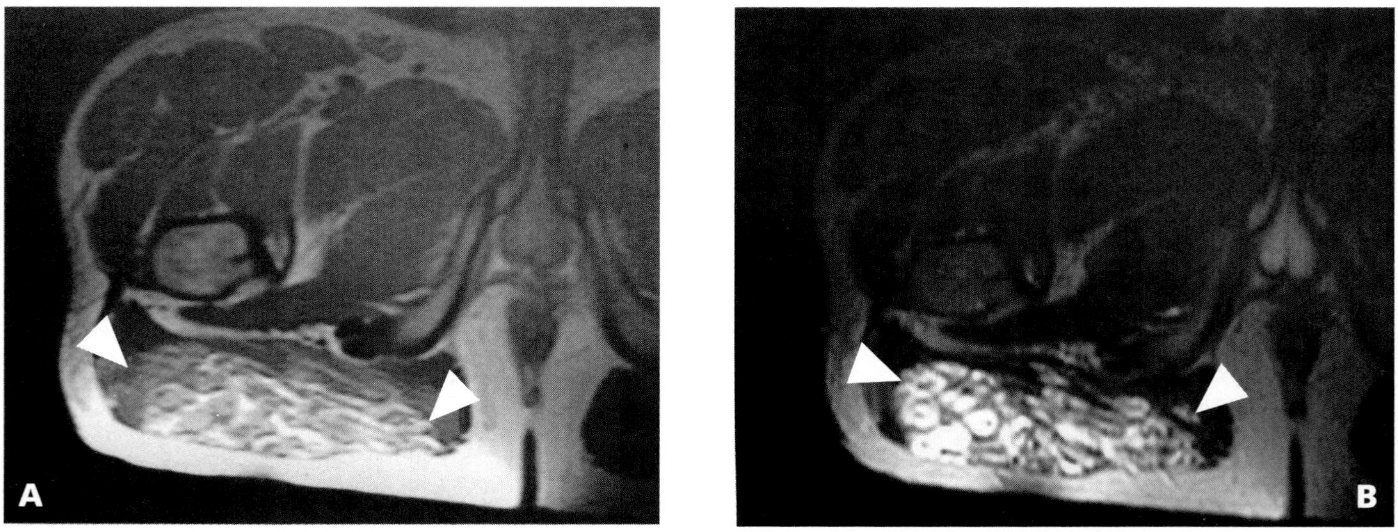

SE 600/11 FSE 3,000/85

Figure 11-15. Venous malformation of the gluteal region in a 31-year-old man with pain. (A) An axial T1-weighted MR image shows an infiltrative, poorly defined mass (arrowheads) enlarging the gluteus maximus muscle. There is heterogeneous signal within the mass, with areas that are isointense relative to muscle and areas of fibrofatty stroma that are isointense relative to subcutaneous fat. (B) An axial T2-weighted image shows the mass (arrowheads) to have increased signal intensity in a serpentine pattern.

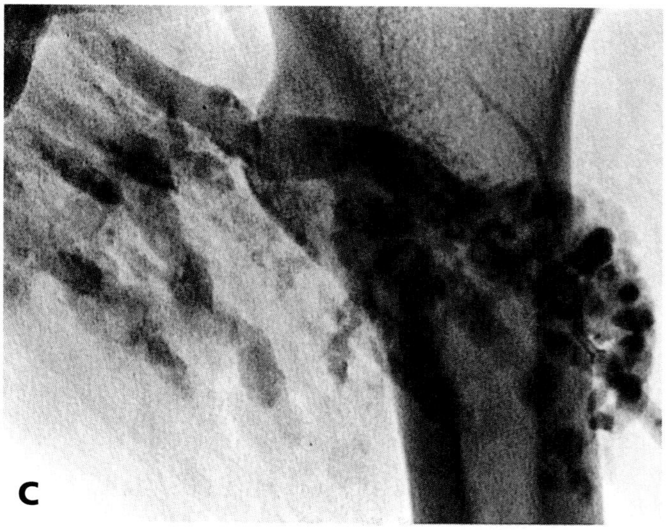

Figure 11-15 (Continued). Venous malformation of the gluteal region in a 31-year-old man with pain. (C) A pericutaneous injection of contrast material with the patient in a prone position during sclerotherapy shows multiple large venous channels, corresponding to the serpentine structures seen in panel B.

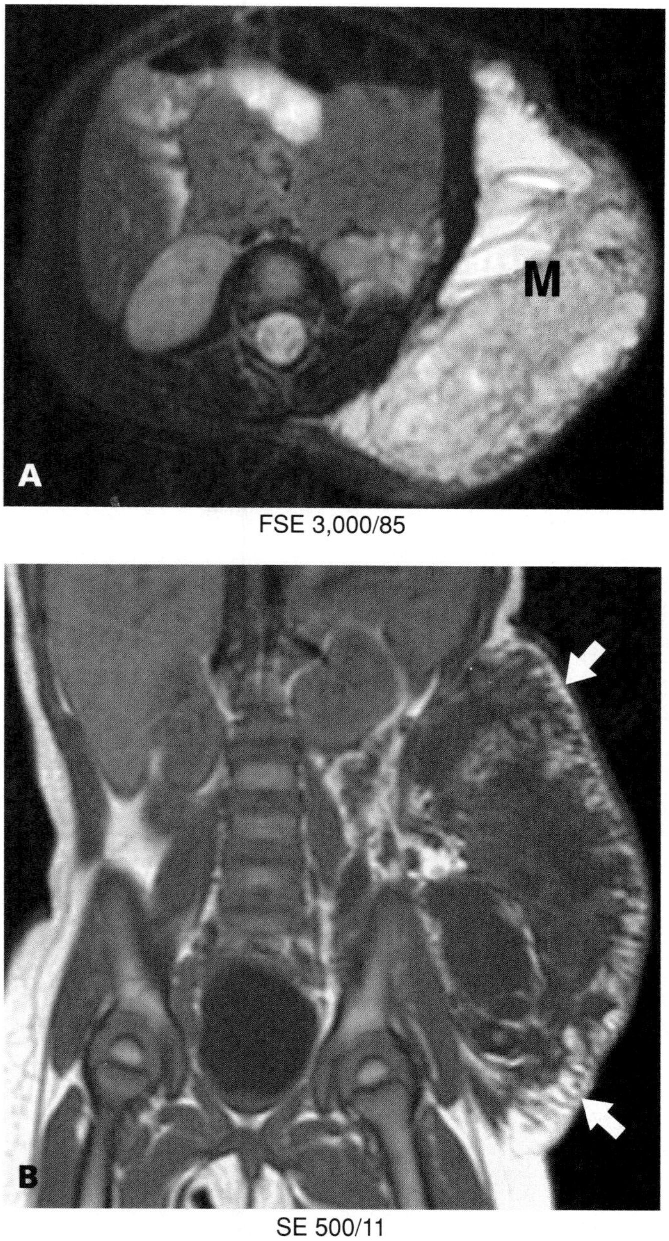

Figure 11-16 Lymphatic malformation in a 18-month-old girl. (A) An axial T2-weighted image shows a large multicystic mass (M) arising from left abdominal wall. The mass is confined to the subcutaneous tissue and does not involve the abdominal wall musculature or intra-abdominal contents. (B) A coronal T1-weighted image shows multi-loculated cysts within mass (arrows). Some of the cysts have a high signal suggesting hemorrhage or proteinacious fluid.

SUGGESTED READINGS

DERMATOMYOSITIS

1. Adams EM, Chow CK, Premkumar A, Plotz PH. The idiopathic inflammatory myopathies: spectrum of MR imaging findings. RadioGraphics 1995; 15:563–574
2. Fraser DD, Frank JA, Dalakas M, Miller FW, Hicks JE, Plotz P. Magnetic resonance imaging in the idiopathic inflammatory myopathies. J Rheumatol 1991; 18:1693–1699
3. Hernandez RJ, Keim DR, Chenevert TL, Sullivan DB, Aisen AM. Fat-suppressed MR imaging of myositis. Radiology 1992; 182:217–219
4. Hernandez RJ, Keim DR, Sullivan DB. Serial magnetic resonance imaging in juvenile dermatomyositis. Arthritis Rheum 1991; 12:1580–1584
5. Hernandez RJ, Sullivan DB, Chenevert TL, Keim DR. MR imaging in children with dermatomyositis: musculoskeletal findings and correlation with clinical and laboratory findings. AJR 1993; 161:359–366
6. Murphy WA, Totty WG, Carroll JE. MRI of normal and pathologic skeletal muscle. AJR 1986; 146:565–574
7. Zagoria RJ, Karstaedt N, Koubek TD. MR imaging of rhabdomyolysis. J Comput Assist Tomogr 1986; 10:268–270

MUSCULAR DYSTROPHY

8. Jehenson P, Leroy-Willig A, de Kerviler E, Duboc D, Syrota A. MR imaging as a potential diagnostic test for metabolic myopathies: importance of variations in the T2 of muscle with exercise. AJR 1993; 161:347–351
9. Liu GC, Jong YJ, Chiang DH, Jaw CH. Duchenne muscular dystrophy: MR grading system with functional correlation. Radiology 1993; 186: 475–480
10. Patrick LE, O'Shea P, Simoneaux SF, Gay BB Jr, Atkinson GO. Fibromatoses of childhood: the spectrum of radiographic findings. AJR 1996; 166:163–169
11. Schreiber A, Smith WL, Ionasescu V, et al. Magnetic resonance imaging of children with Duchenne muscular dystrophy. Pediatr Radiol 1987; 17: 495–497

PLEXIFORM NEUROFIBROMA

12. Bass JC, Korobkin M, Francis IR, Ellis JH, Cohan RH. Retroperitoneal plexiform neurofibromas: CT findings. AJR 1994; 163:617–620
13. Bhargava R, Parham DM, Lasater OE, Chari RS, Chen G, Fletcher BD. MR imaging differentiation of benign and malignant peripheral nerve sheath tumors: use of the target sign. Pediatr Radiol 1997; 27:124–129
14. Elster AD. Radiologic screening in the neurocutaneous syndromes: strategies and controversies. AJNR 1992; 13:1078–1082
15. Matsuki K, Kakitsubata Y, Watanabe K, Tsukino H, Nakajima K. Mesenteric plexiform neurofibroma associated with Recklinghausen's disease. Pediatr Radiol 1997; 27:255–256
16. Suh JS, Abenoza P, Galloway HR, Everson LI, Griffiths HJ. Peripheral (extracranial) nerve tumors: correlation of MR imaging and histologic findings. Radiology 1992; 183:341–346

VASCULAR MALFORMATION AND HEMANGIOMA

17. Bissett GS III. MR imaging of soft-tissue masses in children. Radiol Clin North Am 1996; 4:697–719

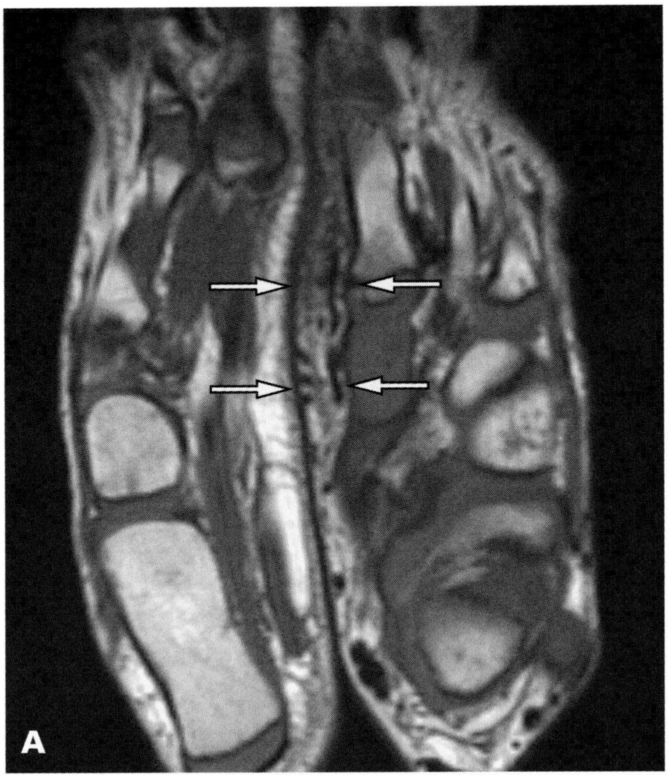

SE 500/11

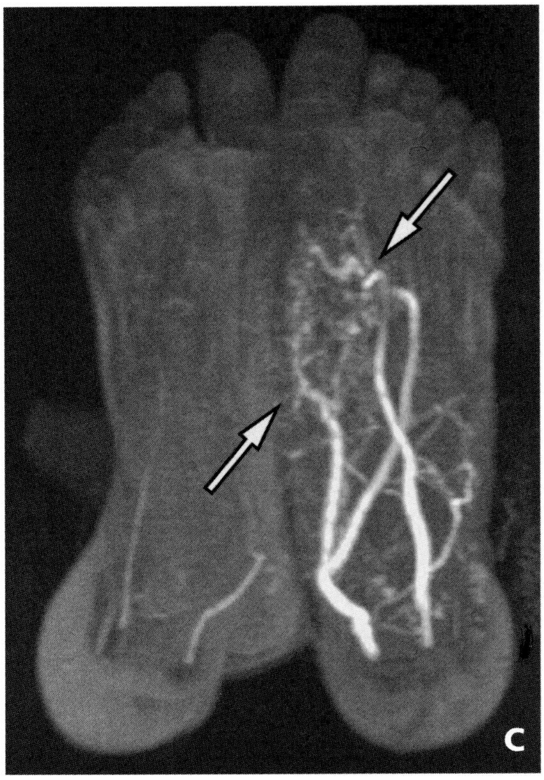

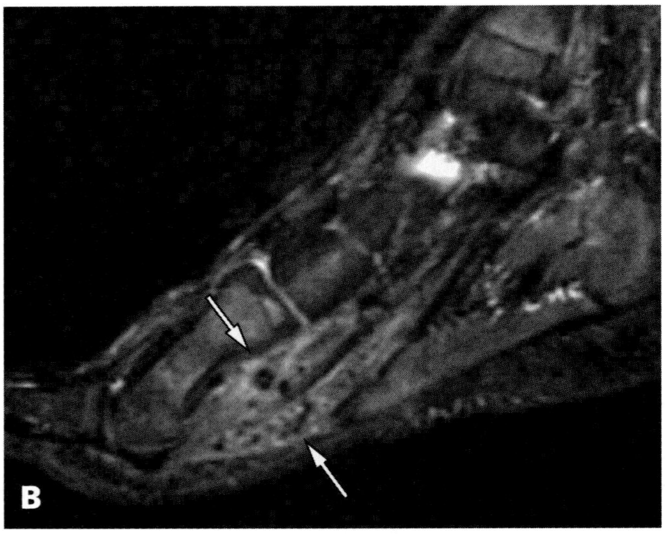

FSE 3,000/85

Figure 11-17. High-flow vascular malformation (arteriovenous malformation) of the left foot in a 4-year-old boy. (A) An axial T1-weighted image shows multiple tubular signal voids (arrows) consistent with vessels medially in the region of left foot. (B) A sagittal T2-weighted image shows multiple tubular signal voids (arrows) consistent with vessels with some surrounding high signal intensity, consistent with edema. (C) A maximum-signal-intensity projection image from two dimensional time-of-flight sequence shows a tangle of high-flow arterial structures (arrows) consistent with a high-flow vascular malformation.

18. Buetow PC, Kransdorf MJ, Moser RP Jr, Jelinek JS, Berrey BH. Radiologic appearance in intramuscular hemangioma with emphasis on MR imaging. AJR 1990; 154:563–567
19. Cohen EK, Kressel HY, Perosio T, et al. MR imaging of soft-tissue hemangiomas: correlation with pathologic findings. AJR 1988; 150:1079–1081
20. Derchi LE, Balconi G, De Flaviis L, Oliva A, Rosso F. Sonographic appearances of hemangiomas of skeletal muscle. J Ultrasound Med 1989; 8:263–267
21. Donnelly LF, Adams DM, Bissett GS III. Vascular malformations and hemangiomas: a practical approach in a multidisciplinary clinic. AJR 2000; 174:597–608
22. Ezekowitz RA, Mulliken JB, Folkman J. Interferon alfa-2a therapy for life-threatening hemangiomas of infancy. N Engl J Med 1992; 326:1456–1463
23. Greenspan A, McGahan JP, Vogelsang P, Szabo RM. Imaging strategies in the evaluation of soft-tissue hemangiomas of the extremities: correlation of the findings of plain radiography, angiography, CT, MRI, and ultrasonography in 12 histologically proven cases. Skeletel Radiol 1992; 21:11–18
24. Jenner G, Söderlund V, Bauer HF, Brosjö O. MR imaging of skeletal muscle hemangiomas: a report of 16 cases. Acta Radiol 1996; 37:140–144
25. Kaplan PA, Williams SM. Mucocutaneous and peripheral soft-tissue hemangiomas: MR imaging. Radiology 1987; 163:163–166
26. Meyer JS, Hoffer FA, Barnes PD, Mulliken JB. Biological classification of soft-tissue vascular anomalies: MR correlation. AJR 1991; 157:559–564
27. Mulliken JB, Glowacki J. Hemangiomas and vascular malformations in infants and children: a classification based on endothelial characteristics. Plast Reconstr Surg 1982; 69:412–422
28. Murphey MD, Fairbairn KJ, Parman LM, Baxter KG, Parsa MB, Smith

WS. From the archives of the AFIP: musculoskeletal angiomatous lesions: radiologic-pathologic correlation. RadioGraphics 1995; 15:893–917

29. Ogita S, Tsuto T, Deguchi E, Tokiwa K, Nagashima M, Iwai N. OK-432 therapy for unresectable lymphangiomas in children. J Pediatr Surg 1991; 26:263–270
30. Rak KM, Yakes WF, Ray RL, et al. MR imaging of symptomatic peripheral vascular malformations. AJR 1992; 159:107–112
31. Sadan N, Wolach B. Treatment of hemangiomas of infants with high doses of prednisone. J Pediatr 1996; 128:141–146
32. Stöver B, Laubenberger J, Niemeyer C, Stahl F, Brandis M, Langer M. Haemangiomatosis in children: value of MRI during therapy. Pediatr Radiol 1995; 25:123–126

CASE 12

Marta Hernanz-Schulman, M.D.

Agenesis of the Corpus Callosum

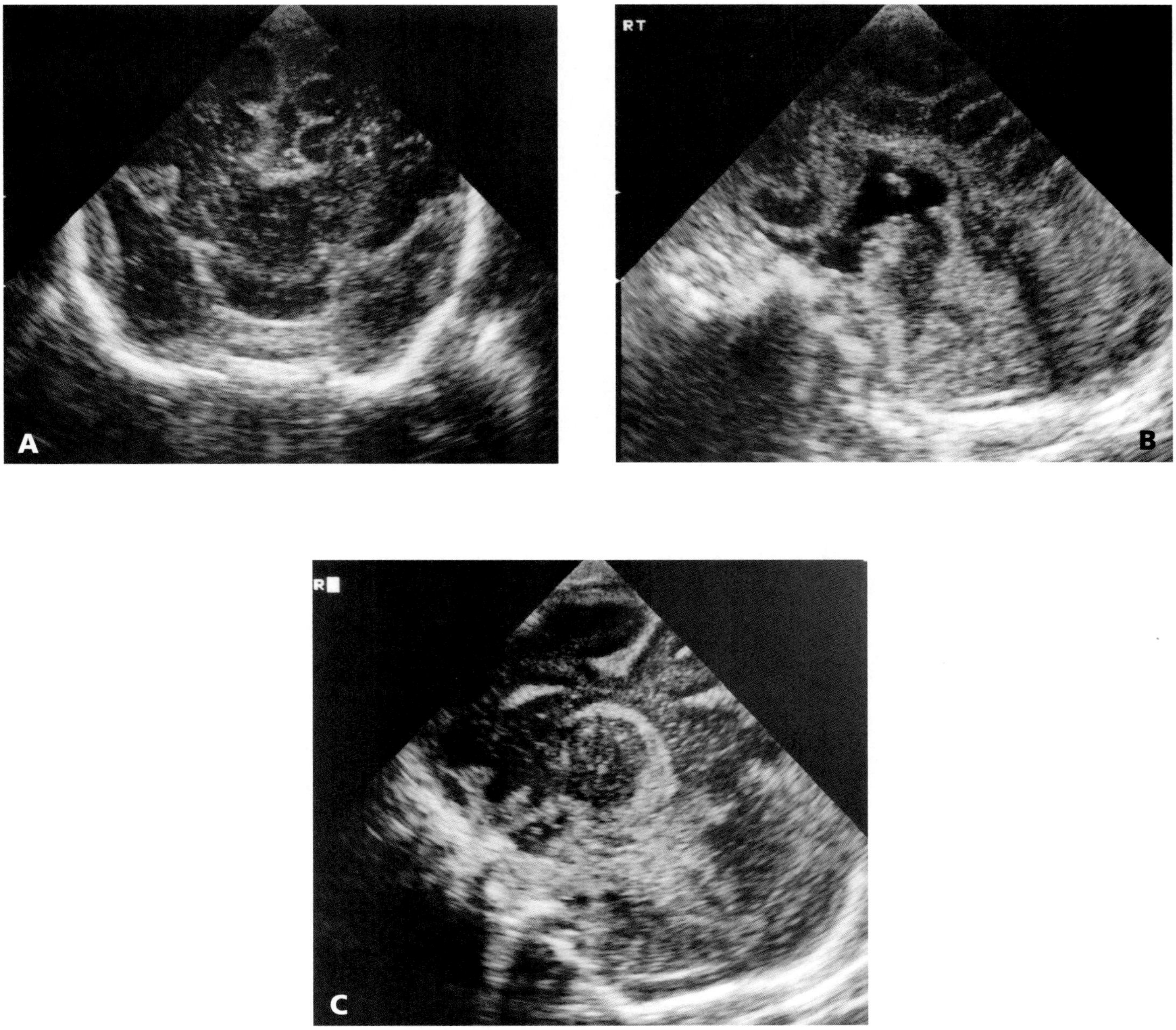

Figure 12-1

Question 61

This term neonate has a diaphragmatic hernia and severe respiratory distress. Cranial ultrasonography was performed before the initiation of extracorporeal membrane oxygenation. You are shown coronal (A), midline sagittal (B), and right parasagittal (C) sonograms.

The test images demonstrate:

(A) holoprosencephaly
(B) agenesis of the corpus callosum
(C) Chiari II malformation
(D) pachygyria
(E) hypoxic-ischemic encephalopathy

The coronal test image (Figure 12-1A) demonstrates widely spaced, normal-sized anterior horns of the lateral ventricles. These are bounded medially by uninverted cingulate gyri, separated from the frontal horns by the longitudinal callosal bundles of Probst (Figure 12-2A). The septum pellucidum and the corpus callosum are absent, consistent with agensis of the corpus callosum **(Option (B) is true)**. The interhemispheric fissure is widened. In addition, the gyral pattern is abnormal; the gyri on the right are abnormally thickened and less numerous than are those on the left. The midline sagittal image (Figure 12-1B), taken just to the left of the widened interhemispheric fissure, confirms the absence of the corpus callosum. It further demonstrates the radial arrangement of the sulcal pattern, which extends from the third ventricle in a "sunburst" configuration, resulting from lack of inversion of the cingulate gyri and subsequent failure of formation of the cingulate sulcus (Figure 12-2B). The parasagittal image angled to the right (Figure 12-1C) illustrates the characteristic dilatation of the occipital horns (colpocephaly) and the widened, abnormal cortical gyri (pachygyria) (Figure 12-2C) **(Option (D) is true)**.

Holoprosencephaly is an abnormality of cleavage of the prosencephalic vesicle, resulting in a failure of all or part of the prosencephalon to separate. The most severe form is the alobar type, in which there is thalamic fusion and a monoventricle surrounded by a dysplastic cerebral mantle, in a mushroomlike configuration (Figure 12-3). Less severe forms include the semilobar and lobar types, which represent a continuum of progressive cleavage dorsoventrally. Thus, the anatomic findings are most severe anteriorly and are characterized by absence of the interhemispheric fissure (Figure 12-4); since an interhemispheric fissure is present and widened in the test patient, holoprosencephaly is not a consideration **(Option (A) is false)**.

The Chiari II malformation is a complex deformity of the hindbrain or rhombencephalon. It is characterized by an abnormally small posterior fossa and caudal herniation of the cerebellar vermis, fourth ventricle, and medulla through the foramen magnum into the spinal canal (Figure 12-5). The midline test image (Figure 12-1B) demonstrates a normal posterior fossa; the fourth ventricle is positioned normally and the vermis appears normal. Thus, the images do not show evidence of the Chiari II malformation **(Option (C) is false)**.

The imaging manifestations of hypoxic-ischemic encephalopathy vary depending on the extent and severity of the initial insult. In term infants with prolonged partial ischemia, the cerebral mantle is most severely affected, especially the watershed areas at the borders of vascular territories. The abnormalities noted at sonography include a diffuse increase in the echogenicity of the involved structures, with indistinctness and eventual loss of definition of anatomic interfaces, loss of gyral gray-white differentiation, and prominence and thickening of the central white matter bands (Figure 12-6A through D).

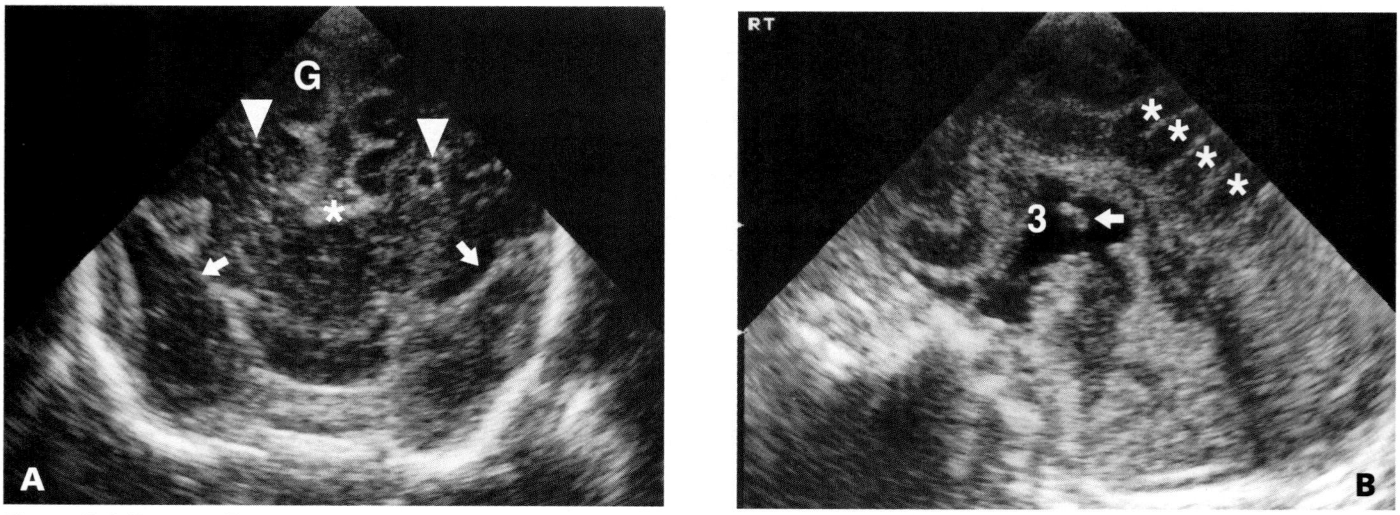

Figure 12-2 (Same as Figure 12-1). Agenesis of the corpus callosum. (A) A coronal sonogram through the plane of the sylvian fissures (arrows) shows that the lateral ventricles (arrowheads) are widely spaced. There is no corpus callosum. (Refer to Figures 12-8B, 12-10A, and 12-13A for comparison.) In this patient, there is little or no elevation of the third ventricle, the roof of which is indicated by the choroid plexus (*). Note the widened abnormal gyri (G) to the right of the widened interhemispheric fissure. (B) A midline sagittal image confirms the absence of the corpus callosum and shows the radial arrangement of the gyri (*) from the roof of the third ventricle (3), with interposed massa intermedia (arrow). (Refer to Figure 12-5B for comparison.)

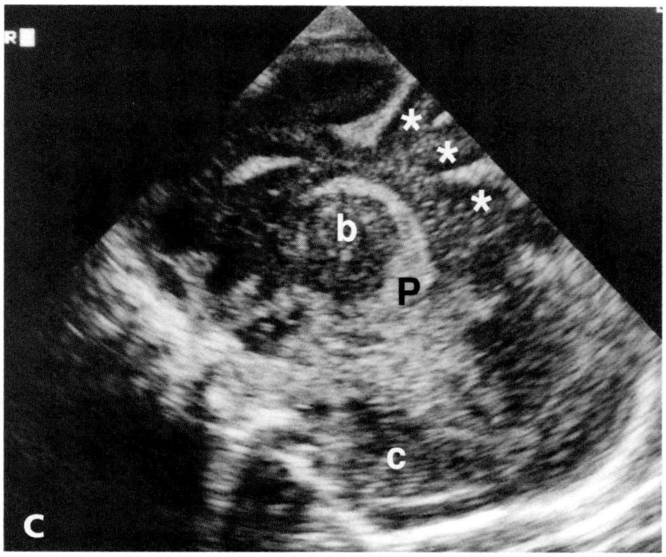

Figure 12-2 (Continued) (Same as Figure 12-1). Agenesis of the corpus callosum. (C) A parasagittal image angled to the right demonstrates the abnormally broad gyri (*) of the pachygyric cortex. P = choroid plexus; b = basal ganglia; c = right cerebellar hemisphere.

None of these findings is present in the test patient (**Option (E) is false**). In patients with severe neuronal injury, autoregulation is lost and both release and failure of reuptake of excitatory amino acids, such as glutamate, are noted. Temporal changes in cerebral blood flow are complex. However, it has been shown that abnormally low resistive indices (RI) obtained close to the time of injury in these infants correlate with a poor prognosis. The normal RI in a term neonate is approximately 0.75 ± 0.10. In patients with severe hypoxic-ischemic encephalopathy, the RI often lies in the range from 0.40 to 0.50 (Figure 12-6E).

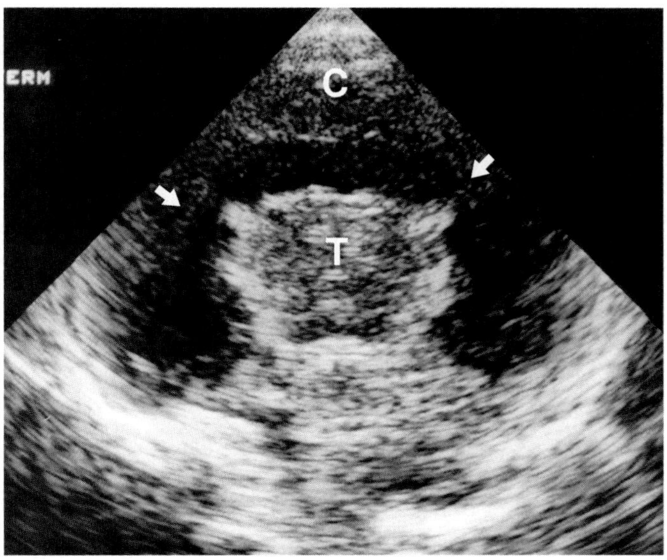

Figure 12-3. Alobar holoprosencephaly. A coronal sonogram of a newborn infant demonstrates fused thalami (T) in the midline, surrounded by a single ventricular cavity (arrows) and a dysplastic, lissencephalic cerebral mantle (C). There is no interhemispheric fissure. (Reprinted with permission from Hernanz-Schulman et al. [7].)

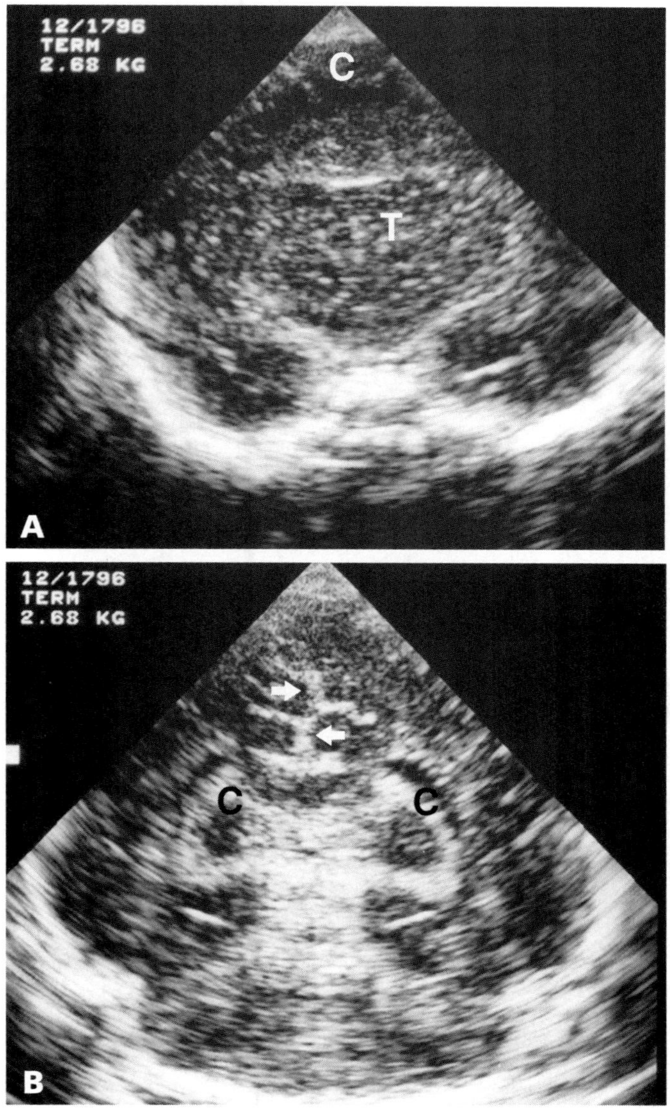

Figure 12-4. Semilobar holoprosencephaly. (A) A coronal sonogram through a very small anterior fontanel in a term infant with multiple congenital anomalies demonstrates anterior fusion of the thalami (T) and of the cerebral cortex (C). The cortical mantle appears abnormally smooth. (B) A posteriorly angled coronal sonogram shows posterior cleavage into two hemispheres and two lateral ventricles. C = choroid plexus in the antrum of each lateral ventricle; arrows point to the developed interhemispheric fissure.

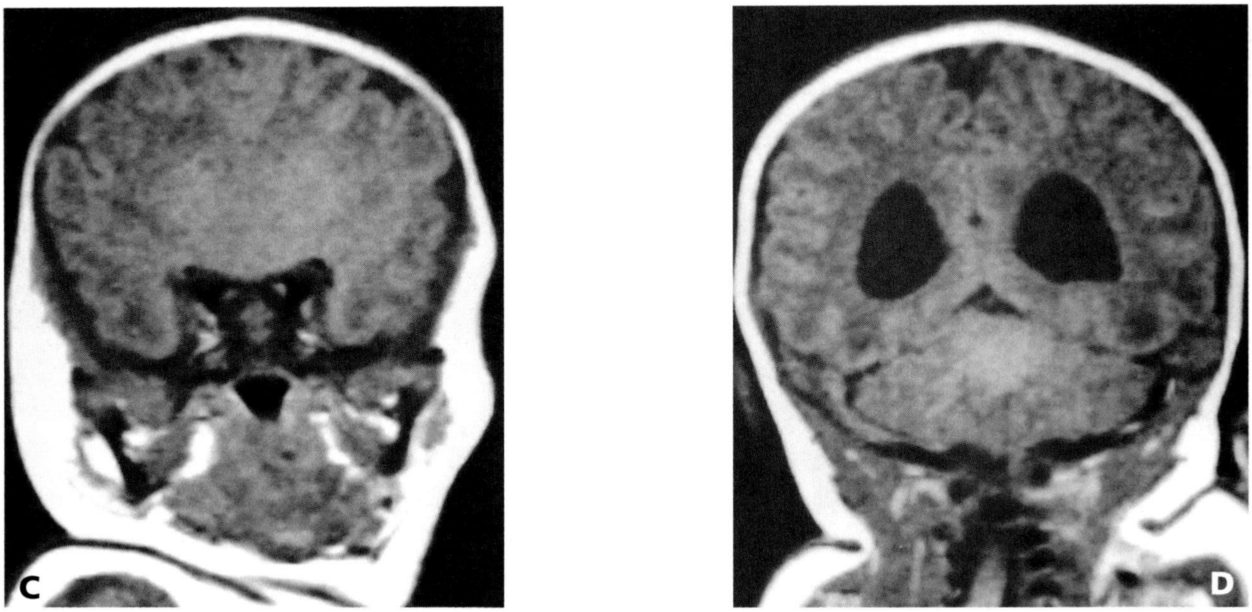

SE 600/15 SE 600/15

Figure 12-4 (Continued). Semilobar holoprosencephaly. (C) A coronal T1-weighted MR image confirms the anterior fusion of the thalami and cerebral cortex, with an abnormally broad gyral pattern. (D) A posterior coronal T1-weighted MR image demonstrates the normal posterior cleavage of the hemispheres and lateral ventricles and reversion to a less smooth gyral pattern.

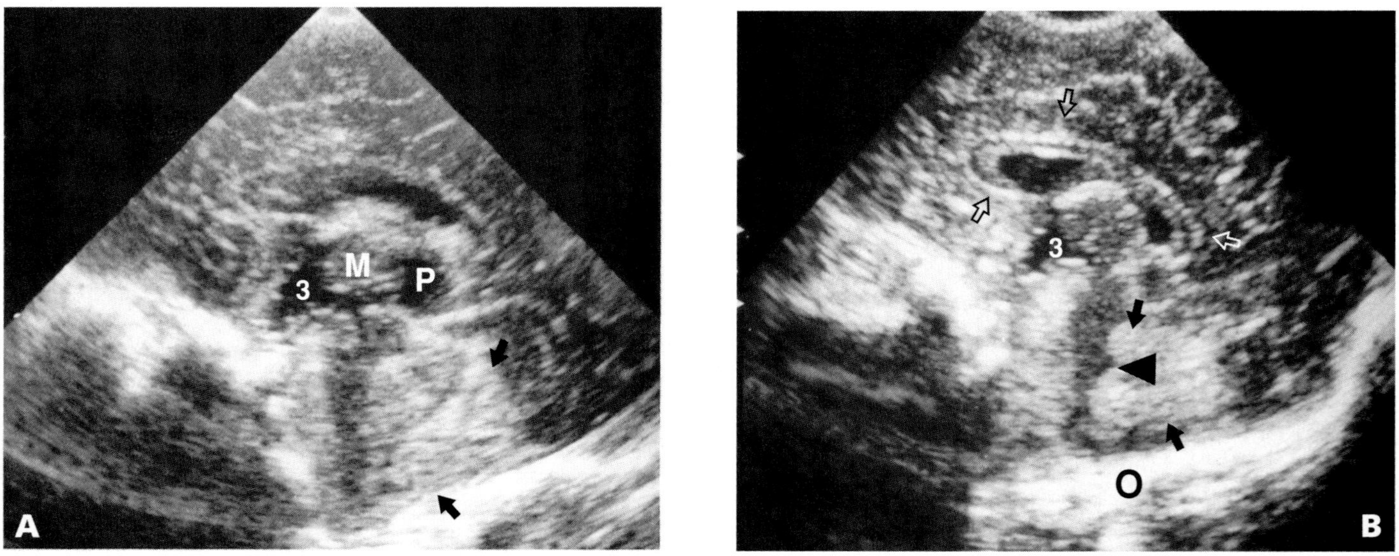

Figure 12-5. Chiari II malformation. (A) A midline sagittal sonogram of a neonate with the Chiari II malformation and myelomeningocele shows inferior displacement of the contents of the posterior fossa (arrows). The third ventricle (3) is enlarged, with prominence of the pineal recess (P). The massa intermedia (M) is likewise enlarged. (B) A midline sagittal sonogram of a normal term infant (for comparison with panel A) shows a normal-appearing cerebellar vermis (solid arrows), separated from the occipital bone (O) by fluid in the cisterna magna, and the normal definition and position of the fourth ventricle (arrowhead). Thalamic tissue protrudes into the normal-sized third ventricle (3) above the optic and infundibular recesses. The open arrows, clockwise from the bottom left, point to the rostrum, genu, and body and splenium of the corpus callosum. (C) A sagittal sonogram of the craniocervical junction in an infant with Chiari II malformation, taken along the dorsal nuchal surface just below the occiput. Note the caudal displacement of the caudal cerebellum (*) and the stretching of the cervical cord and medulla. (D) A sagittal sonogram of the craniocervical junction in a normal infant (for comparison with panel C) shows that the posterior fossa elements are absent from the fluid-filled cervical canal; the cervical cord (c) appears normal. (E) A sagittal T1-weighted MR image of the craniocervical junction in another patient with Chiari II malformation, for comparison with panels C and D. (F) A coronal sonogram in a neonate with Chiari II malformation shows the characteristic "squaring" of the superolateral angles of the frontal horns and inferior beaking of their floor (arrows). (G) A midline T1-weighted MR image of an infant with Chiari II malformation and partial agenesis of the corpus callosum shows absence of the splenium posteriorly and the rostrum anteriorly (compare with panel B). An enlarged massa intermedia (M), tectal beaking (*), stenogyria (thin, closely spaced gyri), and characteristic posterior fossa abnormalities are also present. (H) A midline sagittal sonogram of an infant with Chiari II malformation demonstrates an enlarged massa intermedia (M), tectal beaking (*), stenogyria, and characteristic posterior fossa abnormalities. (Reprinted with permission from Hernanz-Schulman et al. [7].)

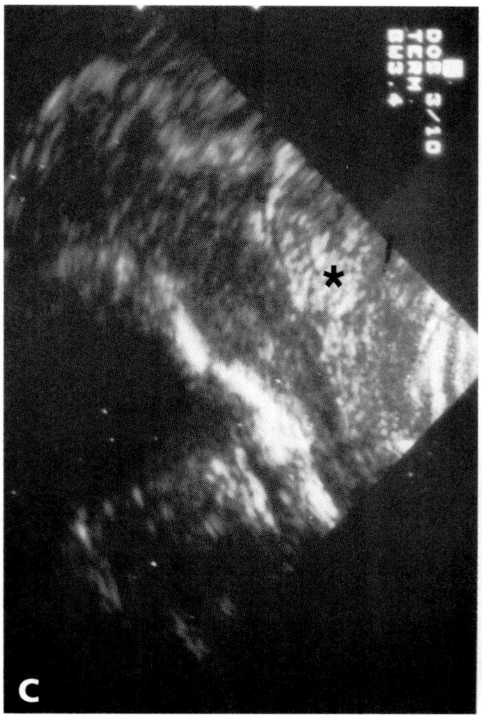

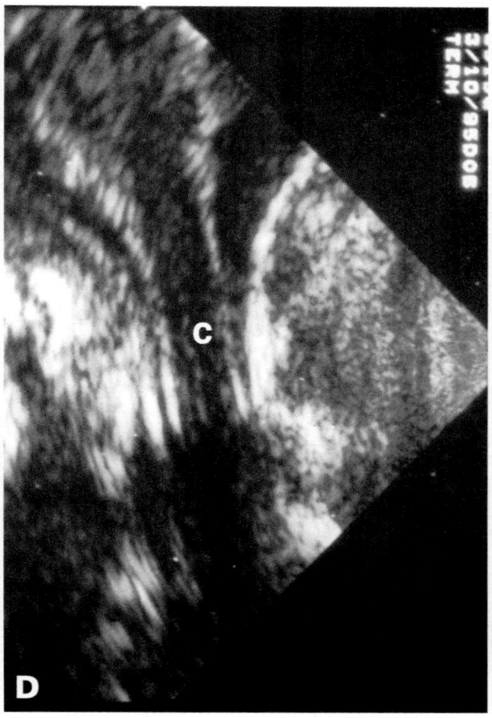

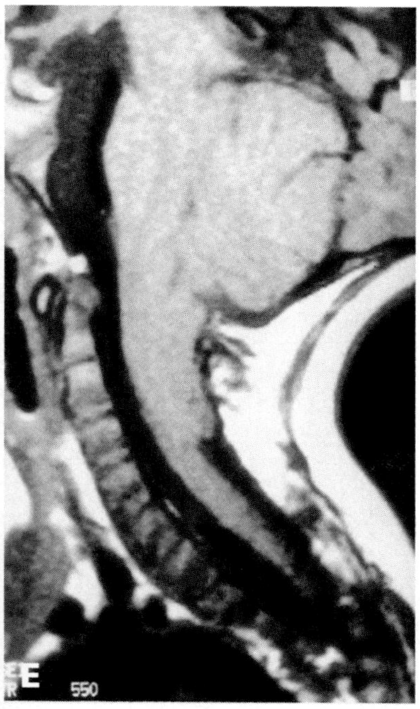

SE 600/15

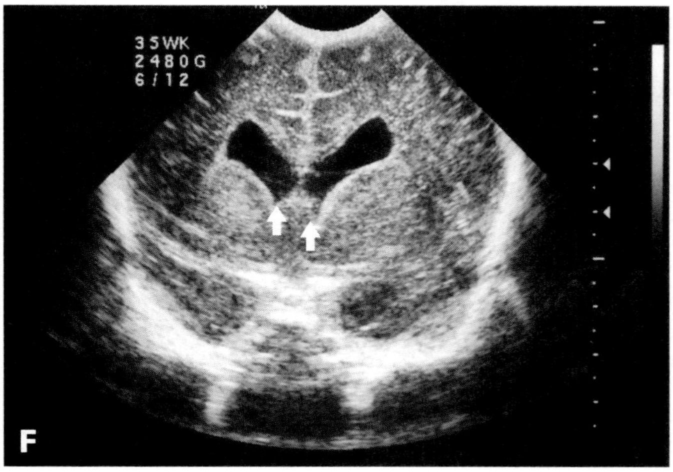

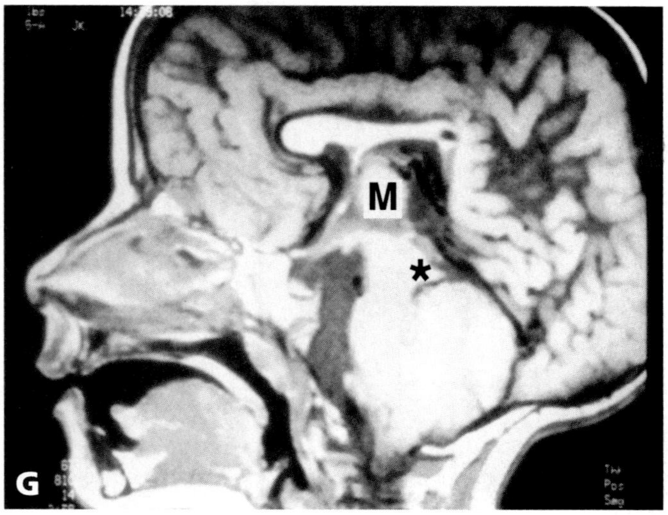

SE 600/15

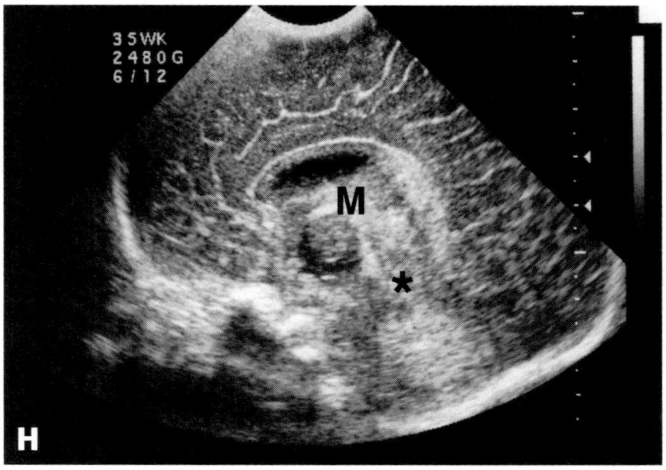

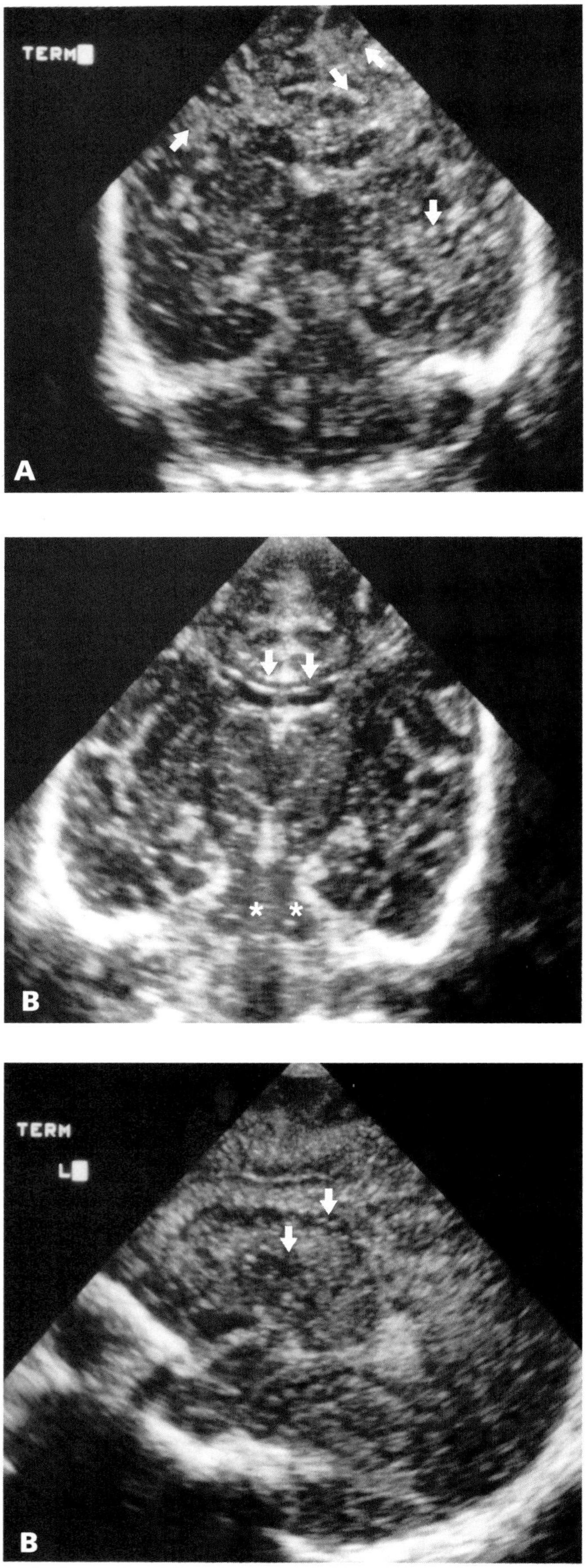

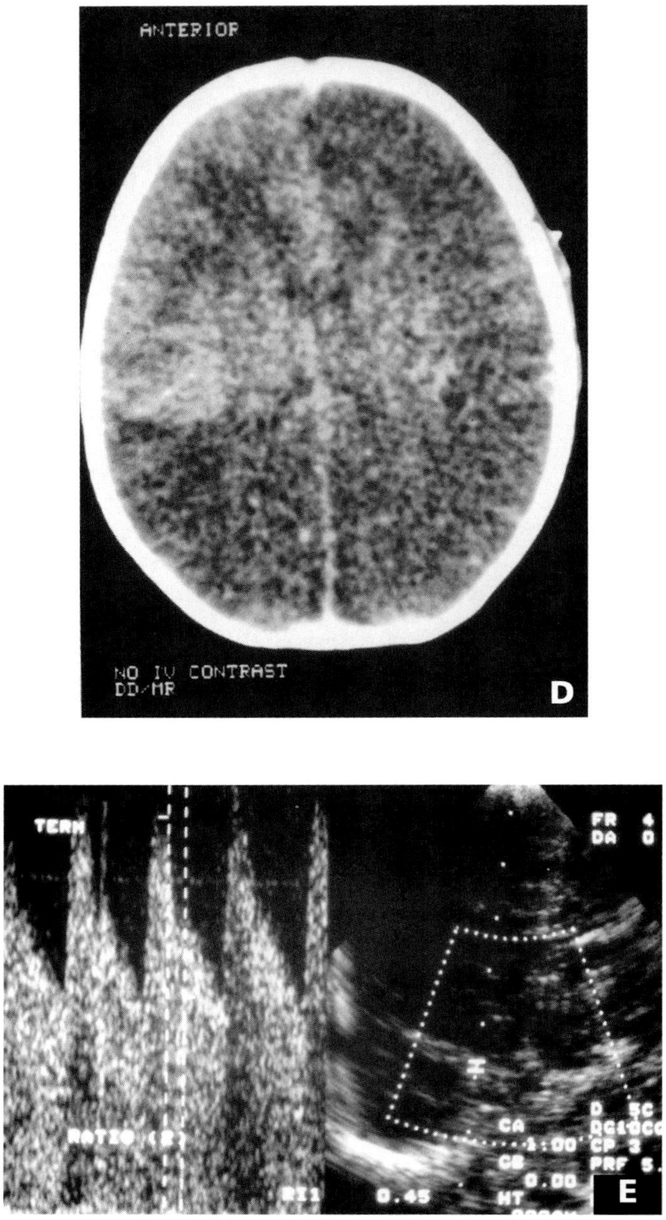

Figure 12-6. Hypoxic-ischemic encephalopathy in a term infant, born at home, who suffered prolonged perinatal asphyxia. (A) A posteriorly angled coronal sonogram shows generalized indistinctness of the cerebral interfaces (compare with panel B) and thickening and increased echogenicity of the central gyral echoes (arrows), more markedly abnormal on the left than on the right. (B) A posteriorly angled coronal sonogram of a normal term infant, taken at a plane slightly more anterior than that in panel A, shows distinct sulcal interfaces and normal cerebral echogenicity. Asterisks denote the cerebellar peduncles. Arrows point to the corpus callosum. (C) A parasagittal sonogram of the patient in panel A again outlines the abnormally thickened central gyral echoes (arrows). (D) A CT scan of the patient in panel A illustrates the intense edema and loss of gray-white differentiation, which are more marked on the left side. (E) A Doppler sonogram obtained at the right carotid bifurcation in the patient in panel A. The RI is 0.45, a markedly abnormal value. (Reprinted with permission from Hernanz-Schulman et al. [7].)

Question 62

Features of semilobar holoprosencephaly include:

(A) agenesis of the anterior portion of the corpus callosum
(B) agenesis of the septum pellucidum
(C) migrational abnormalities of the cerebral cortex
(D) abnormal anterior falx
(E) azygous anterior cerebral artery
(F) cerebellar hypoplasia

Holoprosencephaly refers to a continuum of anomalies characterized by variable failure of cleavage of the prosencephalon into two distinct hemispheres, a process that occurs during weeks 5 and 6 of gestation. The severity of this anomaly ranges along a spectrum from complete failure of cleavage to isolated absence of the septum pellucidum, a condition that overlaps with or encompasses the syndrome known as septo-optic dysplasia. This wide spectrum has been subdivided by DeMyer into three very broad and overlapping categories: alobar, semilobar, and lobar, in order of progressively decreasing severity. This classification is widely used and accepted in the literature and in clinical practice.

In patients with alobar holoprosencephaly, the telencephalic and diencephalic structures do not separate and the thalami are fused (Figure 12-3). The third ventricle does not develop, and the lateral ventricles form a single monoventricle continuous posteriorly with the occiput as a dorsal cyst and the membranous roof of the third ventricle. The monoventricle is in turn enveloped by a thin mantle of dysplastic cortex, which architecturally resembles the hippocampus and other limbic structures, with failure of development of the supralimbic cortex. Since there is no separation of telencephalon or diencephalon, it is obvious that there are no corpus callosum, no septum pellucidum, and no falx cerebri. Absence of the falx, failure of cleavage of the thalami, and absence of a third ventricle are features that help to distinguish this condition from hydranencephaly (Figure 12-7) and from very severe hydrocephalus. However, it must be noted that absence of the septum pellucidum, although a constant feature of all of the holoprosencephalies, is not a distinguishing feature among these various conditions, since it is obviously absent in patients with hydranencephaly and is secondarily obliterated in patients with very severe hydrocephalus.

Since the inductive interactions that direct the differentiation of the forebrain also influence the development of the face, it is not surprising that facial anomalies are present in many of these patients. In patients with the most severe forms, there may be absence of the eyes or a single eye (cyclopia) and a rudimentary nasal structure (proboscis) situated above the orbit. Progressively less severe facial deformities include hypotelorism with a proboscis (ethmocephaly), hypotelorism with cleft lip and palate and single nostril (cebocephaly), or hypotelorism alone. Severe facial anomalies are associated with the more severe forms of holoprosencephaly; however, the converse is not

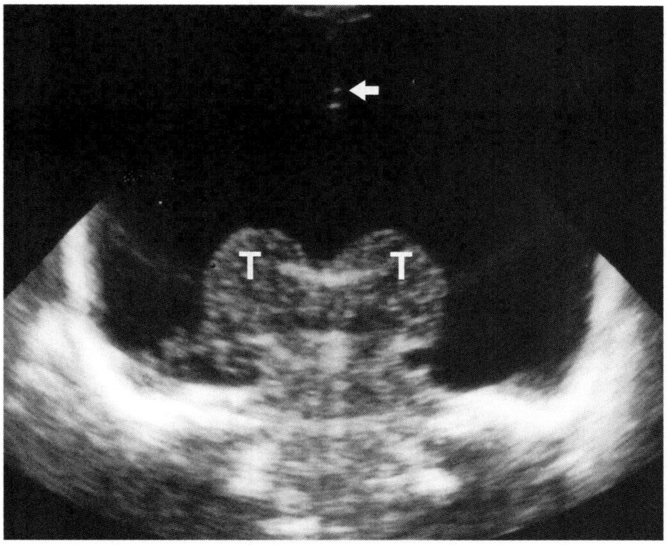

Figure 12-7. Hydranencephaly. A coronal sonogram shows cleavage of the thalami (T). The interhemispheric fissure is clearly visible in the midline (arrow). Compare with Figure 12-3. (Reprinted with permission from Hernanz-Schulman et al. [7].)

true, and approximately 30% of patients with the more severe forms of holoprosencephaly will have a normal or nearly normal face. Abnormalities of other organ systems, notably the skeletal, cardiac, genitourinary, and gastrointestinal systems, occur in approximately 75% of patients. In some cases, holoprosencephaly appears to be part of a chromosomal disorder, notably of chromosomes 13 and 18, as well as of chromosomes 2, 3, 7, and 21. Familial cases also have been reported. Although the limbic structures representative of the rhinencephalon are present, there is universal absence of the olfactory bulbs and thus this anomaly has at times been termed arrhinencephaly.

Within the spectrum of the semilobar and lobar types, cleavage occurs to a variable degree. This cleavage proceeds in a dorsoventral direction. The classification of semilobar holoprosencephaly is generally applied to brains in which there has been partial or complete cleavage of the thalami, with formation of a rudimentary third ventricle, and a variable degree of dorsal telencephalic partitioning, with variable formation of the posterior portion of the falx cerebri and the splenium of the corpus callosum, whereas the septum pellucidum and anterior falx are absent (**Options (B) and (D) are true**) (Figure 12-4). By definition, the anterior portion of the corpus callosum has not formed (in contradistinction to isolated partial callosal agenesis, in which the posterior portion and rostrum of the corpus callosum, the last to form, are absent) (Figure 12-5B and G) (**Option (A) is true**). The hippocampal formation is typically hypoplastic in these patients, and gyral anomalies, such as pachygyria, can be present (Figure 12-4B and D) (**Option (C) is true**). The anterior cerebral circulation, supplying the fused frontal brain, is nearly always a single vessel, the azygous anterior cerebral artery (**Option (E) is true**). An unusual form of this semilobar holoprosencephaly has been described in which failure of cleavage is limited to the central portion of the brain, with fusion of the cerebral hemispheres and absence of the corpus callosum confined to this central area but with normal cleavage anteriorly and posteriorly. Since holoprosencephaly is an abnormality of the prosencephalon, the rhombencephalon does not participate in this anomaly, and the cerebellum in these patients is typically normal (**Option (F) is false**).

Lobar holoprosencephaly, in which the failure of cleavage is limited to the most anterior portion of the telencephalon, is the least severe form of these anomalies. The anterior portion of the falx is present but is usually hypoplastic. The anterior portion of the corpus callosum (genu and rostrum) can be absent. The septum pellucidum is always absent, and thus the frontal horns lack separation. There may be associated abnormalities of one or both optic nerves and of the pituitary gland, overlapping with de Morsier's syndrome, or septo-optic dysplasia (Figure 12-8).

Question 63

Anatomic findings associated with agenesis of the corpus callosum include:

(A) colpocephaly
(B) reduced distance between the frontal horns
(C) malpositioned cingulate gyri
(D) inferiorly displaced third ventricle
(E) gray matter heterotopias

The corpus callosum represents the largest telencephalic commissure of decussating interhemispheric axons. It is seen on sagittal imaging as a crescent-shaped band of white matter that roofs the lateral ventricles and the septum pellucidum (Figure 12-5B). Its superior surface consists of the pericallosal sulcus and the paired, inverted cingulate gyri, which course cocircumferentially above the pericallosal sulcus.

After closure of the anterior end of the neural tube, the midline lamina terminalis forms; at approximately 7 weeks of gestation, a cellular, thickened ridge, in which glial cells provide a "bridge" for interhemispheric axonal decussation, begins to form. Formation of the corpus callosum begins at approximately 10 to 12 weeks of gestation and is completed by 18 to 20 weeks. The growth of the corpus callosum rotates and defines the cingulate gyri in their normal parallel configuration. The septum pellucidum, which is thought to represent a remnant of the commissural plate, forms the medial walls of the frontal horns and lies superior to the third ventricle. Bridged by the corpus callosum, the cerebral hemispheres lie in close apposition at the midline along the interhemispheric fissure.

In patients with complete callosal agenesis, the corpus callosum fails to form. The cingulate gyri do not invert, so that the cingulate sulcus does not form, and are laterally displaced (**Option (C) is true**). Because the malformation often involves the limbic system, both the cingulate and hippocampal gyri may be dysplastic to some degree (Figure 12-9A). The laterally displaced cingulate gyri dislocate and separate the frontal horns of the lateral ventricles (**Option (B) is false**), elongating the foramina of Monro into a horizontal configuration. The leaves of the septum pellucidum, forming the medial walls of the frontal horns, also become deviated, attenuated, or absent. Furthermore, the hemispheres are permitted to separate, with consequent variable widening of the interhemispheric fissure. The undecussated axons that would have formed the corpus callosum, the bundles of Probst, lie in close apposition to the roofs of the lateral ventricles, lateral to the displaced cingulate gyri. In the absence of its superior bordering structures, the roof of

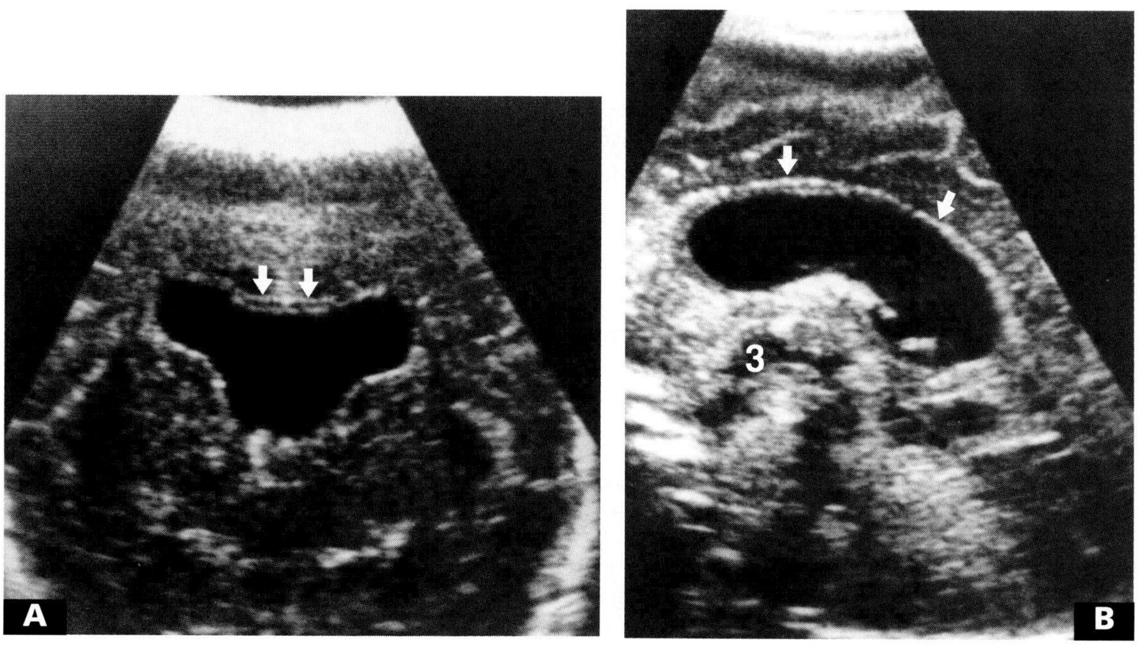

Figure 12-8. Absence of the septum pellucidum. (A) A coronal sonogram in a term infant demonstrates continuity of the two lateral ventricles across the midline, bordered superiorly by the corpus callosum (arrows). (B) A midline sagittal image demonstrates that the corpus callosum (arrows) is present over the lateral ventricles. A distinct third ventricle (3) is seen inferiorly.

the third ventricle is permitted to elevate and does so to a variable degree; in approximately 50% of patients, it reaches the inferior surface of the falx (**Option (D) is false**). The term "corpus callosum" derives from Latin and means "hard body"; the structure is firm, and its mechanical presence contributes to the normal size and shape of the lateral ventricles. The absence of the corpus callosum permits the posterior portion of the lateral ventricles to invaginate the surrounding white matter, allowing persistence of the dilated fetal conformation termed "colpocephaly" (**Option (A) is true**). Anteriorly, the gray matter of the caudate and lentiform nuclei prevents the development of this ectatic configuration and confines the frontal horns to a relatively normal size.

These alterations can be appreciated on several types of imaging studies, but are better depicted by modalities that permit imaging in the coronal and sagittal planes than by those that do not. On coronal images (Figure 12-2A), the characteristic separation of the frontal horns is appreciated, although it is variable in degree and need be manifested only by straightening of the normally medially convex medial walls. The normal septum pellucidum, bridged superiorly by the corpus callosum, is absent, and the midline instead contains the laterally displaced, everted cingulate gyri, with variable separation of the cerebral hemispheres. The third ventricle is no longer bordered superiorly by the septum pellucidum but, rather, is demarcated by the choroid plexus in its roof and by the anomalous gyri

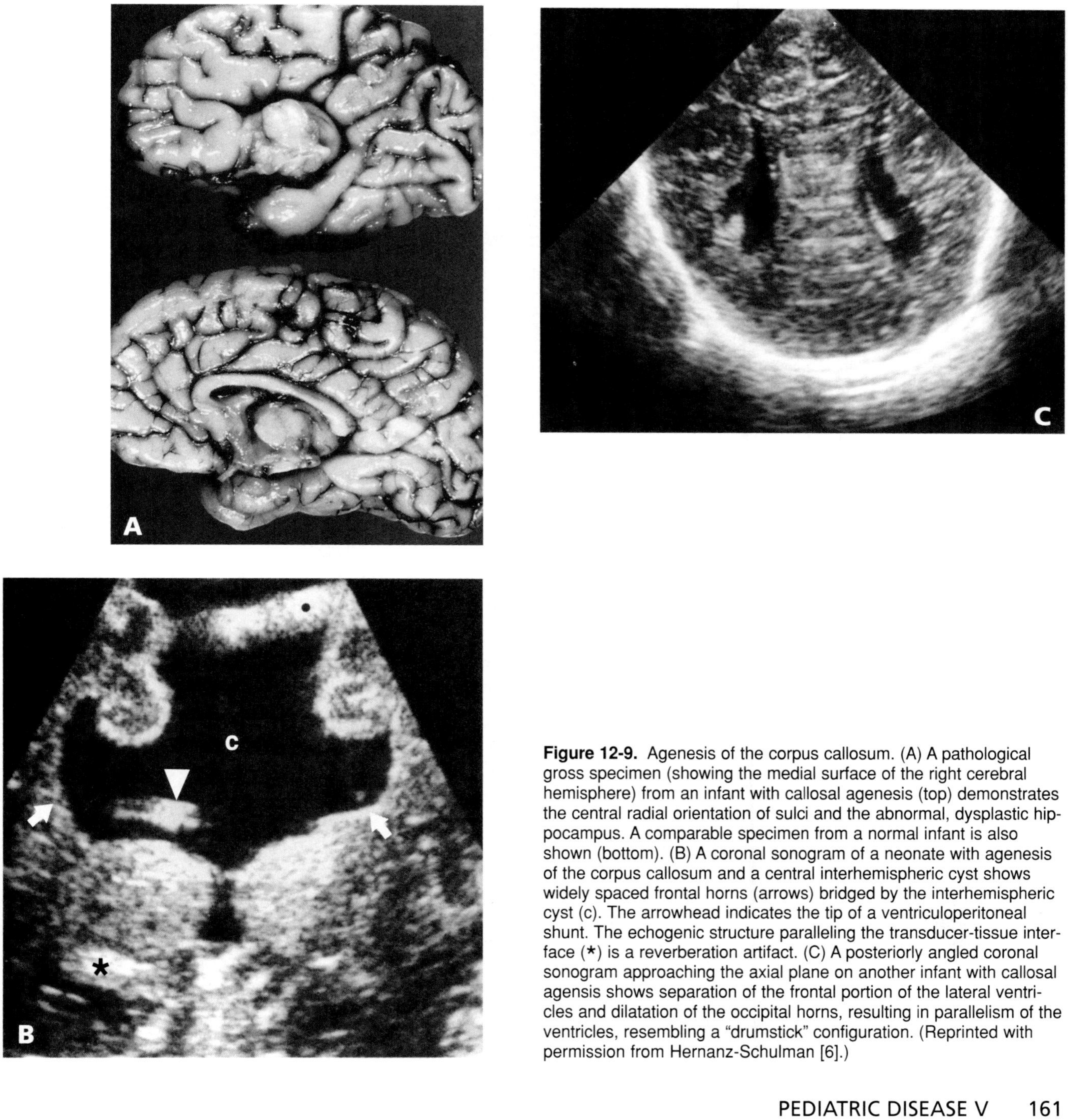

Figure 12-9. Agenesis of the corpus callosum. (A) A pathological gross specimen (showing the medial surface of the right cerebral hemisphere) from an infant with callosal agenesis (top) demonstrates the central radial orientation of sulci and the abnormal, dysplastic hippocampus. A comparable specimen from a normal infant is also shown (bottom). (B) A coronal sonogram of a neonate with agenesis of the corpus callosum and a central interhemispheric cyst shows widely spaced frontal horns (arrows) bridged by the interhemispheric cyst (c). The arrowhead indicates the tip of a ventriculoperitoneal shunt. The echogenic structure paralleling the transducer-tissue interface (*) is a reverberation artifact. (C) A posteriorly angled coronal sonogram approaching the axial plane on another infant with callosal agensis shows separation of the frontal portion of the lateral ventricles and dilatation of the occipital horns, resulting in parallelism of the ventricles, resembling a "drumstick" configuration. (Reprinted with permission from Hernanz-Schulman [6].)

and variably displaced hemispheres (Figure 12-2A). As discussed above, the third ventricle may extend superiorly to abut the falx; an interhemispheric cyst, which may or may not be multiloculated and may communicate with the third or the lateral ventricles, may be present (Figure 12-9B). If this cyst is sufficiently large, it can lead to impaired drainage of cerebrospinal fluid and result in hydrocephalus. Dilated occipital horns do not denote hydrocephalus but are an integral part of the malformation and are seen well on coronal, axial, and parasagittal images. On axial images, the variably superiorly displaced third ventricle can lie interposed between the lateral ventricles. The separation of the frontal horns leads to a parallel orientation of the lateral ventricles, which, in conjunction with the dilatation of the occipital horns, conveys an appearance resembling a "drumstick" (Figure 12-9C). The corpus callosum is absent on sagittal images. Because the pericallosal sulcus is absent and because of the abnormal conformation of the cingulate gyrus and the cingulate sulcus, the cerebral gyri and sulci seem to radiate from the roof of the third ventricle in a sunburst configuration (Figure 12-2B).

As in the test patient, agenesis of the corpus callosum is often associated with other central nervous system anomalies, notably migrational disorders, such as pachygyria, polymicrogyria (Figure 12-10), and gray matter heterotopias (**Option (E) is true**). The variable severity of these associated malformations typically explains the variable clinical symptoms of patients with callosal agenesis. It is important to search for these anomalies on imaging studies. On sonography, CT, and MRI, close attention should be paid to the size and number of gyri, and gray matter heterotopias should be actively sought.

Question 64

Concerning the Chiari II malformation,

(A) it is associated with failure of the neural tube to close in nearly all patients
(B) the posterior fossa is usually normal in size
(C) the severity of hydrocephalus often increases after repair of the myelomeningocele
(D) abnormalities of the corpus callosum are present in fewer than 10% of patients

The Chiari II or Arnold-Chiari malformation is a dysgenesis of the rhombencephalon that is nearly always found in association with open neural tube defects (**Option (A) is true**). The lesion consists of multiple anomalies, including inferior displacement of the fourth ventricle, medulla, and cerebellum through the foramen magnum into the cervical canal, with elongation and thinning of the medulla and pons. In patients with this malformation, the posterior fossa is small, with an abnormally low tentorial attachment (**Option (B) is false**). The cerebellum is forced caudally, with caudal stretching of the pons, medulla, and cervical cord. The cerebellum also can extend along the coronal plane, encircling the posterolateral brain stem.

Supratentorial anomalies are common. Enlargement of the third ventricle is variable but is nearly always proportionally less than that of the lateral ventricles, and there is often disproportionate enlargement of the pineal recess. The massa intermedia is enlarged to a variable degree (Figure 12-5A, G, and H). The occipital horns are disproportionately large (colpocephaly). The frontal horns are beaked inferiorly, with flatten-

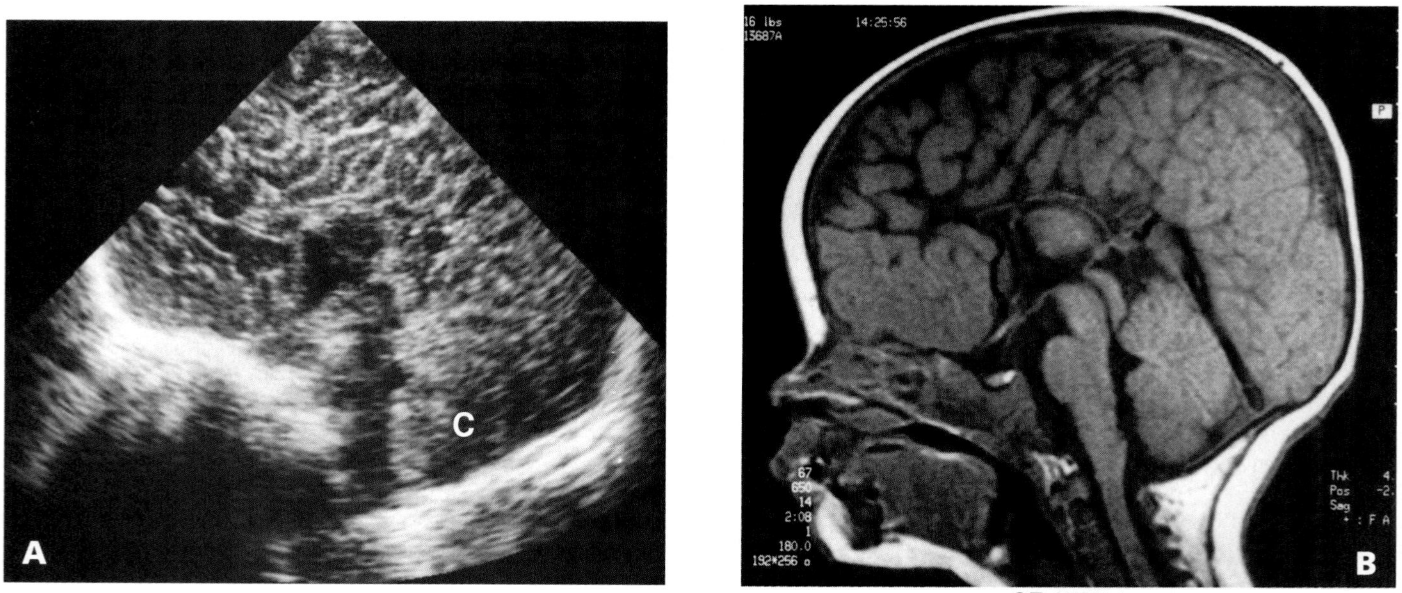

SE 650/14

Figure 12-10. Agenesis of the corpus callosum with polymicrogyria. (A) A midline sagittal sonogram demonstrates several findings similar to those illustrated in Figure 12-2B. However, the gyri are small and closely spaced, consistent with polymicrogyria. C = cerebellar vermis. (B) A midline sagittal T1-weighted MR image illustrates callosal agenesis and polymicrogyric cortex. (Reprinted with permission from Hernanz-Schulman et al. [7].)

ing of the superolateral angles, an appearance resembling a bat wing (Figure 12-5F); this beaking is thought to be due to prominence of the head of the caudate nuclei and can persist despite considerable ventricular dilatation. Hydrocephalus is present in the large majority of patients after closure of the myelomeningocele and may worsen or first become apparent at this time in some patients. The reason for this is postulated to be the closure of the neural tube defect which, prior to closure, provides an outlet for cerebrospinal fluid drainage (**Option (C) is true**). Caudal stretching leads to beaking of the quadrigeminal plate (Figure 12-5G).

Anomalies of the corpus callosum usually consist of hypoplasia or dysgenesis and are seen in up to 90% of patients (Figure 12-5G) (**Option (D) is false**).

Stenogyria, characterized by thin, closely spaced gyri, is present in as many as 40% of patients (Figure 12-5G and H), although a true polymicrogyric migrational anomaly may be present in some of these patients. Hypoplasia and fenestration of the falx lead to apposition of gyri at the midline (Figure 12-11).

These intracranial features are associated with mesodermal defects involving the skull and spinal column. In infants, the skull can have an irregular appearance termed "lückenschädel" (Figure 12-12), a transient abnormality that can be confused with calvarial change resulting from increased intracranial pressure. Scalloping of the petrous bones also can be present.

Clinically, patients present with an obvious myelomeningocele. If the brain stem is compressed by the caudal herniation of the posterior fossa contents, patients can present with stridor, weak crying, and feeding difficulties.

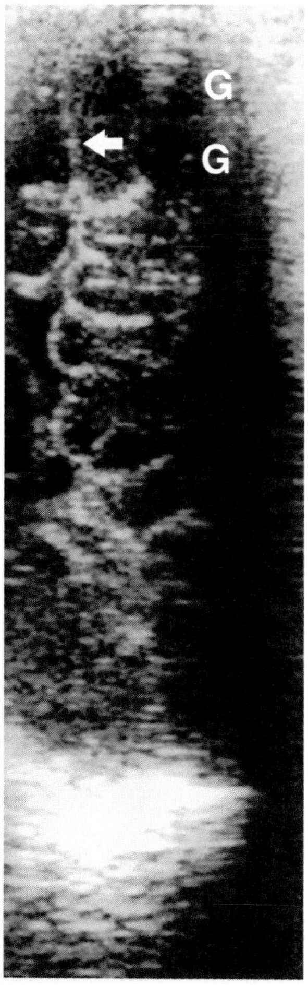

Figure 12-11. Falx fenestration in a patient with Chiari II malformation. A posteriorly angled sonogram approaching the axial plane demonstrates gyral interdigitation (G) across the midline. The arrow points to the falx.

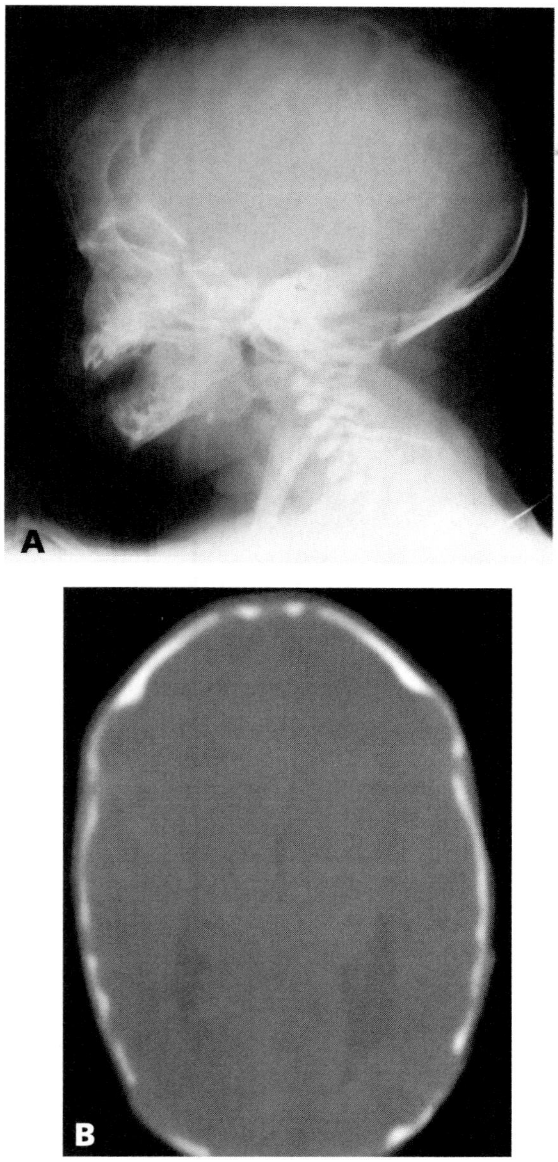

Figure 12-12. Lückenschädel in an infant with Chiari II malformation. (A) A lateral radiograph of the skull shows the characteristic irregularities along the skull vault. (B) A CT scan, photographed at bone-window settings, demonstrates the typical scalloping of the calvarium.

Question 65

Concerning pachygyria,

(A) it is a generalized abnormality of the cerebral cortex
(B) it is characterized by an increased number of gyri
(C) disorganization of neuronal architecture is characteristic
(D) the cortical signal intensity is usually increased on T2-weighted MR images

Pachygyria is a disorder of cortical neuronal migration and organization that is closely related to and believed to be part of the spectrum of lissencephaly. Polymicrogyria is another disturbance of the normal gyral development of the brain with disorganization of the underlying cortex. Although these entities are characterized by variable disorganization of the cortical neuronal layers (**Option (C) is true**), they are named and categorized by the superficial appearance of the cerebrum in the affected areas. Lissencephaly is the term applied to a smooth brain, in which there is total failure of sulcation (Figure 12-13). In patients with pachygyria, the gyri are abnormally broad and present in smaller numbers (Figures 12-2 and 12-4) (**Option (B) is false**). Polymicrogyria, as the name implies, consists of an increased number of small, narrow gyri (Figure 12-10).

Neuronal migration is a complex process, whereby neurons arising in the germinal matrix of the ventricular subependyma migrate along radially oriented glial fibers to populate the cortex in an orderly progression. The initial, or preplate, cellular layer splits to permit passage of the first, or superficial, layer of neurons. Additional migrating waves of neuronal layers, in a deep to superficial sequence, eventuate in a final, normal columnar arrangement. Disturbances of neuronal migration alter the final sulcal configuration of the cerebrum. Neuronal migration is complete by 20 to 24 weeks of gestation, a time when the cerebral cortex is agyric. The stresses resulting from the growth of normally migrated neurons result in the final normal gyral pattern of the cerebrum. The period of most rapid gyral development is 26 to 28 weeks, although the process continues postterm.

The histology of the abnormal cortex is variable. In patients with type I lissencephaly, there is a thin outer cellular layer of neurons separated from a thicker, disorganized inner mantle by a cell-sparse layer. The pachygyric cortex is somewhat better organized, with less prominence of the cell-sparse layer. Thus, the difference between type I lissencephaly and pachygyria is one of degree. Polymicrogyria is characterized by disorganization of the migrating neurons and an abnormally laminated cortex, which can contain four or six layers. In patients with type II lissencephaly, the meninges are thickened and the neurons are arranged in circular groups separated by glial and vascular septa.

The nature of the insult that disrupts normal migration is unknown, but it is believed that vascular insults or infectious processes, such as cytomegalovirus infection and toxoplasmosis, can interfere with the normal organization of the radial glial fibrillary apparatus. There is also a genetic basis, linked to a genetic locus in chromosome 17. Type I lissencephaly is also a component of Miller-Dieker syndrome, characterized by the presence of typical facial anomalies and a deletion in the short arm of chromosome 17. Type II lissencephaly is a component of Walker-Warburg syndrome and may be characterized by typical facies, vermian cerebellar abnormalities, and hydrocephalus. As in the test patient and the patient in Figure 12-14, agenesis or hypoplasia of the corpus callosum is associated with these anomalies. This is not surprising, since the organization of interhemispheric communication is related to normal development of the cerebral cortex; furthermore, the development of the interhemispheric commissure is temporally linked to normal cerebral migration, so that a putative insult would be coincident with both processes.

On imaging studies, all types of lissencephalic brains demonstrate a smooth surface incongruent with the patient's gestational age. Typically, there is incomplete opercularization (Figure 12-13A and C). Patients with type II lissencephaly and with Walker-Warburg syndrome (microphthalmia, lissencephaly, callosal and cerebellar anomalies, and hypotonia) may be distinguished from those with other types of lissencephaly by their associated cerebellar anomalies (vermian hypogenesis and polymicrogyria) and hydrocephalus. The cortical signal intensity is not usually affected, since the underlying abnormality is that of an abnormal organization of neurons; therefore, the signal intensity on MRI is usually normal, although a prolonged T2 relaxation time is seen in the subjacent white matter in a few patients (**Option (D) is false**). Areas of abnormal cortex can coexist with normal cortex (Figure 12-4), and areas of lissencephaly can be present in association with areas of pachygyria (**Option (A) is false**). Therefore, it is particularly important to scrutinize the cerebral surfaces in order to detect these abnormalities, especially in infants with conditions known to be associated with cortical dysplasias, such as congenital infections (Figure 12-14), agenesis of the corpus callosum, or associated clinical syndromes.

SUGGESTED READINGS

AGENESIS OF THE CORPUS CALLOSUM

1. Atlas SW, Shkolnik A, Naidich TP. Sonographic recognition of agenesis of the corpus callosum. AJR 1985; 145:167–173
2. Atlas SW, Zimmerman RA, Bilaniuk LT, et al. Corpus callosum and limbic system: neuroanatomic MR evaluation of developmental anomalies. Radiology 1986; 160:355–362
3. Babcock DS. The normal, absent, and abnormal corpus callosum: sonographic findings. Radiology 1984; 151:449–453
4. Barkovich AJ. Apparent atypical callosal dysgenesis: analysis of MR findings in six cases and their relationship to holoprosencephaly. AJNR 1990; 11:333–339
5. Fischer M, Ryan SB, Dobyns WB. Mechanisms of interhemispheric transfer and patterns of cognitive function in acallosal patients of normal intelligence. Arch Neurol 1992; 49:271–277

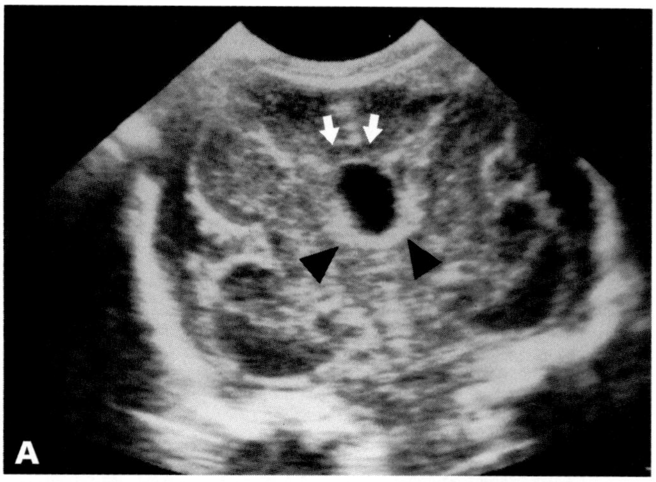

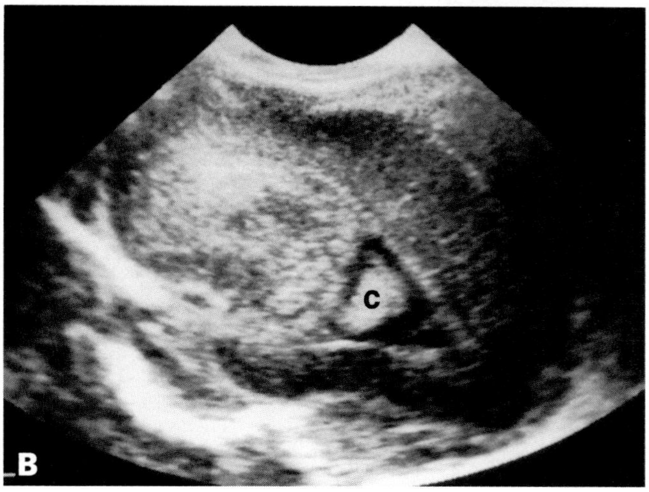

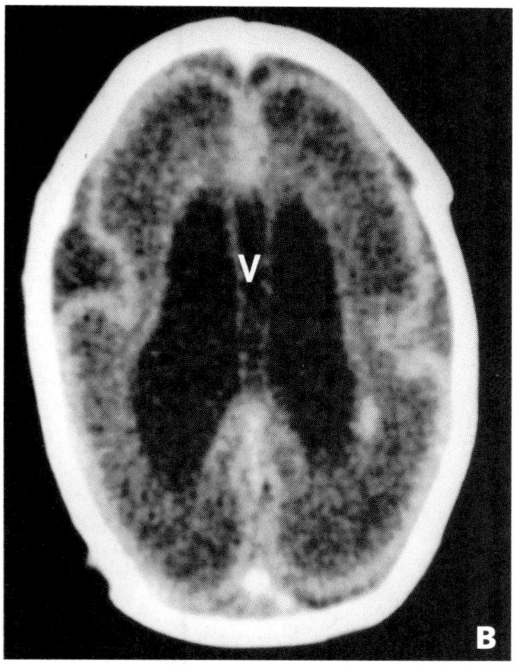

Figure 12-13. Lissencephaly. (A) A coronal sonogram of a term infant presenting with apnea demonstrates a smooth cortical mantle and enlarged cerebrospinal fluid spaces around the brain, with failure of opercularization. The corpus callosum (arrows) is present above a persistent cavum vergae. Arrowheads point to echoes of choroid plexus in the floor of the lateral ventricles and the roof of the third ventricle. (B) A parasagittal sonogram outlines the smooth cortical mantle. Choroid plexus (c) lies within the lateral ventricle. (C) A CT scan of the same patient demonstrates a lissencephalic cortex, enlarged lateral ventricles, and the cavum vergae (V). (Reprinted with permission from Hernanz-Schulman et al. [7].)

6. Hernanz-Schulman M. Neurosonography. In: Merritt CRB (ed), Diagnostic ultrasound categorical course syllabus. Leesburg, Va: American Roentgen Ray Society; 1998:1–10
7. Hernanz-Schulman M, Dohan FC Jr, Jones T, Cayea P, Wallman J, Teele RL. Sonographic appearance of callosal agenesis: correlation with radiologic and pathologic findings. AJNR 1985; 6:361–368
8. Jinkins JR, Whittemore AR, Bradley WG. MR imaging of callosal and corticocallosal dysgenesis. AJNR 1989; 10:339–344
9. Lena G, van Calenberg F, Genitori L, Choux M. Supratentorial interhemispheric cysts associated with callosal agenesis: surgical treatment and outcome in 16 children. Child's Nerv Syst 1995; 11:568–573
10. Serur D, Jeret JS, Wisniewski K. Agenesis of the corpus callosum: clinical, neuroradiological and cytogenetic studies. Neuropediatrics 1988; 19: 87–91
11. Warren ME, Cook JV. Agenesis of the corpus callosum. Br J Radiol 1993; 66:81–85

HOLOPROSENCEPHALY

12. Barkovich AJ, Norman D. Absence of the septum pellucidum: a useful sign in the diagnosis of congenital brain malformations. AJR 1989; 152: 353–360
13. Barkovich AJ, Quint DJ. Middle interhemispheric fusion: an unusual variant of holoprosencephaly. AJNR 1993; 14:431–440
14. Castillo M, Bouldin TW, Scatliff JH, Suzuki K. Radiologic-pathologic correlation. Alobar holoprosencephaly. AJNR 1993; 14:1151–1156
15. Cohen MM Jr, Sulik KK. Perspectives on holoprosencephaly. Part II. Central nervous system, craniofacial anatomy, syndrome commentary, diagnostic approach, and experimental studies. J Craniofac Genet Dev Biol 1992; 12:196–244
16. DeMyer W. Holoprosencephaly (cyclopia-arrhinencephaly). In: Klawans H, Vinken P, Bruyn G, Myrianthopoulos N (eds), Malformations. New York: Elsevier Science; 225–244
17. Fitz CR. Holoprosencephaly and related entities. Neuroradiology 1983; 25:225–238
18. Fitz CR. Holoprosencephaly and septo-optic dysplasia. Neuroimaging Clin North Am 1994; 4:263–281
19. Oba H, Barkovich AJ. Holoprosencephaly: an analysis of callosal formation and its relation to development of the interhemispheric fissure. AJNR 1995; 16:453–460

CHIARI II MALFORMATION

20. DiPietro MA, Venes JL, Rubin JM. Arnold-Chiari II malformation: intraoperative real-time US. Radiology 1987; 164:799–804
21. el Gammal T, Mark EK, Brooks BS. MR imaging of Chiari II malformation. AJR 1988; 150:163–170
22. McLone DG, Naidich TP. Developmental morphology of the subarachnoid space, brain vasculature, and contiguous structures, and the cause of the Chiari II malformation. AJNR 1992; 13:463–482
23. Naidich TP, Pudlowski RM, Naidich JB. Computed tomographic signs of the Chiari II malformation. II. Midbrain and cerebellum. Radiology 1980; 134:391–398
24. Naidich TP, Pudlowski RM, Naidich JB. Computed tomographic signs of the Chiari II malformation. III. Ventricles and cisterns. Radiology 1980; 134:657–663
25. Naidich TP, Pudlowski RM, Naidich JB, Rodriguez FJ. Computed tomographic signs of the Chiari II malformation. Part I. Skull and dural partitions. Radiology 1980; 134:65–71
26. Wolpert SM, Anderson M, Scott RM, Kwan ES, Runge VM. Chiari II malformation: MR imaging evaluation. AJR 1987; 149:1033–1042

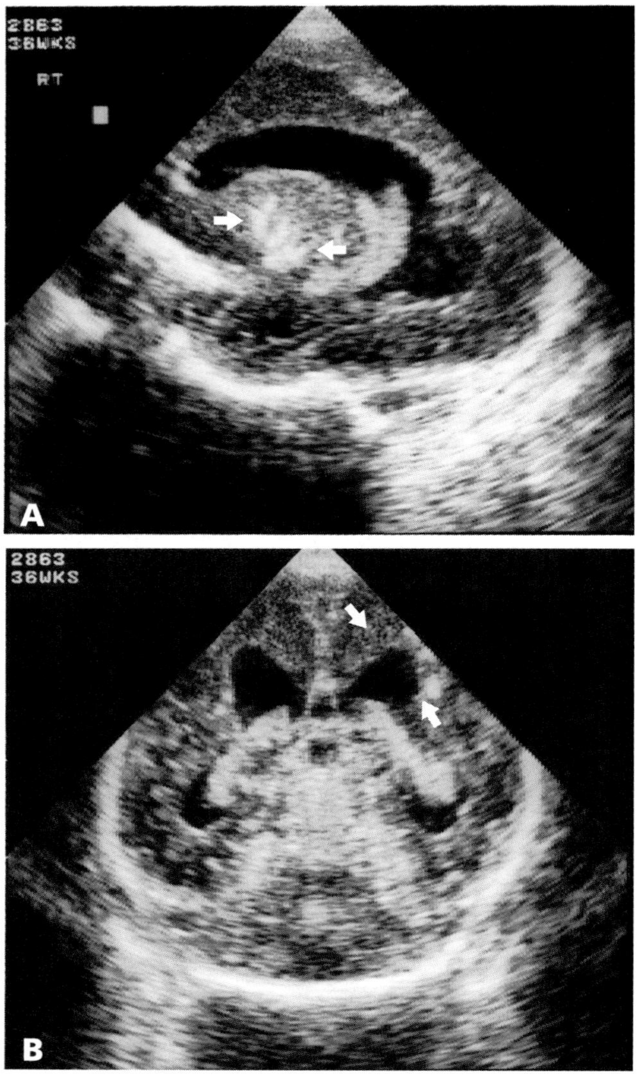

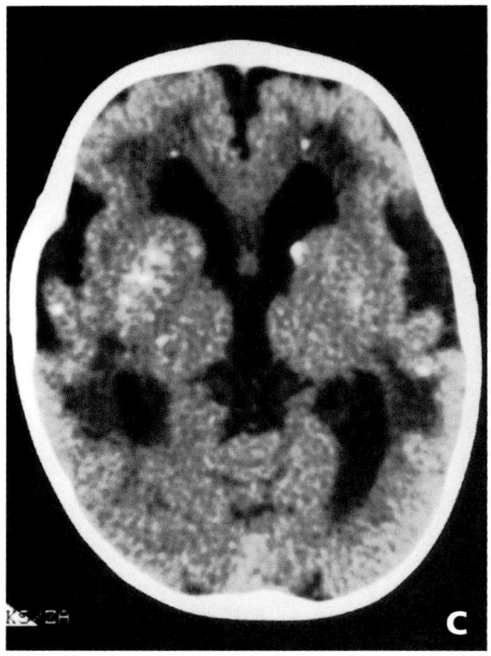

Figure 12-14. Congenital cytomegalovirus infection. (A) A parasagittal sonogram angled to the right in a 36-week-gestation infant with congenital cytomegalovirus infection demonstrates increased echogenicity resulting from the characteristic mineralizing vasculopathy of the basal ganglia (arrows). (B) A posteriorly angled coronal sonogram approaching the axial plane at the level of the bodies of the lateral ventricles shows echogenic calcifications in the periventricular white matter (arrows). The cortex is abnormally smooth. (C) A CT scan shows multiple calcifications and gyral abnormalities.

GYRAL ANOMALIES

27. Aicardi J. The agyria-pachygyria complex: a spectrum of cortical malformations. Brain Dev 1991; 13:1–8
28. Barkovich AJ, Chuang SH, Norman D. MR of neuronal migration anomalies. AJR 1988; 150:179–187
29. Barkovich AJ, Koch TK, Carrol CL. The spectrum of lissencephaly: report of ten patients analyzed by magnetic resonance imaging. Ann Neurol 1991; 30:139–146
30. Barkovich AJ, Lindan CE. Congenital cytomegalovirus infection of the brain: imaging analysis and embryologic considerations. AJNR 1994; 15:703–715
31. Byrd SE, Osborn RE, Bohan TP, Naidich TP. The CT and MR evaluation of migrational disorders of the brain. Part I. Lissencephaly and pachygyria. Pediatr Radiol 1989; 19:151–156
32. Dobyns WB. The neurogenetics of lissencephaly. Neurol Clin 1989; 7:89–105
33. Hayward JC, Titelbaum DS, Clancy RR, Zimmerman RA. Lissencephaly-pachygyria associated with congenital cytomegalovirus infection. J Child Neurol 1991; 6:109–114

HYPOXIC-ISCHEMIC ENCEPHALOPATHY

34. Babcock DS, Ball WJ. Postasphyxial encephalopathy in full-term infants: ultrasound diagnosis. Radiology 1983; 148:417–423
35. Bode H, Strassburg HM, Pringsheim W, Kunzer W. Cerebral infarction in term neonates: diagnosis by cerebral ultrasound. Child's Nerv Syst 1986; 2:195–199
36. Deeg KH, Rupprecht T, Zeilinger G. Doppler sonographic classification of brain edema in infants. Pediatr Radiol 1990; 20:509–514
37. Hernanz-Schulman M, Cohen W, Genieser NB. Sonography of cerebral infarction in infancy. AJR 1988; 150:897–902
38. Seibert JJ, McCowan TC, Chadduck WM, et al. Duplex pulsed Doppler US versus intracranial pressure in the neonate: clinical and experimental studies. Radiology 1989; 171:155–159
39. Stark JE, Seibert JJ. Cerebral artery Doppler ultrasonography for prediction of outcome after perinatal asphyxia. J Ultrasound Med 1994; 13:595–600

CASE 13

Donald P. Frush, M.D.

Sacrococcygeal Teratoma

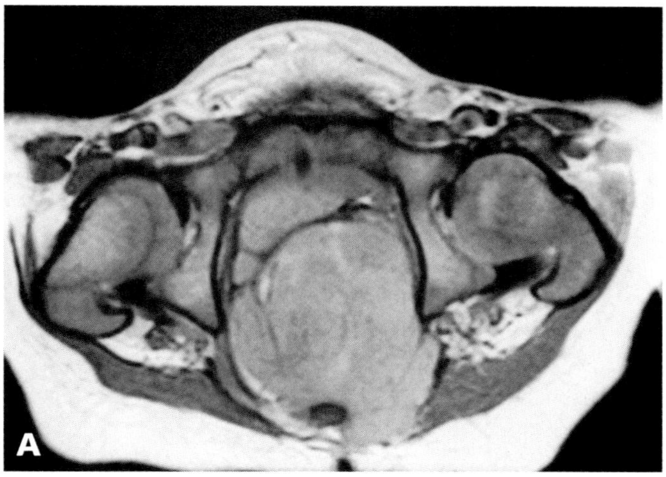

SE 500/20

Question 66

This 13-month-old girl has a pelvic mass. You are shown T1-weighted axial (A) and midline sagittal (B) and fat-suppressed T2-weighted sagittal (C) pelvic MR images (Figure 13-1).

Which *one* of the following is the MOST likely diagnosis?

(A) Neuroblastoma
(B) Rhabdomyosarcoma
(C) Sacrococcygeal teratoma
(D) Lymphoma
(E) Anterior meningocele

The test images (Figure 13-1) demonstrate a large pelvic mass localized in the presacral region; the mass abuts the sacrum and coccyx and displaces the rectum anteriorly (and to the left) (Figure 13-2). The sagittal images demonstrate that the bladder is displaced anteriorly and superiorly. There is a heterogeneous mixture of low, intermediate, and high signal intensities on the T1-weighted images (Figure 13-2A and B).

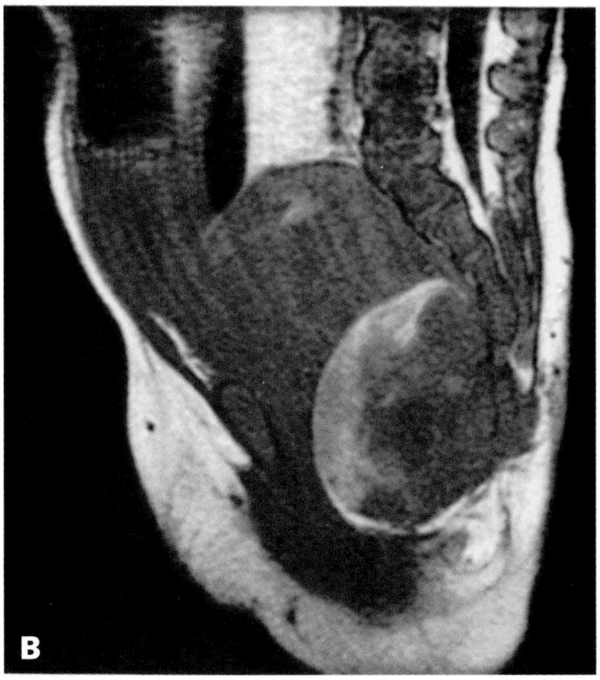

SE 500/20

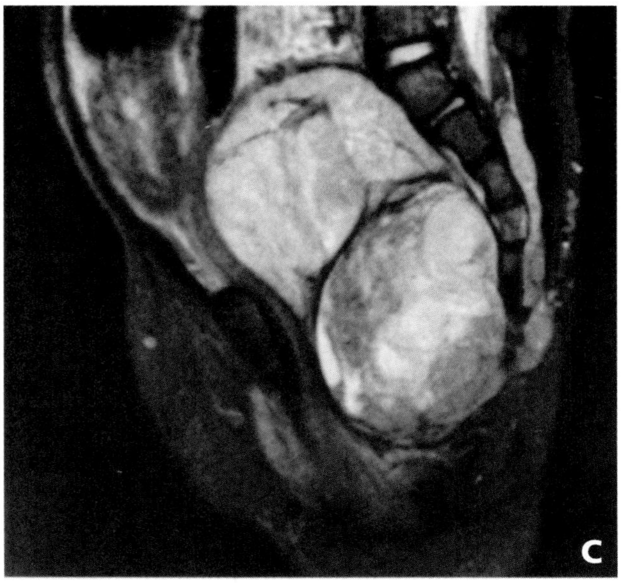

SE 4,000/95

Figure 13-1

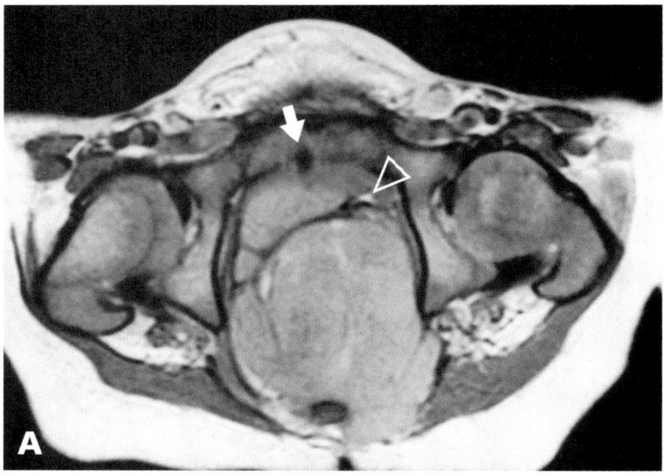

SE 500/20

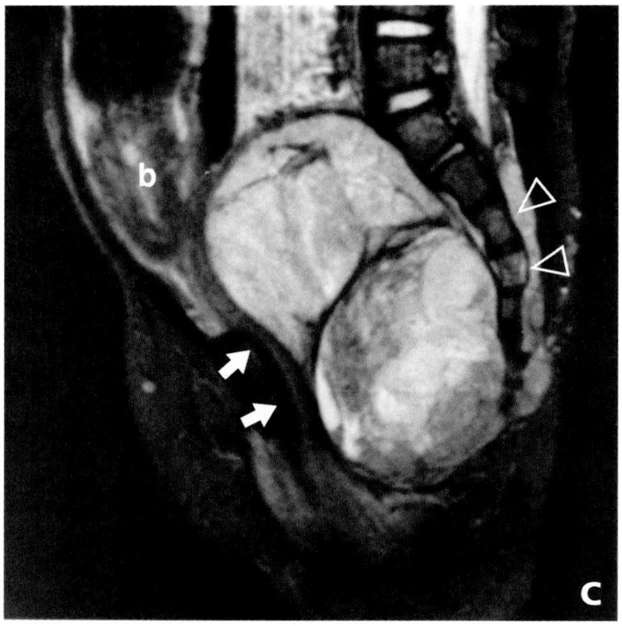

SE 4,000/95

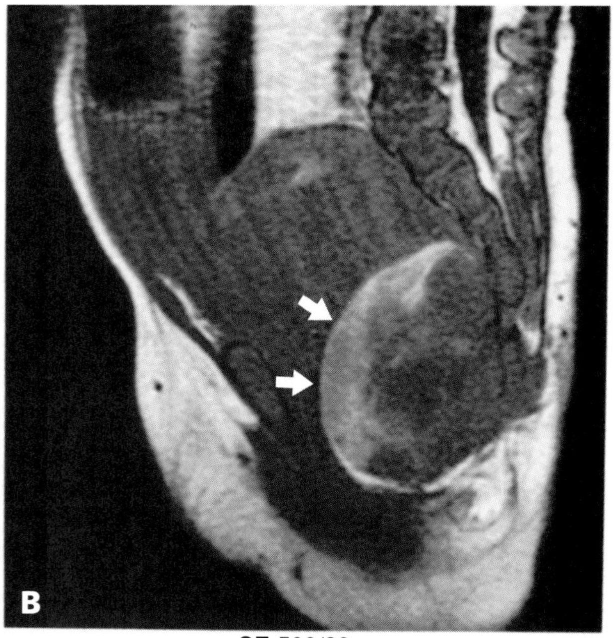

SE 500/20

Figure 13-2. (Same as Figure 13-1). Sacrococcygeal teratoma. (A) A T1-weighted axial MR image through the pelvis demonstrates a presacral mass filling the pelvis and extending dorsal to the sacrum. The mass is predominantly of intermediate signal intensity, except for low-intensity linear regions and several areas of high intensity. The urethra containing the Foley catheter (arrowhead) and the rectosigmoid (arrow) are both displaced anteriorly. (B) A midline sagittal T1-weighted image better illustrates a region of high signal intensity located anteriorly (arrows). (C) A T2-weighted fat-suppressed MR image demonstrates that this area anteriorly has mostly low signal intensity, indicating fat. The large mass causes anterior displacement and stretching of the vagina and uterus (arrows). The bladder (b) is also displaced superiorly and anteriorly. This sagittal view clearly demonstrates the extension posterior to the sacrum and abnormal increased signal intensity of the third and fourth sacral bodies (arrowheads).

Either fat or subacute hemorrhage (extracellular deoxyhemoglobin) could account for the regions of high signal intensity. With T2 weighting and fat suppression, the same area is dark, indicating fat (Figure 13-2C). Of the available options, only a sacrococcygeal teratoma contains fat **(Option (C) is correct).** The T2-weighted sagittal image also demonstrates that the mass is predominantly of high signal intensity, with abnormally increased signal intensity in the marrow of the lower sacrum and coccyx (Figure 13-2C). On both the T1- and T2-weighted sequences, the mass wraps around the lower sacrum and coccyx. Coccygeal involvement is also a feature typical of sacrococcygeal teratoma.

Discussion of the lesions involving the presacral region in children and their imaging features is enhanced by an understanding of the anatomy of this region. The presacral region (also known as the retrorectal space) is located within the true pelvis and is bordered posteriorly by the sacrum and coccyx and anteriorly by the rectum. The presacral region extends from the level of S1 (the pelvic peritoneal reflection) to the levator sling and is bordered laterally by the iliac vessels and ureters. Histologically, the presacral region can be defined by Waldeyer's fascia, which covers the anterior sacrum, and the fascia propria of the posterior rectum. The tissues within the presacral region include mesenchyma, nerves, vasculature, and lymphatics.

Localizing a lesion to an organ or region of origin is critical for limiting the differential diagnosis of a pelvic mass. Imaging is invaluable in this regard. Although either radiography or fluoroscopy can demonstrate the presence of a pelvic mass, the imaging evaluation generally begins with sonography since abnormalities of the ovaries and uterus are frequent causes of pelvic masses. When the sonographic diagnosis is uncertain or more information is needed for surgical planning or staging purposes, cross-sectional imaging is appropriate. CT is best performed with the use of both intravenous and oral contrast agents. The size and extent of the mass and its relationship to adjacent structures are better displayed by CT than by sonography. In particular, adenopathy and osseous involvement are well demonstrated. Superior soft tissue resolution, particularly with contrast enhancement, enables the identification of fat, calcification, soft tissue, vascularity, and fluid. Presacral teratomas are therefore well demonstrated. An abscess can be diagnosed by CT, especially when gas is present, a feature not easily discriminated by sonography or MRI. CT also can demonstrate the fluid attenuation and associated bony abnormality attributable to an anterior meningocele. A primary bone tumor with presacral extension is readily displayed by CT. When these features are not present, the specificity of CT for masses is low. MRI is also excellent for depicting the origin and extent of pelvic masses. It is especially well suited for evaluation of the presacral and parasacral regions by use of a combination of axial and sagittal sequences. The excellent soft tissue contrast resolution helps define the relationship of the mass to other pelvic structures and organs and does not depend on the use of intravenous or oral contrast agents. As with other processes, neural and marrow evaluation of a mass in a paravertebral location is best performed by MRI.

Developmental sacrococcygeal abnormalities account for a relatively high proportion of disorders in this region in children; a few of these disorders present as presacral masses (Table 13-1). Embryologically, this caudal region is formed when neural folds (ectodermal derivative) fuse to form the neural canal, anterior to which is the notochord (Figure 13-3). A normal transient invagination of the notochord connects with the embryonic endoderm. Neurenteric cysts and associated anomalies result when this connection fails to regress. This embryologic relationship between the structures of the presacral region also helps explain the association of neural, bony, and hindgut anomalies, which include Currarino's triad (discussed below).

Not all neural masses of the presacral region are attributable to developmental malformations. Neuroblastoma (Option (A)) is a malignant neural neoplasm and is the most common non-central nervous system (CNS) tumor of childhood. It originates from the neural crest and therefore can be found anywhere along the spinal sympathetic chain, as well as in the adrenal gland. Pelvic neuroblastomas account for only 2% to 5% of cases; the pelvis is the fifth most common site of origin after the adrenal gland, other abdominal sites, and thoracic and cervical paraspinal locations.

Up to one third of all patients present in infancy, and 70% to 80% of cases occur by 5 years of age. Approximately 60% of neuroblastomas are disseminated at presentation. Sites of metastases include the lymph nodes, liver, bone marrow, and skin. A subgroup of patients with metastatic disease limited to the liver, skin, or bone marrow have been traditionally classified as stage IV-S. There are several staging systems, including the Evans system, the Pediatric Oncology Group system, and the International Staging System. Most cases of stage IV-S disease occur in infants, and the prognosis is very good. Symptoms of neuroblastoma are typically systemic and include malaise, weight loss, and fever. Systemic symptoms can be attributable to marrow replacement, resulting in anemia or bruising. The neoplasm also can secrete catecholamines or other hormones, resulting in paraneoplastic syndromes consisting of diarrhea, flushing, tachycardia, or sweating at presentation. This type of presentation is rare; symptoms related to mass effect are much more common. Local manifestations of neuroblastoma in the pelvis include pain, as well as the consequences of mass effect on the bladder (cystitis, urinary retention or frequency), the rectum (constipation), or adjacent nerves (weakness). Alternatively, the patient may be asymptomatic, with the tumor being discovered during a physical examination.

The imaging features of pelvic neuroblastoma are similar to those of neuroblastomas that originate in other locations. Because the tumor arises from ganglion cells, which are most common in a paraspinal plexus, pelvic neuroblastoma originates from and is predominantly centered in the presacral space. Radiography and gastrointestinal or genitourinary contrast studies

Table 13-1: Presacral masses in children

Neural:	**Lymphatic:**	**Other:**
Developmental	lymphangioma	*Inflammatory*
anterior meningocele	lymphoma	perirectal abscess
lipoma	metastasis	inflammatory bowel disease
		granuloma
Nerve	**Mesenchymal:**	
neuroblastoma	rhabdomyosarcoma	*Secondary to sacral abnormalities*
ganglioneuroma	fibroma (including fibromatosis)	hematoma from trauma
neurofibroma		primary bone tumors (Ewing's sarcoma, osteogenic sarcoma, aneurysmal bone cyst)
Schwannoma	**Intestinal:**	metastasis
	duplication	
Embryologic:		*Extension*
germ cell tumor		lesions arising in other pelvic locations
epidermoid		
Vascular:		
vascular malformation		
hemangioma		
hemangiopericytoma		

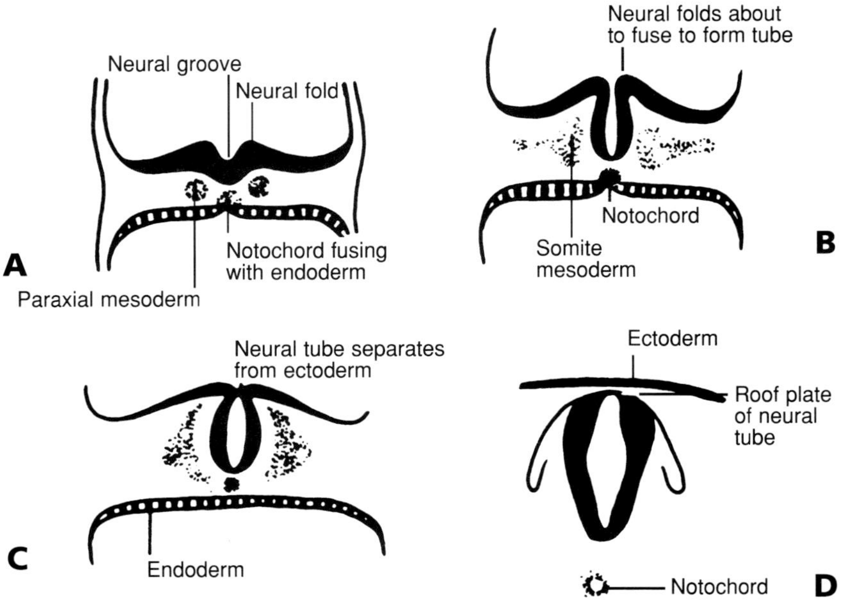

Figure 13-3. Neural tube and notochord development. Schematic diagrams of transverse sections of embryo at 18 and 21 days (A and B) and 5 to 6 weeks (C and D). Note the fusion of the notochord with endoderm (A), which persists as the neural tube begins to form (B). There is eventual separation of the notochord from endoderm (C). Failure of separation of the notochord and endoderm results in various anomalies in the "tail" region, including neurenteric cysts and Currarino's triad. (Reproduced with permission from Bale [1].)

may demonstrate the mass effect on the genitourinary or gastrointestinal organs. Calcification is seen more readily by CT (in up to 90% of patients with abdominal neuroblastoma) and is very suggestive of neuroblastoma (Figure 13-4A). Neuroblastoma can be detected as a mass by sonography, but more definitive diagnosis and surgical planning require either CT or MRI. Neuroblastoma can be either homogeneous or heterogeneous on sonography, CT, or MRI. Heterogeneity is more typically apparent on CT or MRI than on sonography. Cystic areas attributable to hemorrhage or necrosis are relatively rare. With MRI, neuroblastoma is usually heterogeneous in signal intensity. T1-weighted sequences typically demonstrate mixed but predominantly intermediate signal intensity. Areas of hemorrhage may appear bright. With T2 weighting, signal intensity is increased and can be very high with cystic areas. When intravenous contrast material is used with either CT or MRI, enhancement is typically heterogeneous (Figure 13-4B). Neuroblastoma can displace or encase adjacent structures, but it does not contain fat; therefore, it is not the most likely diagnosis in the test patient.

Pelvic rhabdomyosarcoma (Option (B)) originates most commonly in the urinary or reproductive tract but also can arise in the presacral region (Figure 13-5). Presenting symptoms of the neoplasm arising in the presacral area are attributable to mass effect, with obstruction of the bowel or urinary tract. A visible or palpable mass can be the only finding. The sonographic appearance of pelvic rhabdomyosarcoma arising from the bladder has a characteristic appearance of a lobulated

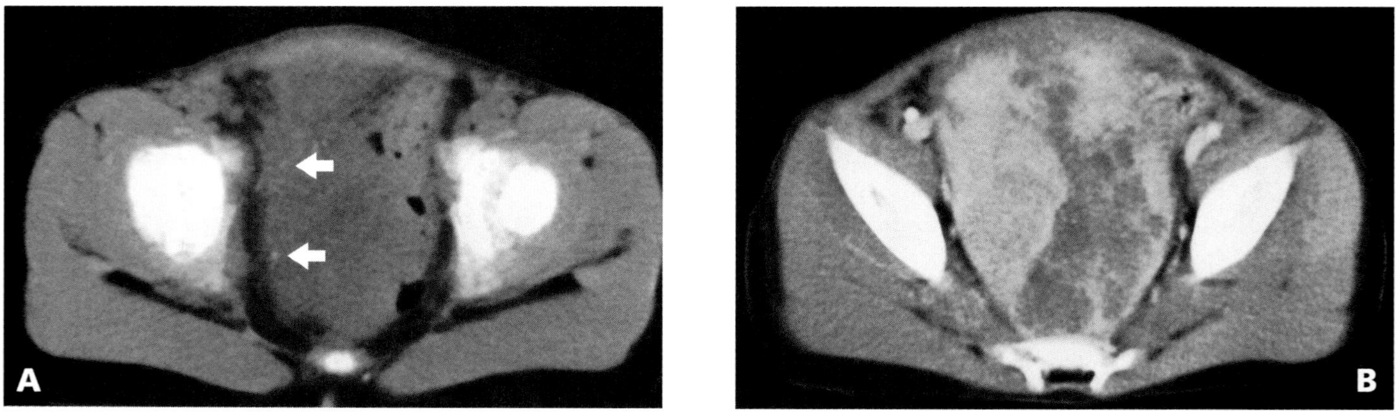

Figure 13-4. Pelvic neuroblastoma discovered incidentally on routine physical examination. (A) A noncontrast axial CT image through the pelvis in a 3-year-old boy depicts a predominantly homogeneous soft tissue mass involving the presacral space and displacing the rectosigmoid colon to the left. Several punctate calcifications are evident on the right side of this mass (arrows). (B) After intravenous contrast agent administration, there is heterogeneous enhancement. The pelvic vasculature is not encased by the tumor. The tumor was completely resected (i.e., stage 1).

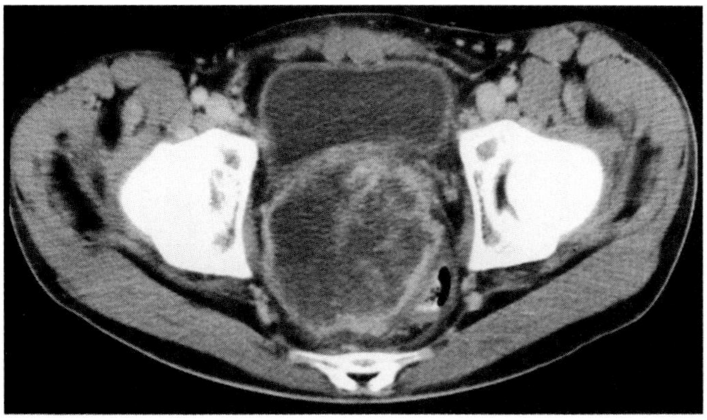

Figure 13-5. Rhabdomyosarcoma. A postcontrast axial CT scan of the pelvis in a 15-year-old boy treated for symptoms of recalcitrant proctitis reveals a presacral mass. Both peripheral enhancement and linear central enhancement are evident in this tumor, which was predominantly necrotic. There is effacement of the posterior aspect of the bladder and displacement of the rectum to the left by this tumor. This tumor was unresectable, and was unresponsive to therapy and rapidly fatal.

mass protruding within the bladder (sarcoma botryoides). Sarcoma botryoides is a term used to describe rhabdomyosarcoma that has a submucosal origin and grows unhindered into a lumen. This type can be found in the bladder, vagina, uterus, and even nasopharynx. For cases that do not display the suggestive botryoides configuration, the sonographic appearance is nonspecific, consisting of a heterogeneously echogenic mass. The bladder may be displaced anteriorly and superiorly by a large pelvic rhabdomyosarcoma. The relationship of the mass to the rectosigmoid (and hence localization to the presacral region) by sonography is difficult. Even if the mass is localized sonographically to the presacral region, CT or MRI is needed to define the full extent and effect on adjacent structures, as well as to detect metastatic disease. The CT appearance of rhabdomyosarcoma is variable. Solid components with attenuation below that of skeletal muscle typically predominate. Calcification is rare. Cystic areas, when present, are attributable to hemorrhage or necrosis. Contrast enhancement is usually heterogeneous. With MRI, the signal intensity of rhabdomyosarcoma is intermediate with T1 weighting and high with T2 weighting. The mass enhances after contrast agent injection, but as with CT, enhancement is usually heterogeneous. Both modalities are excellent for identify involvement of adjacent cortical bone. Marrow and spinal canal invasion is best depicted by MRI. In addition, involvement of complex pelvic anatomy is best displayed with multiplanar MRI. Fat is not a finding in patients with rhabdomyosarcoma, and coccygeal involvement and dorsal extension are also more consistent features of sacrococcygeal germ cell tumors. Therefore, rhabdomyosarcoma is not the most likely diagnosis.

Lymphoma (Option (D)) in children younger than about 10 years of age is more often non-Hodgkin's lymphoma (NHL) than Hodgkin's disease. The histopathologic features of NHL in children are different from those in adults. In children, undifferentiated NHL is most common (40%), followed by lymphoblastic (28%) and large cell (26%) types. NHL in children is more often extranodal in location and more frequently high grade than in adults. In contrast to the three major types of NHL in children, adult NHL is more variable in histologic subtype. NHL is evident most often as a mass or adenopathy. Undifferentiated (also known as small cell) types (which include Burkitt's lymphoma) and large cell types of NHL are encountered most frequently in the abdomen and pelvis. In contrast, most lymphoblastic lymphoma is found above the diaphragm, especially within the thorax. Symptoms can be systemic and include weight loss, anorexia, and other constitutional symptoms, or they can be related to local effects at sites involved by tumor. For example, the presenting features can be related to mediastinal involvement (such as airway compromise), bowel involvement (obstruction, diarrhea, or intussusception), or CNS disease.

When lymph nodes are involved, they can become discretely enlarged or confluent. Nodal heterogeneity can occur in patients with NHL, but high signal intensity on T1-weighted sequences is not a feature of lymphoma. In addition, an isolated presacral location of adenopathy is rare in patients with NHL or Hodgkin's disease; iliac nodes are more often involved when lymphoma occurs in the pelvis. Therefore, lymphoma is not the most likely diagnosis.

Cystic masses of the presacral region include sacrococcygeal germ cell tumors, neurenteric cysts, and anterior meningoceles (Option (E)). Although the presacral germ cell tumor is the most common presacral mass in children, the anterior (or presacral) meningocele is most common when there are associated anomalies of the sacrum. The meninges (dura and arachnoid) herniate through an anterior defect in the sacral vertebral body. The cystic nature is attributable to cerebrospinal fluid (CSF). The mass does not contain solid elements, although microscopic amounts of both neural and fatty tissues can be found in the wall. Therefore, anterior meningocele is not the most likely diagnosis. MRI is the best imaging modality for demonstration of an anterior sacral meningocele. The defect in the sacrum and other associated sacral anomalies (hypoplasia, scalloping, "scimitar" appearance), when present, are well seen with sagittal imaging. Connection of the cyst with the thecal sac is best demonstrated with MRI, confirming that a cyst is an anterior meningocele. The fluid content of the sac is that of CSF on MRI. The relationship of the fluid-filled mass to other pelvic structures, such as the rectum, bladder, and reproductive organs, is well seen with MRI. This modality is also the most useful for detecting associated anomalies, such as a tethered cord or occult dysraphism.

The differential diagnosis for pelvic masses in children is extensive considering the array of tissues and organs present in the pelvis, as well as the types of disorders that can affect these structures. Masses with congenital, developmental, neoplastic, inflammatory, or traumatic etiologies can arise from reproductive, urinary, intestinal (including mesenteric and omental), muscular, neural (Figure 13-6), vascular (Figure 13-7), lymphatic, mesenchymal (Figure 13-8), or osseous (Figures 13-9 and 13-10) structures within or adjacent to the pelvis (Table 13-1).

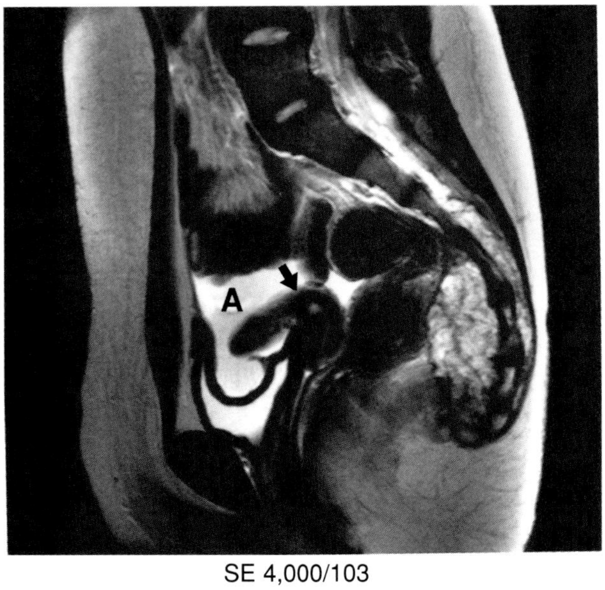

Figure 13-6. Neurofibromatosis. A T2-weighted sagittal MR image of the pelvis in a 16-year-old girl with neurofibromatosis shows a mass with heterogeneous, but predominantly high, signal intensity directly anterior to the sacrum. A small amount of tumor with increased signal intensity extends dorsal to the sacrum as well. The patient had additional extension of these plexiform neurofibromas into the left lower extremity. Ascites (A) between the uterus (arrow) and anterior abdominal wall is also present.

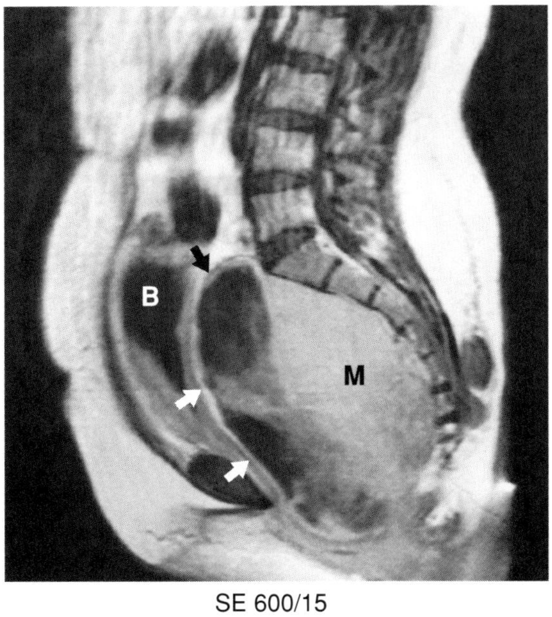

Figure 13-8. Ewing's sarcoma. A sagittal T1-weighted MR image of a 14-year-old girl with hip pain clearly depicts a presacral mass (M) with homogeneous signal intensity. The rectosigmoid (arrows) and bladder (B) are displaced anteriorly. Although there appears to be a slight amount of cortical disruption in the lower anterior sacral segments, the bones were intact. A small amount of the mass extends dorsal to the sacrum. This was a presacral extraosseous Ewing's sarcoma.

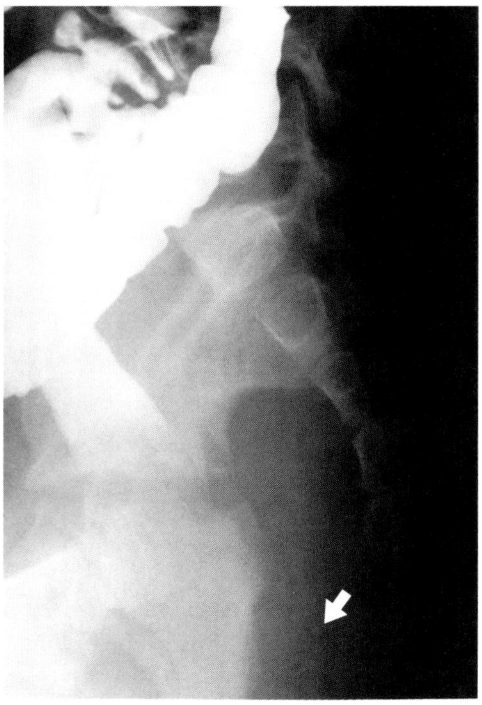

Figure 13-7. Hemangioma. A lateral radiograph of the pelvis was obtained during a barium enema in a 6-year-old child with a large hemangioma of the left thigh treated with steroids. The postcontrast study was performed to evaluate new-onset rectal bleeding. The rectosigmoid colon is displaced anteriorly (and slightly narrowed) by new extension of the hemangioma into the presacral space. The lesion contains a phlebolith (arrow). The sacrum appears normal.

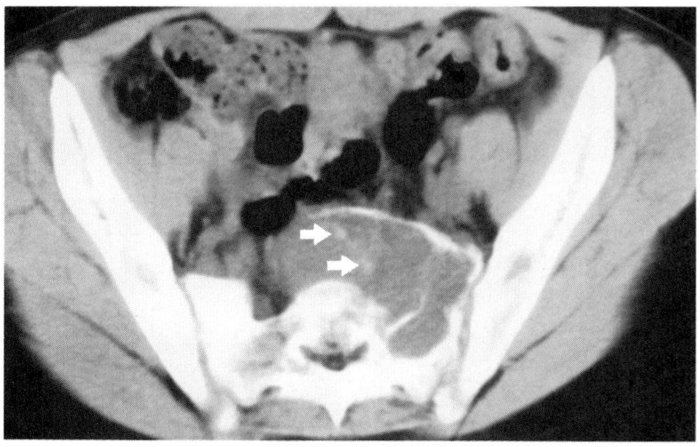

Figure 13-9. Chordoma. An anteroposterior radiograph of the pelvis (not shown) in a 14-year-old girl with back and hip pain was normal despite the presence of an expansile sacral chordoma with cortical disruption and presacral extension readily evident on this postcontrast CT scan at the midlevel of the sacroiliac joints. This lesion exhibited mild central enhancement and was limited to the left aspect of the sacrum. Calcification is present centrally (arrows).

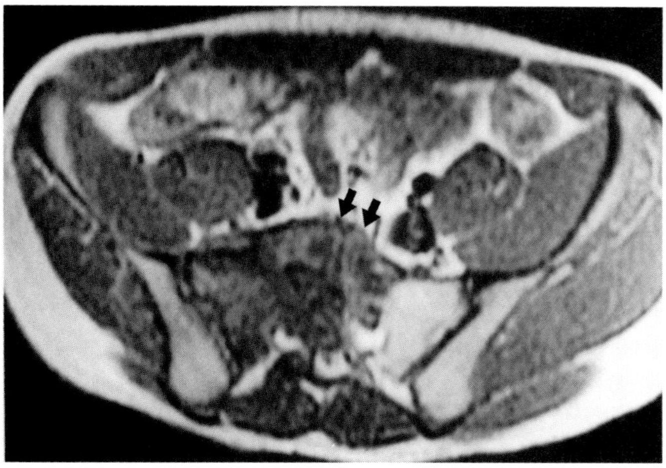

Figure 13-10. Osteogenic sarcoma. A T1-weighted axial MR image through the pelvis at the midlevel of the sacroiliac joints in a 6-year-old boy with back and hip pain demonstrates low signal intensity replacing the normal high-intensity marrow of the right sacral ala and the sacral body. The cortical margin anteriorly is indistinct, and there is extension of this osteogenic sarcoma into the presacral space (arrows). The sacroiliac joint is indistinct, but there is no obvious involvement of the adjacent right iliac bone or dorsal neural canal.

Question 67

Concerning pelvic rhabdomyosarcomas,

(A) most arise in the presacral region
(B) central calcification is characteristic
(C) those arising from the genitourinary tract have a better prognosis than those arising from most other locations
(D) most are diagnosed in infancy
(E) radiation therapy is the treatment of choice

Rhabdomyosarcoma is a neoplasm that is found almost exclusively in children. It is the third most common non-CNS solid neoplasm of childhood, after Wilms' tumor and neuroblastoma, and is the fifth overall leading cause of childhood cancer when brain tumors and leukemia or lymphoma are included. The age of peak occurrence is 3.5 years, and there is a second, smaller cluster in adolescence. Only 4% to11% are diagnosed within the first year of life **(Option (D) is false).** Rhabdomyosarcoma is metastatic in up to 20% of patients at the time of presentation; the most common sites are the lungs, bone and bone marrow, and lymph nodes.

Rhabdomyosarcomas are classified histologically as embryonal or alveolar. Rarely, rhabdomyosarcoma is pleomorphic (also called adult type), mixed, or undifferentiated. The embryonal type is the most common, accounting for about 80% of all rhabdomyosarcomas. Rhabdomyosarcoma is one of the "small round blue cell" tumors of childhood. This classification also includes Ewing's sarcoma, primitive neuroectodermal tumor, NHL, desmoplastic tumor, and neuroblastoma. These tumors contain cells that are all characterized by their small size, deep blue staining, and small nuclear to cytoplasmic ratio. Immunocytochemistry and electron microscopy are often necessary to distinguish among these tumor types. Strict classification into one of the types of small round blue cell tumors is not always possible, supporting the notion of a common origin from a primitive nerve cell origin, with variable degrees of differentiation.

Rhabdomyosarcoma arises from primitive mesenchyma, which eventually gives rise to striated muscle. However, rhabdomyosarcoma is not typically found in locations where skeletal muscle is found. Similarly, cross-striations are not always found histologically. Rhabdomyosarcoma can be found virtually anywhere in the body, but the most frequent sites of origin are the head and neck (22% to 55%), the genitourinary tract (21% to 31%), and the extremities (14% to 20%). Most pelvic rhabdomyosarcomas arise from genitourinary organs, including the bladder, prostate, uterus, vagina, and, occasionally, urachus and adnexa. Extragenitourinary pelvic sites are less common (accounting for less than 5% of all rhabdomyosarcomas). These include tumors arising from the pelvic musculature (e.g., iliopsoas muscle) and those in the presacral region **(Option (A) is false).** Symptoms of rhabdomyosarcomas at these nongenitourinary sites include a palpable mass and symptoms attributable to mass effect on the adjacent bladder (frequency, urgency, or retention) or rectosigmoid colon (constipation). Rhabdomyosarcomas that arise in the urinary bladder also can cause hematuria, whereas those that originate in the vagina present as vaginal bleeding or as a prolapsing mass. When rhabdomyosarcoma arises from the pelvic musculature, such as the iliopsoas muscle, the tumor is asymmetrically positioned in the pelvis (Figure 13-11). In the rare circumstances when rhabdomyosarcoma arises in the presacral region, the differential diagnosis includes neuroblastoma and solid sacrococcygeal germ cell tumor. Although all of these may occur in infancy and children, a pre-

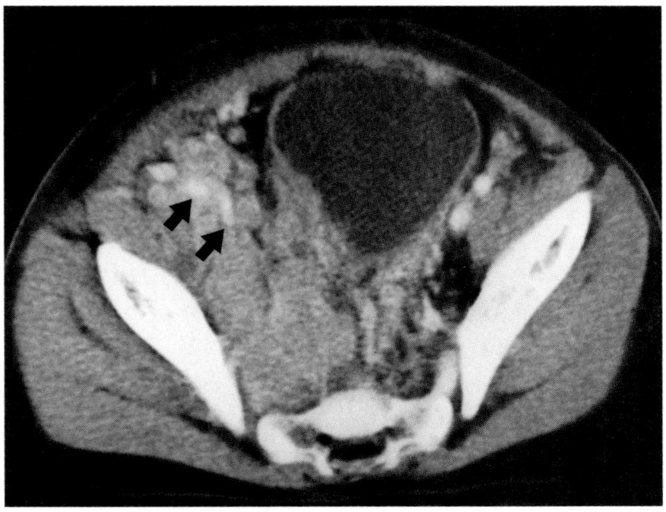

Figure 13-11. Rhabdomyosarcoma of iliopsoas muscle in a 2-year-old boy. The tumor was discovered during repair of what was thought to be a right inguinal hernia. Postcontrast CT shows that the mass extends into the right presacral region, and adenopathy surrounds the contrast-enhanced iliac vessels (arrows). The bladder is also effaced on the right side and displaced slightly to the left.

sacral mass in a child more than about 8 years old is more likely a rhabdomyosarcoma.

CT is an excellent method for identifying the presence and extent of a pelvic rhabdomyosarcoma. Calcification is very uncommon (**Option (B) is false**). The attenuation of the tumor is heterogeneous on CT, especially when there are areas of hemorrhage or necrosis. The enhancement of the mass is also heterogeneous and typically less than that of muscle. CT is useful for staging purposes, especially for detection of metastases to regional lymph nodes as well to the lungs or other solid organs. The features of rhabdomyosarcoma on MRI are also nonspecific. On T1-weighted MR images, the signal intensity of the lesion is intermediate and heterogeneous, and the enhancement is heterogeneous when intravenous contrast agents are used. On T2-weighted images, the signal intensity is high and also heterogeneous, an appearance indistinguishable from that of a wide variety of neoplasms.

The prognosis of rhabdomyosarcoma depends on the histology (embryonal histology with a botryoides configuration is the most favorable), primary site (orbital and genitourinary lesions have the best prognosis), and stage at the time of diagnosis (**Option (C) is true**). More specifically, the 5-year survival rate is greatest with the botryoid embryonal type (90%), followed by other embryonal types (70%) and the alveolar type (50%). Histology is associated with site of origin. Embryonal histology is found with 70% of head and neck as well as genitourinary rhabdomyosarcomas. Alveolar types occur in less than 20% of tumors originating in these locations. Hyperdiploidy and some cytogenetic features (e.g., translocations) also are correlated with a poorer outcome.

Treatment of rhabdomyosarcoma depends on the location and stage. The tumor is generally radiosensitive, but radiotherapy is used only when the tumor is unresponsive to chemotherapy (**Option (E) is false**). Because of these nonoperative options, radical surgical intervention is now performed less often than in the past. The timing and contribution of each of these three modalities in the treatment of rhabdomyosarcoma are evolving.

Question 68

Concerning sacrococcygeal germ cell tumors,

(A) most are diagnosed at birth
(B) an intrapelvic location favors malignancy
(C) they are predominantly cystic
(D) the highest frequency of malignancy is in children older than 1 year
(E) sacral erosion is typical

Sacrococcygeal germ cell tumors, the vast majority of which are benign teratomas, are encountered most frequently in neonates and infants and are the most frequent cause of presacral masses in this population. They are still relatively rare, occurring in only 1 in 40,000 live births. There is a female/male ratio of up to 4:1, but the gender distribution is nearly equal when only malignant tumors are considered. Up to 90% of these tumors are diagnosed in the neonatal period (**Option (A) is true**). However, up to 17% may present between 5 and 15 years of age. Sacrococcygeal teratoma is the most common tumor in newborns.

Newborns with sacrococcygeal germ cell tumors are typically asymptomatic. A mass is evident either on abdominal palpation or on visual inspection if there is an exophytic component (Figure 13-12). In 1974, the Surgical Section of the American Academy of Pediatrics classified these tumors on the basis of the degree of abdominal and pelvic extension, including exophytic components (Altman classification) (Figure 13-13). Associated anomalies are present in up to 18% of children with germ cell tumors. The most clearly recognized association is with anorectal malformations, including Currarino's triad: presacral mass (i.e., teratoma), sacral bony anomalies, and rectalano malformations.

Several factors are associated with malignancy of germ cell tumors, the most compelling of which is the age of the child. The frequency of malignant sacrococcygeal germ cell tumors in children younger than 4 months is less than 10%, as opposed to 50% to 90% in children older than 4 months (**Option (D) is true**). The location of the tumor is another factor associated with malignancy. Tumors with exophytic components are less likely to be malignant (less than 20%) than those that are purely intrapelvic or intra-abdominal (34% to 38%) (**Option (B) is true**). Tumor size is not a factor predictive of malignancy, but the composition can be suggestive. Tumors with predominantly solid components have been shown in some series to be more likely to be malignant. Calcification can be seen on radiographs in up to 50% of sacrococcygeal germ cell tumors and is not an indicator of malignancy. Coccygeal destruction or erosion is most often attributable to malignant extension but can be attributable to pressure from large benign tumors. Overall, sacral abnormalities are rare (**Option (E) is false**). Even with malignant lesions, bony changes are not invariably present.

Germ cell tumors contain all three germ cell layers (ectoderm, mesoderm, and endoderm) in various amounts and with various degrees of differentiation. Teratomas are differentiated forms of these embryonic tumors. They have in common with extraembryonic tumors (e.g., endodermal sinus or yolk sac tumors and choriocarcinomas) and seminiferous germ cell tumors (e.g., seminomas) an origin from primordial germ cells. Because of this common origin, elements of other germ cell tumors can occur in teratomas. Teratomas composed only of mature elements are benign. The hallmark of the mature teratoma is the presence of fluid, calcification, fat, and small amounts of soft tissue. Neural tissue is the predominant solid component. The presence of large amounts of immature tissue appears to be related to the malignant potential of a teratoma; malignant teratomas contain immature elements, and local recurrence of tumors is in-

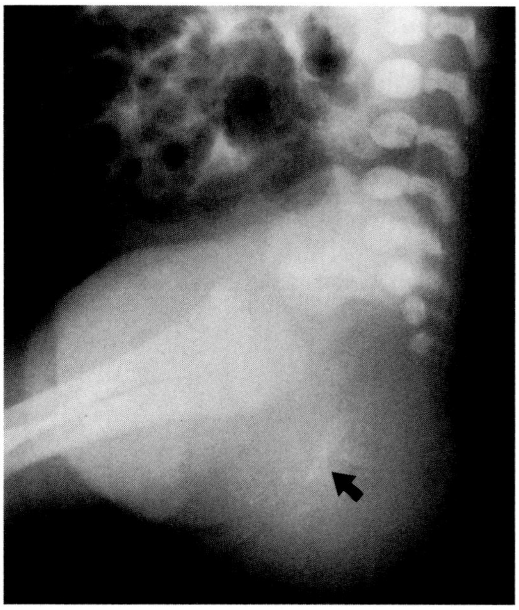

Figure 13-12. Benign sacrococcygeal teratoma with a large exophytic component in a newborn. A shardlike calcification (arrow) is evident inferiorly on this lateral radiograph. There is also deficiency of the distal sacrococcygeal region.

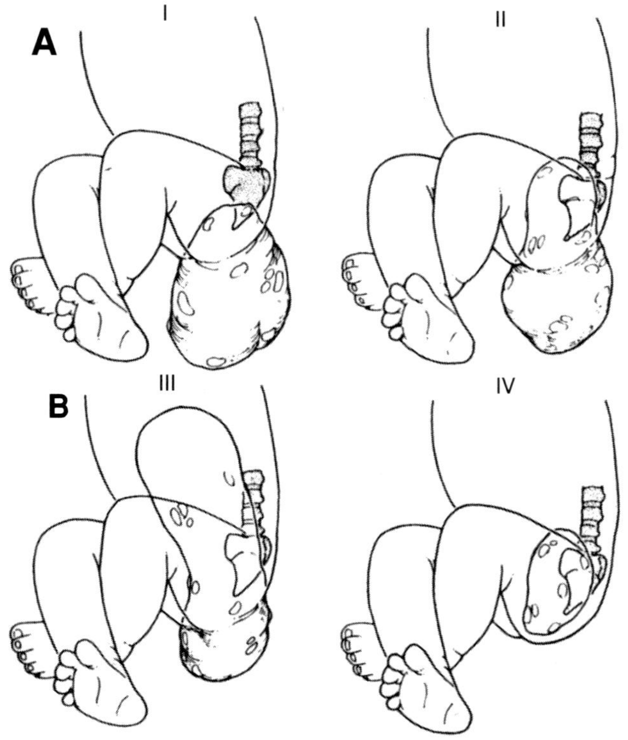

Figure 13-13. Altman classification of sacrococcygeal teratomas. Row A illustrates teratomas with primarily exophytic components. The "dumbbell" appearance in type II lesions is also seen with type III lesions. Row B illustrates sacrococcygeal teratomas with predominantly intrapelvic locations. (Reproduced with permission from Grosfeld and Billmire [3].)

creased in teratomas with immature components. The immature component is mostly primitive neuroectodermal tissue.

Overall, malignant teratomas are relatively rare, accounting for only about 3% of childhood cancers. The sacrococcygeal region is the most common location of origin of teratomas (up to 70%) and is followed by ovarian or testicular (30%), mediastinal (5%), and retroperitoneal (4%) sites.

The most important goals of imaging after detection of the mass are characterization of the type of mass, its extent (including distant metastases), and involvement of adjacent structures for treatment planning. Imaging helps in establishing the location of a mass, such as in the presacral area. Because of the presence of the three germ cell layers, a large variety of tissues can be present, particularly in differentiated tumors; thus, fluid, calcification, and fat, in addition to other soft tissues, can be detected by radiography, CT, MRI, or sonography. Both fetal and postnatal sonography can detect the presence of a sacrococcygeal germ cell tumor. When mixed solid and large cystic areas and calcification are visible, the diagnosis is more certain. However, sonography is not sufficient for surgical planning and should be followed by either CT or MRI. CT is the best modality for detecting calcification or ossification and is excellent for demonstrating fat, fluid (including fluid-fluid levels), and soft tissue components. Most teratomas are predominantly cystic, and thus large fluid collections are typically present (**Option (C) is true**) (Figure 13-14). The extent and involvement of adjacent bowel, vascular, and osseous structures are also well displayed for surgical planning. MRI best displays the presacral location of the germ cell tumor and the relationship to the adjacent sacrum and coccyx. Both foraminal involvement and marrow abnormalities are best displayed by MRI, and this information is essential for determining the level of sacrococcygeal resection and the need for neurosurgical assistance during surgery. Fat, other soft tissues, and fluid are all well demonstrated by MRI. The presence of large calcifications can be inferred by the finding of signal voids. Sacrococcygeal germ cell tumors can cause compression of the rectum (resulting in obstruction) or ureters. During evaluation of any large pelvic mass, the kidneys should be included to determine if an obstruction is present. Even when the subjacent coccyx is not directly involved, it is removed because of the otherwise high rate of local recurrence.

Malignant teratomas and tumors without obvious malignancy but containing immature elements are treated by both local resection and chemotherapy with close follow-up. Elevated alpha-fetoprotein levels are associated with malignancy, and this carcinoembryonic protein can be a useful marker for monitoring response to therapy as well as for detecting recurrence. Imaging is critical for the diagnosis and follow-up of all patients with teratomas, since even those tumors with mature (benign) histology occasionally reoccur. Infants and children with mature teratomas do not receive chemotherapy.

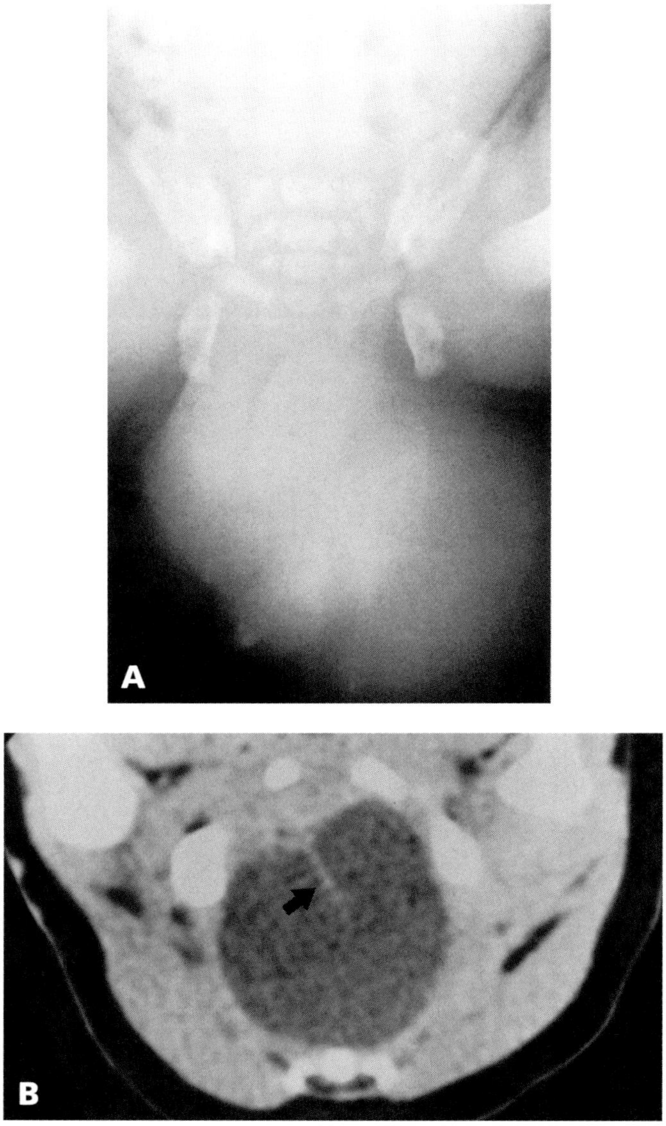

Figure 13-14. Sacrococcygeal teratoma. (A) An anteroposterior pelvic radiograph in a newborn with a large exophytic mature teratoma shows that the ischia are widely spread by the mass. (B) An axial CT scan through the upper aspect of the presacral mass demonstrates a water-attenuation region, indicating the predominantly cystic nature of this teratoma. There is also a central septation (arrow).

Question 69

Features associated with anterior meningocele include:

(A) sacral anomalies
(B) presacral mass
(C) neurofibromatosis type 2
(D) Currarino's triad (imperforate anus, sacral anomaly, presacral mass)
(E) tethered cord

An anterior meningocele is a fluid-filled prevertebral mass (**Option (B) is true**). Sacral anterior meningoceles occur when there is herniation of the sac consisting of meninges enclosing CSF through the anterior aspect of the sacrum, often with associated osseous abnormalities of the sacrum (**Option (A) is true**). Anterior meningoceles may contain nerve roots and are associated with occult spinal dysraphism, including a tethered spinal cord (**Option (E) is true**). Overall, these meningoceles are found about four times as frequently in female patients. Imaging features reflect the osseous and neural soft tissue abnormalities, as well as the relationship to and effect on adjacent organs and structures in the pelvis.

The imaging appearance of the vertebral defect depends upon the type and extent of sacral involvement. Osseous defects range from deficiency of a single vertebral level or scalloping (attributable to dural ectasia) to hypoplasia (including a comma- or scimitar-shaped sacrum) and aplasia. The neck connecting the meningocele to the rest of the thecal sac is typically small. The sac may contain only CSF, but nerve roots also may be present. This is an important feature to identify before surgical repair. An anterior meningocele is suggested when sonography demonstrates a predominantly fluid-filled presacral mass. Osseous anomalies of the sacrum also may be demonstrated. CT better depicts the bony abnormalities and the neck of the low-attenuation CSF-containing sac. If a connection with the thecal sac is not obvious, CT myelography may be helpful. However, because of superior anatomic depiction (primarily attributable to multiplanar capabilities), MRI is the preferred modality for evaluation of anterior meningoceles.

The sagittal projection is optimal for evaluating anterior meningoceles. In this plane, the sacral defects, neck, and sac can be precisely displayed. Nerve roots are best seen with T2 weighting as intermediate signal intensity within the bright signal intensity of CSF. MRI best depicts associated dysraphism, including tethered cord or lipoma, when present.

Anterior meningoceles are associated with other anomalies, including malformations of the uterus, anorectal malformations, and Marfan's syndrome. Anterior meningoceles are also associated with neurofibromatosis type 1 (von Recklinghausen's disease). Neurofibromatosis type 1 consists of cutaneous, skeletal, soft tissue, and CNS (i.e., optic gliomas) manifestations. Thoracic meningoceles are more common than sacral lesions and account for about 85% of all meningoceles. Symptoms are predominantly attributable to the mass effect on genitourinary (incontinence, dysmenorrhea, childbirth), gastrointestinal (constipation), or nervous (headache or, rarely, sciatic pain or bladder dysfunction) systems. Neurofibromatosis type 2 is not associated with meningoceles (**Option (C) is false**), but is associated with acoustic neuromas and other CNS neoplasms.

The constellation of anorectal malformations (A), sacral anomalies (S), and a presacral mass (including anterior meningoceles) (P) is known as ASP association or Currarino's triad (**Option (D) is true**) (Figure 13-15). This triad of anomalies was reported in three infants in 1981. Each had rectal stenosis and sacral anomalies. The presacral masses consisted of an anterior meningocele in one, a teratoma in the second, and an enteric cyst in the third. Since that time, there has been additional confirmation of this unique constellation of findings.

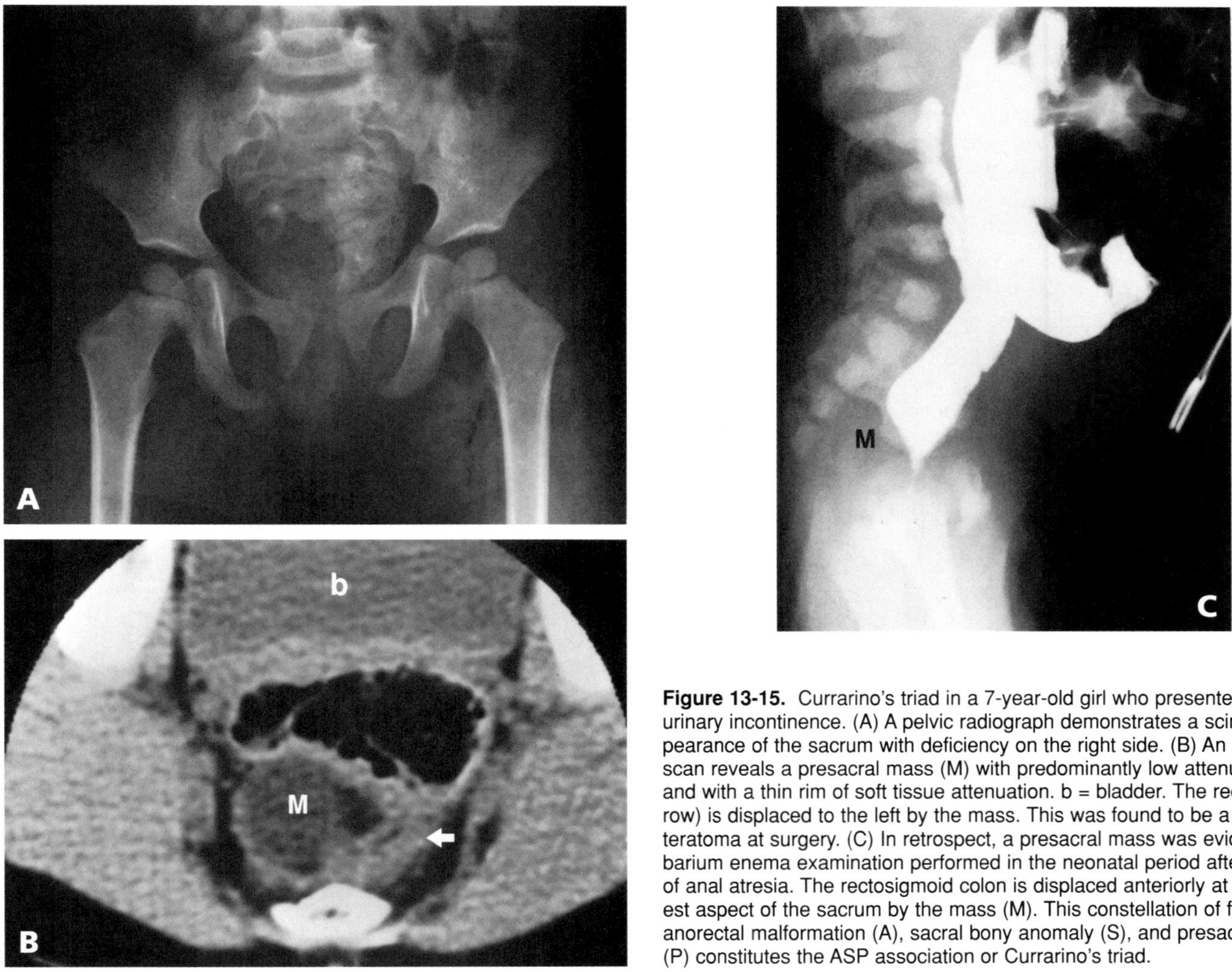

Figure 13-15. Currarino's triad in a 7-year-old girl who presented with urinary incontinence. (A) A pelvic radiograph demonstrates a scimitar appearance of the sacrum with deficiency on the right side. (B) An axial CT scan reveals a presacral mass (M) with predominantly low attenuation and with a thin rim of soft tissue attenuation. b = bladder. The rectum (arrow) is displaced to the left by the mass. This was found to be a benign teratoma at surgery. (C) In retrospect, a presacral mass was evident on a barium enema examination performed in the neonatal period after repair of anal atresia. The rectosigmoid colon is displaced anteriorly at the lowest aspect of the sacrum by the mass (M). This constellation of findings of anorectal malformation (A), sacral bony anomaly (S), and presacral mass (P) constitutes the ASP association or Currarino's triad.

The triad is postulated to result from disordered separation of the neuroectoderm and endoderm and a subsequent displaced or split notochord. Failure of the somite to fuse normally results in communication of the neural tube and ventrally located primitive hindgut. The fistulous communication can therefore consist of predominantly hindgut (duplication), neural elements (anterior meningocele), or intermediate germ cell tissue (teratoma). In 44 patients reviewed by Kirks et al., the soft tissue masses consisted of meningocele, teratoma, enteric duplication, or a combination of these lesions. A teratoma was present in 40% of these masses and was always benign. Anterior meningoceles were reported most frequently, in 50% of the patients. Enteric duplication was present in 5% of the patients.

The anomaly is rare, has an approximately equal gender distribution, and is associated with an autosomal dominant pattern of inheritance, with incomplete penetrance in about 50% of patients; thus, survey pelvic radiography of family members has been recommended by some authors. The symptoms depend on the time of diagnosis, which can vary from birth to the seventh decade. Patients presenting later in life mostly have incomplete forms with minor anomalies of the triad. Constipation is the most frequent symptom, present in 43 of 44 patients in the review of the literature by Kirks et al. Anorectal malformations are chiefly responsible for the constipation. Rectal narrowing also can be attributable to either mass effect or infiltration of the rectal wall, but this does not usually cause constipation. Urinary tract abnormalities, including reflux, voiding difficulties, and incontinence, are also frequent and can be attributable to mass effect or neural involvement. Infection and abscess formation represent the next most frequent presentation. A patient with an anterior meningocele can present with low back pain, headache, or meningitis.

The osseous anomaly in this triad ranges from asymmetric hypoplasia, resulting in a scimitar or crescent appearance, to hypoplasia of the entire distal sacrum and coccyx. Other associations include spinal dysraphism, e.g., tethered cord, lipomas, and lipomeningoceles; uterine and vaginal septation abnormalities; and rectovaginal fistula.

Imaging of patients with this complex should be directed at preoperative evaluation, specifically to determine the location and extent of the mass, the type and severity of anorectal malformations, and the presence of associated genitourinary anomalies. Although the genitourinary tract evaluation can be accomplished by sonography, MRI is best suited for evaluation of the mass, given the potential involvement of neural structures and association with dysraphism. In addition, teratomas can coexist with anterior meningoceles.

Anterior meningoceles can occur independently of the ASP association. They are most often discovered in older children and young adults. Overall, anterior meningoceles are rare, occurring in 1 in 40,000 individuals. Approximately 80% are diagnosed in the first decade, with incomplete forms tending to be recognized in later life. Although up to about 85% of anterior meningoceles are found in females, this may reflect serendipitous detection during pelvic evaluation. The frequency in pediatric series approaches a more even gender split. Associated conditions include uterine developmental anomalies and anorectal malformations (independent of the ASP association). Individuals can be asymptomatic, and their masses are discovered serendipitously. When present, symptoms can be attributable to mass effect (chronic constipation, urinary obstruction, obstetric difficulties, or back pain), neurologic compromise (lower extremity sensory deficits, sciatic pain, neurogenic bladder, or other sphincter dysfunction), or alterations in intracranial pressure (headache, nausea, or vomiting). Neurologic symptoms are present in 10% of patients. The most common physical finding is a pelvic mass. If an abdominal radiograph is obtained and demonstrates a sacral anomaly, MRI is indicated for preoperative evaluation. Radiographic findings in the sacrum range from subtle enlargement of a sacral foramen or a defect in one or more of the sacral bodies to agenesis. A crescentic anomaly (scimitar) of the sacrum is considered pathognomonic. The sacral body anomalies are generally in the midsacrum. Displacement of bowel gas can be seen when the meningocele is large. If a contrast study is performed for evaluation of gastrointestinal symptoms, the contrast column is deviated superiorly, laterally, and anteriorly with an increase in the presacral space thickness.

The diagnosis of an anterior meningocele can be suspected when pelvic sonography demonstrates a simple cyst in the presacral region. Sonography is not sufficient for preoperative planning. CT likewise demonstrates the cystic nature of this mass in the presacral region. The bony defect is seen well, and the diagnosis is virtually limited to an anterior meningocele. However, MRI is necessary for reliable identification of the stalk connecting the sac to the meningocele. MRI is also warranted because neural elements and the filum terminale occasionally course into the sac. Myelography alone or in conjunction with CT can demonstrate the CSF content of the cystic mass only when the connection is sufficiently large. There is no advantage in using myelography (especially in children) if MRI is available.

SUGGESTED READINGS

SACROCOCCYGEAL GERM CELL TUMORS

1. Bale PM. Sacrococcygeal developmental abnormalities and tumors in children. Perspect Pediatr Pathol 1984; 8:9–56
2. Ein SH, Mancer K, Adeyemi SD. Malignant sacrococcygeal teratoma–endodermal sinus, yolk sac tumor–in infants and children: a 32-year review. J Pediatr Surg 1985; 20:473–477
3. Grosfeld JL, Billmire DF. Teratomas in infancy and childhood. Curr Probl Cancer 1985; 9:1–53
4. Keslar PJ, Buck JL, Suarez EC. From the archives of the AFIP. Germ cell tumors of the sacrococcygeal region: radiologic–pathologic correlation. RadioGraphics 1994; 14:607–620
5. Khanna S, Arya NC, Singhal GD. Sacrococcygeal tumours in children. J Postgrad Med 1987; 33:109–114
6. Mahour GH. Sacrococcygeal teratomas. CA Cancer J Clin 1988; 38: 362–367
7. Wells RG, Sty JR. Imaging of sacrococcygeal germ cell tumors. RadioGraphics 1990; 10:701–713

NEUROBLASTOMA

8. Black CT, Atkinson JB. Neuroblastoma. Semin Pediatr Surg 1997; 6:2–10
9. Cohen MD. Imaging of children with cancer. St. Louis: Mosby-Year Book; 1992:134–169
10. Grosfeld JL, Baehner RL. Neuroblastoma: an analysis of 160 cases. World J Surg 1980; 4:29–37
11. Halperin EC, Constine LS, Tarbell NJ, Kun LE (eds). Pediatric radiation oncology. 2nd ed. New York: Raven Press; 1994:171–206
12. Kushner BH, Cheung NK. Neuroblastoma. Pediatr Ann 1988; 17:269–284

RHABDOMYOSARCOMA

13. Agrons GA, Wagner BJ, Lonergan GJ, Dickey GE, Kaufman MS. Genitourinary rhabdomyosarcoma in children: radiologic–pathologic correlation. RadioGraphics 1997; 17:919–937
14. Cohen MD. Imaging of children with cancer. St. Louis: Mosby-Year Book; 1992:308–337
15. Geoffray A, Couanet D, Montagne JP, Leclere J, Flamant F. Ultrasonography and computed tomography for diagnosis and follow-up of pelvic rhabdomyosarcomas in children. Pediatr Radiol 1987; 17:132–136
16. Halperin EC, Constine LS, Tarbell NJ, Kun LE (eds). Pediatric radiation oncology. 2nd ed. New York: Raven Press; 1994:303–340
17. McManus AP, Gusterson BA, Pinkerton CR, Shipley JM. The molecular pathology of small round-cell tumours—relevance to diagnosis, prognosis, and classification. J Pathol 1996; 178:116–121
18. Tannous WN, Azouz EM, Homsy YL, Kiruluta HG, Grattan-Smith D. CT and ultrasound imaging of pelvic rhabdomyosarcoma in children. A review of 56 patients. Pediatr Radiol 1989; 19:530–534

LYMPHOMA

19. Cohen MD. Imaging of children with cancer. St. Louis: Mosby-Year Book; 1992:89–126
20. Hamrick-Turner JE, Saif MF, Powers CI, Blumenthal BI, Royal SA, Iyer RV. Imaging of childhood non-Hodgkin lymphoma: assessment by histologic subtype. RadioGraphics 1994; 14:11–28

ANTERIOR MENINGOCELE

21. Barkovich AJ. Pediatric neuroimaging. 2nd ed. New York: Raven Press; 1995:508–509
22. Chamaa MT, Berney J. Anterior-sacral meningocele: value of magnetic resonance imaging and abdominal sonography. A case report. Acta Neurochir (Wien) 1991; 109:154–157
23. Jabre A, Ball JB Jr, Tew JM Jr. Anterior sacral meningocele. Current diagnosis. Surg Neurol 1985; 23:9–13
24. Mellion BT, George RE, Fischer DK, Lidsky MD, Baskin DS. Anterior sacral meningocele and tuberculous spondylitis of the sacrum in a patient with neurofibromatosis. Case report and review of the literature. Neurofibromatosis 1989; 2:299–308

25. Simpson BA, Glass RE, Mann CV. Anterior sacral meningocoele: magnetic resonance imaging and surgical management. Br J Surg 1987; 74: 1185
26. Skinner DW, Jacobson I. Anterior sacral meningoceles. J R Coll Surg Edinb 1983; 28:229–232
27. Villarejo F, Scavone C, Blazquez MG, et al. Anterior sacral meningocele: review of the literature. Surg Neurol 1983; 19:57–71

CURRARINO'S TRIAD

28. Currarino G, Coln D, Votteler T. Triad of anorectal, sacral, and presacral anomalies. AJR 1981; 137:395–398
29. Kirks DR, Merten DF, Filston HC, Oakes WJ. The Currarino triad: complex of anorectal malformation, sacral bony abnormality, and presacral mass. Pediatr Radiol 1984; 14:220–225
30. Kochling J, Pistor G, Marzhauser Brands S, Nasir R, Lanksch WR. The Currarino syndrome—hereditary transmitted syndrome of anorectal, sacral and presacral anomalies. Case report and review of the literature. Eur J Pediatr Surg 1996; 6:114–119
31. O'Riordain DS, O'Connell PR, Kirwan WO. Hereditary sacral agenesis with presacral mass and anorectal stenosis: the Currarino triad. Br J Surg 1991; 78:536–538
32. Pfluger T, Czekalla R, Koletzko S, Munsterer O, Willemsen UF, Hahn K. MRI and radiographic findings in Currarino's triad. Pediatr Radiol 1996; 26:524–527

SACROCOCCYGEAL LESIONS: GENERAL

33. Bale PM. Sacrococcygeal developmental abnormalities and tumors in children. Perspect Pediatr Pathol 1984; 8:9–56
34. Cohen MD, Bugaieski EM, Haliloglu M, Faught P, Siddiqui AR. Visual presentation of the staging of pediatric solid tumors. RadioGraphics 1996; 16:523–545
35. Levine E, Batnitzky S. Computed tomography of sacral and perisacral lesions. Crit Rev Diagn Imaging 1984; 21:307–374
36. Wagner M, Zastrow R, Reasa DA. Presacral tumors: case report, review of the literature. Clin Anat 1995; 8:227–230
37. Wang JY, Hsu CH, Changchien CR, et al. Presacral tumor: a review of forty-five cases. Am Surg 1995; 61:310–315
38. Wechsler RJ, Schilling JF. CT of the gluteal region. AJR 1985; 144:185–190
39. Wetzel LH, Levine E. Pictorial essay. MR imaging of sacral and presacral lesions. AJR 1990; 154:771–775

Lane F. Donnelly, M.D.

Tarsal Coalition

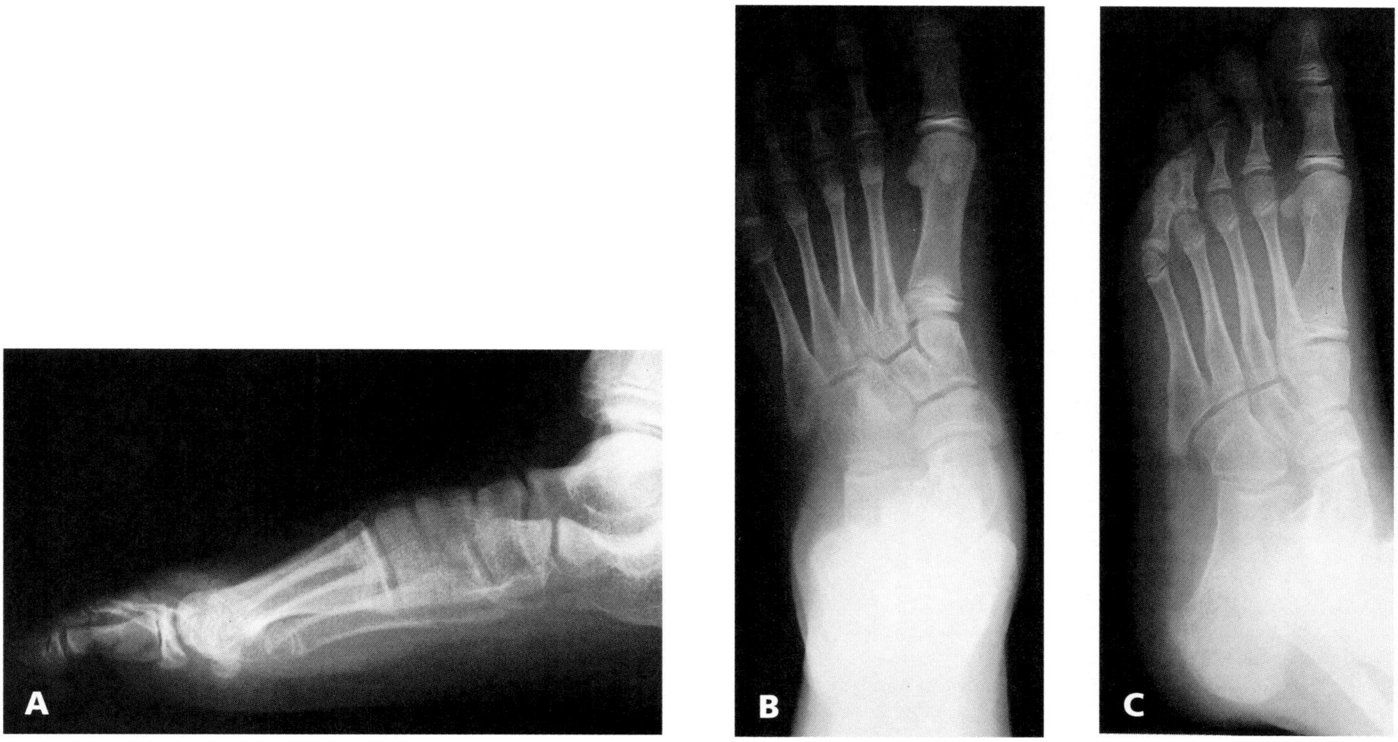

Figure 14-1

Question 70

This 13-year-old boy has chronic foot pain. You are shown a series of three radiographs of the foot (Figure 14-1).

Which *one* of the following is the MOST likely diagnosis?

(A) Stress fracture
(B) Nonopaque foreign body
(C) Tarsal coalition
(D) Osteochondritis dissecans
(E) Jones' fracture

The lateral view from the series of radiographs of the foot in the test patient (Figure 14-1A) shows pes planus, talar beaking, prominence of the lateral process of the talus, and poor visualization of the talocalcaneal joint (Figure 14-2). There is a C-shaped overlap of the talus and calcaneus in the region of the subtalar joint. No other abnormalities are present. On the basis of these findings, talocalcaneal coalition is the most likely diagnosis (**Option** (C) **is correct**).

Tarsal coalitions represent abnormal fusion of one or more of the tarsal bones. In patients with talocalcaneal coalition, one of the more common types of coalition, visualization of the actual fusion on standard radiographic views is unusual and the diagnosis must be based on secondary signs of the coalition, as are seen in the test patient. The diagnosis in this patient was subsequently confirmed by CT (Figure 14-3).

A stress fracture (Option (A)) is defined as an area of microinjury and reactive change that results from a repetitive stress. When repeated stress leads to such an injury in normal bone, it is referred to as a fatigue fracture. When the stress fracture is predisposed by an underlying bone abnormality, such as

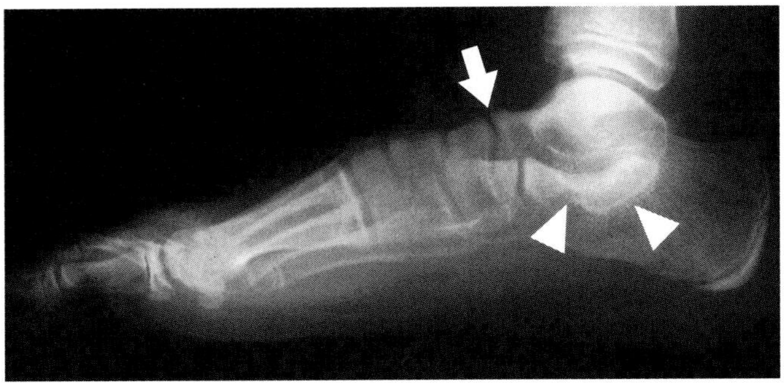

Figure 14-2 (Same as Figure 14-1A). Talocalcaneal coalition. A lateral view from the series of radiographs of the foot in the test patient shows pes planus, talar beaking (arrow), and prominence of the lateral process of the talus. The talocalcaneal joint is not well visualized. There is a C-shaped overlap of the talus and calcaneus (arrowheads) in the region of the subtalar joint.

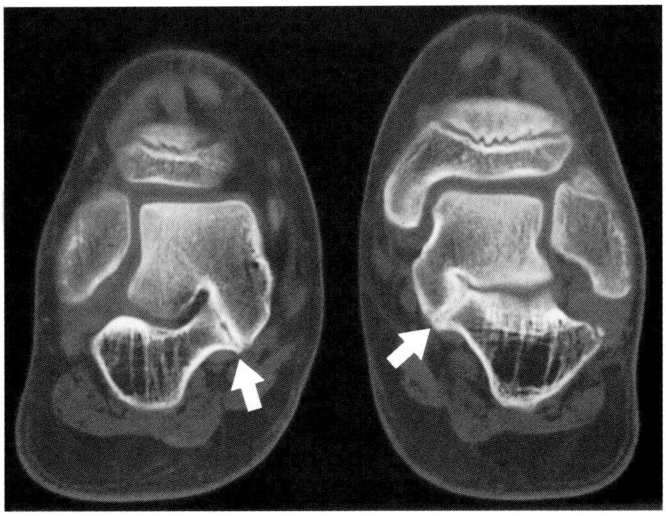

Figure 14-3. Same patient as in Figures 14-1 and 14-2. Talocalcaneal coalition. A CT scan obtained in the coronal plane shows nearly complete bony fusion of both middle talocalcaneal joints (arrows), with adjacent sclerotic, irregular bone.

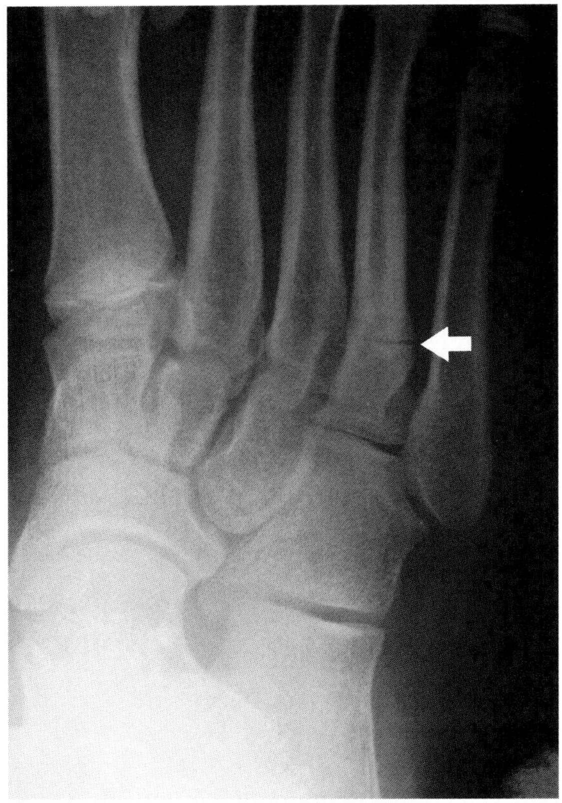

Figure 14-4. Stress fracture of the fourth metatarsal in a 12-year-old soccer player with foot pain. A radiograph shows an incomplete fracture line (arrow) through the lateral cortex, with surrounding sclerosis.

osteoporosis, the injury is referred to as an insufficiency fracture. Clinically, children with stress fractures present with localized pain, which often subsides with rest; when the stress fracture involves the lower extremities, patients can present with a limp. Localized tenderness, swelling, and warmth are often present. Any child can develop a stress fracture, but athletes and children with underlying bony abnormalities are predisposed to this condition. One common scenario is the child with disuse osteoporosis, related to immobilization for a fracture, who develops a stress fracture upon resuming normal activity.

On radiographs, a stress fracture typically appears as a small area of cortical resorption or low density. There is often adjacent periosteal reaction or cortical thickening. A transverse band of increased density can be present in the adjacent medullary portion of the bone secondary to osteoblastic repair (Figures 14-4 and 14-5). An incomplete fracture line is sometimes visualized. Stress fractures that are not treated with rest can progress to complete fractures. Common locations of stress fractures in the foot include the proximal metatarsals (Figure 14-4), calcaneus (Figure 14-5), and cuboid. When the calcaneus is involved, the stress fracture appears on the lateral view as a vertical band of sclerosis aligned parallel to the posterior cortex of the calcaneus. Bone scintigraphy can demonstrate abnormalities related to stress fractures 2 to 3 weeks before findings are apparent on radiographs (Figure 14-6). MRI also demonstrates abnormally increased signal intensity of the marrow and cortex of involved areas of bone on T2-weighted images (Figure 14-7) and decreased intensity on T1-weighted images before abnormalities are apparent on radiographs. Such abnormalities are seen on MRI with high frequency in long-distance runners and other high-performance athletes.

The test images contain no bands of sclerosis, periosteal reaction, or incomplete fracture lines to suggest stress fracture as the cause of the pain in the test patient.

Children are notorious for walking barefoot in places where they should not do so. This behavior predisposes them to a penetrating injury that can result in the introduction of a foreign body into the foot (Option (B)). If the foreign body is not detected at the time of injury, the child may present at a later time with infection, unexplained chronic pain, or a palpable mass (Figure 14-8). On radiographs, potential findings include identification of a radiopaque foreign body, soft tissue swelling or focal mass, or evidence of osteomyelitis or chronic remodeling of bone. None of these findings is present in the test images.

Osteochondritis dissecans (Option (D)) is a transchondral

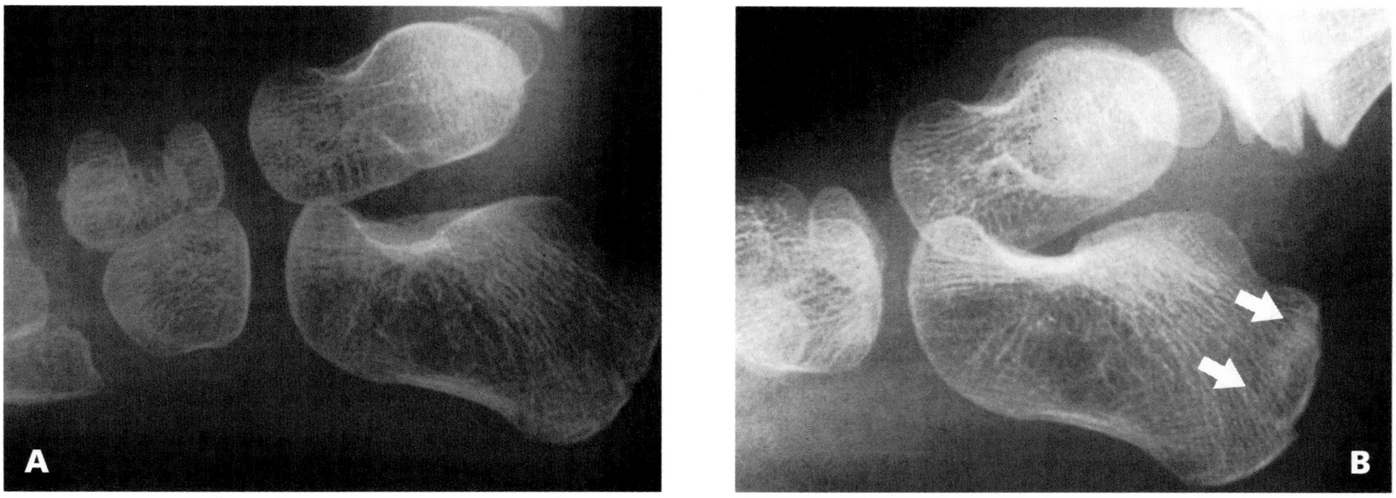

Figure 14-5. Stress fracture of the calcaneus in a 3-year-old girl with foot pain and limp. (A) An initial lateral radiograph of the foot is normal. (B) A lateral radiograph obtained 7 days later, when the patient returned with persistent pain, shows a new band of sclerosis (arrows) parallel to the posterior cortex of the calcaneus.

fracture that splits the articular cartilage from or extends through the subjacent bone. As a result, there is a flap of cartilage, with or without an attached fragment of underlying bone, that is attached at one edge or exists as a free fragment. The terminology is misleading because it implies an inflammatory process. However, current opinion holds that the lesion is attributable to trauma, either one major traumatic event or the summation of multiple repetitive minor events. Because the lesions occur in predicted locations and are often bilateral and symmetric, it is believed that local ischemia or poor blood supply to cartilage predisposes these areas to chondral fracture with minor trauma. Commonly involved areas in children include the elbow (capitellum), knee (femoral condyles) (Figure 14-9), and ankle (talar dome) (Figure 14-10). Other regions of the foot and ankle are not typical sites of osteochondritis dissecans.

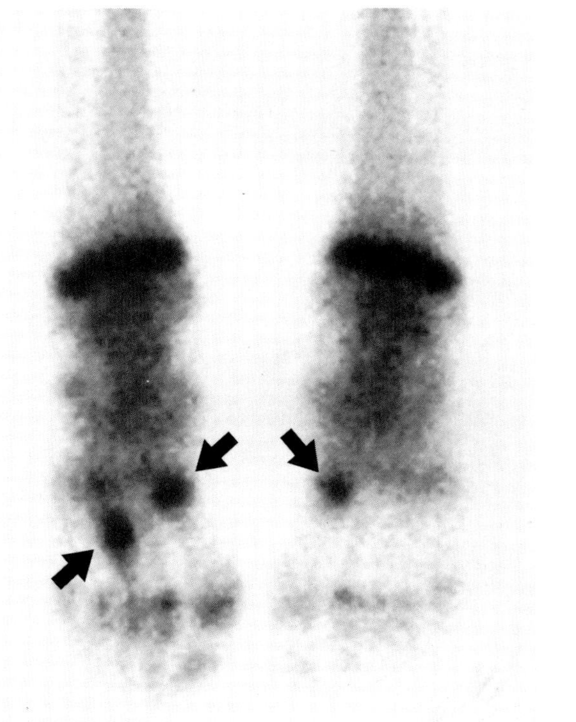

Figure 14-6. Stress injury of multiple metatarsals in a 13-year-old runner. Dorsal Tc-99m methylene disphosphonate scintigrams show increased uptake (arrows) in the proximal ends of both first metatarsals and the midshaft of the right third metatarsal. Radiographs obtained at that time (not shown) were normal.

Osteochondral lesions that involve the talar dome can present with chronic pain. However, the lesions can be asymptomatic. A history of major trauma is frequently absent, but there is often a history of previous ankle injury or lax ankle ligaments. Osteochondritis dissecans is three times more common in boys than in girls, and when the talar dome is involved, presentation is most common during the second decade.

Radiographically, a fossalike defect or occasionally a lucent line involving the medial or lateral talar dome is visualized (Figure 14-10). The defect is often surrounded by bony sclerosis. Reactive sclerosis is sometimes seen involving the opposing tibial articular surface. A fragment of bone (loose body *in situ*) often can be identified within the defect. In contrast to adults, free loose bodies in association with osteochondritis dissecans are rare in children. In the rare event that an osteochondral fragment does become free, it can lead to secondary degenerative arthritis. The radiographic appearance is often stable for years.

In a patient with osteochrondritis dissecans, the status of the overlying cartilage can be evaluated by arthrography or MRI (Figure 14-11). In children, the overlying cartilage is often intact. This implies that the injury to the subchondral bone is related to a compressive force transmitted through but not injuring the cartilage. When an osteochondral lesion is visualized on CT, the defect is often larger than would have been predicted by radiography.

No defect is seen in the dome of the talus in Figure 14-1, making osteochondritis dissecans unlikely in the test patient.

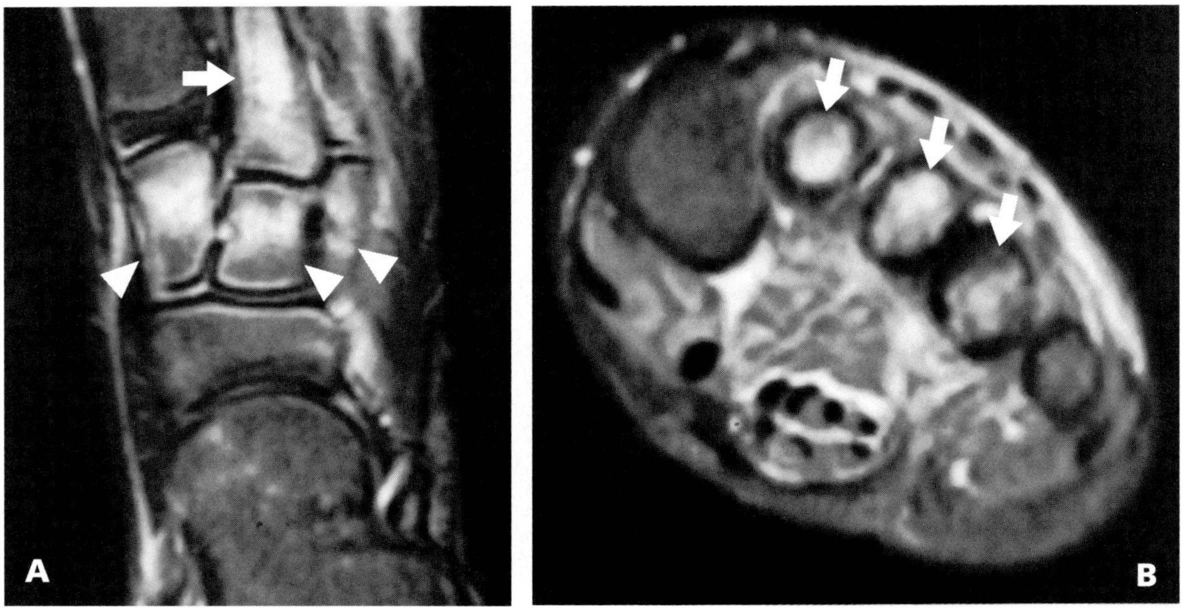

FSE 2,000/80 FSE 2,000/80

Figure 14-7 (Left). Stress injury involving the metatarsals and cuneiforms in a 12-year-old football player with pain. Axial (long-axis) (A) and coronal (short-axis) (B) fast spin-echo, fat-saturated, T2-weighted MR images show abnormal increased signal intensity in all of the cuneiforms (arrowheads) and in the second through fourth metatarsal bones (arrows).

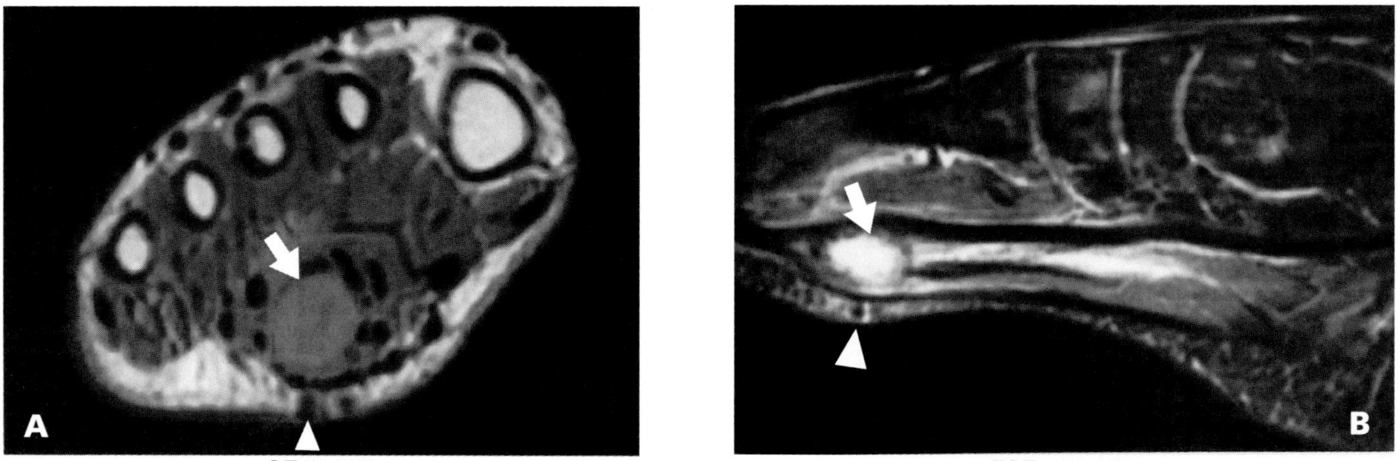

SE 600/11 FSE 2,000/80

Figure 14-8. Chronic foreign body (foreign body granuloma) presenting as a palpable mass in the foot of a 7-year-old boy. (A) A coronal T1-weighted MR image shows a well-defined heterogeneous mass (arrow) immediately adjacent to the plantar flexor tendons. A low-intensity tract is seen in the subcutaneous tissues (arrowhead) extending from the skin surface to the mass. (B) A sagittal fast spin-echo, T2-weighted MR image demonstrates heterogeneous high signal intensity within the mass (arrow) and small amounts of surrounding edema. The tract extending through the subcutaneous tissues (arrowhead) is again noted. At surgery, a small piece of rubber was found to be the foreign body. The child had stepped on a nail, which went through his shoe, 1 year earlier. The injury had introduced part of the rubber sole into the soft tissues. (Reprinted with permission from Donnelly et al. [16].)

A Jones' fracture (Option (E)) is defined as a transverse fracture of the proximal portion of the fifth metatarsal at the insertion of the peroneus brevis tendon. The mechanism of injury is a plantar flexion and inversion stress. The appearance of the normal apophysis of the base of the fifth metatarsal must be differentiated from fracture. Most avulsion fractures of the base of the fifth metatarsal are oriented transversely relative to the long axis of the bone (Figure 14-12). The typical apophysis is oriented obliquely relative to the long axis of the metatarsal shaft, with its proximal end more medial than its distal end (Figure 14-13). The orientation of the lucency reliably differentiates fracture from normal apophysis in most patients. There is, however, a great deal of variation in the appearance of this apophysis, and when the radiographic diagnosis is in doubt, tenderness on physical examination is the most helpful finding in differentiating fracture from normal apophysis. There is no transverse lucency through the base of the fifth metatarsal to suggest a Jones' fracture in the test patient.

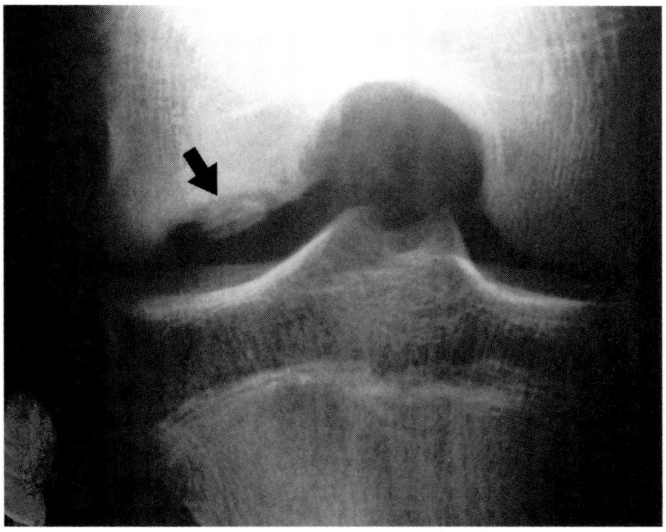

Figure 14-9. Osteochondritis dissecans of the distal femur in a 14-year-old boy. A radiograph shows a fossa-like defect (arrow) in the lateral femoral condyle, with surrounding sclerosis and a loose body *in situ.*

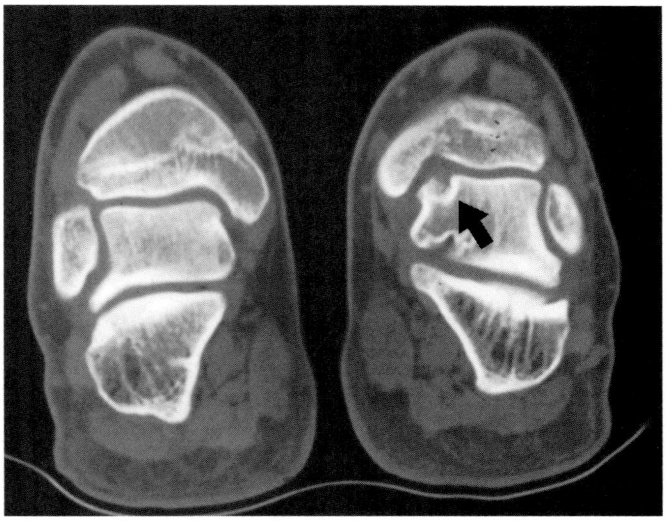

Figure 14-10. Osteochondritis dissecans of the talar dome in a 15-year-old boy with foot pain. A CT scan was ordered to exclude tarsal coalition. The coronal CT image shows a fossalike defect (arrow) in the medial talar dome, with surrounding sclerosis and a loose body *in situ.*

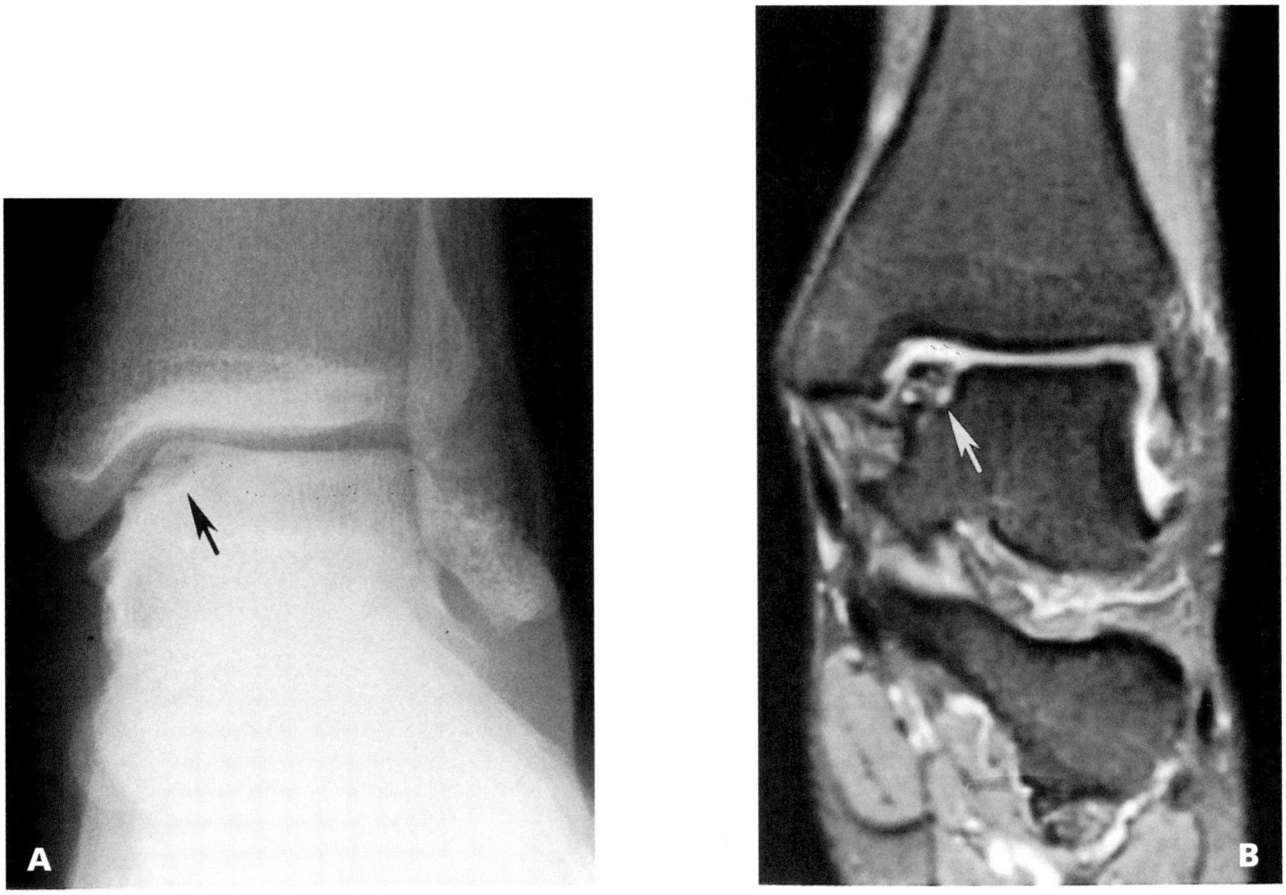

SE 3,000/19

Figure 14-11. Osteochondritis dissecans of the talar dome in an 18-year-old girl with foot pain. (A) A frontal radiograph of the left ankle shows an area of lucency (arrow) in the medial talar dome. (B) A proton-density-weighted coronal MRI image shows a loose body *in situ* (arrow). The overlying cartilage appears intact.

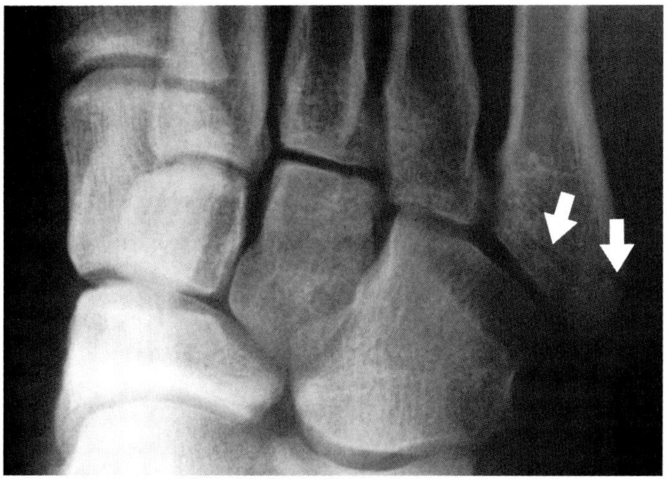

Figure 14-12. Jones' fracture. A radiograph shows a transverse lucency (arrows) through the base of the fifth metatarsal. The fracture is oriented transversely with respect to the axis of the metatarsal shaft.

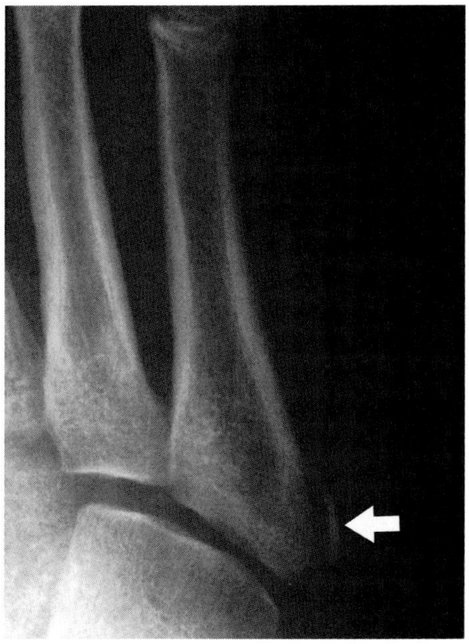

Figure 14-13. Normal appearance of the apophysis of the proximal fifth metatarsal. A radiograph shows that the apophysis (arrow) is oriented obliquely with respect to the shaft of the fifth metatarsal.

Question 71

Concerning foreign bodies in the feet,

(A) sonography reliably detects radiolucent foreign bodies
(B) most nonleaded glass is radiolucent on conventional radiographs
(C) MRI usually shows findings specific for a foreign body in patients who present with a soft tissue mass
(D) bone scintigraphy is generally indicated in a patient with a chronic foreign body

Penetrating injuries of the foot in children are often associated with the introduction of foreign bodies. The most common scenario occurs when a barefoot child steps on glass. When a child presents with a wound resulting from such an injury, imaging plays an important role in identifying the foreign body and, when necessary, assisting in its removal. Radiographs of the feet and other extremities are often obtained to exclude the presence of a radiopaque foreign body. Although it is often stated that only leaded glass is radiopaque, almost all glass is radiopaque and even very small fragments are usually identified radiographically (Figure 14-14) **(Option (B) is false).** Metal-containing foreign bodies are also radiopaque, whereas plastic foreign bodies usually are not identifiable on radiographs. When a radiopaque foreign body is identified on radiography but cannot be located on physical inspection of the wound, fluoroscopy can be used for imaging-guided removal of the foreign body.

When a radiolucent foreign body is suspected, sonography is accurate in identifying foreign bodies, which appear as hyperechoic foci associated with acoustic shadowing or reverberation artifacts (Figure 14-15) **(Option (A) is true).** Sonographic guidance has also been advocated to be useful in the removal of foreign bodies.

An occult foreign body within the soft tissues can incite the formation of a foreign body granuloma and present as a mass long after the original penetrating injury is forgotten. Patients may be referred for MRI because of a clinical suspicion of a primary soft tissue neoplasm (Figure 14-8). Foreign bodies consisting of wood, plastic, glass, or metal appear as signal void, and the overall appearance of the inflammatory mass on MRI is nonspecific **(Option (C) is false).** Metallic foreign bodies may be associated with susceptibility artifacts. Therefore, when a mass evaluated by MRI is located in an area predisposed to foreign body deposition, such as the sole of the foot, foreign body and the resultant inflammatory response should be considered in the differential diagnosis.

With the exception of the evaluation of the orbit, CT plays only a minor role in the evaluation of foreign bodies. Likewise, bone scintigraphy plays no role in the evaluation of foreign bodies, unless underlying osteomyelitis is suspected. A

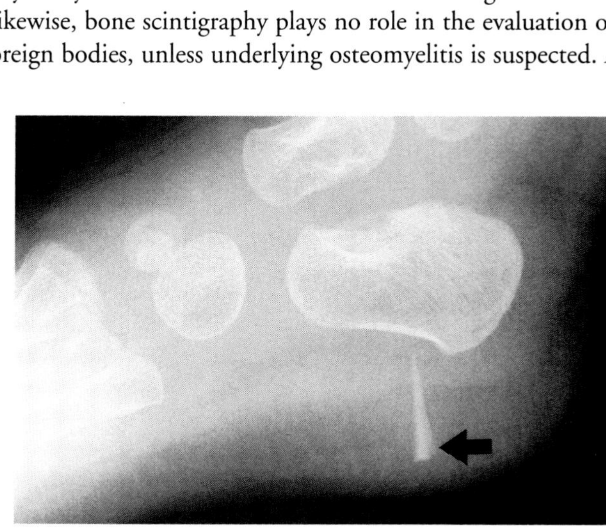

Figure 14-14. Foreign body. A lateral radiograph of the foot in a 2-year-old girl who stepped on glass while walking barefoot shows a piece of glass (arrow). (Reprinted with permission from Donnelly et al. [16].)

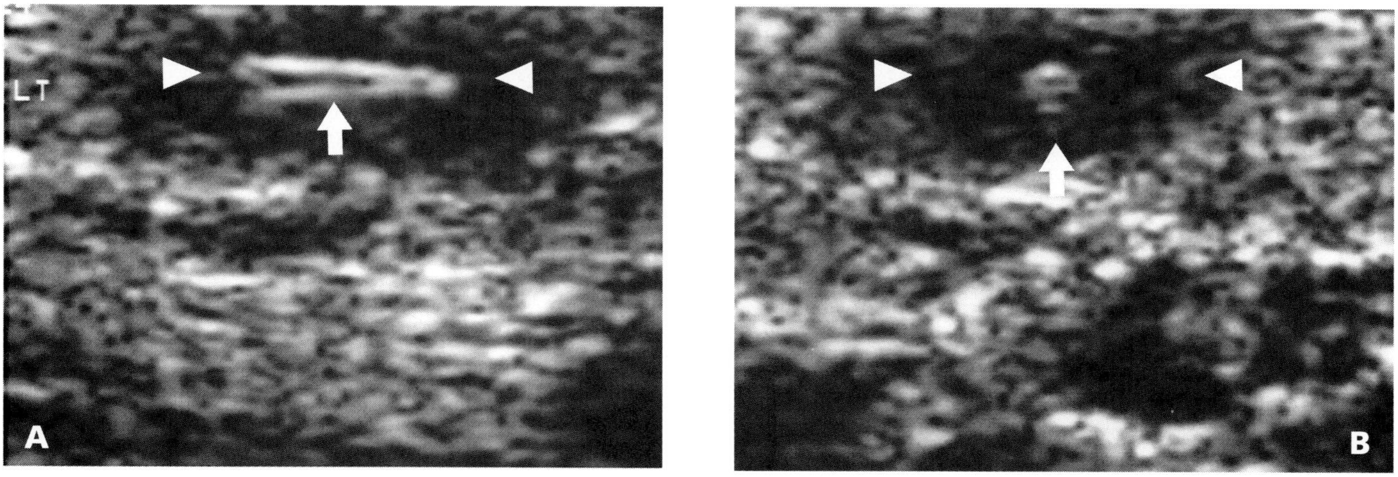

Figure 14-15. Foreign body. A radiolucent splinter in the foot of a 7-year-old girl is demonstrated by sonography. Longitudinal (A) and transverse (B) sonograms demonstrate an echogenic linear structure (arrow) with a reverberation artifact, consistent with a wood splinter. There is a surrounding zone of hypoechogenicity (arrowheads) consistent with edema and inflammation. (Reprinted with permission from Donnelly et al. [16].)

chronic foreign body is not in itself an indication for bone scintigraphy (**Option (D) is false**).

Question 72

Concerning tarsal coalition,

(A) most patients are asymptomatic
(B) the most common types involve the calcaneus
(C) in patients with talocalcaneal coalition, fusion most commonly involves the posterior facet
(D) distinguishing osseous from fibrous coalition is important for planning surgical management
(E) fibrous coalitions are delineated better by MRI than by CT

Tarsal coalitions represent an abnormal fusion of one or more of the tarsal bones. Although the fusion can occur secondary to acquired causes, such as surgery, infection, and trauma, developmental causes are thought to be more common. The lesions can be truly congenital, since such abnormalities have been identified in fetuses. There is a familial history in some cases.

The most common type of tarsal coalition is reported in various sources as either talocalcaneal or calcaneonavicular coalition (**Option (B) is true**). Together, these two types represent nearly 90% of tarsal coalitions. Other, less common types include calcaneocuboid and talonavicular coalitions. Multiple tarsal bones can be fused in patients with some syndromes. This feature has been found in patients with otopalatodigital syndrome, hand-foot-uterus syndrome, hereditary symphalangism, arthrogryposis, and Apert's syndrome. A coalition can be fibrous, cartilaginous, or osseous; although this characteristic affects the radiographic appearance, it does not have a bearing on management decisions (**Option (D) is false**). The decision to perform surgical repair is based upon both the presence of a coalition and clinical symptoms.

Symptoms of tarsal coalition usually begin in the second or third decade of life. Most patients develop symptoms (**Option (A) is false**). The symptoms include restricted motion and vague pain, often exacerbated by prolonged standing or exercise. Patients with tarsal coalition are also prone to ankle injury, related to the abnormal mechanics of the hindfoot, and they can present with a history of multiple or recurrent ankle fractures or injuries. On physical examination, limited range of motion of the subtalar joint, pes planus, and intermittent spasm of the peroneal muscles are noted.

In patients with talocalcaneal coalition, the fusion involves the middle facet of the talocalcaneal joint, between the talus and sustentaculum tali. Fusion of the posterior facet is extremely uncommon (**Option (C) is false**). Boys are much more commonly affected than girls, and talocalcaneal coalitions are bilateral in up to 50% of patients.

Direct visualization of the talocalcaneal coalition on standard radiographic views of the foot is very uncommon. A penetrated axial radiograph (Harris-Beath view) will demonstrate the coalition in some cases. The diagnosis therefore must be considered on the basis of secondary radiographic signs. Most patients with talocalcaneal coalition have pes planus (Figures 14-2 and 14-16). Another reliable secondary sign of talocalcaneal coalition is talar beaking (Figures 14-2 and 14-16). This finding is visualized on the lateral view. Production of the talar beak is related to subperiosteal proliferation; this condition is attributable to abnormal dorsal subluxation of the navicular bone as a result of subtalar rigidity and consequent elevation of the periosteum. A similar overgrowth can be present in the adjacent portion of the navicular bone (Figure 14-16), although it is less consistently present than the talar beak. Other conditions that predispose to abnormal talonavicular motion can result in similar findings, and so the finding is not specific.

Another secondary finding of talocalcaneal coalition is poor

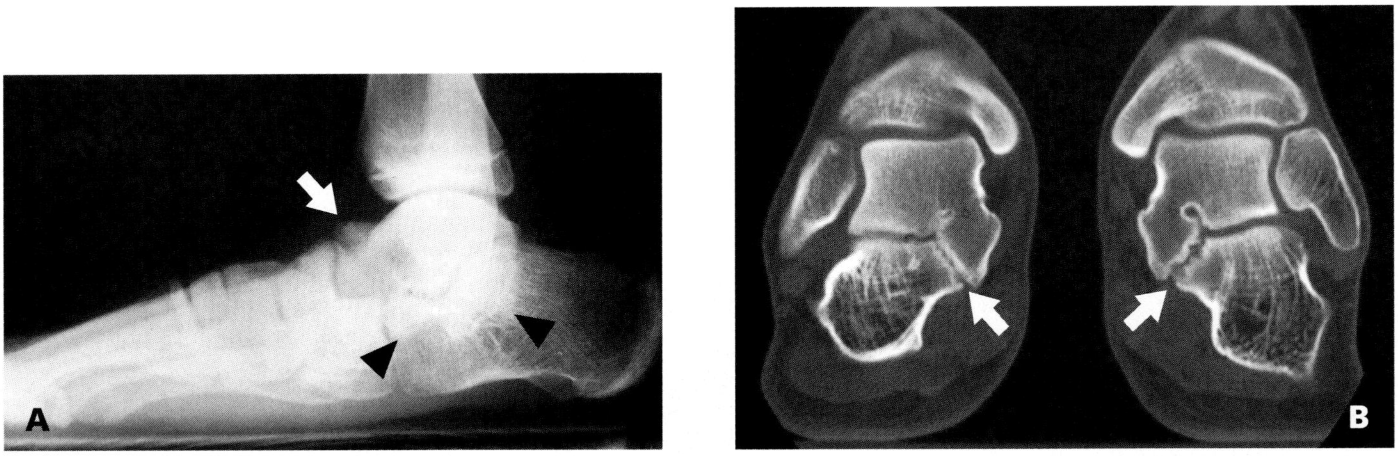

Figure 14-16. Bilateral talocalcaneal fibrous coalitions in a 16-year-old boy with pain. (A) A radiograph of the right foot shows pes planus. Talar beaking (arrow) and a similar prominence of the adjacent navicular bone are also visible. The talocalcaneal joint is poorly visualized, and there is a C-shaped bony overlap (arrowheads) of the talus and calcaneus. The left foot (not shown) had identical findings. (B) A coronal CT image shows narrowing, adjacent irregularity, and sclerosis of the middle facets (arrows) of both subtalar joints.

visualization of the subtalar joint (Figures 14-2 and 14-16), in particular the middle facet, on a true lateral view. An appropriately positioned lateral view of the foot should be directed down the plane of the subtalar joint, and therefore the joint should be well visualized. In patients with talocalcaneal coalition, this joint is poorly visualized. Unfortunately, the subtalar joint also can be poorly visualized if the radiograph is obtained with the x-ray beam angled cranially or caudally (Figure 14-17). In association with the poor visualization of the subtalar joint, a C-shaped overlap of the talus and calcaneus, which is not seen normally, can occur. Other secondary signs of talocalcaneal coalition include broadening of the lateral process of the talus and a "ball-and-socket" appearance of the tibiotalar joint.

When talocalcaneal coalition is suspected clinically or radiographically, a definitive diagnosis can be made by CT. The subtalar joint is best visualized on the coronal (short-axis) view of the foot. When a bony coalition is present, the coronal images show a bony bridge connecting the talus to the sustentaculum tali of the calcaneus (Figure 14-18), bridging the middle facet of the subtalar joint. With a cartilaginous or fibrous coalition, the middle facet is narrowed and irregular, with adjacent sclerosis on both sides of the joint (Figure 14-18). Although MRI also can demonstrate these coalitions, it has no demonstrated advantage over CT (Figure 14-18) (**Option (E) is false).** Emery et al., in a blinded review of both CT and MRI studies obtained in 20 children with tarsal coalitions, found that all coalitions identified on MRI were also identified on CT. In fact, one incomplete condition that was identified on CT was not seen on MRI.

In contrast, calcaneonavicular coalition, the other com-

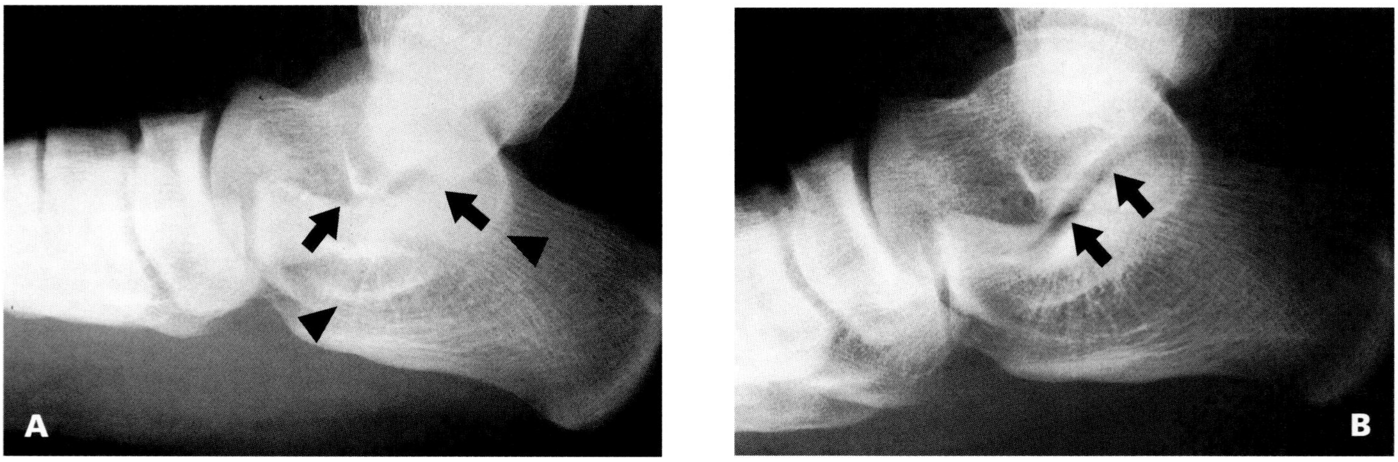

Figure 14-17. Variability of appearance of the subtalar joint with angulation of the x-ray beam. (A) A lateral radiograph of a 15-year-old boy with foot and ankle injury shows pes planus, poor visualization of the subtalar joint (arrows), and the C-shaped bony overlap of the talus and calcaneus (arrowheads). The findings are suspicious for talocalcaneal coalition. (B) A lateral radiograph, obtained as part of the evaluation of the ankle, shows a well-visualized subtalar joint (arrows) that appears normal. The findings suspicious for talocalcaneal coalition on the other radiograph are artifactual. Also, note the normal appearance of the relationship between the calcaneus and the navicular bone, in contrast to the findings of calcaneonavicular coalition shown in Figure 14-19.

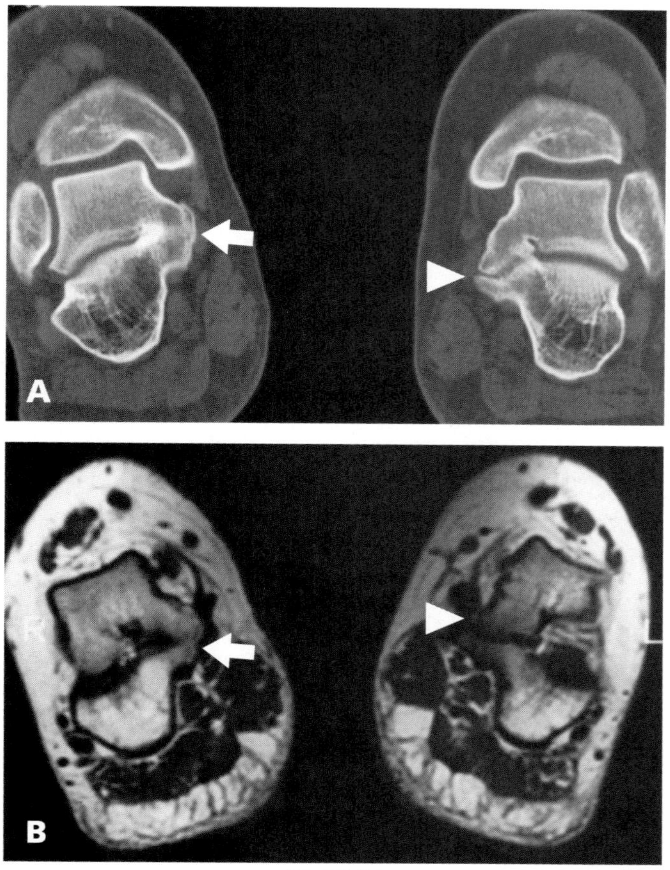

SE 600/11

Figure 14-18. Bilateral talocalcaneal coalition in a 13-year-old girl. (A) A coronal CT scan shows complete bony bridging (arrow) of the middle subtalar facets in the right foot, consistent with bony coalition. Narrowing, adjacent irregularity, and sclerosis of the middle subtalar facets (arrowhead), consistent with fibrous coalition, are visible in the left foot. (B) A coronal T1-weighted MR image also shows the right bony coalition (arrow) and left fibrous coalition (arrowhead).

mon type of coalition, is usually directly visualized on standard radiographs of the foot. Calcaneonavicular coalitions tend to be associated with less severe symptoms than talocalcaneal coalitions and are less likely to be bilateral.

A 45° oblique view of the foot of a patient with bony calcaneonavicular coalition shows a bony bar extending between the calcaneus and the navicular bone (Figure 14-19). Normally, there is no articulation between the calcaneus and the navicular bone. In patients with a fibrous or cartilaginous coalition, the space between these two bones is abnormally narrow and adjacent sclerosis and cortical irregularity are present. On the lateral view, extension of the neck of the calcaneus is visualized in the direction of the navicular bone. The appearance has been referred to as an "anteater nose" (Figure 14-19). Other diagnostic imaging tests are usually not necessary in patients with calcaneonavicular coalition. However, if the diagnosis is in question, these coalitions are well depicted on axial (long axis of the foot) CT images (Figure 14-20).

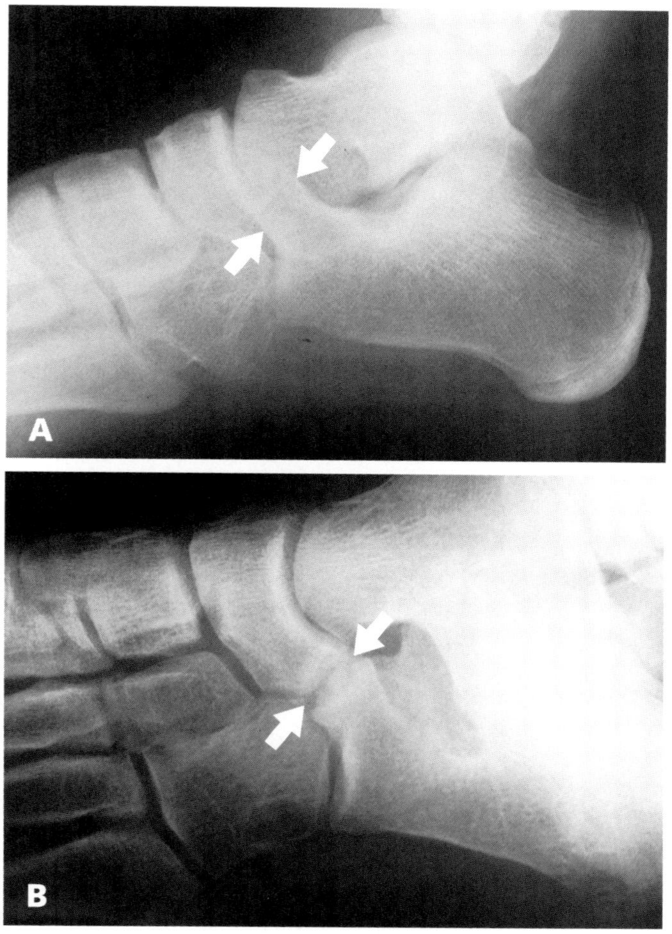

Figure 14-19. Calcaneonavicular coalition in a 14-year-old boy with pain and a history of repeated injuries. (A) A lateral radiograph shows extension of the neck of the calcaneus (arrows) in the direction of the navicular bone, i.e., the "anteater nose" sign. (B) A 45° oblique radiograph shows narrowing of the calcaneonavicular junction (arrows), irregularity, and sclerosis of the calcaneal and navicular surfaces at the site of the coalition.

Question 73

Concerning the anatomy of the foot,

(A) the calcaneonavicular joint has three facets
(B) the sinus tarsi separates the anterior and middle facets of the talocalcaneal joint
(C) the talocalcaneal joint is best demonstrated in the axial plane (long axis of the foot)
(D) the calcaneonavicular joint is best demonstrated in the coronal plane (short axis of the foot)

There are some controversy and confusion about the naming of the anatomic planes with respect to the foot. By convention, imaging planes are named as if the body part were in the anatomic position. When in the anatomic position, the foot is at a 90° angle relative to the leg and is thus neither dorsiflexed nor plantar flexed. The position of the feet is identical to that in a standing individual. The coronal plane of the foot is the short axis, and the toes are seen in cross section. The axial

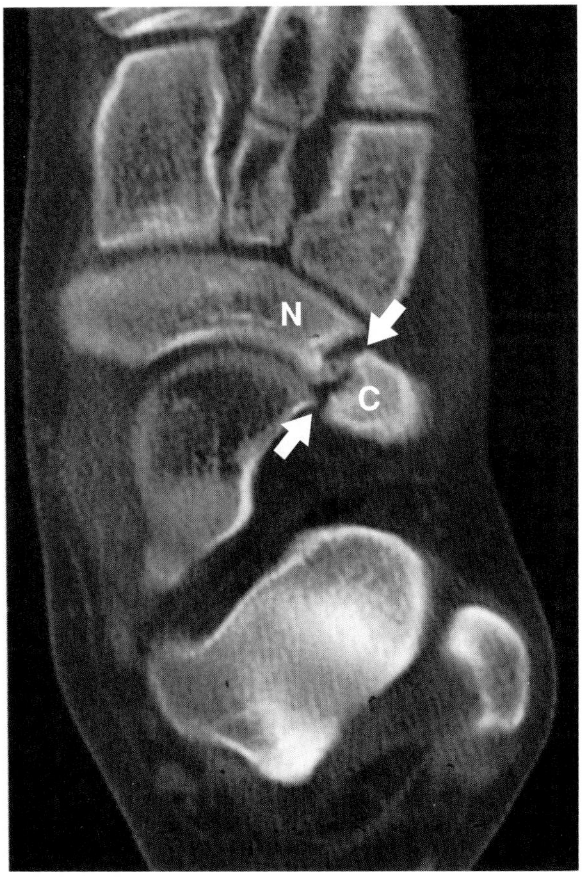

Figure 14-20. Calcaneonavicular coalition in a 13-year-old boy. A CT scan shows narrowing of the space (arrows) between the calcaneus (C) and the navicular bone (N), with adjacent cortical irregularity and sclerosis.

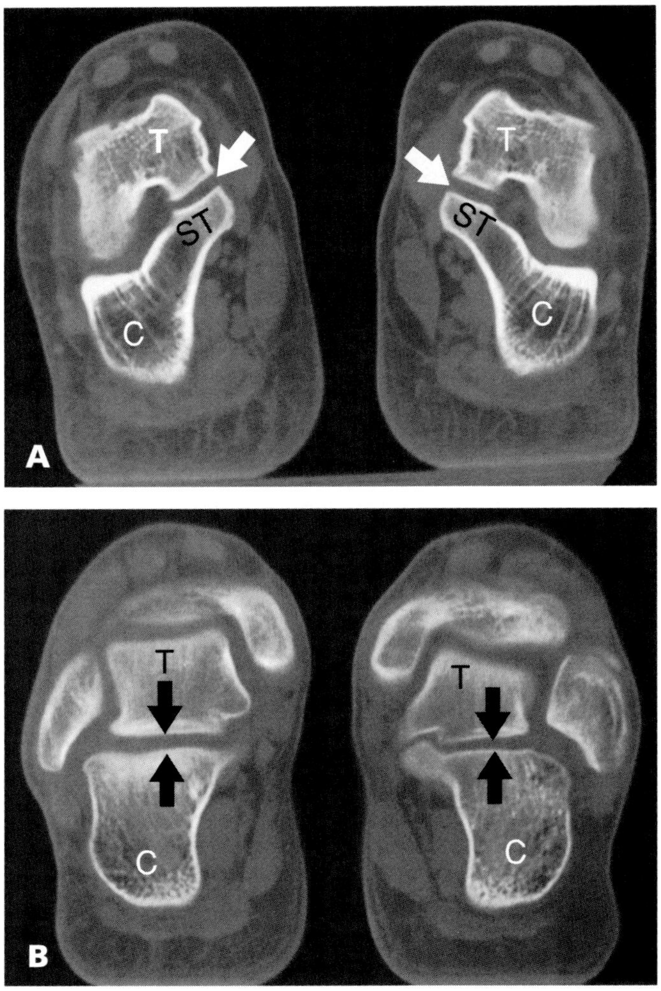

Figure 14-21. Normal appearance of the subtalar joint on coronal CT. (A) The facets of the middle subtalar joint normally demonstrate a smooth cortex and a symmetric joint space. The middle facet rests medially on top of the medially extending process of the calcaneus (C) called the sustentaculum tali (ST). (B) The posterior subtalar joint (arrows) rests on the body of the calcaneus (C). It and the anterior facet (not shown), which also rests on the body of the calcaneus, are positioned more laterally than the middle facet. T = talus.

plane of the foot is the long axis, and the toes are seen in longitudinal section. Misunderstanding of these planes can lead to problem, both when directing technologists to perform CT or MRI studies of the foot and when communicating results to referring physicians. For CT scanning, the feet are imaged in the coronal plane by positioning the patient with the knees flexed and the feet flat on the CT bed. The axial plane is imaged with the patient's legs straight and the feet in the anatomic position.

The talocalcaneal articulations are complex, and an understanding of their anatomy is essential for the accurate identification of talocalcaneal coalitions. There are three articulating facets between the talus and calcaneus: anterior, middle, and posterior. The posterior talocalcaneal articulation is between the posterior calcaneal facet of the talus and the posterior talar facet of the calcaneus (Figure 14-21). The posterior facet is separated from the middle facet by the sinus tarsi (**Option (B) is false**). The anterior and middle articulations are contiguous and are not identified by CT as two truly discrete joints. The middle articulation is between the sustentaculum tali of the calcaneus and the middle facet of the talus. The sustentaculum tali is a plateau of the calcaneus that extends medially from the body of the calcaneus (Figure 14-21). Therefore, the middle facet of the subtalar joint sits on top of the sustentaculum tali and is positioned more medially than the anterior and posterior facets, which rest on the body of the calcaneus (Figure 14-21). The subtalar joints are oriented approximately 45° to the plantar surface of the standing foot and are best visualized in the coronal (short axis of the foot) plane (Figure 14-21) (**Option (C) is false**).

Normally, there is no articulation between the calcaneus and the navicular bone. Therefore, there are no articulating facets (**Option (A) is false**). The relationship between the two bones is best seen in the axial (long axis of the foot) plane (**Option (D) is false**). Normally, there is space between these two bones and the bones demonstrate a normal-appearing cortex (Figure 14-22). In patients with coalition, either there is a bony bar connecting the two bones or the space separating the bones is narrowed, with adjacent sclerosis and irregularity (Figure 14-20).

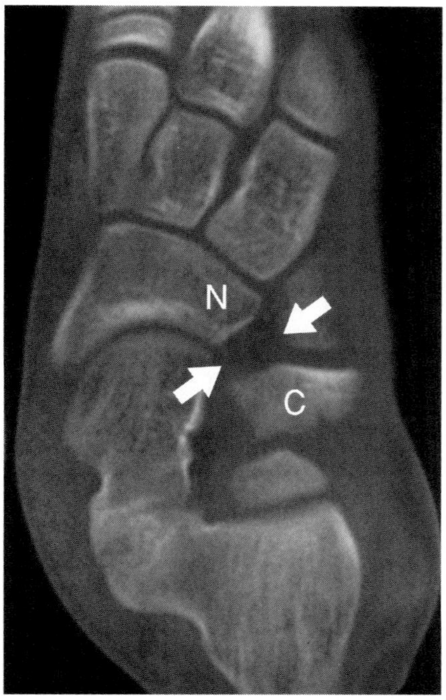

Figure 14-22. Normal appearance of the relationship between the calcaneus (C) and navicular bone (N) on CT. The calcaneonavicular space (arrows) is best seen on axial (long-axis) images. There are normally no articulation and some space between the two bones.

SUGGESTED READINGS

TARSAL COALITION

1. Beckly DE, Anderson PW, Pedegana LR. The radiology of the subtalar joint with special reference to talo-calcaneal coalition. Clin Radiol 1975; 26:333–341
2. Conway JJ, Cowell HR. Tarsal coalition: clinical significance and roentgenographic demonstration. Radiology 1969; 92:799–811
3. Downey MS. Tarsal coalitions: a surgical classification. J Am Podiatr Med Assoc 1991; 81:187–197
4. Emery KH, Bisset GS III, Johnson ND, Nunan PJ. Tarsal coalition: a blinded comparison of MRI and CT. Pediatr Radiol 1998; 28:612–616
5. Herschel H, von Ronnen JR. The occurrence of calcaneonavicular synosteosis in pes valgus contractus. J Bone Joint Surg [Am] 1950; 32:280
6. Ho CP. Magnetic resonance imaging of the ankle and foot. Semin Roentgenol 1995; 30:294–303
7. Oestreich AE, Mize WA, Crawford AH, Morgan RC Jr. The "anteater nose": a direct sign of calcaneonavicular coalition on the lateral radiograph. J Pediatr Orthop 1987; 7:709–711
8. Pachuda NM, Lasday SD, Jay RM. Tarsal coalition: etiology, diagnosis, and treatment. J Foot Surg 1990; 29:474–488
9. Shaffer HA Jr, Harrison RB. Tarsal pseudo-coalition—a positional artifact. J Can Assoc Radiol 1980; 31:236–237
10. Wechsler RJ, Karasick D, Schweitzer ME. Computed tomography of talocalcaneal coalition: imaging techniques. Skeletal Radiol 1992; 21: 353–358

STRESS FRACTURES

11. Aerts P, Disler DG. Abnormalities of the foot and ankle: MR imaging findings. AJR 1995; 165:119–124
12. John SD, Moorthy CS, Swischuk LE. Expanding the concept of the toddler's fracture. RadioGraphics 1997; 17:367–376
13. Swischuk LE. Painless limp. Pediatr Emerg Care 1992; 8:105–106
14. Swischuk LE. Leg pain with activity. Pediatr Emerg Care 1993; 9:53–54
15. Umans H, Pavlov H. Stress fractures of the lower extremities. Semin Roentgenol 1994; 29:176–193

FOREIGN BODIES

16. Donnelly LF, Frush DP, Bisset GS III. The multiple presentations of foreign bodies in children. AJR 1998; 170:471–477
17. O'Driscoll SW. Glass is detectable on plain radiographs. CMAJ 1988; 139:643–644
18. Monu JU, McManus CM, Ward WG, Haygood TM, Pope TL Jr, Bohrer SP. Soft-tissue masses caused by long-standing foreign bodies in the extremities: MR imaging findings. AJR 1995; 165:395–397
19. Roberts WC. Radiographic characteristics of glass. AJR 1972; 115:636–640
20. Shiels WE II, Babcock DS, Wilson JL, Burch RA. Localization and guided removal of soft-tissue foreign bodies with sonography. AJR 1990; 155: 1277–1281
21. Tandberg D. Glass in the hand and foot. Will an X-ray film show it? JAMA 1982; 248:1872–1874

FOOT ANATOMY

22. Herring C. Nomenclature for imaging planes of the feet. AJR 1997; 168: 277–278
23. Moore KL. Clinically oriented anatomy. 3rd ed. Baltimore: Williams & Wilkins; 1992:4–30
24. Preidler KW, Wang YC, Brossmann J, Trudell D, Daenen B, Resnick D. Tarsometatarsal joint: anatomic details on MR images. Radiology 1996; 199:733–736

CASE 15

Marta Hernanz-Schulman, M.D.

Lipomyelocele

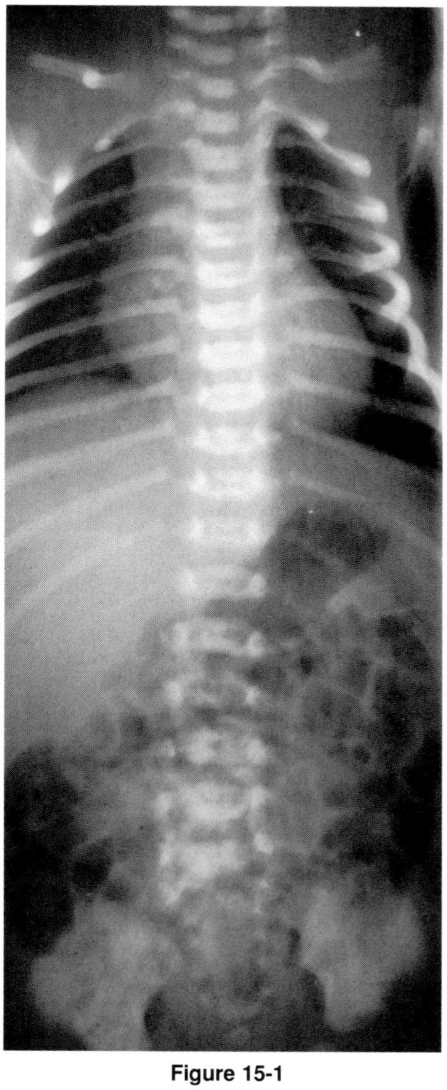

Figure 15-1

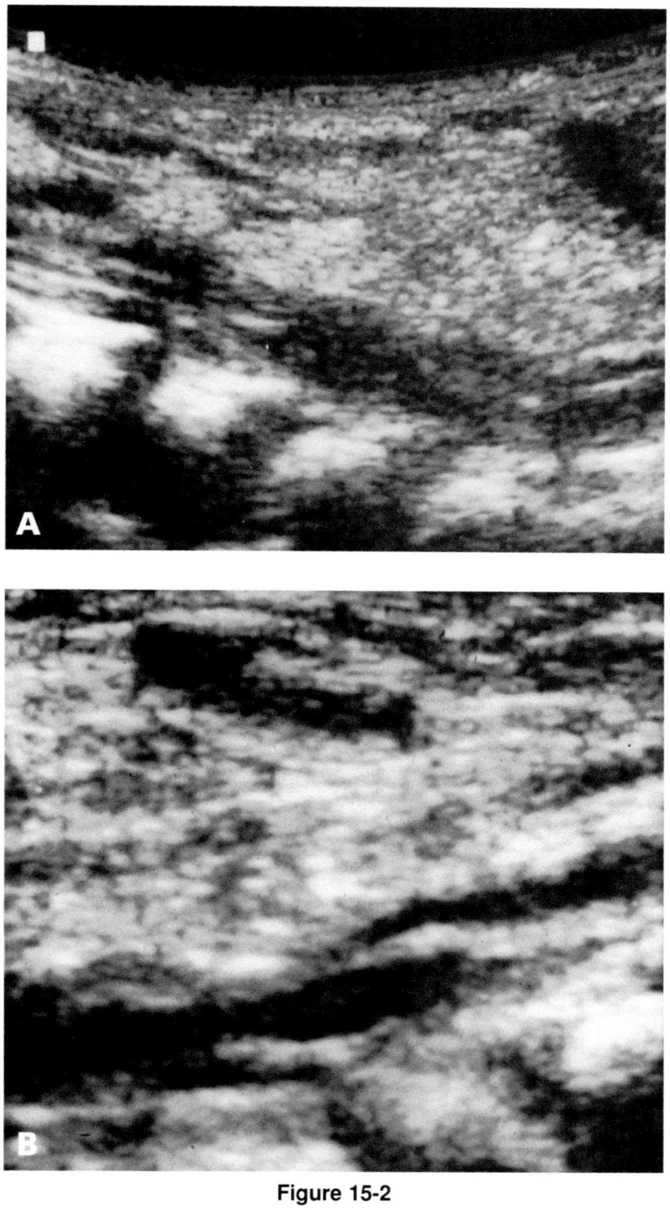

Figure 15-2

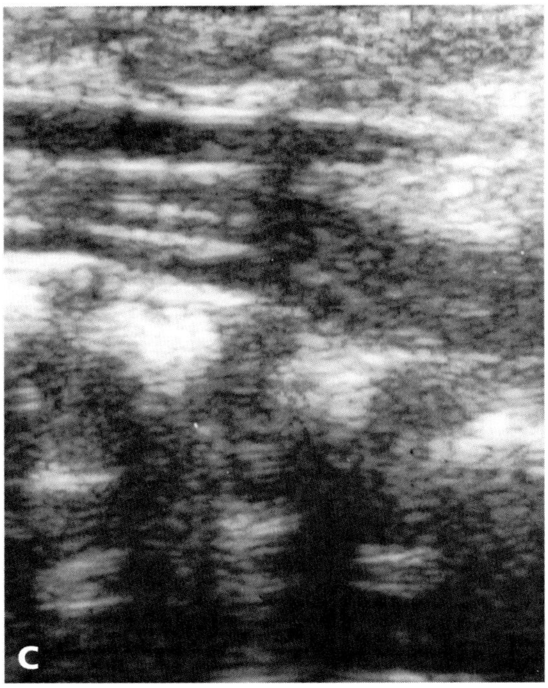

Figure 15-2 (Continued)

Question 74

This newborn infant has soft tissue fullness of the lower back on physical examination. You are shown a radiograph (Figure 15-1) and three longitudinal sonograms of the spine (Figure 15-2).

Which *one* of the following is the MOST likely diagnosis?

(A) Hemangioma
(B) Lipomyelocele
(C) Myelocystocele
(D) Myelomeningocele
(E) Sacrococcygeal teratoma

The test patient's frontal abdominal radiograph (Figure 15-1) demonstrates mild widening of the spinal canal at L4 and L5 (Figure 15-3). A longitudinal sonogram of the lumbosacral spinal canal (Figure 15-2A) taken with a 3.75-MHz transducer illustrates highly echogenic material, consistent with fat, extending from the subcutaneous tissue into the spinal canal and flattening the unneurulated neural tissue, or placode, against the vertebral bodies along the ventral boundary of the spinal canal (Figure 15-4A). The L5-S1 junction can be recognized by the characteristic lumbosacral lordotic curve described by the vertebral bodies. The image (Figure 15-2B) obtained with a 7.5-MHz linear transducer outlines the termination of the tethered cord at the S1-S2 level (Figure 15-4B). More rostrally, the superior extension of the fatty mass within the spinal canal above the area of bony defect is outlined (Figures 15-2C and 15-4C). These findings are characteristic of lipomyelocele **(Option (B) is correct)**. A CT scan (Figure 15-5) clearly demonstrates the fatty mass extending into the spinal canal through the dorsal bony defect. A T1-weighted MR image (Figure 15-6) from a subsequent MRI examination, performed to further assess the abnormality, demonstrates the short T1 relaxation time of the fatty lesion and the extension of this high-intensity tissue into the spinal canal.

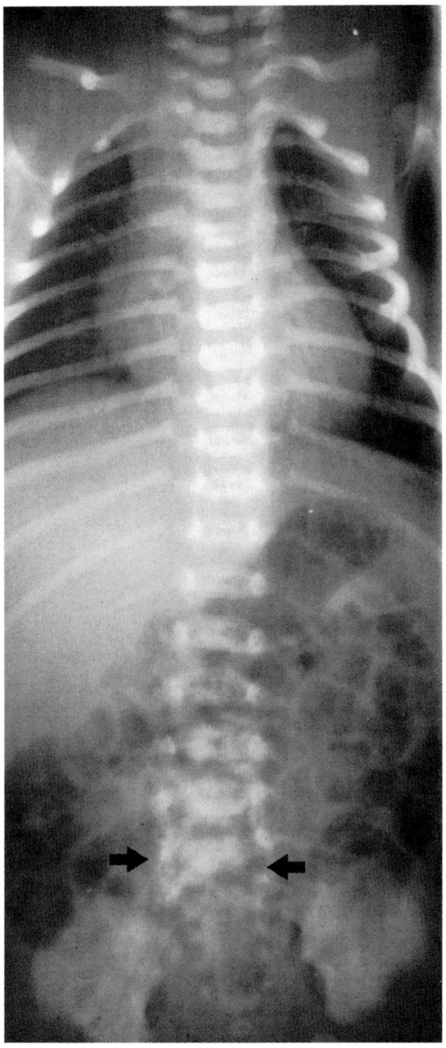

Figure 15-3 (Same as Figure 15-1). Lipomyelocele. A frontal radiograph of the chest and abdomen shows subtle, but definite, widening of the spinal canal at the lumbosacral junction (arrows).

Embryologically, central mesodermal cells coalesce into the notochordal process during the third week of gestation. This structure induces the differentiation of the overlying ectoderm into a thick plate of columnar pseudostratified neuroepithelium or neuroectoderm, the neural plate. The neural plate appears near the cranial end of the embryo and differentiates craniocaudally (Figure 15-7). During the fourth week of gestation, the flat neural plate infolds into the neural tube by a process termed neurulation. A central neural cleft or groove (Figure 15-7), thought to be induced by the notochord and by the longitudinal growth of the embryo, acts as a hinge around which the thickened lateral edges of the neural plate infold and come into contact in the midline. The dorsal surface of the neural plate now becomes the central portion of the neurulated

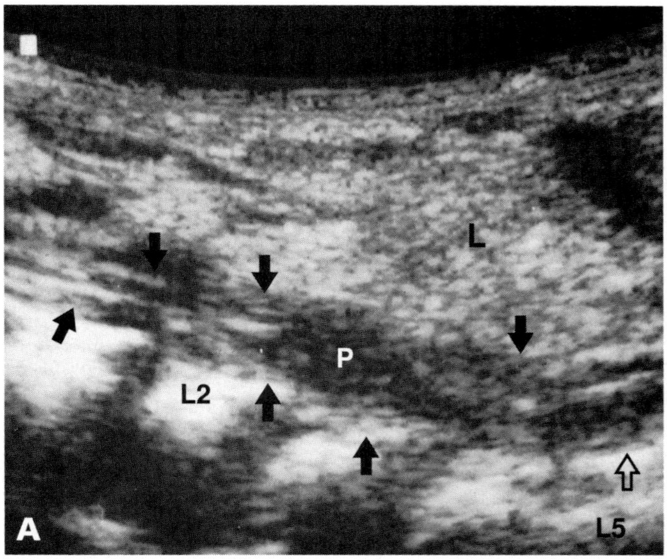

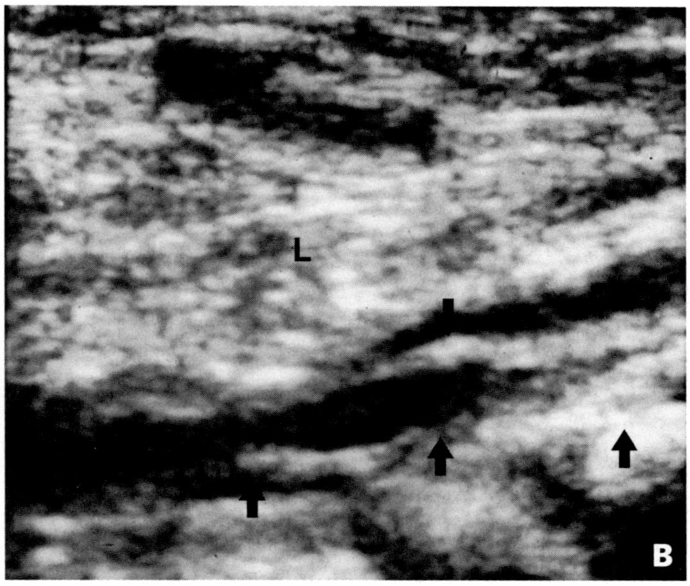

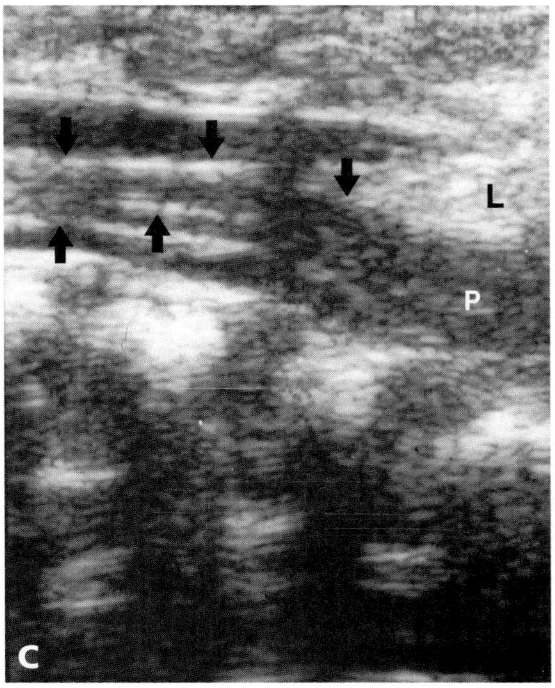

Figure 15-4 (Same as Figure 15-2). Lipomyelocele. (A) A longitudinal sonogram (3.75-MHz curvilinear transducer) along the back of the infant shows the lesion suggested by the clinical findings and by the frontal radiograph. Highly echogenic material consistent with fat (lipoma, L) extends from the subcutaneous tissues into the spinal canal. The cord (solid arrows) is tethered beyond L5 (open arrow). Note that the echogenic line in the central portion of the cord is not seen at the level of the placode (P), which begins at approximately L2. (B) A longitudinal sonogram (7.5-MHz linear transducer) just caudal to that in panel A outlines the termination of the tethered cord (arrows) at S1-S2, with lipoma (L) dorsally. (C) A longitudinal sonogram (7.5-MHz linear transducer) just cephalad to that in panel A illustrates more clearly the invasion of the spinal canal by lipoma (L) and the loss of the echogenic central line of the cord (arrows) at the placode (P).

cord, enclosing the neural canal. As the lips of the neural tube fuse by a process of cell recognition, the overlying ectoderm is pulled dorsally and its lateral margins fuse, detaching the neural tube from the overlying surface ectoderm, a process known as disjunction (Figure 15-8). Neurulation is thought to begin at the craniocervical junction and to progress bidirectionally.

The caudal end of the neural tube, filum terminale, and caudal neural coverings are formed by a related, but separate, process called secondary neurulation or retrogressive differentiation. In the caudal end of the embryo, the notochord and overlying neuroepithelium fuse, dorsal to the cloaca. During the fifth week of gestation, the cells of this caudal cell mass form multiple microcysts; these cavities fuse along their central axis, and the resultant lumen joins with the neural canal.

Abnormalities in the formation of the spinal cord and its investing structures are termed spinal dysraphism. This heterogeneous group of anomalies can be subdivided into several categories. One system, outlined by Barkovich, is based on their embryologic origin. Abnormalities of neurulation include nondisjunction, which results in failure of closure of the neural tube and of separation from overlying ectoderm (e.g., meningocele, meningomyelocele). Premature disjunction results from premature separation of the neuroectoderm from the overlying ectoderm, allowing the surrounding mesenchyma to migrate into the overlying neural plate, where it differentiates into fat and prevents closure of the neural tube (e.g., lipomyelocele, lipomeningomyelocele). Both of these types of anomalies result in failure of neurulation of the neural tube, and the resultant

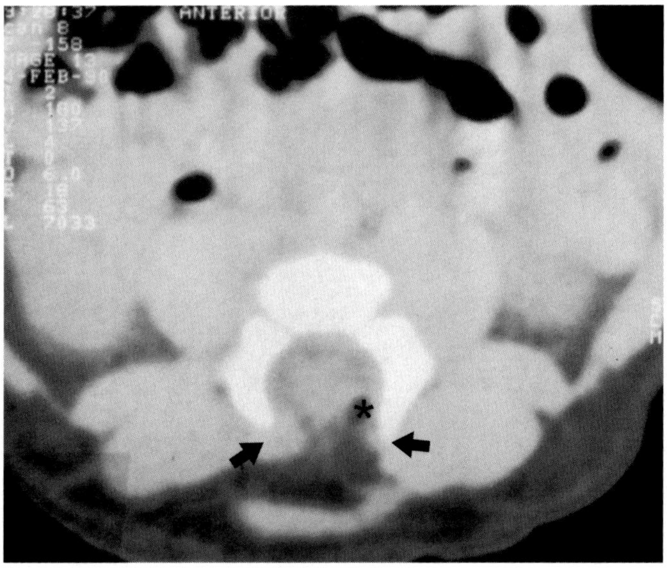

Figure 15-5. Same patient as in Figures 15-1 through 15-4. Lipomyelocele. A CT image obtained at the lumbosacral junction demonstrates the spinal dysraphism (arrows) and the subcutaneous fat (*) in the spinal canal.

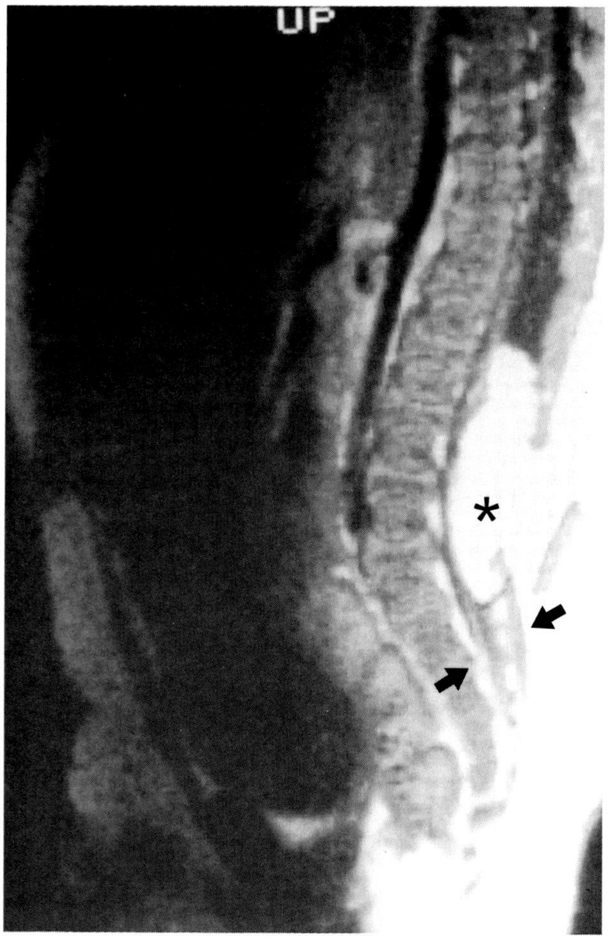

Figure 15-6. Same patient as in Figures 15-1 through 15-5. Lipomyelocele. A sagittal T1-weighted MR image confirms the fatty mass (*) encroaching into the spinal canal and the cord termination at S2 (arrows).

neural tissue is termed the neural placode. The third broad type of abnormality encompasses anomalies of the caudal cell mass, including abnormalities of the filum (tight filum, lipoma of the filum, caudal regression syndrome, and terminal myelocystocele).

Another classification, outlined by Byrd et al., is based on the clinical manifestations of the lesion. The first type includes those lesions that lack a skin covering (myelocele and myelomeningocele). The second type includes those lesions that are skin covered and associated with a subcutaneous mass (lipomyelocele, lipomyelomeningocele, and myelocele). The last type are those cases of spinal dysraphism that are clinically occult (including diastematomyelia, anterior sacral meningocele, hydromyelia, lateral thoracic meningocele, and the continuum of sacral agenesis).

The normal conus terminates at L2 or above at term. Termination at L3 is indeterminate as an isolated finding; termination below L3 is unequivocally abnormal. The normal conus is thicker than the remainder of the cord, but tapers rapidly, resembling a sharpened pencil (Figure 15-9). The normal cauda equina is echogenic, but its linear, closely apposed echoes representing the nerve roots are easily differentiated from the amorphously echogenic material seen in the soft tissue mass of the test patient.

Hemangiomas (Option (A)) are benign tumors that are common in young infants, occurring in approximately 2% to 3% of newborns. They typically undergo a period of rapid growth, followed by involution. Approximately 40% occur in the head and neck region and 30% occur in the trunk. Hemangiomas in the lumbosacral region, on or about the midline, undergo involution in a manner similar to that of those found elsewhere; however, these lesions are considered harbingers of occult spinal dysraphism, and affected patients are at high risk for underlying cord tethering. Therefore, it is important to recognize the significance of a lumbosacral hemangioma in an infant, even if the patient is asymptomatic, since the lesion may no longer be present when the child grows and symptoms of tethering are manifested. In the clinical setting of the test case, a hemangioma would be manifested as a typical cutaneous abnormality, which in this location would be an indicator of underlying spinal dysraphism. The test patient has imaging findings characteristic of lipomyelocele and, although this is a type of spinal dysraphism, a hemangioma was not present at physical examination of this neonate.

Myelocystocele (Option (C)) refers to a cystic dilatation of the central canal of the spinal cord that protrudes through a spinal defect as a skin-covered mass. A myelocystocele occurring at the termination of the cord is known as a terminal myelocystocele. These lesions are characterized by variable dilatation, or meningocele, of the distal subarachnoid space, traversed by the cord, which in turn terminates in a large cyst that is lined by ependyma and is continuous with the central canal of the cord (Figure 15-10). Although there can be a variable amount of extradural fat associated with the sac of a myelocystocele, the diagnosis is made by demonstration of hydromyelia, continuous

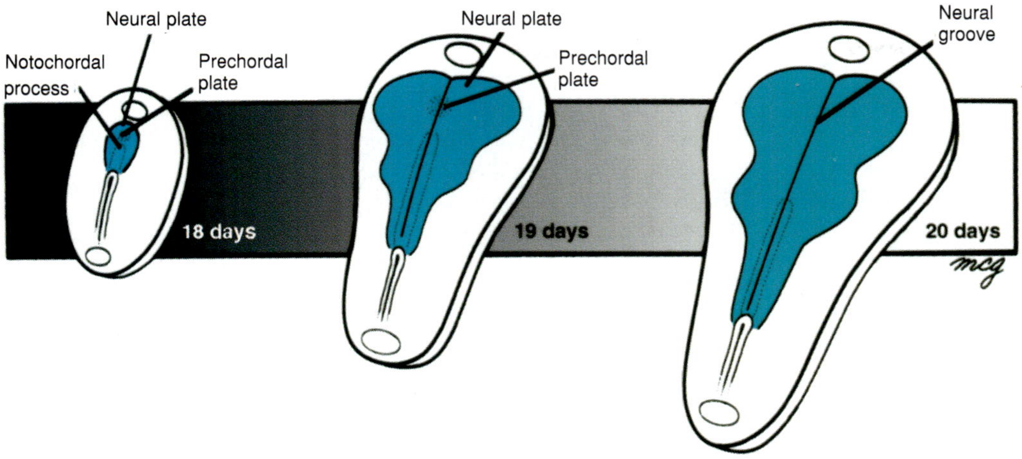

Figure 15-7. Central neural cleft. Schematic diagram illustrating the unneurulated neural plate and neural groove and their relationship to the notochordal process. (Reprinted with permission from Larsen [1].)

with the dilated fluid-filled sac, coursing through the variably distended distal subarachnoid space, or meningocele. These findings are not present in the test images.

Myelomeningocele (Option (D)) is a lesion that results from nondisjunction and failure of neurulation of the neural plate. As a result, this lesion is not covered with skin, but consists of exposure of the neural placode, which is visible and attached laterally to the edges of the surrounding skin surfaces. In patients with myelomeningocele, there is ventral accumulation of cerebrospinal fluid (CSF), elevating the placode above the plane of the patient's back. In patients with myelocele, ventral accumulation of CSF is lacking, resulting in the placode being located along the plane of the patient's back (Figure 15-11). In the test images, the lesion is covered with skin.

Sacrococcygeal teratoma (Option (E)) is a caudal neoplasm characterized by pluripotential cells giving rise to a wide variety of tissues at various stages of maturation. These represent approximately 40% of germ cell tumors. They are located caudal to the sacrum and can extend into the pelvis and abdomen, between the sacrum and rectum. Sacrococcygeal teratomas are grouped into four major types according to their size and location. Type I teratomas are largely external, with a

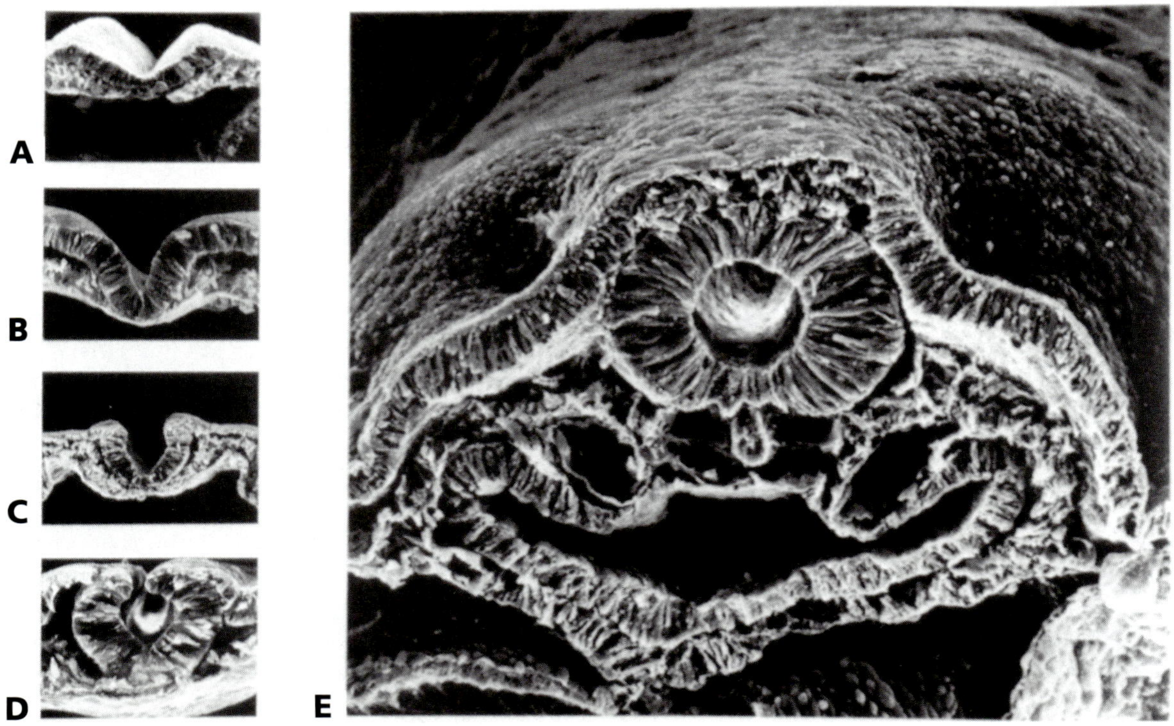

Figure 15-8. Disjunction. Scanning photomicrographs illustrate the sequence of neurulation (A to C) and disjunction (D to E). The infolding of the neural plate about the neural groove and the separation and subsequent union of the superficial ectodermal layer are well seen. (Reprinted with permission from Larsen [1].)

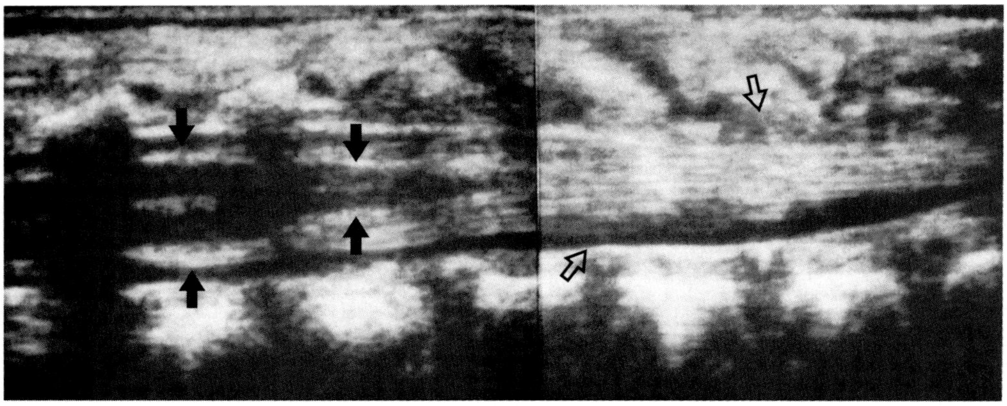

Figure 15-9. Normal cord and spine. A composite sonogram of the normal cord (solid arrows) in an infant (7.5-MHz linear transducer). Note the gradual distal tapering of the cord and the orderly linear arrangement of nerve roots in the cauda equina more distally (open arrows).

minimal intrapelvic component; type II teratomas contain a large external component, but have significant presacral extension; type III teratomas are characterized by a large intrapelvic and abdominal portion, with a smaller external component (Figure 15-12); type IV teratomas are entirely presacral, without an external component (Figure 15-13). Types with an external component present as skin-covered mass lesions below the coccyx in the neonate; the soft tissue fullness over the lower back present in the test case is not typical of teratomas. Approximately 2% can extend into the sacral canal (Figure 15-14). Unlike the abnormality in the test images, most of these lesions are either cystic or both solid and cystic, and cord tethering does not occur. Furthermore, the bulk of the teratoma extends into the pelvis anterior to the sacrum, rather than along the dorsal surface of the placode, as in the test patient.

Microscopically, teratomas are composed of mature, immature, or malignant elements. The mature lesions contain well-differentiated tissues, such as brain, gastrointestinal elements, skin, and bone. Immature lesions contain embryonic neuroglial or neuroepithelial cells. These are subdivided into four grades, 0 through 3, depending on their mitotic activity and the number of immature elements present. Malignant tumors contain one or more of the malignant germ cell types, such as embryonal carcinoma or endodermal sinus tumor, in addition to mature or immature elements. In general, younger patients with immature teratomas tend to have a better prognosis than older patients. Although most sacrococcygeal tumors are benign at birth, a delay in diagnosis permits malignant degeneration. The frequencies of malignancy when the

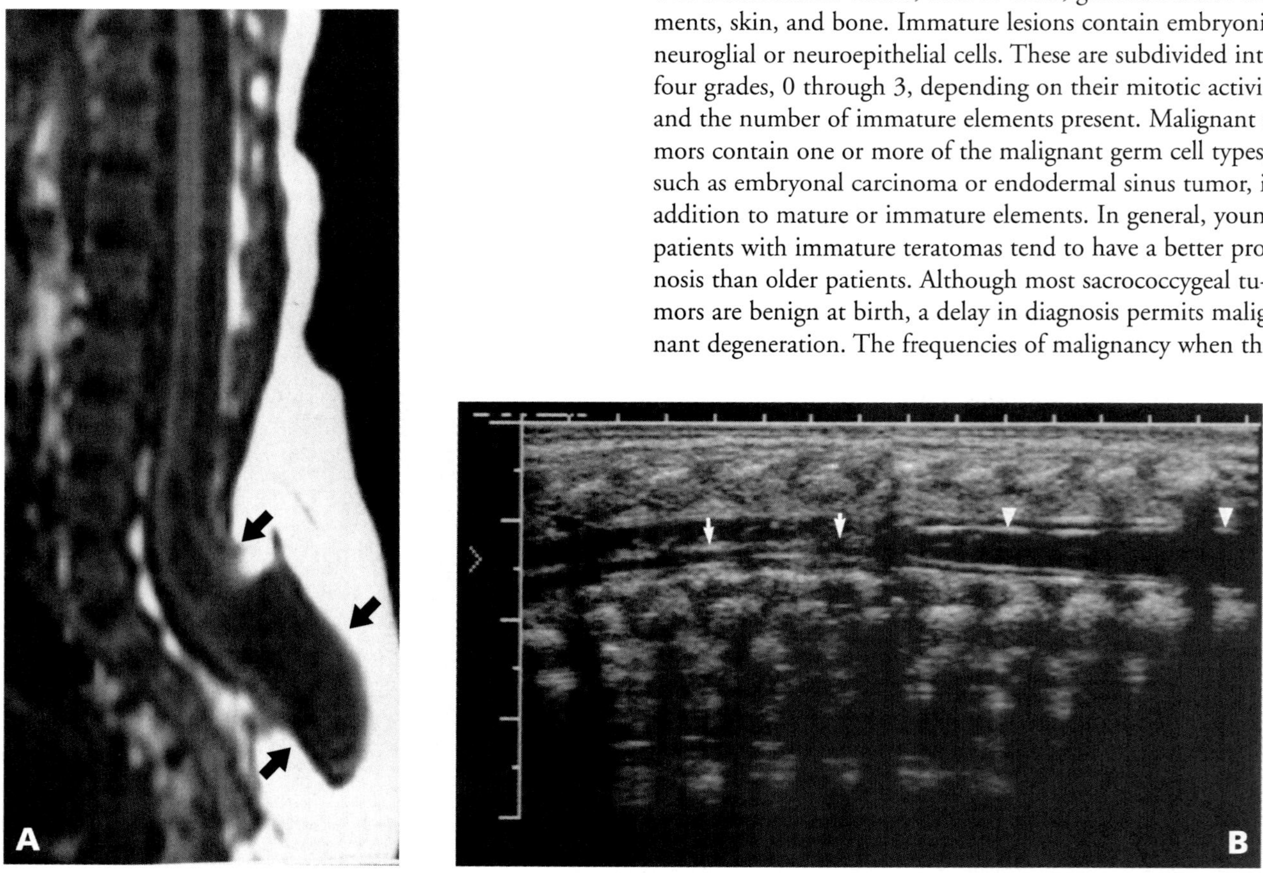

Figure 15-10. Myelocystocele. (A) A longitudinal T1-weighted image in 1-month-old infant with cloacal exstrophy demonstrates progressive caudal dilatation of the central canal of the cord, which surrounds the cystic protrusion into the back in a "trumpetlike" configuration (arrows). (Case courtesy of Patrick Barnes, Boston Children's Hospital, Boston, Mass.; reprinted with permission from Appignani et al. [16]). (B) A longitudinal composite sonogram of another patient with terminal myelocystocele demonstrates the junction of the normal cord (arrows) with hydromyelic cord (arrowheads), cephalad to the terminal cyst.

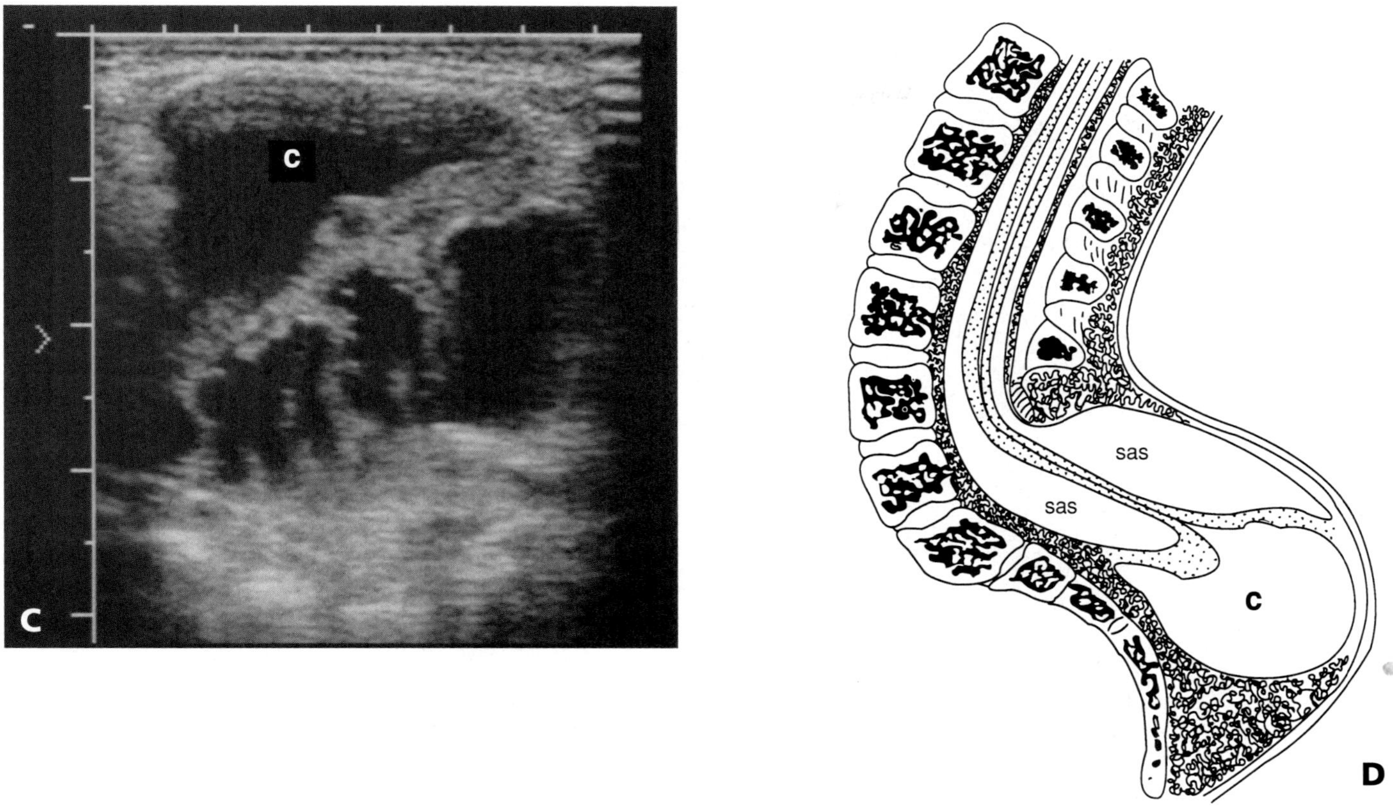

Figure 15-10 (Continued). Myelocystocele. (C) Same patient as in panel B. Longitudinal sonogram of terminal cyst (c). (D) Diagrammatic illustration of the components of terminal myelocystocele. c = terminal cystic expansion of the central canal of the tethered cord (stippled). The expansion of the subarachnoid space or meningocele (sas) surrounds the distal cord. Note that the defect is skincovered. (Reprinted with permission from Barkovich [17].)

diagnosis is made before the age of 2 months are approximately 10% in boys and 7% in girls; however, if the diagnosis is made after the age of 2 months, the frequencies increase to 67% in boys and 47% in girls.

Staging of extragonadal germ cell tumors differentiates them into four groups. Stage I refers to completely resected lesions limited to one organ or structure; stage II includes completely resected lesions extending to more than one adjacent organ or structure, including tumors requiring more than one excision for removal, accomplished without tumor spillage; stage III refers to incompletely resected tumors, including those with tumor spillage during surgery; stage IV indicates disseminated disease. Treatment is surgical and can require both transsacral and abdominal approaches for large tumors with extensive intrapelvic and abdominal extension. Removal of the coccyx is mandatory in order to prevent tumor recurrence.

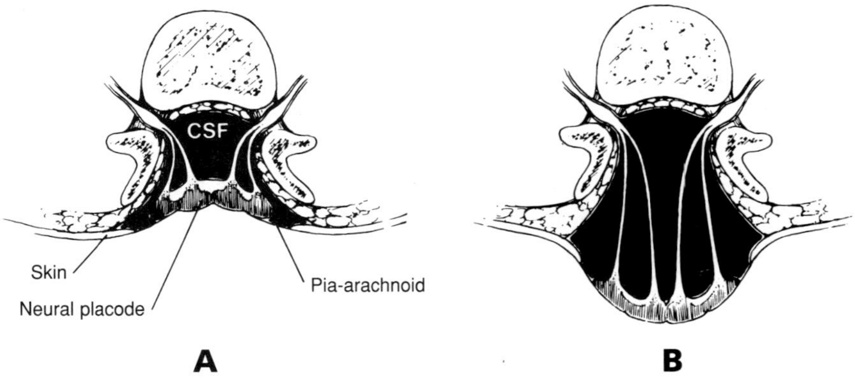

Figure 15-11. Meningocele and myelomeningocele. (A) Meningocele. Diagrammatic representation of the neural placode and the lack of meningeal and cutaneous investment of the flat neural tissue, which is exposed to the external environment. The nerve roots arise from the ventral surface of the placode, and the dorsal roots are placed laterally with respect to the more medially oriented ventral roots. (B) Myelomeningocele. Diagrammatic representation illustrating the expansion of the ventral subarachnoid space, leading to protrusion of neural elements above the plane of the patient's back. (Reprinted with permission from Barkovich [17].)

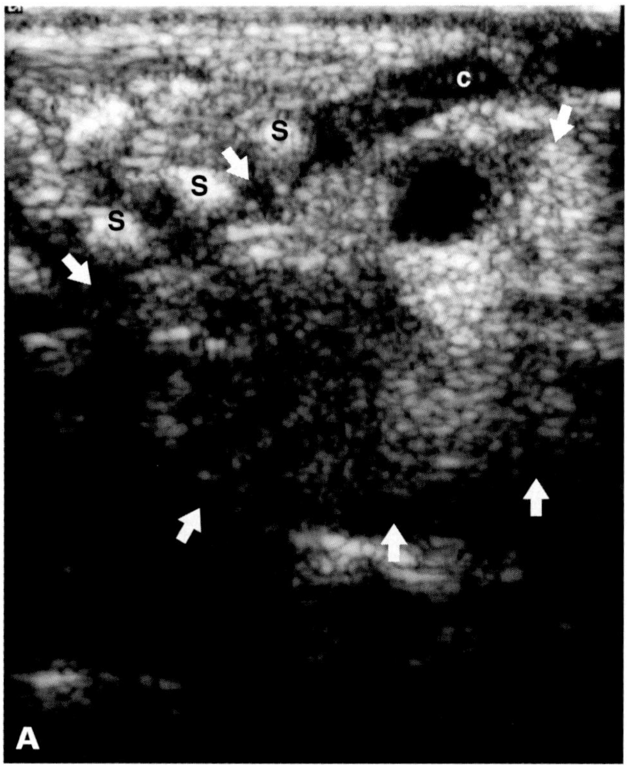

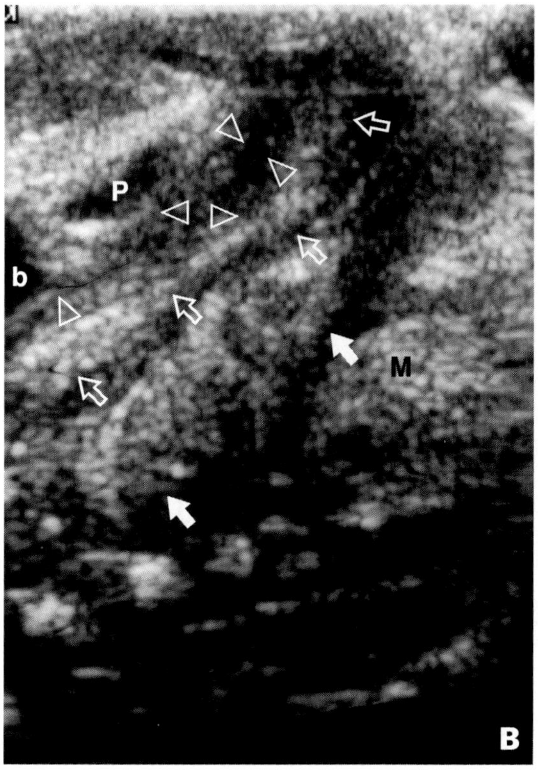

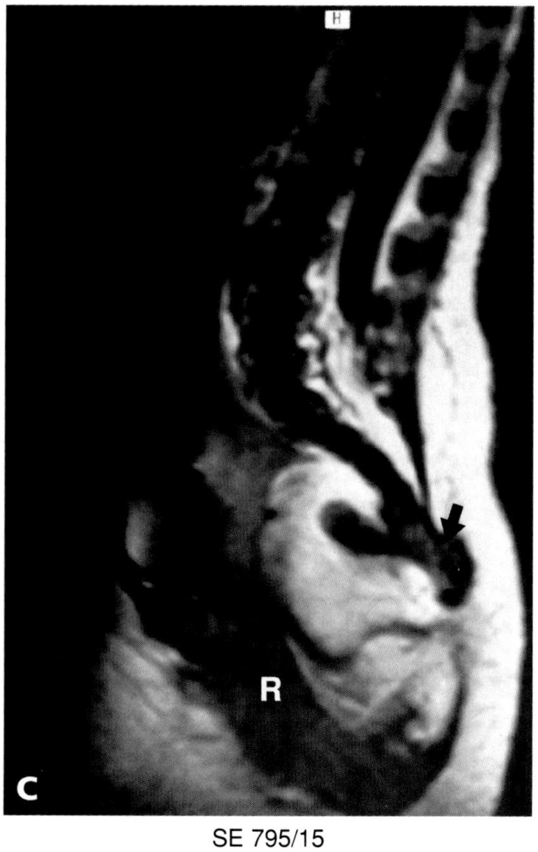

SE 795/15

Figure 15-12. Type III sacrococcygeal teratoma. (A) A longitudinal sonogram (7- to 10-MHz linear transducer) along the back of a newborn premature infant in the neonatal intensive care unit, with a very small, skin-covered mass between the buttocks, shows extension of the lesion (arrows) deep relative to the cartilaginous coccyx and sacrum. S = sacral vertebrae; c = coccyx. (B) A transperineal sonogram outlines the relationship of the mass (M) to the rectum (solid arrows), vagina (open arrows), bladder (b), urethra (arrowheads), and cartilaginous symphysis pubis (P). (C) A sagittal T1-weighted MR image clearly demonstrates the presacral extension of the lipomatous and cystic mass and its relationship to the coccyx (arrow). This examination was performed 7 months after the images in panels A and B were obtained, at a corrected gestational age of approximately 4 months. At this time, the mass was not palpable. R = rectum.

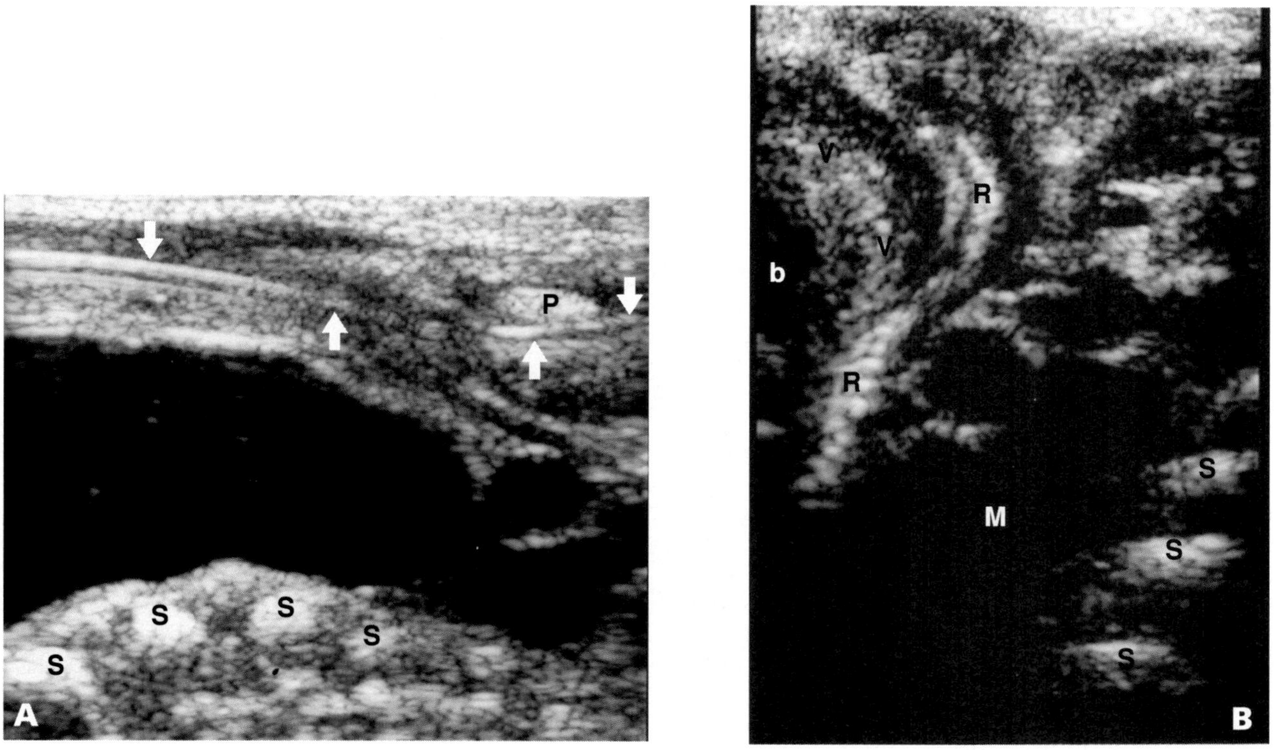

Figure 15-13. Type IV sacrococcygeal teratoma. (A) A midline longitudinal sonogram (7- to 10-MHz linear transducer) was obtained for a premature infant diagnosed *in utero* with bilateral hydronephrosis and a cystic pelvic mass. There was no visible extrapelvic component to the lesion. The examination outlines the symphysis pubis (P) and an echogenic catheter introduced through the urethra (arrows) to decompress the bladder, which is displaced superiorly above the image plane. The cystic mass contains internal septation and lies apposed to the lumbar and sacral vertebrae (S). (B) A transperineal sonogram clearly demonstrates the multiple septations of the mass (M), with some intervening echogenic components, and its location between the sacral vertebrae (S) and the rectum (R). b = bladder; V = vagina.

Question 75

Concerning lipomyelocele,

(A) it most often occurs in the lower thoracic region
(B) it is invariably associated with cord tethering
(C) surgery is not indicated in asymptomatic patients
(D) vertebral segmentation anomalies are present in nearly all patients
(E) it is synonymous with lipoma of the filum terminale

Lipomyeloceles and lipomyelomeningoceles are lesions in which a lipomatous mass extends in continuity from the subcutaneous tissues to the dorsal surface of the neural placode through an open vertebral defect (Figure 15-15A). These lesions are postulated to occur as a result of premature disjunction of the neural tube from the overlying ectoderm, before closure. Normally, disjunction does not occur until after the neural tube has closed; surrounding mesenchyma then migrates into this space and is induced to form meninges, neural arches, and paraspinal musculature. Premature disjunction, before closure of the neural tube, permits migrating mesenchyma to contact the interior of the neural tube, where it is induced to become fat.

Lipomyelomeningocele differs from lipomyelocele in that

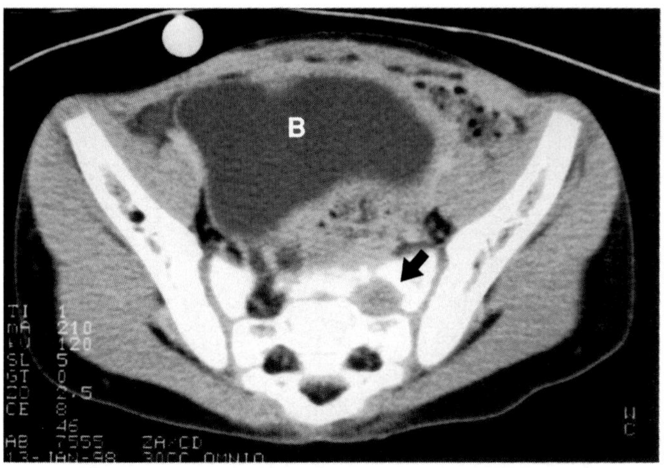

Figure 15-14. Recurrent teratoma. A CT scan of a 6-year-old patient with recurrence of sacrococcygeal teratoma demonstrates invasion into the sacral foramina on the left (arrow). B = bladder.

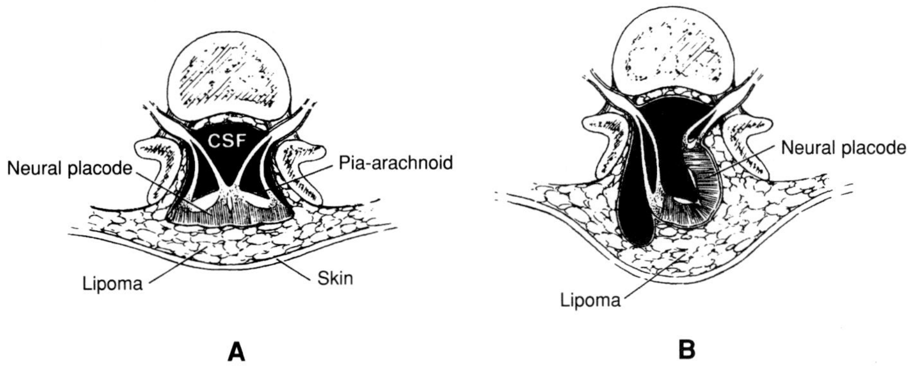

Figure 15-15. Lipomyelocele and lipomyelomeningocele. (A) Diagrammatic representation of lipomyelocele illustrating the neural placode and its investment by lipoma and intact skin. Note that the nerve roots arise from the ventral surface of the placode, with lateral positioning of the dorsal nerve roots with respect to the medial placement of the ventral nerve roots. (B) Diagrammatic representation of lipomyelomeningocele. Expansion of the subarachnoid space leads to elevation of the lesion above the plane of the back. Note asymmetric protrusion of the meningocele. (Reprinted with permission from Barkovich [17].)

there is also dilatation of the underlying CSF spaces, elevating the lesion and leading to a more clinically obvious subcutaneous mass. These lesions occur in the lumbosacral region **(Option (A) is false),** account for approximately 20% of skin-covered lumbosacral masses and 50% of occult spinal dysraphism, and are approximately one fourth as common as meningomyeloceles. The lipoma is attached to the dorsal surface of the placode, which is lined by fibrous tissue and neuroglia, rather than ependyma. The dura is dorsally open at this level and the cord is invariably tethered, with a junction of dura, fibrous tissue, neural tissue, and lipoma at the lateral margins of the placode; fibrovascular bands are also present above and below the boundaries of the spina bifida defect, contributing to the tethering of the cord **(Option (B) is true).** The cord can terminate at the level of the placode (Figure 15-16) or can be reconstituted distally. The lipoma can extend cephalad along the central canal of the spinal cord or along its dorsal surface (Figure 15-2C and 15-4C). Failure of neurulation with persistence of the placode leads to the exit of the dorsal nerve roots laterally and the ventral nerve roots medially from the ventral aspect of the placode (Figure 15-15). If the lipoma is asymmetric, the placode is rotated so that the dorsal surface, in contact with the lipoma, is rotated toward the side of the lipoma, consequently rotating the site and direction of the exiting nerve roots and bringing the contralateral dorsal roots toward the midline, where they could be damaged during surgical repair. In patients with lipomyelomeningocele, the meningocele is rotated toward the contralateral side to protrude dorsally, adjacent to the lipoma (Figure 15-15B).

In approximately 75% to 90% of cases, cutaneous or subcutaneous abnormalities alert the clinician to the possibility of an underlying occult dysraphic state. Lesions that suggest a high probability of underlying spinal dysraphism include subcutaneous nodules (lipoma, neural tissue, or cyst), skin tags or "taillike" appendages, hypertrichosis, hemangioma, dermal pits, or aplasia cutis. In patients with lipomyelocele without lipomyelomeningocele, the lipomatous mass can be subtle; in older patients, an alerting hemangioma can have undergone involution if not detected during infancy. Although urodynamic testing reveals abnormal lower urinary tract function in about one third of newborns, most patients are asymptomatic at birth. On the other hand, 92% of patients older than 3 years have evidence of an upper or lower motor neuron lesion on urodynamic testing or show neurologic signs of lower-extremity dysfunction. Typical symptoms in these older patients include gait abnormalities with hammertoes and highly arched feet (pes cavus), ankle weakness, asymmetry in strength and muscle mass between the lower extremities, urinary and fecal incontinence after an initial period of successful toilet training, absent perineal sensation, and back and testicular pain. Once neurologic symptoms occur, the potential for reversibility is dependent on the promptness of surgical release and is in the range of 25% to 50%. The progression of symptoms can be insidious or

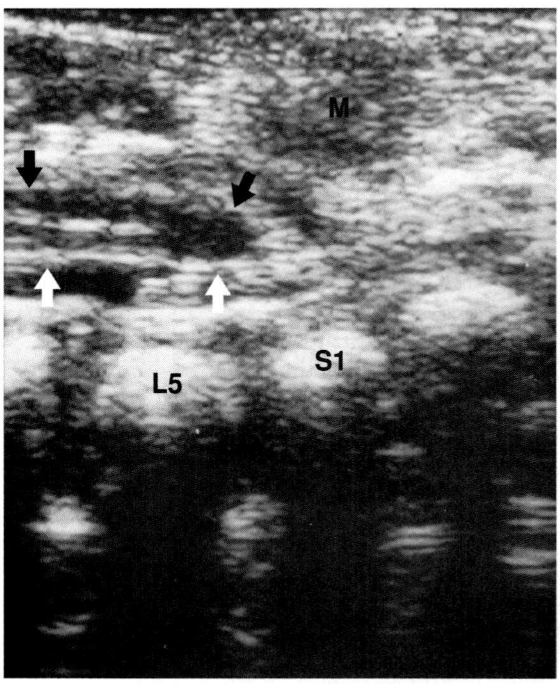

Figure 15-16. Lipomyelocele. A longitudinal midline sonogram of a neonate with a skin-covered lumbrosacral mass shows a lack of posterior bony elements. A heterogeneous soft tissue mass (M) extends into the spinal canal at the termination of the cord (arrows) at the L5-S1 junction, identified by the lordotic spinal curvature.

precipitous. Older patients are at a greater risk of irreversible neurologic damage. Thus, although surgical repair is not urgent in the neonate, it should be undertaken early, prior to the onset of symptoms (**Option (C) is false**). Experimental data in human and animal subjects suggest that electrophysiologic dysfunction is related to impairment of mitochondrial oxidative metabolism in the tethered cord. Approximately 10% to 25% of patients may have no cutaneous stigmata to alert the clinician to the presence of occult spinal dysraphism, and the condition in these patients is unlikely to be detected before the onset of symptoms.

Patients who have typical lesions undergo imaging examinations to evaluate the extent of spinal dysraphism. Radiographs typically show a widening of the spinal canal at the level of the posterior spinal defect, as in the test patient. Sacral agenesis and segmentation anomalies can be seen in as many as 50% of patients (**Option (D) is false**).

Sonography is advocated in many centers as a useful, inexpensive, and noninvasive tool in the screening of infants suspected of having occult spinal dysraphism. The current literature indicates that a negative sonographic examination is highly predictive of a normal cord and spinal canal. MRI is considered the gold standard and is the examination of choice for the complete evaluation of these lesions. T1-weighted, thinly collimated (2- to 3-mm) images in the sagittal and axial planes are best for the preoperative delineation of these lesions.

The filum terminale is a thin band of fibrous tissue that originates at the conus and inserts along the roof of the spinal canal, at the dorsal surface of C1. Lipoma of the filum terminale refers to a variable amount of fat within either the intradural or extradural portion of the filum terminale or along its entire length. The conus lies in the normal position, and the patients are asymptomatic. Isolated lipomas of the filum terminale can be identified in as many as 6% of normal individuals at autopsy, and an area within the filum of low density on CT or high intensity on T1-weighted MRI is usually an incidental finding in patients being imaged for other reasons. Lipoma or fibrolipoma of the filum terminale, as an isolated finding, is not associated with myeloschisis and is not synonymous with lipomyelocele or lipomyelomeningocele (**Option (E) is false**).

The tight filum syndrome is a symptomatic lesion associated with cord tethering. The conus is typically low-lying and the filum is abnormally short and thickened, measuring more than the normal 2 mm at the L5-S1 junction. The patients become symptomatic during periods of growth spurts through the mechanisms discussed earlier. Symptoms are typically worse after exercise and upon awakening. This situation is believed to be secondary to stretching of the cord during exercise and to lengthening of the spinal column by accumulation of water within intervertebral discs while supine during sleep. Nearly one half of the patients demonstrate alerting cutaneous stigmata, such as hypertrichosis and hemangioma, as previously discussed. Radiographs will often detect failure of posterior bony closure of one or several lumbosacral vertebrae. Sonography, MRI, or myelography will outline the typically low-lying position of the conus. The filum is thickened, and as many as one fourth of these patients may demonstrate an associated lipoma within the abnormal filum.

Question 76

Concerning myelocystocele,

(A) hydromyelia is present in more than 90% of patients
(B) it most often occurs at the caudal termination of the spinal cord
(C) vertebral anomalies are invariably present
(D) associated cloacal anomalies are present in most patients
(E) the cystocele usually communicates directly with the subarachnoid space

Myelocystocele is defined as a cystic dilatation of the central canal of the spinal cord that protrudes through a vertebral defect as a skin-covered mass (Figure 15-10). Therefore, hydromyelia is always present (**Option (A) is true**). Most myelocystoceles occur at the caudal end of the cord and are termed "terminal myelocystoceles" (**Option (B) is true**). These uncommon lesions represent approximately 4% to 8% of skin-covered lumbosacral masses.

Embryologically, the lesion has been postulated to arise from an obstruction to the passage of CSF in the central canal, leading to dilatation of the ventriculus terminalis. The expanding central canal disrupts the overlying mesenchyma, sparing the more distant, or superficial, ectoderm. Thus, there are failure of development and fusion of the overlying bony canal (i.e., spina bifida) (**Option (C) is true**), variable aggregates of lipomatous tissue, and an intact skin cover. The distended central canal spreads the surrounding spinal cord in a "trumpet-like" fashion and can extend distally beyond the sac of the meningocele into the extra-arachnoidal space. The overlying arachnoid is distended by the enlarging cyst, forming a meningocele (Figure 15-10).

In embryogenesis, development of the caudal end of the spinal canal is spatially and temporally related to the formation of the distal gastrointestinal and urinary tracts, which are formed from a common cloaca during the second month of gestation. The caudal cell mass lies dorsal to the cloaca and includes the notochord and cells destined to become the distal spinal cord. This temporal and spatial relationship leads to an association of these lesions with the spectrum of caudal regression syndrome, including sacral abnormalities, anal atresia and cloacal exstrophy with ambiguous and bifid genitalia, and the OEIS complex (omphalocele, exstrophy, imperforate anus, and spinal deformities). The terminal myelocystocele and other types of caudal dysgenesis of the cord can be seen as a spectrum of anomalies resulting from dysgenesis of the hind end of the embryo. Terminal myelocystocele has a high association (50% to 70%) with cloacal exstrophy (**Option (D) is true**). The presence and severity of cord anomalies correlate with the severity of the caudal abnormality. In a series of 92 patients with caudal anomalies, the prevalences of spinal lesions were as follows: 17% in patients with low imperforate anus; 34% in patients with high imperforate anus; 46% in patients with cloacal malformations; and 100% in patients with cloacal exstrophy.

Myelocystoceles are sporadic lesions with no proven teratogenic cause, although agents such as loperamide hydrochloride and retinoic acid can be implicated. Despite the frequency of sacral anomalies in patients with these lesions, maternal diabetes is not considered an etiologic or concurrent factor.

On imaging studies, the dilatation of the central canal in continuity with the cyst must be demonstrated for diagnosis of myelocystocele. The cystic dilatation of the canal extends into the skin-covered lesion. In terminal myelocystocele, the cystic central canal extends distally into the spinal canal beyond the confines of the expanded subarachnoid space, i.e., meningocele (Figure 15-10). On myelographic studies, the meningocele communicating with the subarachnoid space is readily demonstrated. However, the dilated central cyst does not directly communicate with the subarachnoid space surrounding the cord and initially appears as a large filling defect (**Option (E) is false**). On delayed CT images, contrast material can be found within the terminal cyst. The availability of MRI, with its detailed depiction of the anatomy, permitting demonstration of the origin of the central cyst, has obviated the more invasive myelographic diagnosis.

Question 77

Concerning myelomeningoceles,

(A) the dorsal surface of the placode corresponds to the central portion of the spinal canal
(B) about 5% are covered with skin
(C) cord tethering usually occurs as a postoperative complication
(D) the primary role of preoperative imaging is to evaluate the extent of the cord lesion

Myeloceles and myelomeningoceles are the most common congenital anomalies of the spine, occurring in approximately 0.2% of live births in the United States and Canada. Myelomeningocele differs from myelocele by the presence of an underlying dilatation of the subarachnoid space ventral to the placode, resulting in elevation of the placode above the skin surface of the infant, in a manner analogous to that of lipomyelomeningocele and lipomyelocele (Figure 15-11).

Myeloceles and myelomeningoceles are believed to occur as a result of nondisjunction of the neural ectoderm from the overlying ectoderm. As a result, there is failure of neurulation of the neural tube, which remains open so that what is normally the central portion of the tube lies along the dorsal surface of the patient; this unneurulated tissue is termed the "neural placode" (**Option (A) is true**). There are consequent failure of mesenchyma to migrate dorsal to the neural tissue and failure of formation of the overlying meninges. The open, interposed neural tissue does not permit closure of the ectodermal structures and, consequently, skin does not cover the lesion (**Option (B) is false**). The spinal canal is widened, and the pedicles are rotated from their normal anteroposterior or sagittal orientation into the coronal plane. The laminae are rotated or hypoplastic, and the spinal musculature is displaced laterally (Figure 15-17).

Cord tethering in these infants is present at birth, as the neural placode and the posterior margins of the incomplete dura blend with the surrounding, open ectodermal tissues (**Option (C) is false**). After repair of the myelomeningocele, patients have a stable neurologic deficit. Neurologic deterioration or development of a new neurologic deficit suggests retethering of the spinal cord, which can be caused by postoperative scarring and adhesions or by an associated malformation, including lipoma, dermoid, and a thickened or tight filum terminale. Approximately one third of infants have the associated diastematomyelia (Figure 15-18). MRI is helpful in diagnosis of associated lesions, although dermoids and epidermoids can be difficult to detect. Cord tethering is suggested if the cord is adherent to the surgical site (Figure 15-19). Analysis of cord motion varying with respiration on real-time sonography also can be helpful, since tethering is unlikely if normal cord motion is detected.

Preoperative spinal imaging is not usually performed in infants with myeloceles or myelomeningoceles, because the presence and extent of the defect are clinically obvious (**Option (D) is false**). Cranial imaging is indicated, either in the preoperative period or soon afterward, to detect the degree of ventriculomegaly associated with the Chiari II malformation, which is nearly always present in affected infants. Since ventriculomegaly is likely to worsen after repair of the cord lesion, postoperative brain imaging is indicated if shunting is not performed initially. Postoperative imaging of the spine is indicated for the detection of associated lesions leading to continued tethering or retethering, as discussed above, or of other lesions that can be present in these infants, including syringomyelia and ischemic changes.

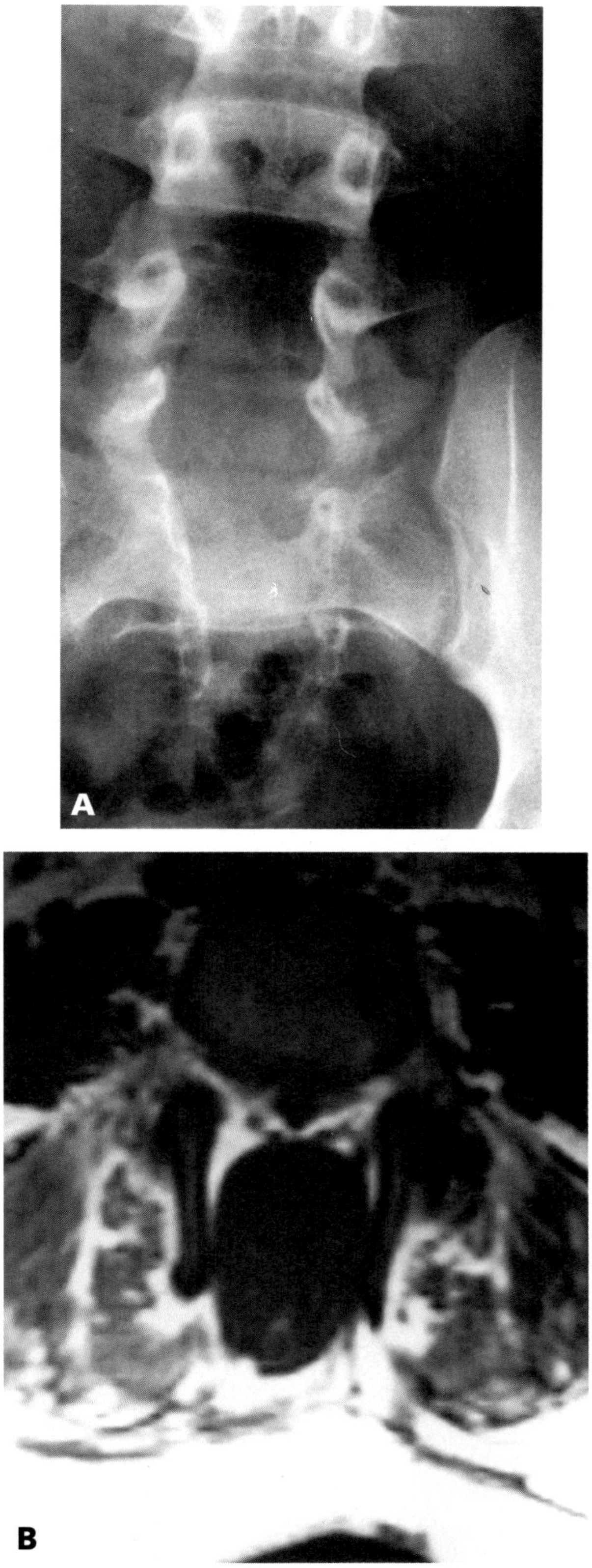

SE 750/15

Figure 15-17. Myelomeningocele. (A) A frontal radiograph of an adolescent patient with low lumbosacral myelomeningocele demonstrates the widening of the bony canal, pedicular rotation, and the absence of posterior laminae and spinous processes. Compare with the two normal lumbar vertebrae above the defect. (B) A T1-weighted MR image illustrates these vertebral abnormalities in the axial plane.

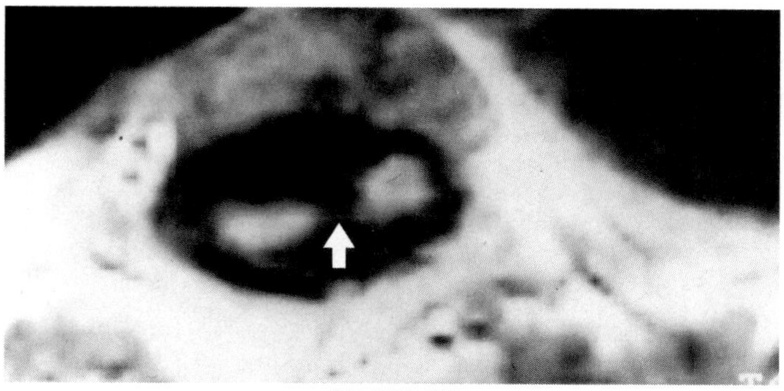

SE 750/15

Figure 15-18. Diastematomyelia. An axial T1-weighted MR image through the thoracic spine in a patient with myelomeningocele demonstrates diastematomyelia (arrow), with separation of the spinal cord into two components.

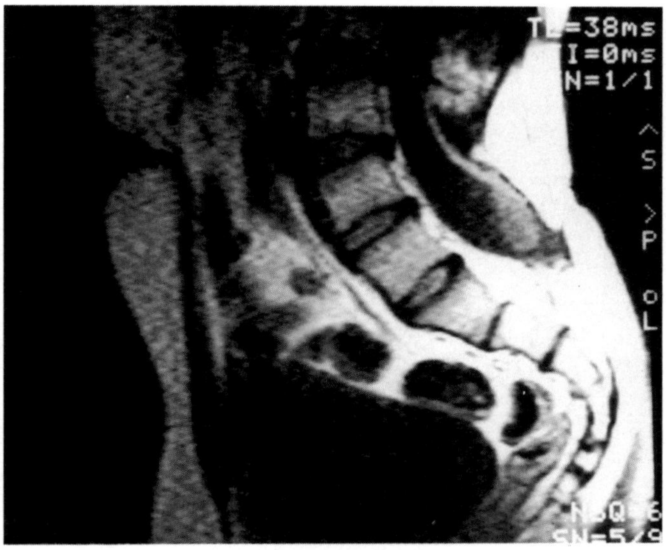

SE 500/38

Figure 15-19. Postsurgical retethering. A T1-weighted sagittal MR image of a teenage boy who underwent surgical repair of myelomeningocele in the neonatal period and who now has worsening symptoms demonstrates juxtaposition of atrophic cord to the dorsal surface of the spinal canal, suggestive of postsurgical retethering.

SUGGESTED READINGS

DEVELOPMENT OF SPINAL CORD AND CANAL

1. Larsen WJ. Human embryology. New York: Churchill Livingstone; 1993

OCCULT SPINAL DYSRAPHISM

2. Albright AL, Gartner JC, Wiener ES. Lumbar cutaneous hemangiomas as indicators of tethered spinal cords. Pediatrics 1989; 83:977–980
3. Altman NR, Altman DH. MR imaging of spinal dysraphism. Am J Neuroradiol 1987; 8:533–538
4. Babcook CJ. Ultrasound evaluation of prenatal and neonatal spina bifida. Neurosurg Clin North Am 1995; 6:203–218
5. Brunberg JA, Latchaw RE, Kanal E, Burk DL Jr, Albright L. Magnetic resonance imaging of spinal dysraphism. Radiol Clin North Am 1988; 26:181–205
6. Byrd SE, Darling CF, McLone DG, Tomita T. MR imaging of the pediatric spine. MRI Clin North Am 1996; 4:797–832
7. Davis DA, Cohen PR, George RE. Cutaneous stigmata of occult spinal dysraphism. J Am Acad Dermatol 1994; 31:892–896

8. Korsvik HE. Ultrasound assessment of congenital spinal anomalies presenting in infancy. Semin Ultrasound CT MR 1994; 15:264–274
9. McLone DG, Mutluer S, Naidich TP. Lipomeningoceles of the conus medullaris. Concepts Pediatr Neurosurg 1983; 3:170–177
10. Naidich TP, McLone DG, Mutluer S. A new understanding of dorsal dysraphism with lipoma (lipomyeloschisis): radiologic evaluation and surgical correction. AJR 1983; 140:1065–1078
11. Naidich TP, McLone DG, Shkolnik A, Fernbach S. Sonographic evaluation of caudal spine anomalies in children. AJNR 1983; 4:661–664
12. Raghavan N, Barkovich AJ, Edwards M, Norman D. MR imaging in the tethered spinal cord syndrome. AJR 1989; 152:843–852
13. Rindahl MA, Colletti PM, Zee CS, Taber P. Magnetic resonance imaging of pediatric spinal dysraphism. Magn Reson Imaging 1989; 7:217–224
14. Satar N, Bauer SB, Shefner J, Kelly MD, Darbey MM. The effects of delayed diagnosis and treatment in patients with an occult spinal dysraphism. J Urol 1995; 154:754–758
15. Yamada S, Zincke D, Saunders D. Pathophysiology of "tethered cord syndrome." J Neurosurg 1981; 54:494–503

MYELOCYSTOCELES AND CAUDAL REGRESSION SYNDROMES

16. Appignani BA, Jaramillo D, Barnes PD, Poussaint TY. Dysraphic myelodysplasias associated with urogenital and anorectal anomalies: prevalence and types seen with MR imaging. AJR 1994; 163:1199–1203
17. Barkovich AJ. Pediatric neuroimaging, 2nd ed. Raven Press: New York; 1995:477–540
18. Byrd SE, Harvey C, McLone DG, Darling CF. Imaging of terminal myelocystoceles. J Natl Med Assoc 1996; 88:510–516
19. Cohen AR. The mermaid malformation: cloacal exstrophy and occult spinal dysraphism. Neurosurgery 1991; 28:834–843
20. McLone D, Naidich T. Terminal myelocystocele. Neurosurgery 1985; 16: 36–43
21. Peacock WJ, Murovic JA. Magnetic resonance imaging in myelocystoceles. Report of two cases. J Neurosurg 1989; 70:804–807

MENINGOMYELOCELE AND ITS COMPLICATIONS

22. Balasubramaniam C, Laurent JP, McCluggage C, Oshman D, Cheek WR. Tethered-cord syndrome after repair of meningomyelocele. Child's Nerv Syst 1990; 6:208–211
23. Liptak GS, Bloss JW. Briskin H, Campbell JE, Hebert EB, Revell GM. The management of children with spinal dysraphism. J Child Neurol 1988; 3:3–20
24. Pang D. Split cord malformation. Part II: clinical syndrome. Neurosurgery 1992; 31:481–500

SACROCOCCYGEAL TERATOMA

25. Altman RP, Randolph JG, Lilly J. Sacrococcygeal teratoma. J Pediatr Surg 1973; 9:389–398
26. Feldman M, Byrne P, Johnson MA, Fischer J, Lees G. Neonatal sacrococcygeal teratoma: multiimaging modality assessment. J Pediatr Surg 1990; 25:675–678
27. Keslar PH, Buck JL, Suarez ES. Germ cell tumors of the sacrococcygeal region: radiologic–pathologic correlation. RadioGraphics 1994; 14:607–620
28. Wells RG, Sty JR. Imaging of sacrococcygeal germ cell tumors. RadioGraphics 1990; 10:701–713

CASE 16

Donald P. Frush, M.D.

Ewing's Sarcoma

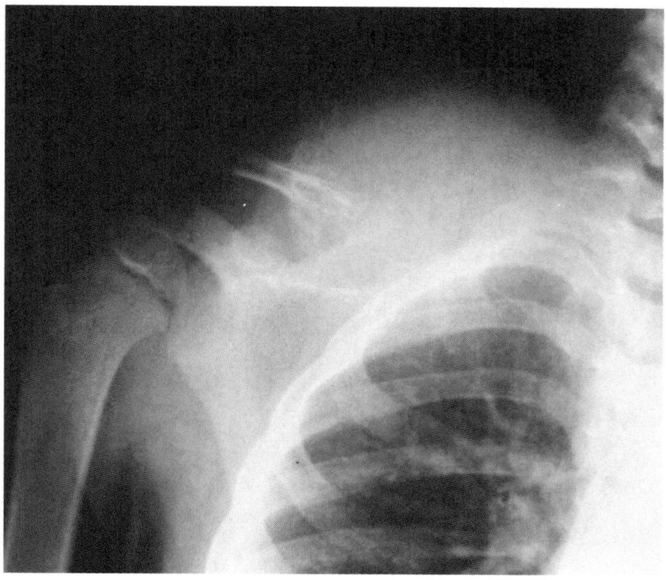

Figure 16-1

Question 78

This 6-year-old boy was diagnosed with a right clavicular fracture 4 months ago. He has persistent clavicular pain. You are shown an anteroposterior radiograph of the right shoulder region (Figure 16-1) and two axial CT images (Figure 16-2).

Which *one* of the following is the MOST likely diagnosis?

(A) Congenital pseudarthrosis
(B) Osteomyelitis
(C) Langerhans cell histiocytosis
(D) Aneurysmal bone cyst
(E) Ewing's sarcoma

The anteroposterior radiograph of the test patient (Figure 16-1) shows disruption of the middle portion of the right clavicle and an associated soft tissue mass (Figure 16-3). The bone and soft tissue abnormalities are better characterized on the noncontrast CT scans (Figure 16-2). Specifically, there are expansion and destruction of the middle portion of the clavicle and a large, homogeneous soft tissue mass. A permeative pattern and subtle periosteal reaction are evident in the medial clavicle. Disordered new bone formation radiates from the center of the lesion. A 3.0-mm nodule is also present in the right

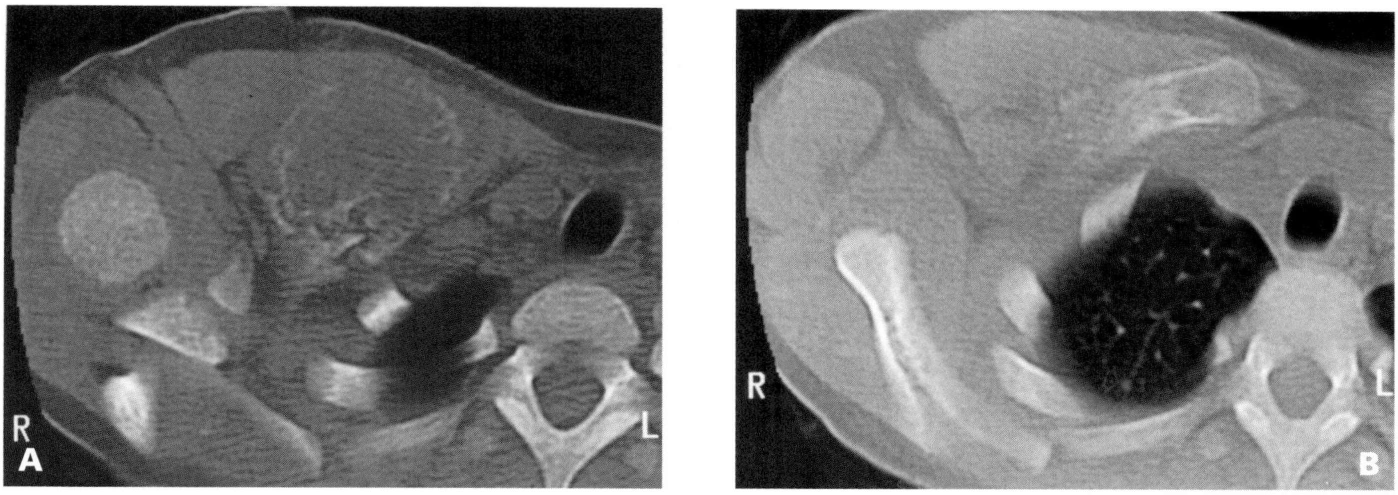

Figure 16-2

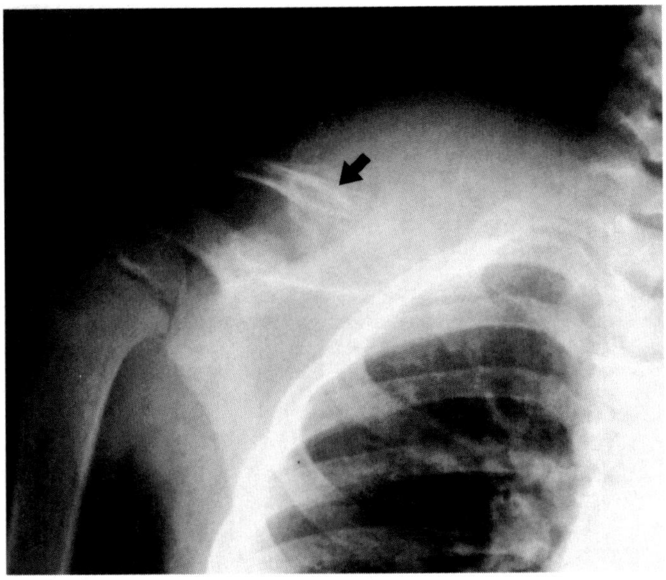

Figure 16-3 (Same as Figure 16-1). Ewing's sarcoma of the right clavicle. An anteroposterior radiograph shows an aggressive lesion involving the clavicle; there is destruction predominantly of the middle portion of the bone and an associated soft tissue mass. Note the periosteal elevation (arrow).

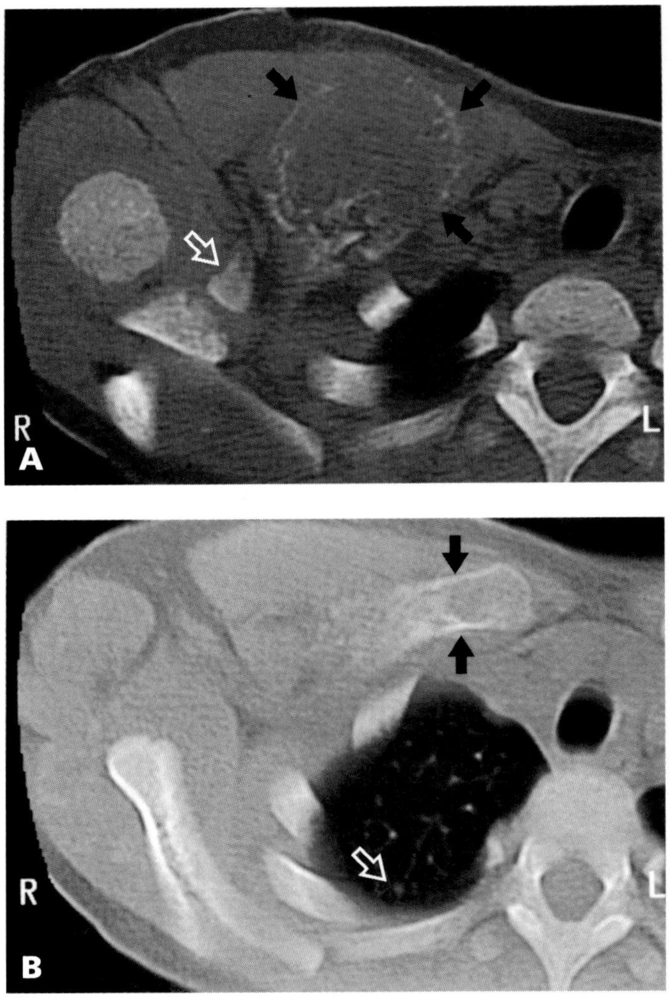

Figure 16-4 (Same as Figure 16-2). Ewing's sarcoma of the right clavicle. Transaxial CT images of the right clavicle were obtained with a bone algorithm. (A) An image obtained at the level of the right pulmonary sulcus demonstrates destruction of the midclavicle and radially oriented new bone formation (solid arrows) surrounding a soft tissue mass. The acromion (open arrow) is preserved. (B) An image obtained at a slightly lower level shows a permeative pattern of involvement in the medial clavicle and faint periosteal reaction (solid arrows). A nodular density, representing a pulmonary metastasis, is present in the posterior aspect of the right upper lobe (open arrow).

upper lobe (Figure 16-4). On the basis of the aggressive CT appearance of the clavicular lesion in the test patient, a primary bone neoplasm with a lung metastasis is the likely explanation. Of the choices listed, Ewing's sarcoma is the most likely diagnosis (**Option (E) is correct**).

Clavicular pseudarthrosis is not an aggressive process and is not associated with bone destruction. Pseudarthrosis can be either acquired, such as with fracture nonunion, or congenital. In patients with congenital clavicular pseudarthrosis (Option (A)), there is a defect in the midclavicle. The ends of the clavicle at the margins of the defect are smooth and corticated (or sclerotic). There is no associated soft tissue mass. Therefore, this is not the most likely diagnosis for the test patient. (Congenital clavicular pseudarthrosis is discussed further in Question 79.)

Acute osteomyelitis of the clavicle (Option (B)) can be either secondary, as a result of hematogenous spread of organisms, or primary, as a result of the spread of organisms from an adjacent area of infection (e.g., cellulitis) or from direct inoculation of the bone. Primary osteomyelitis can occur in patients with an open clavicular fracture, after surgery to the clavicle, or after interventions such as subclavian venipuncture. A patient with osteomyelitis presents clinically with local pain, erythema, and swelling. The patient may be febrile and may have leukocytosis and an elevated erythrocyte sedimentation rate.

Irrespective of the site involved, the radiographic findings associated with osteomyelitis are similar. Periosteal reaction and osteopenia are seen early in the infection, and trabecular and cortical bone destruction occurs in more advanced cases. Sclerosis, mixed lucency and sclerosis, or sequestrum formation is typical of more chronic infection. Soft tissue changes associated with osteomyelitis include fascial and muscle edema attributable either to reactive inflammation or to spread of infection (myositis, cellulitis, or frank abscess formation). The presence of marked expansion and radially oriented new bone formation in the test images is more typical of a rapidly growing and aggressive bone neoplasm than of osteomyelitis. Furthermore, although osteomyelitis can cause septic pulmonary emboli, the resultant opacities are usually ill defined, unlike the small, well-defined pulmonary nodule in the test images. Therefore, acute osteomyelitis is not the most likely diagnosis.

Langerhans cell histiocytosis (LCH) (Option (C)) is the preferred term now used for histiocytosis X. LCH is a disorder of unknown cause, characterized pathologically by granuloma formation attributable to proliferation of histiocytes of the Langerhans cell type. The defining feature is the demonstration by electron microscopy of cytoplasmic organelles called

Burbeck granules.

LCH can be localized or diffuse and can involve the bone, reticuloendothelial system, soft tissues, lymph nodes, or lungs. Bone pain is the usual presenting symptom in patients with skeletal involvement. Osseous LCH occurs in 60% to 80% of patients and is the most common type. However, skeletal lesions represent less than 1% of all the tumorlike conditions of bone. In patients with skeletal disease, the skull is most often involved (approximately 40% of cases). Long bone involvement is next in frequency (20% of cases), followed by the spine (15%), ribs (10%), and pelvis (8%). In a 1996 series of children with LCH, Van Nieuwenhuyse et al. noted that the clavicle is one of the rarest sites of involvement by LCH (4%).

The radiographic appearance of LCH is highly variable. The most easily recognized lesion is a well-defined lucent lesion. In the skull, different extents of involvement of the inner and outer tables result in a characteristic beveled-edge appearance. When there is a central inclusion of calcification or bone, a "button sequestrum" can be seen. Lesions also can be sclerotic or mixed lytic and sclerotic. The margins can be ill defined, expansile, or destructive (Figure 16-5), and an accompanying soft tissue mass can be present. In the spine, LCH can result in vertebral collapse (vertebra plana). On bone scintigraphy, lesions can show either increased or decreased uptake, depending on the balance between lytic destruction and new bone formation.

Both CT and MRI are excellent methods for demonstrating the presence and extent of osseous LCH. Diagnosis and follow-up of LCH in children are best performed by a radiographic skeletal survey or bone scintigraphy. There is no optimal single imaging method for evaluating the entire skeleton. Radiography misses up to 25% of lesions, and the reported sensitivity of bone scintigraphy ranges from 35% to 100%. Often, both modalities are used for initial evaluation, with subsequent imaging being performed by the study that best displays the lesions in a particular patient.

In addition to the musculoskeletal system, LCH can involve the skin, reticuloendothelial system (liver, spleen, and lymph nodes), central nervous system, and lungs. Pulmonary LCH appears as bilaterally symmetric interstitial lung disease with small (typically less than 1.0 cm) nodules and thin-walled cysts, varying in size from less than 1.0 cm to several centimeters. Because LCH rarely involves the clavicle and asymmetric lung involvement in a 6-year-old child would be even rarer, LCH is not the most likely diagnosis for the test patient.

An aneurysmal bone cyst (ABC) (Option (D)) is a bone lesion of uncertain etiology that occurs most often in older children and young adults. The lesion is very rare in children younger than 6 years. ABC consists primarily of blood products, along with bony and fibrous trabeculae. The lesion is not a primary neoplasm, but is probably a reactive process in bone, often associated with trauma. An ABC is associated with other primary tumors that can occur in childhood, including nonossifying fibroma, giant cell tumor, and osteoblastoma. ABC is seen most frequently in the long bones, pelvis, and spine. In

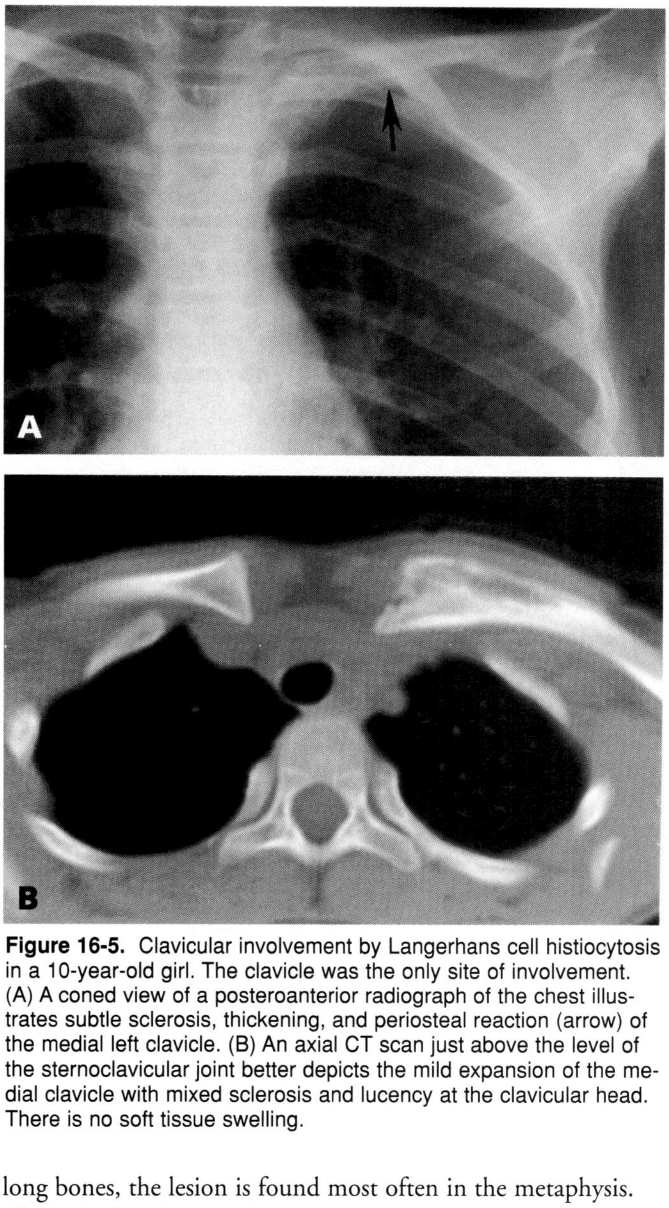

Figure 16-5. Clavicular involvement by Langerhans cell histiocytosis in a 10-year-old girl. The clavicle was the only site of involvement. (A) A coned view of a posteroanterior radiograph of the chest illustrates subtle sclerosis, thickening, and periosteal reaction (arrow) of the medial left clavicle. (B) An axial CT scan just above the level of the sternoclavicular joint better depicts the mild expansion of the medial clavicle with mixed sclerosis and lucency at the clavicular head. There is no soft tissue swelling.

long bones, the lesion is found most often in the metaphysis. Clavicular involvement is rare.

On radiographs, an ABC is typically expansile, often with a thin covering of cortical bone, periosteum, or calcification. Centrally there are bony septations, giving a cystic appearance with little or no matrix (Figure 16-6). Because of the age of the test patient, the permeative and destructive nature of the lesion, and the presence of a lung nodule, ABC is not a consideration.

Among malignant bone tumors in children, Ewing's sarcoma is second only to osteosarcoma in frequency. Ewing's sarcoma is a primary bone tumor and is most common in patients between 10 and 15 years of age, but it does occur in younger children and in adults. However, it is very rare in children younger than 2 years of age. The frequency of occurrence is slightly higher in girls (3:2). Ewing's sarcoma is one of the pediatric cancers characterized by small, round, blue-staining cells. Bone pain, often with a history of trauma, is the most frequent complaint and occurs in nearly 80% of patients. Neurologic symptoms can accompany Ewing's sarcoma of the

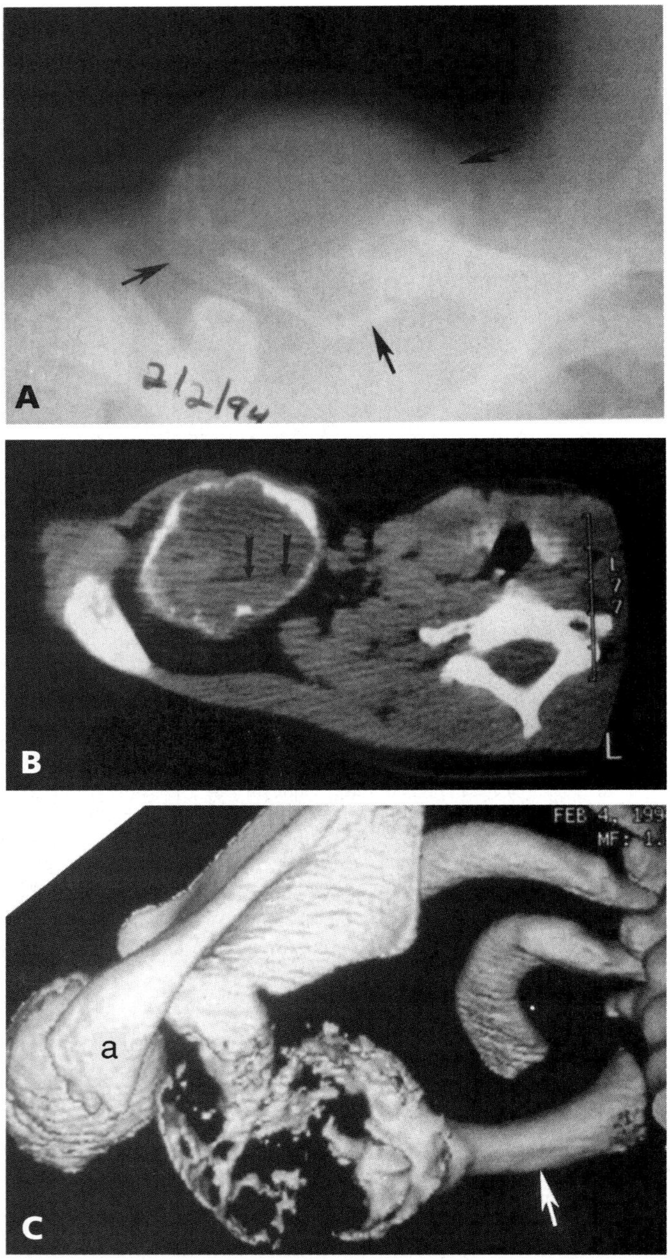

Figure 16-6. Aneurysmal bone cyst. The patient is a 10-year-old boy with a painless, expansile right clavicular mass, which was monitored for 18 months. (A) A posteroanterior radiograph demonstrates an expansile mass of the lateral half of the right clavicle. Note the peripheral ossification (arrows). (B) An axial CT scan through the right midclavicle better demonstrates the peripheral ossification surrounding a central region with predominantly soft tissue attenuation values. Note the subtle fluid-fluid level (arrows). (C) A three-dimensional reconstruction of the right clavicular mass as viewed from above illustrates the peripheral ossification and the relationship of the mass to the acromion (a) and the normal proximal clavicle (arrow). (Case courtesy of Sara O'Hara, MD, Children's Hospital Medical Center, Cincinnati, OH.)

spine. Ewing's sarcoma also can present with local inflammatory signs and symptoms, including erythema and swelling. Fever, elevated leukocyte count, and elevated erythrocyte sedimentation rate occur in a minority of patients with Ewing's sarcoma, making distinction from osteomyelitis difficult.

Ewing's sarcoma is found in long bones in more than 50% of patients, with 35% to 45% of cases occurring in the femur, tibia, or fibula. The pelvis is the most common site of flat bone involvement, accounting for up to 17% of lesions. The clavicle is affected in only 2% of patients.

Ewing's sarcoma is an aggressive bone tumor that originates in the bone marrow. There is a wide range of radiographic findings, including permeative, lytic, sclerotic, and mixed patterns. Cortical changes include thickening and disruption. Periosteal reaction occurs in at least 50% of patients and includes an "onion skin" or "sunburst" appearance. The latter pattern, seen with rapidly growing tumors, indicates that new bone formation is radially oriented along Sharpey's fibers. Extraosseous findings consist of a soft tissue mass in 80% of patients. The soft tissue component can be large.

Ewing's sarcoma of bone is clearly seen by scintigraphy with either Tc-99m methylene diphosphonate or Ga-67 citrate. CT scans depict the trabecular and cortical abnormalities as well as the periosteal reaction. The soft tissue component is also clearly seen by CT. The extent of marrow and soft tissue involvement associated with primary malignant bone neoplasms, including Ewing's sarcoma, is best appreciated by MRI (Figures 16-7 and 16-8). The high signal intensity of fatty marrow on T1-weighted images is replaced by intermediate signal intensity, similar to that of muscle. The bone and soft tissue abnormalities are seen on T2-weighted images as heterogeneous lesions with predominantly increased signal intensity.

Sites of metastasis of Ewing's sarcoma include the lungs, bone, lymph nodes, and brain. Pulmonary metastases are most common, and up to 50% of patients have imaging evidence of metastases to the lungs at the time of presentation. The prognosis depends on (1) the size of the tumor (tumors smaller than 8 cm in diameter or 100 mL in volume have a more favorable prognosis), (2) location as an indicator of resectability (unresectable pelvic lesions have a poorer prognosis than resectable extremity lesions), (3) extent of metastatic disease and (4) response to chemotherapy. The tumor is radiosensitive, and so radiation therapy is often combined with chemotherapy before resection. For resectable lesions, the 5-year survival rate is approximately 75%.

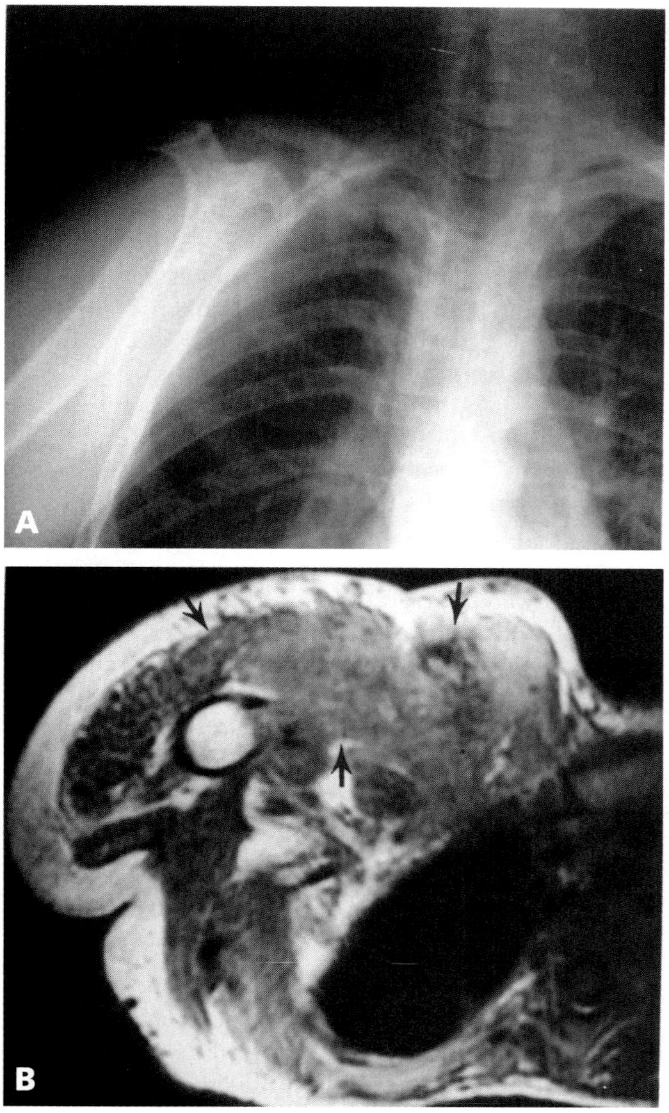

SE 2,000/12

Figure 16-7. Osteosarcoma of the clavicle in an 18-year-old girl. This tumor was induced by local irradiation for lymphoma 13 years earlier. (A) A coned radiograph of the right shoulder demonstrates a destructive lesion of the clavicle. The margins of the clavicle are poorly seen. (B) An axial proton-density-weighted MR image at the level of the right clavicle illustrates the destruction of the bone and an associated soft tissue mass. The mass (arrows) has completely replaced the right clavicle and has mixed signal intensity.

Question 79

Concerning congenital clavicular pseudarthrosis,

(A) it is usually right sided
(B) it is easily distinguished radiographically from an acute fracture
(C) it often heals spontaneously
(D) it is associated with ipsilateral Erb's palsy
(E) it occurs at any point along the clavicle

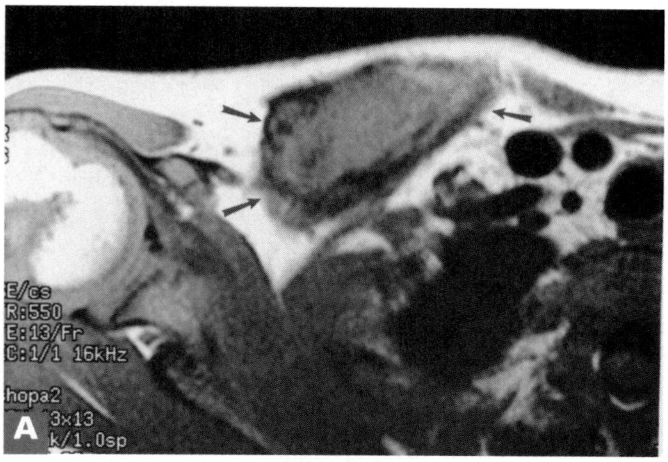

SE 550/13

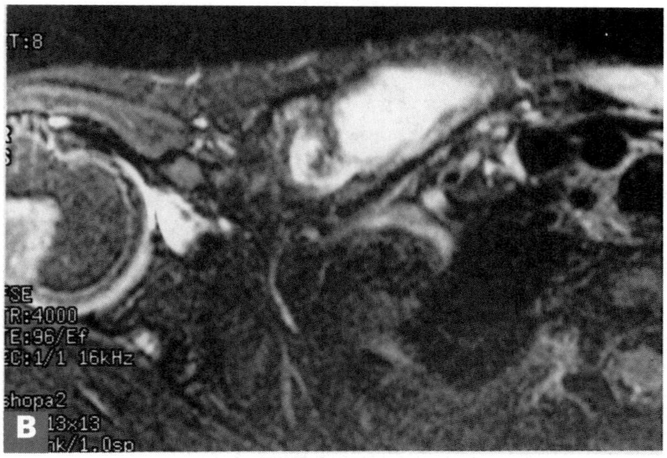

FSE 4,000/96

Figure 16-8. Same patient as in Figures 16-1 through 16-4. Ewing's sarcoma. These images were obtained 3 months after diagnosis. (A) An axial T1-weighted MR image of the right clavicle demonstrates a soft tissue mass (arrows) with intermediate signal intensity; the lesion has decreased in size since the time of diagnosis. (B) An axial T2-weighted fast spin-echo MR image shows the extent of the predominantly high-signal-intensity residual sarcoma. No bony anatomy was evident except at the most medial and lateral aspects of the right clavicle (not shown).

There are two types of clavicular pseudarthrosis: post-traumatic and congenital. Most congenital pseudarthroses are sporadic, but an autosomal dominant transmission has been noted in some families.

The pathogenesis of congenital pseudarthrosis of the clavicle probably relates to the embryology of the clavicle. The developing embryologic clavicle is composed of two ossification centers that typically fuse *in utero* at 5 to 6 weeks. The most credible explanation of congenital pseudarthrosis is that the two centers fail to fuse. Other investigators argue that the clavicle has essentially one ossification center and that congenital pseudarthrosis results from abnormal separation of this ossification center. A third explanation, also related to abnormal separation of a single ossification center, implicates the proximity of the developing clavicle to the subclavian artery. Almost all cases of congenital pseudarthrosis are in the right clavicle (**Op-**

tion (A) **is true**) and in the middle of the bone (**Option** (E) **is false**). On the right, the course of the subclavian artery is directly below the middle of the clavicle. Further supporting this vascular relationship is the fact that the rare left-sided pseudarthrosis is usually associated with anomalies of the aortic branch vessels, such as a right-sided aortic arch with mirror-image branching of the vessels from the arch. Finally, an association with cervical ribs has been reported. In up to 25% of patients, a fibrous connection between the first rib and a cervical rib has been noted. It is proposed that the subsequent elevation of the first rib results in a higher location of the subclavian artery and the development of pseudarthrosis.

Congenital pseudarthrosis can be a serendipitous finding on neonatal radiography performed for unrelated reasons (Figure 16-9). Alternatively, radiographs may be obtained for evaluation of a mass in the supraclavicular region or because a clavicular fracture is suspected. Congenital pseudarthrosis is most often detected in the first few months of life. The most common finding is a painless mass in the right clavicle. The mass may enlarge slowly. The lesion is usually painful only if it is traumatized; however, discomfort can be caused by contact with clothing, including straps. There is no association with birth trauma, including Erb's palsy (**Option** (D) **is false**). Movement at the pseudarthrosis can be detected on physical examination, and the clavicle can be foreshortened, but the range of motion of the upper extremity is normal. Vascular symptoms, in particular, thoracic outlet syndrome, have been reported in adults with congenital pseudarthrosis.

Right clavicular involvement occurs in about 95% of patients. Isolated left-sided involvement occurs in fewer than 5% of patients, and bilateral involvement occurs in less than 10%. The nonossified portion usually is localized in the middle of the clavicle and usually is short (1.0 to 2.0 cm). The ends of the bone adjoining the pseudarthrosis are rounded, with a continuous cortex. There also can be sclerosis and slight expansion of these ends. The medial aspect of the clavicular pseudarthrosis is usually larger than the acromial end and is oriented anteriorly and superiorly. The lateral aspect is usually directed superiorly and slightly posteriorly. The superior orientation at the pseudarthrosis is responsible for the visible protrusion in the supraclavicular region. These features, together with the absence of trauma and callus formation, help to distinguish pseudarthrosis from acute or subacute clavicular fracture. Clavicular fractures usually occur in the middle third of the clavicle, but the fracture site does not have corticated, smooth, or sclerotic ends (**Option** (B) **is true**).

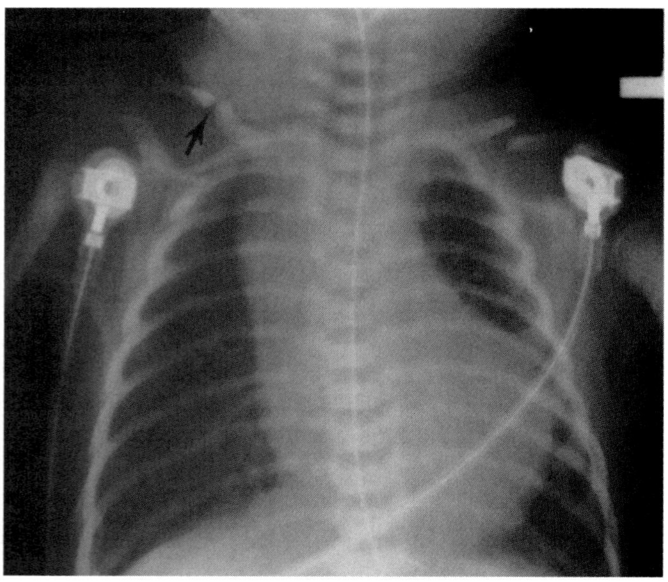

Figure 16-9. Congenital clavicular pseudarthrosis in a 10-day-old girl. A radiograph shows congenital pseudarthrosis in the right clavicle and a birth-related fracture in the left clavicle. Typical findings of clavicular pseudarthrosis include right-sided location and involvement of the midportion. The ends are relatively well defined (arrow), and there is superior orientation of the medial aspect of the clavicle. These findings are in contrast to those on the left, where there is the typical superior positioning of the medial fracture fragment.

Other than an acute fracture, the differential diagnosis of congenital clavicular pseudarthrosis includes a fracture nonunion and cleidocranial dysostosis. Fracture nonunion can be distinguished from congenital pseudarthrosis by its lateral location, presence of callus, history of trauma, and more rapid enlargement and pain. In cleidocranial dysostosis, the clavicle is usually absent or partially hypoplastic. In patients with partial involvement, the bone is usually tapered and the lateral aspect is most often involved. Isolated medial involvement is rare. In addition to the clavicular abnormalities, patients with cleidocranial dysostosis typically exhibit abnormalities of the scapulae, hypoplasia of the pubic bones, and wormian (intrasutural) bones in the skull.

Congenital clavicular pseudarthrosis does not heal spontaneously (**Option** (C) **is false**). Most individuals are evaluated for surgical intervention either for cosmetic reasons or because of symptoms. Surgical correction requires removal of the cartilaginous pseudarthrosis and direct apposition of residual clavicle, insertion of a bone graft, or plate fixation. Rare complications include infection, nonunion, and brachial plexus trauma.

Question 80

Concerning clavicular osteomyelitis in children,

(A) most patients are immunodeficient
(B) the clavicle is commonly involved in patients with chronic recurrent multifocal osteomyelitis
(C) the responsible organism is identified in fewer than 30% of patients
(D) radiographs are usually normal

Overall, only about 3% of clavicular disorders in children are nontraumatic. Of these nontraumatic clavicular disorders, 75% are equally divided between neoplastic and infectious causes and the remaining 25% are congenital. Congenital abnormalities include pseudarthrosis, duplications (Figure 16-10), and anomalies associated with dysplasias such as cleidocranial dysostosis. Normal variations also can mimic disease. These include irregularity of the medial end of the clavicle and prominent rhomboid fossa (Figure 16-11).

The clavicle is the site of infection in fewer than 7% of children with osteomyelitis. The metaphyses of bones are the more typical sites for osteomyelitis, and the long bones are most often involved.

Immunocompromised children are at greater risk for a variety of infections, including osteomyelitis; however, most cases of clavicular osteomyelitis occur in children with normal immune status **(Option (A) is false)**. The most frequent clinical manifestations of clavicular osteomyelitis are pain, swelling, and fever. In a 1997 series of five children reported by Lowden and Walsh, all three of these findings, as well as elevation of the erythrocyte sedimentation rate, were present. *Staphylococcus aureus* is the most frequent organism isolated (in about 75% of cases). *Streptococus pneumoniae*, group A *Streptococcus*, and mixed organisms also can be responsible for infection. In most cases of acute clavicular osteomyelitis in children (at least 50%), an organism is cultured from aspirates, biopsy specimens, or blood **(Option (C) is false)**. Clavicular infection can be either primary (e.g., from surgical intervention) or hematogenous. In children, infection is usually attributable to hematogenous spread. Infectious foci, including pneumonia and tonsillitis, are found in about 50% of these patients.

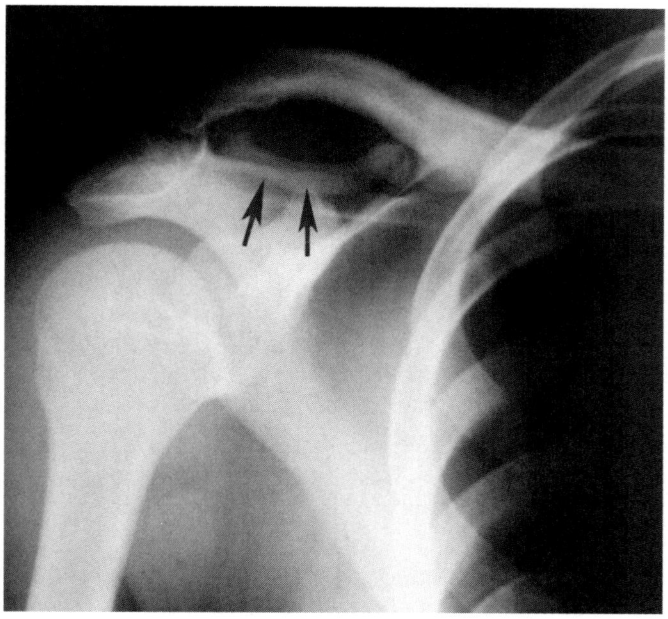

Figure 16-10. Duplication of the clavicle in a 20-year-old man. Note the hypoplastic duplication (arrows) inferior to the lateral aspect of the clavicle. The radiographic examination, which was otherwise normal, was obtained following trauma to the right shoulder.

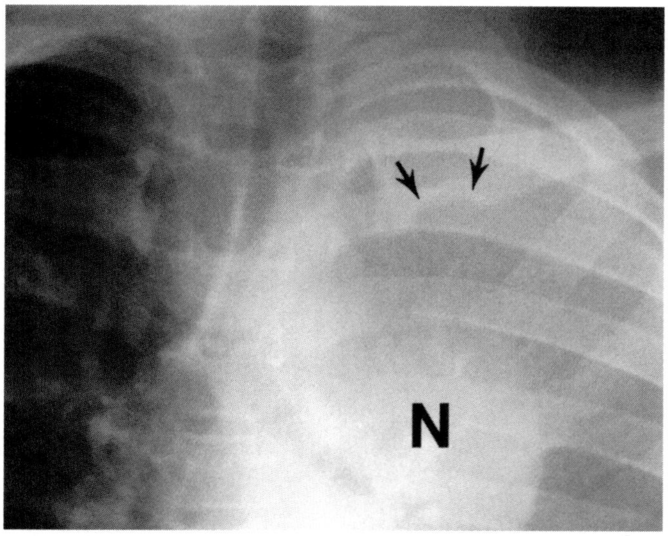

Figure 16-11. Prominent rhomboid fossa of the left clavicle in a 7-year-old boy. Note the typical scalloped irregularity of the inferior aspect of the medial clavicle (arrows). The left upper lobe opacity is attributable to atelectasis secondary to central compression of the left upper lobe bronchus by tuberculous adenopathy (N).

Diagnostic imaging plays an important role in the detection and delineation of clavicular osteomyelitis. Conventional radiography is usually the initial imaging study. Radiographs are typically normal in the first week after onset of symptoms, and early changes of osteomyelitis can be difficult to see on radiographs because of overlapping bony anatomy. Because clavicular osteomyelitis is often not initially suspected clinically, children may be misdiagnosed as having a more common entity, such as a fracture (even with normal radiographs). Therefore, most cases of clavicular osteomyelitis have accompanying bone changes **(Option (D) is false)**.

Radiographic changes are usually either predominantly sclerotic or lytic, and these varieties occur with equal frequency, together accounting for about 75% of cases. In the remaining 25% of cases, mixed sclerosis and lysis are seen. The middle or medial portion of the clavicle is involved in most patients (Figure 16-12). Periosteal reaction is evident in only about one third of patients. Acromioclavicular or sterno-clavicular joint involvement can ensue by direct extension of infection from the lateral or medial aspects of the clavicle, respectively. Joint involvement has been noted in about 50% of cases in adults and children. Acute osteomyelitis of the clavicle can result in a pathologic fracture. In such cases, medial resorption of the clavicle can result (despite successful treatment) if the main blood supply for the clavicle, which enters the bone laterally, is disrupted.

Scintigraphy, CT, and MRI are additional modalities for the detection of clavicular osteomyelitis. Hyperperfusion and hyperemia are seen on radionuclide angiography and immediate images, and there is marked tracer accumulation on delayed static images. Bone scintigraphy with Tc-99m phosphonates is helpful in distinguishing osteomyelitis from cellulitis. Osseous destruction or sclerosis, periosteal reaction, and soft tissue abnormalities, including acromioclavicular and sternoclavicular joint involvement, cellulitis, and abscess, are well seen by CT. However, these changes and the bone and marrow abnormalities are best delineated by MRI. CT also can be used to localize areas for surgical or percutaneous biopsy. Sonography has a limited role in osteomyelitis, but it can be used to identify subperiosteal fluid.

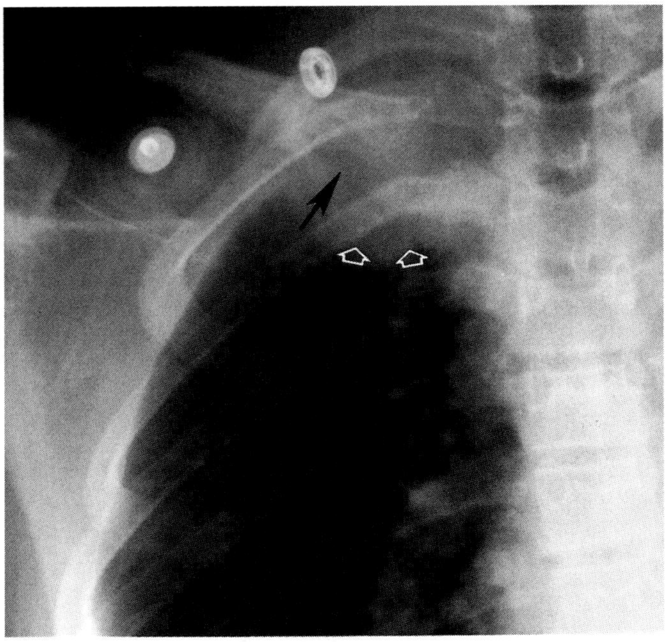

Figure 16-12. Staphylococcal osteomyelitis of the clavicle in a 14-year-old boy. A coned view of a posteroanterior chest radiograph demonstrates that the inferior cortical margin of the medial clavicle is indistinct (black arrow). There also is a soft tissue mass in this area (open arrows), indicating extraosseous extension of inflammation. These features are not specific and can be associated with other aggressive disorders, such as primary or secondary malignant bone tumors.

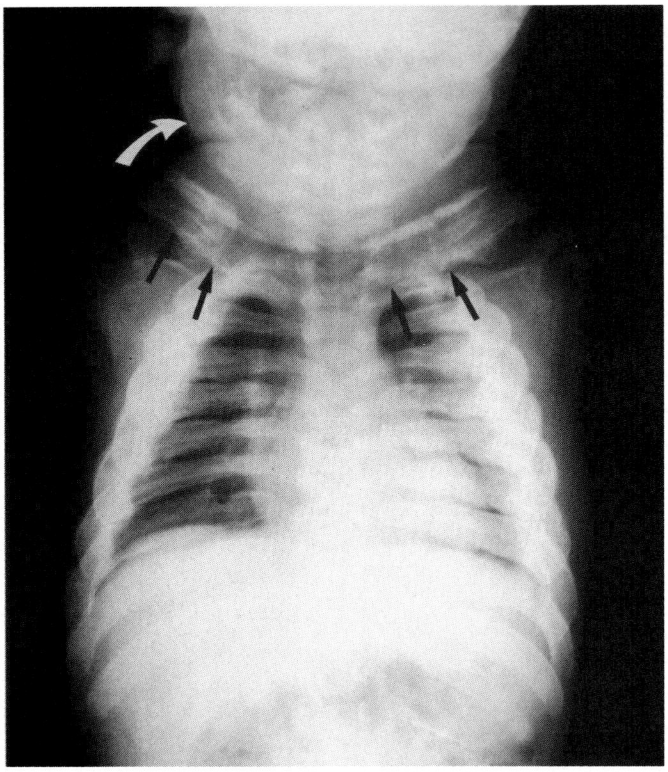

Figure 16-13. Infantile cortical hyperostosis (Caffey's disease) in a 3-month-old infant. Note the marked cortical thickening with periosteal new bone formation in both clavicles (straight arrows). Similar changes are seen in the ribs as well as the mandible, most evident on the right (curved arrow).

The features of osteomyelitis are clearly shown on a combination of spin-echo T1- and T2-weighted MR images. Decreased signal intensity may not be evident on T1-weighted images in children and some adults if there is a predominance of red marrow. The marrow signal intensity is abnormally increased on T2-weighted images, especially when fat suppression techniques are used. Sinus tracts, periosteal abnormalities, and soft tissue abnormalities of adjacent muscles, fasciae, and subcutaneous fat, as well as focal fluid collections, also are best seen on T2-weighted images. These collections show peripheral enhancement after intravenous administration of gadolinium chelates. Use of intravenous contrast material is not routinely necessary, since in children most solitary clavicular lesions that are not clearly traumatic should be biopsied.

Clavicular osteomyelitis can be mimicked clinically and radiographically by several other conditions. Infantile cortical hyperostosis (Caffey's disease), which commonly involves the clavicle, can have a similar clinical presentation, with irritability, fever, and soft tissue swelling. Involvement of other bones (in particular, the mandible and one or more ribs) and osseous sclerosis attributable to marked cortical thickening favor the diagnosis of Caffey's disease (Figure 16-13). In older children, Ewing's sarcoma, eosinophilic granuloma, and osteosarcoma have a radiographic appearance similar to that of osteomyelitis. Sclerosis also is seen in patients with osteoid osteoma. The distinction between osteoid osteoma and low-grade or chronic osteomyelitis can be difficult unless the nidus characteristic of osteoid osteoma is demonstrated. Osteitis condensans, clavicular avascular necrosis, sternocostoclavicular hyperostosis (Figure 16-14), and Garré's sclerosing osteomyelitis are extremely uncommon causes of clavicular sclerosis in children.

Chronic recurrent multifocal osteomyelitis (CRMO) can also mimic osteomyelitis. CRMO is a poorly understood inflammatory disorder of bone. The etiology of this disorder is unknown, but it may be an immune system phenomenon or attributable to an occult viral or bacterial pathogen. CRMO is more common in girls (2:1) and usually occurs near the end of the first decade, with approximately 50% of cases occurring between 7 and 12 years of age. The signs and symptoms include pain and swelling of the affected regions. Fever and other systemic symptoms are rare. Elevations in both antistreptolysin and antistapholysin titers have been reported. Pustulosis palmaris et plantaris occurs in about 20% of patients with CRMO. The distribution is multifocal and symmetric in 66% of patients and involves the metaphyses of the tubular bones, most often the distal tibia. Other common sites for CRMO, in decreasing order of frequency, are the distal femur, proximal tibia, and clavicle. The clavicle is involved in about one third of cases in children **(Option (B) is true).** In patients with clavicular involvement, the medial ends are most often involved. The pattern of multifocal involvement is either simultaneous or sequential. There are up to five lesions in two thirds of individuals, and patients with as many as 20 sites of involvement have been reported.

Radiographically, CRMO is characterized by sclerosis and osteolysis, most often with at least two adjacent lucent lesions. Periostitis and cortical thickening also can be found (Figure 16-15 and 16-16). Lesions demonstrate increased activity on bone scintigraphy. CT better displays these features than does radiography. A biopsy (or course of antibiotics) is usually undertaken early in the course of disease, when there is sufficient overlap between the clinical or radiographic features of CMRO and pyogenic osteomyelitis. If the clinical findings do not resolve after about 3 months of treatment, CRMO is the presumed diagnosis. Treatment of CRMO with antibiotics, steroids, nonsteroidal anti-inflammatory agents, and curettage has not been consistently effective. CRMO is almost always self-limited, and the symptoms and radiographic changes resolve over several years. The radiographic features resolve more slowly than the clinical features.

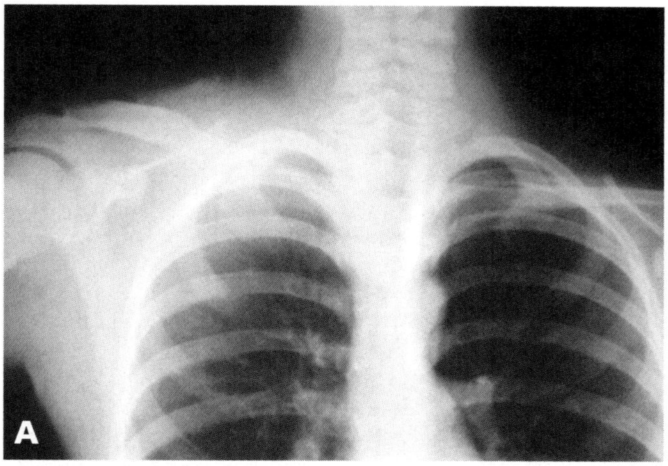

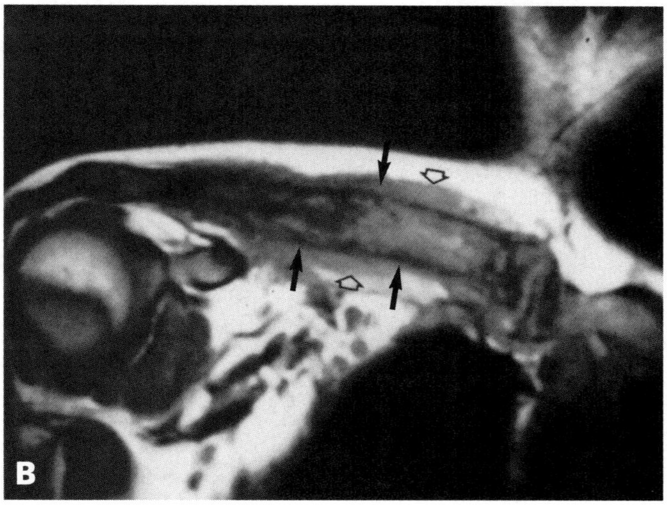

SE 500/20

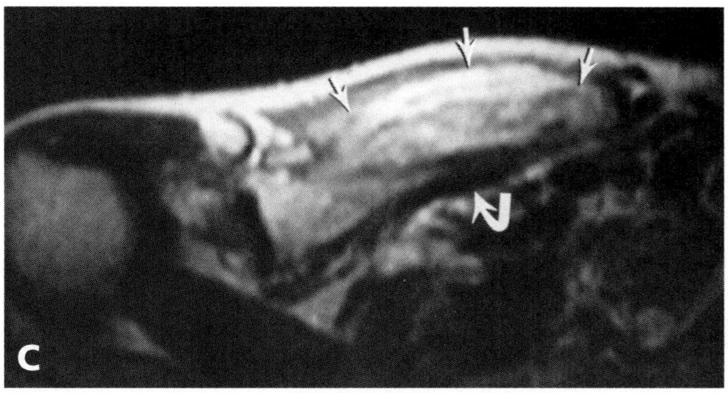

SE 2,000/80

Figure 16-14. Sternocostoclavicular hyperostosis in a 12-year-old girl. (A) A coned view of a posteroanterior chest radiograph shows thickening and sclerosis of the right clavicle with sparing of its lateral aspect. (B) A coronal T1-weighted MR image demonstrates the thickening of the clavicle (black arrows) with sparing of the lateral aspect. Areas of intermediate signal intensity in the periosteal region (open arrows) may be attributable either to periosteal reaction or to inflammation of adjacent soft tissues. There is no soft tissue mass. (C) An axial T2-weighted MR image through the middle of the right clavicle demonstrates heterogeneous but predominantly high signal intensity within the marrow. This finding is probably attributable to a mixture of medullary fibrosis and inflammation. Some of this abnormal signal superficially is likely attributable to extraosseous inflammation (straight arrows). Cortical thickening (curved arrow) is evident posteriorly.

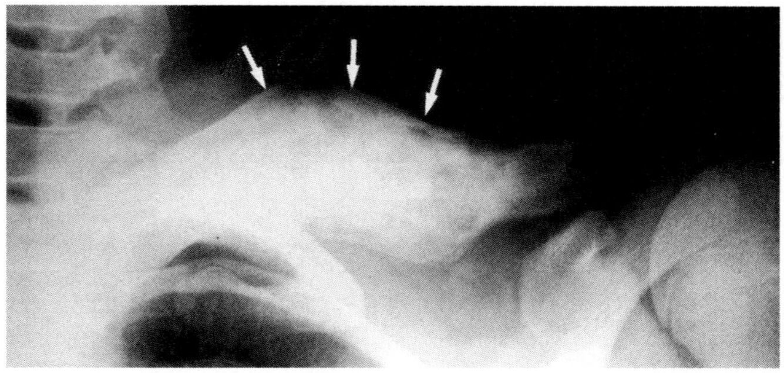

Figure 16-15. Chronic recurrent multifocal osteomyelitis in an 8-year-old girl. A radiograph shows an expansile sclerotic lesion involving all but the most lateral aspect of the left clavicle (arrows). Bone scintigraphy (not shown) demonstrated increased activity in the affected clavicle, as well as in the left tibia. The tibia was radiographically normal.

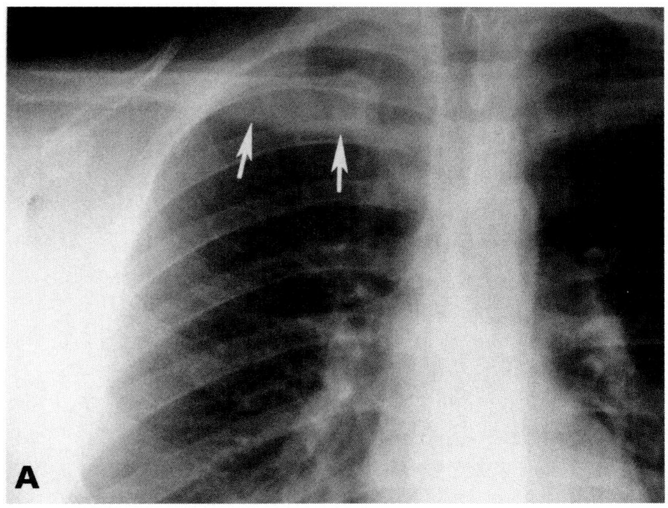

Figure 16-16. Chronic recurrent multifocal osteomyelitis in a 17-year-old boy. (A) A coned view of a posteroanterior radiograph of the chest illustrates subtly increased density and expansion of the medial right clavicle (arrows).

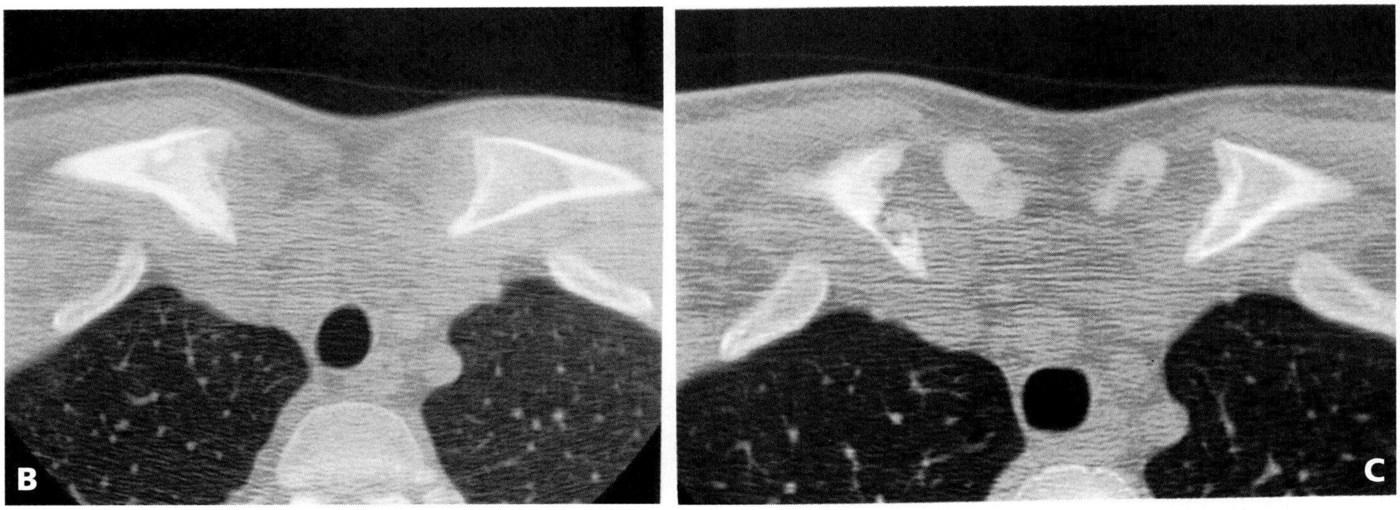

Figure 16-16 (Continued). Chronic recurrent multifocal osteomyelitis in a 17-year-old boy. (B) An axial CT scan of the medial clavicle better demonstrates the sclerosis and irregularity of the medial aspect of the right clavicle. (C) A CT image closer to the level of the sternoclavicular joint shows fragmentation of the medial right clavicle. There is no soft tissue abnormality. There also is minimal irregularity of the medial aspect of the left clavicle; the patient had no symptoms at this site, and this is a normal appearance.

Question 81

Concerning clavicular fracture in children,

(A) the lateral fragment is usually displaced inferiorly
(B) osteolysis is an occasional sequela
(C) in an infant, it strongly suggests child abuse
(D) nonunion is rare
(E) the lateral third is least commonly involved
(F) acromioclavicular joint separation is commonly associated

The clavicle is one of the most frequently fractured bones in children. In children of all ages, clavicular fractures account for 4% to 15% of all fractures. Affected children typically present with pain and limited motion of the ipsilateral upper extremity. Clavicular fractures usually result either from a direct force or, more commonly, from a compressive force that pushes the shoulder medially or medially and anteriorly. Lateral fractures result from vertical loads near the acromioclavicular joint, whereas medial fractures are usually the result of direct trauma. Fractures of the clavicle typically have straightforward clinical presentations and radiographic appearances, are usually not associated with other regional injuries, and heal completely without sequelae. However, recognition of atypical cases is important, since the prognosis may be worse and further imaging evaluation may be required.

In most isolated clavicular fractures, the disruption is near the junction of the middle and lateral thirds of the bone, where the bone is structurally the weakest. The lateral segment of the clavicle is fixed by the coracoclavicular ligaments and remains in the normal position; it is not displaced inferiorly (Figure 16-17) (**Option (A) is false**). The medial aspect of the clavicle is relatively unsupported, and the axis is directed cephalad.

Fractures of the clavicle occur during 0.2% to 5% of births and are more common with large infants, shoulder dystocia, and breech presentations. The true frequency of birth-related clavicular fractures is probably higher than reported, since many healing fractures are detected incidentally during radiography for unrelated reasons in infants. Clavicular fractures are found in 9% to 13% of newborns, with Erb's palsy secondary to shoulder dystocia.

Other entities that can be mistaken for clavicular fracture include "pseudofracture" (Figure 16-18) and congenital pseudarthrosis. A pseudofracture appearance occurs with lordotic positioning for the radiographic examination. The midclavicle appears sclerotic and lacks its usual smooth contour. As noted earlier, congenital pseudarthrosis is nearly always on the right side, with sclerotic ends at the point of osseous discontinuity, differentiating this entity from the irregular margins of a neonatal clavicular fracture (Figure 16-9).

Nonaccidental trauma (child abuse) is a consideration in the setting of an acute clavicular fracture later in infancy. According to Kleinman, a clavicular fracture alone is not highly specific for nonaccidental trauma in the infant (**Option (C) is**

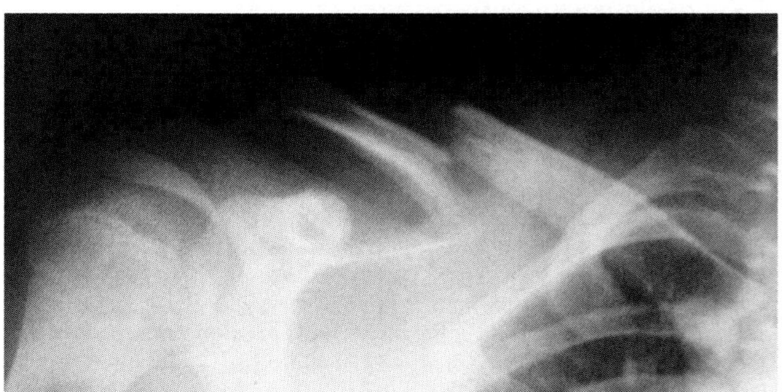

Figure 16-17. Acute fracture of the midclavicle in a 13-year-old boy. The displacement of the medial fragment is typical, since the lateral fragment remains fixed by the coracoclavicular ligaments.

false). Fractures considered highly suspicious for child abuse (i.e., those with high specificity) include fractures of the posterior vertebral elements, sternum, scapulae, or posterior ribs, as well as the classic transmetaphyseal fractures (also called bucket-handle or corner fractures). Moderate-specificity findings include the presence of fractures of different ages, digit fractures, and complex skull fractures. Low-specificity injuries include clavicular fractures, simple skull fractures, and long bone fractures.

The Allman classification of clavicular fractures divides fractures into types based on location and displacement. Type 1 fractures involve the middle clavicle and are the most common type (65% to 85%); type 2 (lateral clavicle) and type 3 (medial clavicle) account for 20% to 25% and 1% to 10% of fractures, respectively (**Option (E) is false**). In adults, when the medial (sternal) portion of the clavicle is injured, the sternoclavicular joint should be evaluated to assess for dislocation or subluxation. In children, rather than actual dislocation or subluxation of the sternal head of the clavicle, medial clavicular disruption represents a physeal injury, with separation of the metaphysis from the epiphysis. The clavicle can be either anteriorly or posteriorly located (Figure 16-19). With posterior location, there is a higher risk for injury to the subjacent aortic arch vessels. Injury at the medial aspect of the clavicle can be difficult to detect by standard radiography. If it is not diagnosed, chronic pain or cosmetic deformity can ensue. Although well seen on both MRI or CT, medial clavicular and sternoclavicular injuries are best evaluated by CT, including three-dimensional reconstructions.

The classification of lateral clavicular fractures is based on the involvement of the coracoclavicular ligaments. One classification for lateral clavicular fractures is the Neer classification. Across all ages, Neer type 1 (intact ligament) fractures account for about 66% of the cases (Figures 16-19 and 16-20), type 2 (disrupted ligament) fractures account for 21%, and type 3 (disruption of the acromioclavicular joint, intact ligaments) fractures account for 13%. In children, the frequency of type 1 fractures is about 50% and the frequencies of the other types are about equal. In adults, type 1 fractures usually heal well with immobilization and type 2 fractures usually are repaired by internal fixation. Sequelae of type 3 fractures include osteolysis and acromioclavicular arthrosis and may require distal clavicular resection. The prognosis for healing of lateral clavicular fractures by conservative treatment is better in children. This is because the inferior periosteum of the clavicle remains adherent to the coracoid and coracoclavicular ligament complex. Therefore, healing with remodeling is usually complete even with disruption of the ligamentous complex by a displaced lateral clavicular fracture.

Since lateral and medial clavicular fractures are much less common than fractures in the midclavicle and since the majority of clavicle fractures in children are nondisplaced or minimally displaced, the vast majority of clavicular fractures heal with immobilization alone. Nonunion of clavicular fractures is rare, occurring in less than 1% at all ages (**Option (D) is true**). Injury to the acromioclavicular joint occurs in only about 1% of all clavicular fractures in children (**Option (F) is false**).

Traumatic clavicular osteolysis occurs after trauma to the shoulder; it can be associated with acromioclavicular dislocation or ligamentous injury. In a minority of cases, it is seen in patients with fractures of the clavicle, particularly the lateral clavicle (**Option (B) is true**). In these cases, there is probably concomitant injury of the acromioclavicular joint. Radiographically, there is resorption or tapering of up to about 3.0 cm of the acromial end of the clavicle, resulting in widening of the distance between the acromion and the remaining clavicle. MRI abnormalities of traumatic osteolysis are localized to the acromioclavicular joint, where increased signal intensity is noted on T2-weighted images. The marrow of the distal clavicle is usually normal.

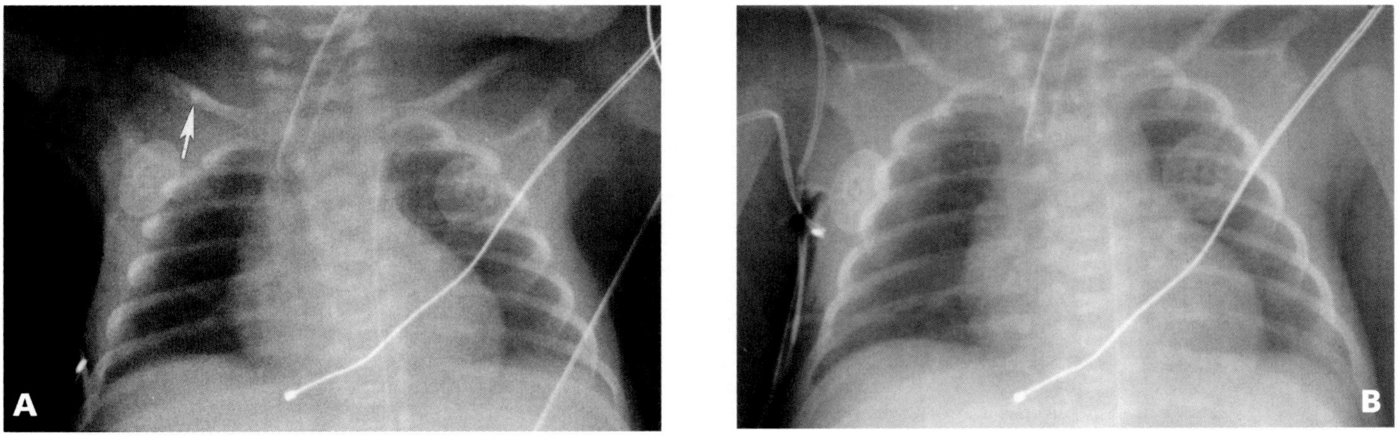

Figure 16-18. Clavicular pseudofracture in a 4-day-old preterm male infant. (A) An anteroposterior radiograph of the chest obtained with slight lordotic positioning shows elevation of the clavicles and an apparent sclerotic region in the right midclavicle (arrow). (B) A true anteroposterior view of the chest obtained 6 hours later demonstrates a more typical S-shaped course of the clavicles without any evidence of fracture.

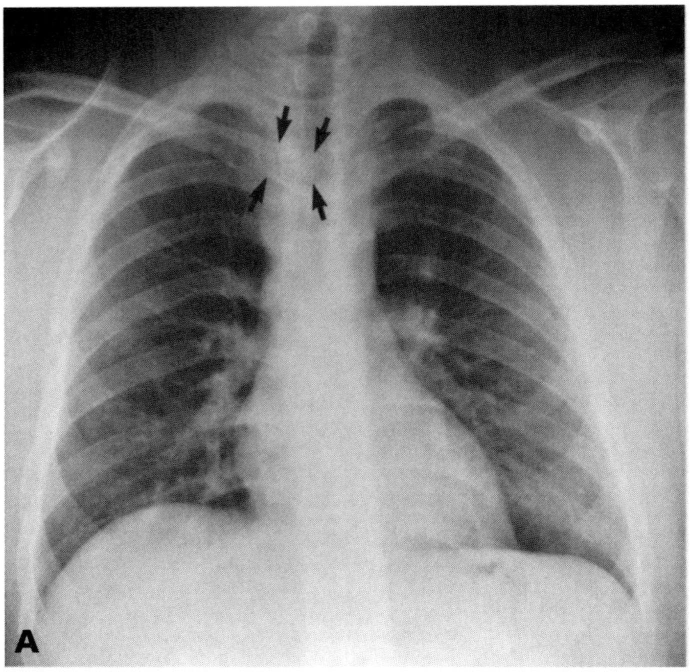

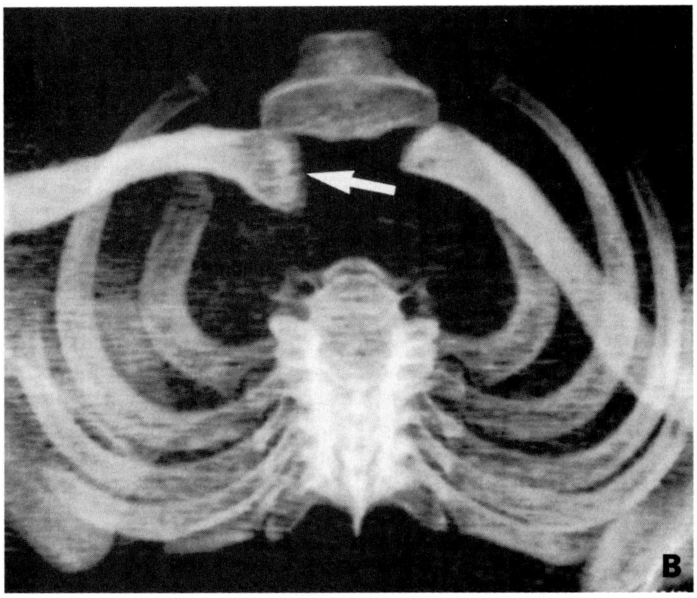

Figure 16-19. Acute posterior subluxation of the right clavicle at the sternoclavicular junction in a 16-year-old boy. (A) A posteroanterior chest radiograph demonstrates the clavicular head displaced superiorly and medially (arrows). (B) A volume-rendered CT examination of the thorax as viewed from above demonstrates the posterior subluxation and slight rotation of the right clavicular head (arrow) compared with the left.

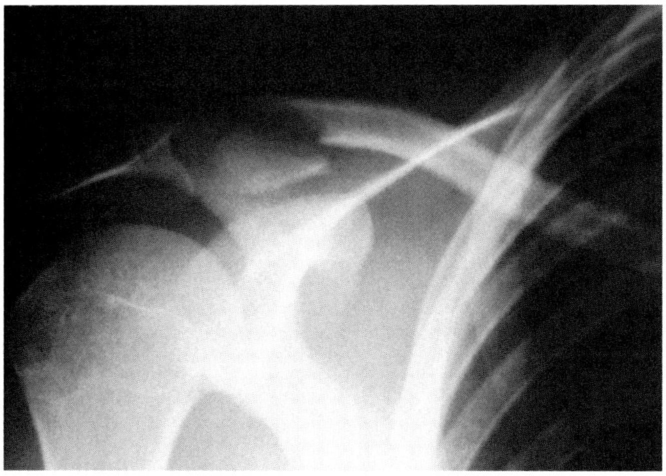

Figure 16-20. Lateral clavicular fracture following trauma in a 16-year-old girl. There is an oblique fracture through the lateral aspect of the right clavicle. Follow-up evaluation revealed that the coroco-clavicular ligaments were intact (Neer type 1 fracture).

SUGGESTED READINGS

EWING'S SARCOMA

1. Cohen MD. Imaging of children with cancer. St. Louis: Mosby-Year Book; 1992:219–238
2. Cotterill SJ, Ahrens S, Paulussen M, et al. Prognostic factors in Ewing's tumor of bone; analysis of 975 patients from the European Intergroup Cooperative Ewing's Sarcoma Study. J Clin Oncol 2000; 18:3108–3114
3. Eggli KD, Quiogue T, Moser RP Jr. Ewing's sarcoma. Radiol Clin North Am 1993; 31:325–337
4. Grier HE. The Ewing family of tumors. Ewing's sarcoma and primitive neuroectodermal tumors. Pediatr Clin North Am 1997; 44:991–1004
5. West DC. Ewing sarcoma family of tumors. Curr Opin Oncol 2000; 12: 323–329

CONGENITAL PSEUDARTHROSIS

6. Alldred AJ. Congenital pseudarthrosis of the clavicle. J Bone Joint Surg [Br] 1963; 45:312–319
7. Hahn K, Shah R, Shalev Y, Schmidt DH, Bajawa T. Congenital clavicular pseudarthrosis associated with vascular thoracic outlet syndrome: case presentation and review of the literature. Catheter Cardiovasc Diagn 1995; 35:321–327
8. Hirata S, Miya H, Mizuno K. Congenital pseudarthrosis of the clavicle. Histologic examination for the etiology of the disease. Clin Orthop 1995; 315:242–245
9. Lloyd-Roberts GC, Apley AG, Owen R. Reflections upon the aetiology of congenital pseudarthrosis of the clavicle. With a note on cranio-cleido dysostosis. J Bone Joint Surg [Br] 1975; 57:24–29
10. Resnick D. Bone and joint imaging. 2nd ed. Philadelphia: WB Saunders; 1996:1185–1186
11. Schoenecker PL, Johnson GE, Howard B, Capelli AM. Congenital pseudarthrosis. Orthop Rev 1992; 21:855–860
12. Shalom A, Khermosh O, Wientroub S. The natural history of congenital pseudarthrosis of the clavicle. J Bone Joint Surg [Br] 1994; 76:846–847

OSTEOMYELITIS

13. Dangman BC, Hoffer FA, Rand FF, O'Rourke EJ. Osteomyelitis in children: gadolinium-enhanced MR imaging. Radiology 1992; 182:743–747
14. Gerscovich EO, Greenspan A. Osteomyelitis of the clavicle: clinical, radiologic, and bacteriologic findings in ten patients. Skeletal Radiol 1994; 23:205–210
15. Lowden CM, Walsh SJ. Acute staphylococcal osteomyelitis of the clavicle. J Pediatr Orthop 1997; 17:467–469
16. Ma LD, Frassica FJ, Bluemke DA, Fishman EK. CT and MRI evaluation of musculoskeletal infection. Crit Rev Diagn Imaging 1997; 36: 535–568
17. Morrey BF, Bianco AJ Jr. Hematogenous osteomyelitis of the clavicle in children. Clin Orthop 1977; 125:24–28
18. Resnick D. Bone and joint imaging. 2nd ed. Philadelphia: WB Saunders; 1996:649–673
19. Schuster T, Bielek J, Dietz HG, Belohradsky BH. Chronic recurrent multifocal osteomyelitis (CRMO). Eur J Pediatr Surg 1996; 6:45–51

LANGERHANS CELL HISTIOCYTOSIS

20. Libicher M, Roeren T, Troger J. Localized Langerhans cell histiocytosis of bone: treatment and follow-up in children. Pediatr Radiol 1995; 25: S134–S137
21. Van Nieuwenhuyse JP, Clapuyt P, Malghem J, et al. Radiographic skeletal survey and radionuclide bone scan in Langerhans cell histiocytosis of bone. Pediatr Radiol 1996; 26:734–738

ANEURYSMAL BONE CYST

22. Capanna R, Campanacci DA, Manfrini M. Unicameral and aneurysmal bone cysts. Orthop Clin North Am 1996; 27:605–614
23 Hecht AC, Gebhardt MC. Diagnosis and treatment of unicameral and aneurysmal bone cysts in children. Curr Opin Pediatr 1998; 10:87–94
24. Leithner A, Windhager R, Lang S, Haas OA, Kainberger F, Kotz R. Aneurysmal bone cyst. A population based epidemiologic study and literature review. Clin Orthop 1999; 363:176–179
25. Oda Y, Tsuneyoshi M, Shinohara N. "Solid" variant of aneurysmal bone cyst (extragnathic giant cell reparative granuloma) in the axial skeleton and long bones: a study of its morphologic spectrum and distinction from allied giant cell lesions. Cancer 1992; 70:2642–2649
26. Sullivan RJ, Meyer JS, Dormans JP, Davidson RS. Diagnosing aneurysmal and unicameral bone cysts with magnetic resonance imaging. Clin Orthop 1999; 366:186–190

CLAVICULAR TRAUMA

27. al-Qattan MM, Clarke HM, Curtis CG. The prognostic value of concurrent clavicular fractures in newborns with obstetric brachial plexus palsy. J Hand Surg [Br] 1994; 19:729–730
28. Apter S, Hertz M, Salai M, Nerubai J, Bubis JJ. Post-traumatic reactive and resorptive lesions of the medial end of the clavicle. Clin Imaging 1992;16:40–42
29. Cahill BR. Atraumatic osteolysis of the distal clavicle. A review. Sports Med 1992; 13:214–222
30. Dameron TB, Rockwood CA. Fractures and dislocations of the shoulder. In: Rockwood CA, Wilkins KA, King RE (eds), Fractures in children. Philadelphia: JP Lippincott; 1984:608–650
31. Hardy JR. Complex clavicular injury in childhood. J Bone Joint Surg [Br] 1992; 74:154
32. Joseph PR, Rosenfeld W. Clavicular fractures in neonates. Am J Dis Child 1990; 144:165–167
33. Kleinman PK. Diagnostic imaging in infant abuse. AJR 1990; 155:703–712
34. Madsen B. Osteolysis of the acromial end of the clavicle following trauma. Br J Radiol 1963; 36:822–828
35. Nordqvist A, Petersson C. The incidence of fractures of the clavicle. Clin Orthop 1994; 300:127–132
36. Nordqvist A, Petersson C, Redlund-Johnell I. The natural course of lateral clavicle fracture. 15 (11–21) year follow-up of 110 cases. Acta Orthop Scand 1993; 64:87–91
37. Oppenheim WL, Davis A, Growdon WA, Dorey FJ, Davlin LB. Clavicle fractures in the newborn. Clin Orthop 1990; 250:176–180
38. Patten RM. Atraumatic osteolysis of the distal clavicle: MR findings. J Comput Assist Tomogr 1995; 19:92–95
39. Post M. Current concepts in the treatment of fractures of the clavicle. Clin Orthop 1989; 245:89–101

MISCELLANEOUS CLAVICULAR LESIONS

40. Azouz EM, Jurik AG, Bernard C. Sternoclavicular hyperostosis in children: a report of eight cases. AJR 1998; 171:461–466
41. Conway WF, Hayes CW. Miscellaneous lesions of bone. Radiol Clin North Am 1993; 31:339–358
42. Oda Y, Hashimoto H, Tsuneyoshi M, Masuda S. Case report 793. Periosteal osteosarcoma of the clavicle. Skeletal Radiol 1993; 22:375–377
43. Tait TJ, Chalmers AG, Bird HA. Condensing osteitis of the clavicle: differentiation from sternocostoclavicular hyperostosis by magnetic resonance imaging. Br J Rheumatol 1994; 33:985–987
44 . Vierboom MA, Steinberg JD, Mooyaart EL, van Rijswijk MH. Condensing osteitis of the clavicle: magnetic resonance imaging as an adjunct method for differential diagnosis. Ann Rheum Dis 1992; 51:539–541

CASE 17

Lane F. Donnelly, M.D.

Lymphoproliferative Disorder

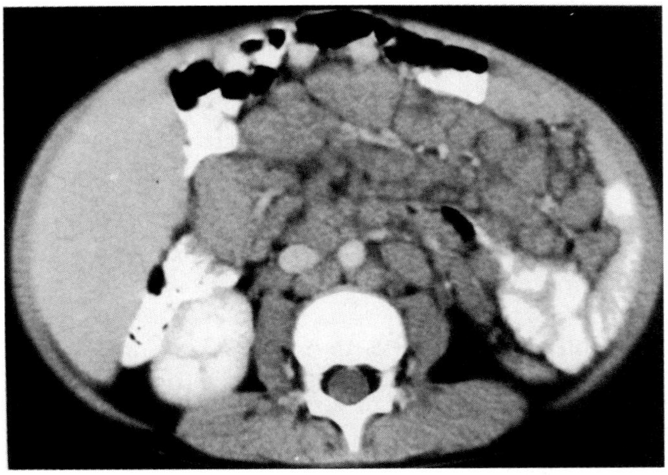

Figure 17-1

Question 82

This 4-year-old boy has an abdominal mass. You are shown a postcontrast abdominal CT image (Figure 17-1).

Which *one* of the following is the MOST likely diagnosis?

(A) Kawasaki disease
(B) Tuberculosis
(C) Chronic granulomatous disease of childhood
(D) Lymphoproliferative disorder
(E) Mesenteric adenitis

The CT image of the test patient (Figure 17-1) shows lymph node enlargement involving the mesenteric and retroperitoneal nodes (Figure 17-2). The attenuation of the nodes is homogeneous and similar in density to that of skeletal muscle. Of the options listed, lymphoproliferative disorder is the most likely explanation for lymphadenopathy with this distribution and this nodal appearance (**Option (D) is correct**). The test patient had an underlying T-lymphocyte deficiency.

The lymphoproliferative disorders are potentially life-threatening conditions occurring in patients with underlying primary or secondary immunodeficiency. The pathogenesis of the lymphoproliferative disorders begins with an Epstein-Barr virus-induced proliferation of B lymphocytes. In hosts with competent immune systems, such proliferation is controlled by T-cell-mediated mechanisms. When these T-cell defenses are deficient, the proliferation of B lymphocytes continues and a polyclonal lymphoproliferative disorder can result. If the lymphocytes continue to proliferate, clonal selection can occur, allowing overgrowth of the fastest-growing, dominant clone. When this situation occurs, the lymphoproliferative disorders can become monoclonal. Lymphoproliferative disorders have been found in solid-organ transplant recipients, bone marrow transplant recipients, patients with primary immunodeficiencies, and patients with AIDS. When the disorder is manifested as lymphadenopathy, the lymph nodes are often large and numerous. As in the test patient, involvement of the lymph nodes of the retroperitoneum and mesentery is common in patients with lymphoproliferative disorder; in one series, it occurred in about 50% of patients with abdominal involvement. Although the appearance of involved nodes in patients with lymphoproliferative disorder can vary and central low attenuation as a result of necrosis has been reported, the lymph nodes usually appear as nodules with homogeneous attenuation, as in the test patient. See the discussion of Question 83 for additional infor-

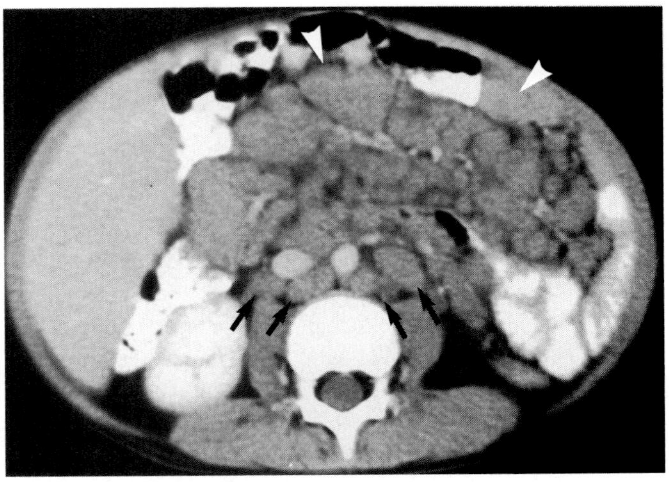

Figure 17-2 (Same as Figure 17-1). Lymphoproliferative disorder in a 4-year-old boy with a history of congenital T-lymphocyte deficiency. A CT image shows extensive lymphadenopathy involving both the mesentery (arrowheads) and the retroperitoneum (arrows). The lymph nodes are of homogeneous attenuation, similar to muscle.

mation about lymphoproliferative disorders.

Kawasaki disease (acute infantile febrile mucocutaneous syndrome) (Option (A)) is an illness related to a systemic vasculitis. It was first described in 1967 and is still of unknown etiology. The associated vasculitis affects the media and adventitia of medium and small arteries, which are infiltrated by lymphocytes and large mononuclear cells. Kawasaki disease predominantly affects children younger than 5 years (the peak incidence is at 1 to 2 years of age). Therefore, the age of the test patient is consistent with this diagnosis.

Kawasaki disease is an acute febrile illness that can be divided into acute, subacute, and convalescent phases. During the acute phase, the diagnostic criteria include fever for 5 days and four or five of the following features: peripheral extremity edema, erythema or desquamation, conjunctivitis, mucosal changes, truncal rash, or cervical lymphadenopathy.

Of the five criteria, cervical lymphadenopathy is the least common, occurring in only 50% to 75% of patients. The other criteria are all seen in approximately 90% of patients. The lymphadenopathy is typically unilateral and confined to the cervical region. Abdominal lymphadenopathy has been found, but it is uncommon. The massive abdominal lymphadenopathy seen in the test patient is not consistent with Kawasaki disease.

Most commonly, Kawasaki disease is a self-limited illness. However, serious morbidity and mortality, usually related to coronary artery disease or myocarditis, can occur if the disease is left untreated. Although the association with coronary artery aneurysms has received the greatest attention in the literature, most morbidity is related to either acute myocarditis (Figure 17-3) or coronary artery stenosis in later years. In a study by Kato et al. of 594 children with Kawasaki disease, 4.7% developed ischemic heart disease, 1.9% developed myocardial infarction, and 0.8% died of cardiac complications. Coronary artery aneurysms have been depicted by echocardiography, arteriography, and MRI (Figure 17-4). Calcifications can be seen within the aneurysms on chest radiographs. The treatment for Kawasaki disease includes intravenous gamma globulin and aspirin. This therapy has been shown to reduce the frequency of development of coronary artery aneurysms from 25% to 5%. The acute febrile illness usually subsides within 48 hours after therapy is initiated.

The most common abdominal imaging feature of Kawasaki disease is gallbladder hydrops. Other imaging features include enterocolitis, splenic infarction, cholangitis, and intussusception.

Human infection with *Mycobacterium tuberculosis* is older than recorded history. Classic spinal changes of tuberculosis have been identified in the skeletons of Neolithic humans. The term "tuberculosis" was first used by Fansiscus Sylvius in 1769 to describe the characteristic lung nodules. It is derived from the Latin *tubercula*, which means "small knots." During the 1800s, tuberculosis (Option (B)) was considered the cause of 20% to 30% of all deaths and was a particularly common cause of death in children. With the advent of antimicrobial therapy in the 1950s, the disease became a much less dominant public health problem, and by the 1960s, its eradication was predicted. Unfortunately, in the late 1980s, there was an alarming increase in the prevalence of the disease worldwide. It is estimated that one of every three persons in the world harbors *M. tuberculosis* and is at risk for developing the disease. There are 8 million new cases annually and 3 million deaths secondary to tuberculosis annually. Although most of these cases are in Africa and Asia, where tuberculosis accounts for up to 16.5% of all deaths, there also has been a rapid increase in the number of cases of tuberculosis in the United States and United Kingdom. This increase is attributable to multiple factors, including increasing drug resistance of *M. tuberculosis*, an aging population, the overcrowding of indigent people in large urban

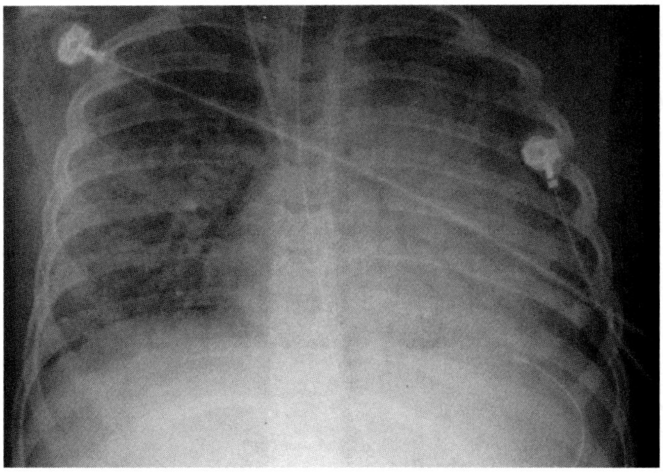

Figure 17-3. Kawasaki disease presenting with shock secondary to myocarditis in a 1-year-old boy. A chest radiograph shows bilateral diffuse lung opacification secondary to pulmonary edema. The child presented with a prolonged febrile illness that progressed to shock and was not responsive to inotropic drugs. Echocardiography initially showed a dilated left ventricle with markedly decreased wall motion. Only later did the child develop the characteristic distal extremity rash, as well as dilated coronary arteries on echocardiography.

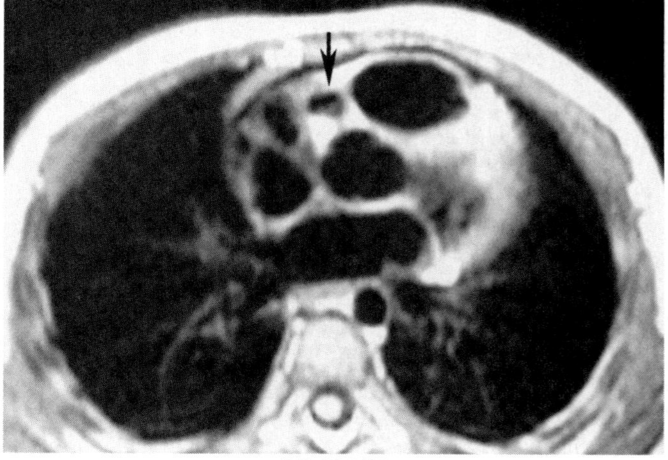

SE 600/10

Figure 17-4. Coronary artery aneurysms secondary to Kawasaki disease in a 3-year-old boy. An axial T1-weighted spin-echo MR image shows aneurysmal dilatation (arrow) of the proximal right coronary artery. (Case courtesy of George S. Bisset III, M.D., Duke University Medical Center, Durham, NC.)

areas, the spread of AIDS, and poor patient and physician compliance with drug therapy. There also has been an alarming increase in the number of tuberculosis cases in children. During the late 1980s and early 1990s, pediatric tuberculosis infections increased by approximately 30% per year.

Because tuberculosis is spread through the respiratory system, the chest is the most common site of involvement. The most common chest radiographic appearance of primary tuberculosis in children is hilar or mediastinal lymphadenopathy in the absence of pulmonary opacification. The hilar lymphadenopathy is usually unilateral (Figure 17-5). When the lung is consolidated, the consolidation has no lobar predilection, unlike the pattern of parenchymal lung involvement in secondary tuberculosis, which most often affects the upper lobes. Other chest radiographic findings include reticulonodular opacities, unexplained pleural fluid, lobar collapse secondary to bronchial compression by enlarged lymph nodes (Figure 17-5), and persistent lung opacity despite antibiotic therapy. CT can be used to further delineate the location of disease (Figure 17-6), detect occult cavitation, characterize the opacities as nodular, and detect bronchiectasis.

Abdominal involvement in tuberculosis can occur either as a result of swallowing sputum harboring the organisms or hematogenous dissemination. Most of the published series of abdominal tuberculosis are from Africa or Asia and include a mixture of pediatric and adult patients. Chest radiographs are normal in up to 65% of patients who have abdominal tuberculosis. The most common manifestation of abdominal tuberculosis is lymphadenopathy; this is the sole abdominal manifestation in up to 55% of patients. The lymph nodes are best imaged by CT and tend to be large and bulky, measuring up to 3 cm in diameter. Compared with other causes of lymphadenopathy, tuberculous lymphadenopathy classically tends to exhibit central low attenuation and peripheral enhancement of involved lymph nodes (Figure 17-7). Histologically, this appearance is related to a peripheral highly vascular inflammatory reaction and central liquefaction and caseating necrosis. It is highly suggestive, but not pathognomonic, of tuberculosis and has been reported to occur in up to 60% of patients with tuberculous lymphadenopathy. The lymph nodes can appear as multiple separate nodes, but often appear as a conglomerate mass. The most common sites of involvement include the mesentery, omentum (Figure 17-7), and peripancreatic groups. Retroperitoneal lymphadenopathy has been reported, but it is uncommon. Tuberculosis is a possibility in the test patient, but the distribution is both mesenteric and retroperitoneal. Additionally, there is no evidence of central low attenuation or peripheral enhancement. The absence of these features would be unusual for tuberculosis with such extensive lymphadenopathy.

Abdominal tuberculosis also can involve the genitourinary system, including the kidneys, ureters, bladder, prostate, and epididymis. Tuberculosis also can involve any part of the gastrointestinal tract, but most commonly affects the cecum and terminal ileum. CT may show bowel wall thickening and irregularity (Figure 17-8), luminal narrowing, and ulceration. The wall thickening may be circumferential or asymmetric. The characteristic appearance is asymmetric thickening of the terminal ileum and medial wall of the cecum (which occurs in 45% of patients) (Figure 17-8). The findings on CT can appear similar to those of lymphoma and Crohn's disease. Barium

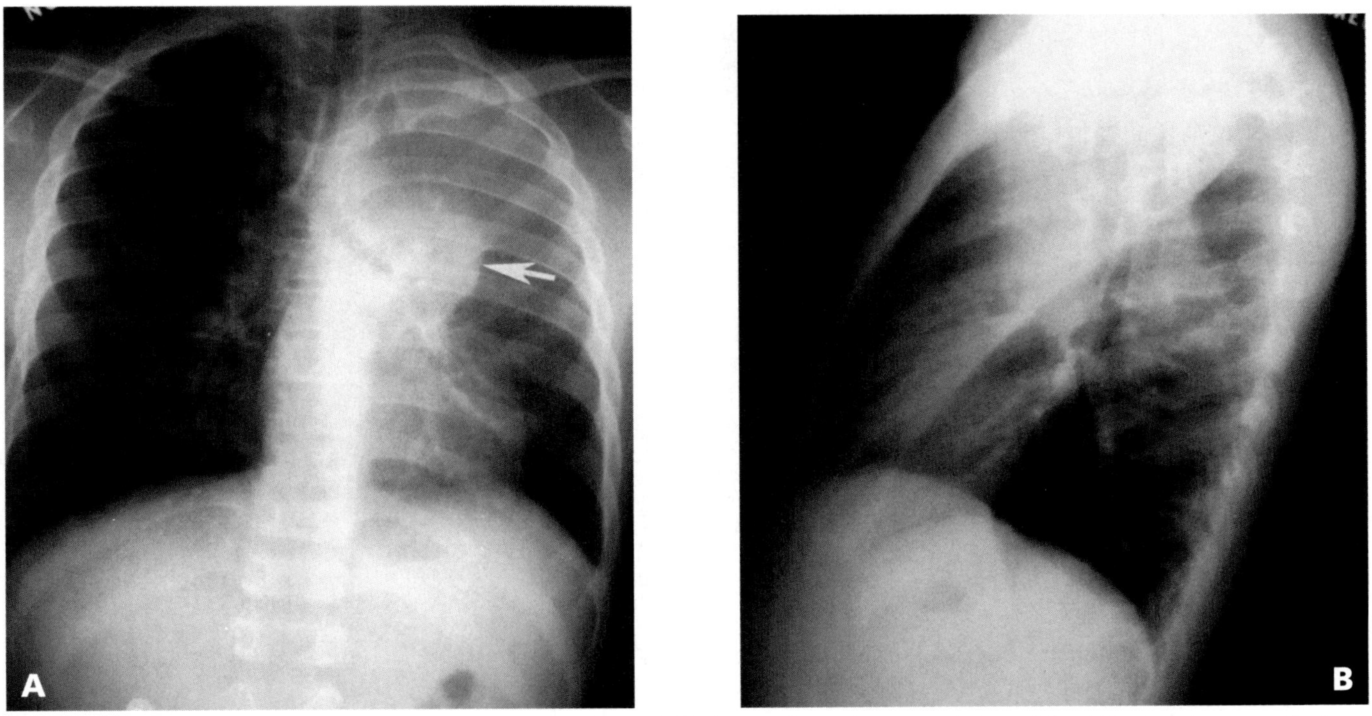

Figure 17-5. Tuberculosis in a 16-year-old boy. Frontal (A) and lateral (B) chest radiographs demonstrate unilateral hilar lymphadenopathy (arrow). There is also left upper lobe collapse, attributable to compression of the left upper lobe bronchus by the enlarged lymph nodes.

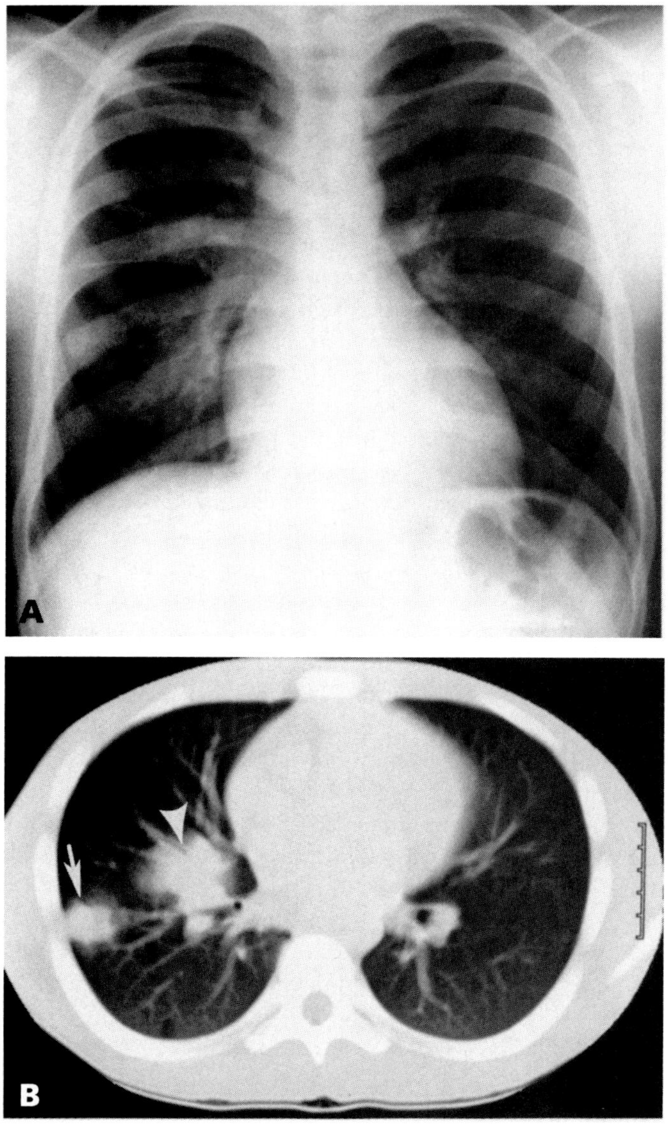

Figure 17-6. Tuberculosis in a 17-year-old boy. (A) A frontal chest radiograph shows poorly defined density in the lateral right lower lung and right hilar region. (B) A CT image shows nodular consolidation in the peripheral right lower lobe (arrow) and right hilar lymphadenopathy (arrowhead).

studies can show luminal narrowing and irregularity (Figure 17-9), ulceration, fistula, or obstruction. Isolated peritoneal involvement occurs in less than 4% of patients. The liver, spleen, and pancreas also can be involved by tuberculosis.

Chronic granulomatous disease of childhood (Option (C)) is a primary immunodeficiency disorder attributable to enzymatic defects in polymorphonuclear leukocytes and a resultant inability to defend against infections by certain bacteria and fungi. The disease is an X-linked recessive disorder. Affected individuals are particularly susceptible to infection by catalase-positive organisms such as *Staphylococcus aureus* and gram-negative bacteria. The remaining components of cellular and humoral immunity are intact. Common manifestations of chronic granulomatous disease include osteomyelitis (Figure 17-10), granulomatous lesions of the skin, chronic or recurrent pneumonia (Figure 17-11), intermittent

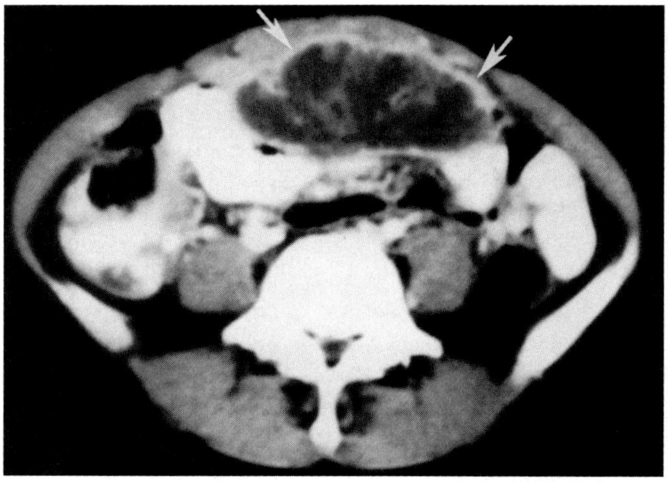

Figure 17-7. Tuberculosis in a 16-year-old girl. A CT scan shows a large omental mass representing a conglomerate of involved lymph nodes (arrows). The lesion demonstrates central low attenuation and peripheral enhancement, characteristic of lymphadenopathy attributable to tuberculosis. (Case courtesy of Ingo O. Rencken. M.D., University of California at San Francisco, San Francisco, CA.)

abdominal pain, cystitis, and esophageal strictures. Although lymphadenopathy can occur, massive mesenteric and retroperitoneal lymphadenopathy, as seen in the test image, would be atypical.

Mesenteric adenitis (Option (E)) is a clinical entity characterized by benign inflammatory lymphadenopathy of the mesentery, sometimes with associated ileitis. The typical CT finding is right lower quadrant lymphadenopathy, most commonly anterior to the right psoas muscle and within the small bowel mesentery. Retroperitoneal lymphadenopathy, as seen in the test image, is not associated with mesenteric adenitis. Mesenteric adenitis is further considered in the discussion of Question 84.

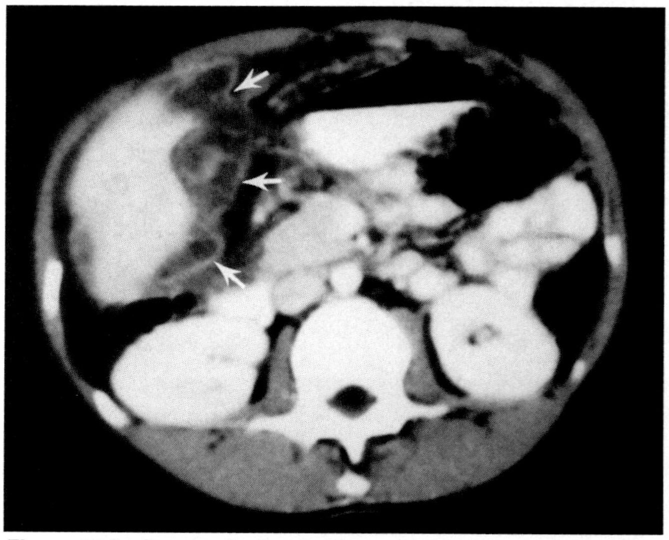

Figure 17-8. Same patient as in Figure 17-7. Tuberculosis in a 16-year-old girl. A CT scan shows thickening of the medial wall of the cecum (arrows). This distribution of wall thickening is characteristic of tuberculosis. (Case courtesy of Ingo O. Rencken, M.D.)

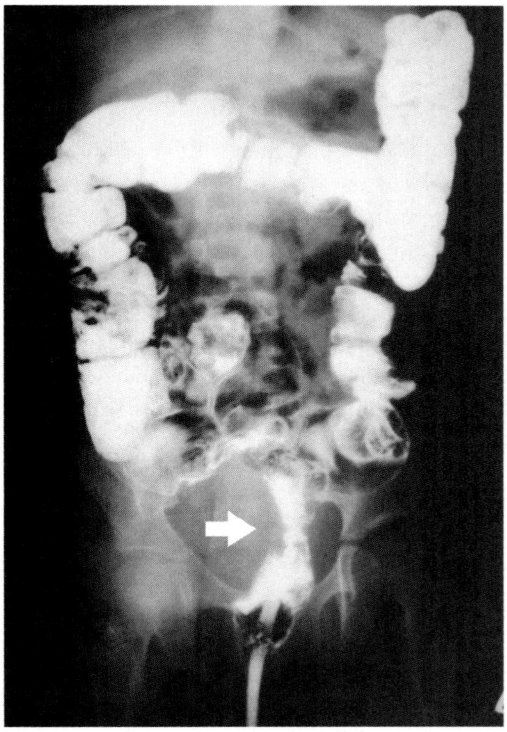

Figure 17-9. Tuberculosis in a 6-year-old girl. A barium enema examination shows narrowing and irregularity of the sigmoid colon (arrow). There is mass effect from adjacent lymphadenopathy. (Case courtesy of Ingo O. Rencken, M.D.)

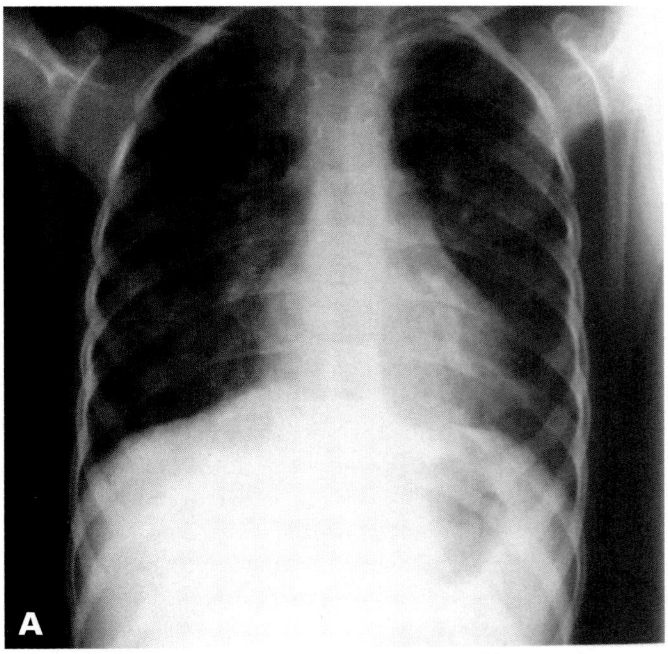

Figure 17-10. Chronic pneumonia and osteomyelitis secondary to *Staphylococcus aureus* infection in a 6-year-old boy with chronic granulomatous disease of childhood. (A) A chest radiograph demonstrates increased peribronchial markings and patchy bilateral lung consolidation; these findings were present on serial radiographs.

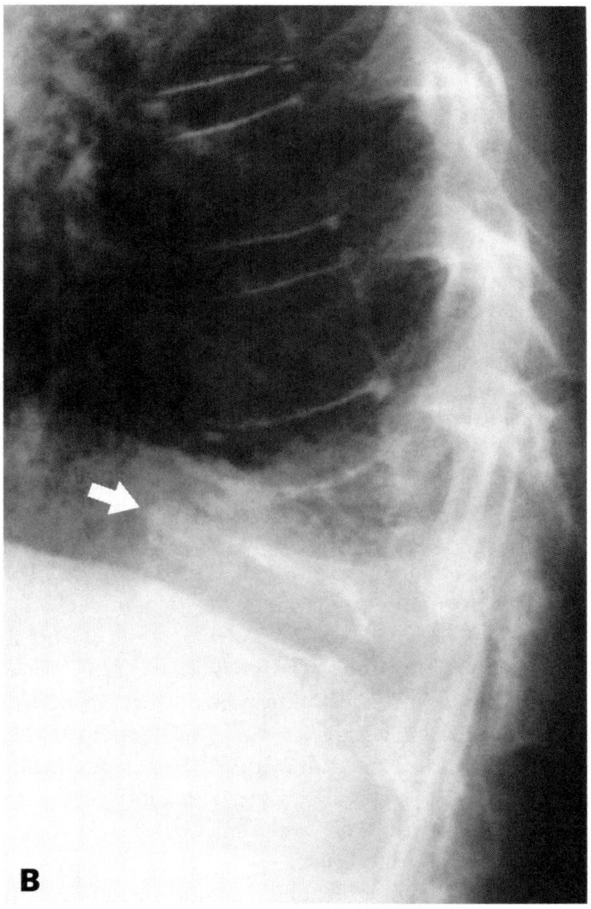

Figure 17-10 (Continued). Chronic pneumonia and osteomyelitis secondary to *Staphylococcus aureus* infection in a 6-year-old boy with chronic granulomatous disease of childhood. (B) A lateral radiograph of the thoracolumbar spine shows collapse with mixed sclerosis and lucency involving the 11th thoracic vertebral body (arrow), consistent with osteomyelitis.

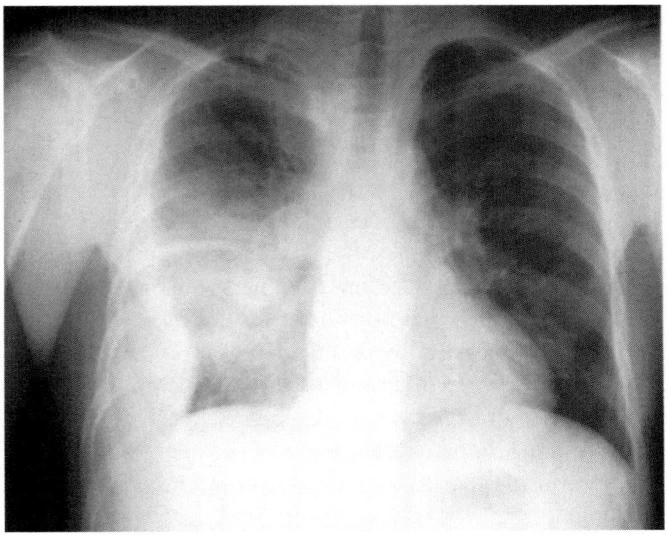

Figure 17-11. *Staphylococcus aureus* pneumonia and empyema in a 15-year-old boy with chronic granulomatous disease of childhood. A chest radiograph shows right pleural thickening, consolidation of the superior segment of the right lower lobe, and right hilar lymphadenopathy.

Question 83

Concerning lymphoproliferative disorder,

(A) it occurs most commonly in bone marrow transplant recipients
(B) the prognosis is more closely related to the cause of the underlying immunodeficiency than to the distribution of the disease
(C) it is caused by Epstein-Barr virus
(D) children with congenital B-cell deficiencies are at high risk for its development
(E) extranodal is more frequent than nodal involvement in the abdomen
(F) the usual initial treatment is chemotherapy

When a primary infection with Epstein-Barr virus occurs in an immunocompetent host, acute infectious mononucleosis can occur. It is essentially a self-limited lymphoproliferative disorder. In patients with mononucleosis, the proliferation of infected B lymphocytes is controlled by cytotoxic T lymphocytes. When the infected host has a deficiency of functional cytotoxic T lymphocytes, the proliferation of infected B cells may not be controlled and an Epstein-Barr virus-induced lymphoproliferative disorder can result (**Option (C) is true**). Lymphoproliferative disorder represents a spectrum of abnormalities including mononucleosis sepsis, polyclonal B-cell hyperplasia, and monoclonal B-cell cancers.

Although lymphoproliferative disorders are most common and have been most thoroughly characterized in solid-organ transplant recipients (**Option (A) is false**), they can occur in patients with immunosuppression from almost any cause. Lymphoproliferative disorder has been found in children with solid-organ transplants, bone marrow transplants, HIV infection, and primary immunodeficiencies. In one series by Donnelly et al., the underlying causes of lymphoproliferative disorders were solid-organ transplantation in 66% of the patients, bone marrow transplantation in 15% of the patients, and primary immunodeficiency in 19% of the patients. Because cytotoxic T lymphocytes control Epstein-Barr virus-infected B lymphocytes, patients with primary immunodeficiencies that most severely impair T-cell function are at the highest risk for developing lymphoproliferative disorder. These immunodeficiencies include Wiskott-Aldrich syndrome, severe combined immunodeficiency syndrome, and other congenital T-lymphocyte deficiencies. Children with congenital B-lymphocyte deficiencies are not at risk for lymphoproliferative disorder (**Option (D) is false**).

The distribution of disease for all children with lymphoproliferative disorder has been described by Donnelly et al.; in their series the abdomen was involved in 63% of the cases, the chest was involved in 37%, the neck (cervical nodes and oropharyngeal lymphatic tissues) was involved in 30%, and the brain was involved in 4%. Approximately one half of the patients had localized disease and one half had involvement of multiple organ systems or anatomic areas. However, in solid-organ transplants, the disease is more likely to occur in the allograft organ itself and within the anatomic region of the transplant (Figures 17-12 through 17-16). It is speculated that the allograft acts as a chronic antigenic stimulus and, like a foreign body, attracts the proliferating B lymphocytes to the region of the transplant. In children with heart transplants, the disease is most likely to involve the chest and neck; isolated abdominal involvement is uncommon. In contrast, in liver transplant recipients, the disease usually occurs in the allograft liver and is often isolated to the abdomen. The likelihood that an abnormality represents a lymphoproliferative disorder can be estimated on the basis of the location of the abnormality in relation to the type of organ transplant that the patient has received. For example, mediastinal lymphadenopathy is much more likely to represent lymphoproliferative disorder in a heart transplant recipient than in a liver transplant recipient.

Much like lymphoma, lymphoproliferative disorder can be manifested in a number of ways, including lymphadenopathy, focal parenchymal masses or nodules, or diffuse infiltration of organs without a focal mass. The imaging appearances of these manifestations are nonspecific. Extranodal involvement is more common than nodal disease in the abdomen (**Option (E) is true**). In one series by Pickhardt and Siegel of both children and adults with abdominal involvement by lymphoproliferative disorder, nodal disease occurred in 34% of the patients, with retroperitoneal and iliac nodes being more commonly involved than intraperitoneal nodes. On CT scans, the nodes most commonly appear solid (Figure 17-2). However, necrosis and central low attenuation have been described. Such necrotic nodes can mimic abscesses.

The liver is the most common abdominal organ affected by lymphoproliferative disorder. Of the 60 patients with abdominal lymphoproliferative disease reported by Pickhardt and Siegel, 69% had liver involvement, followed by bowel and splenic involvement in 28% and 22%, respectively. In 17 cases reported by Donnelly et al., the liver was involved in 71%, the spleen was involved in 35%, and the bowel was involved in 17%. On CT scans, the findings of the disease in the liver are variable, ranging from a discrete mass or masses (Figure 17-12) to diffuse hepatomegaly without a focal mass. Periportal low attenuation (Figure 17-12) has been reported in about one third of patients. One unique characteristic of lymphoproliferative disorder involving the liver is that the masses tend to surround and engulf the portal venous structures; in contrast, most hepatic masses of other causes displace the portal venous structures (Figure 17-12). This appearance and the prevalence of periportal low attenuation may reflect the fact that the lymphoproliferative masses tend to arise in the periportal lymphatic tissues, whereas most other hepatic masses tend to arise in the hepatic parenchyma and secondarily involve portal structures. Hepatic masses in lymphoproliferative disorder appear as areas of low attenuation on CT scans and are hypoechoic on sonography.

The most common appearance of splenic involvement is a focal discrete mass (Figure 17-12) or masses. However, splenomegaly without an identifiable focal mass can occur. As in the

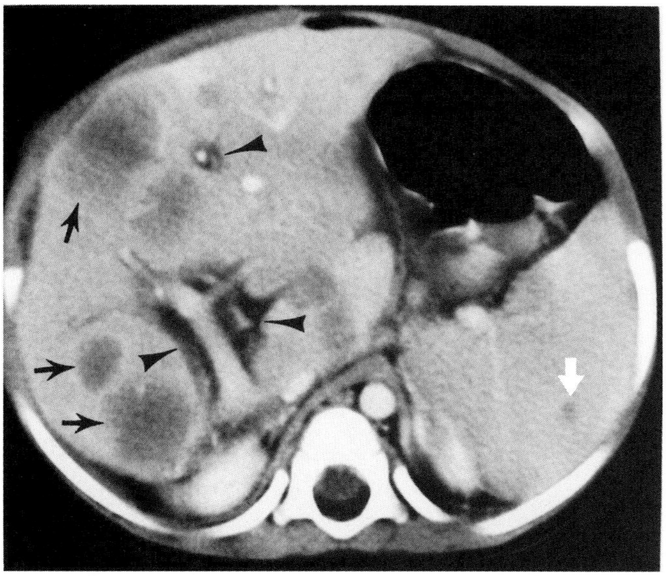

Figure 17-12. Lymphoproliferative disorder in a 1-year-old boy after liver transplantation. A CT scan shows multiple low-attenuation masses (black arrows) in a left-lobe segmental liver transplant. Periportal low attenuation (arrowheads) and a splenic lesion (white arrow) are also seen.

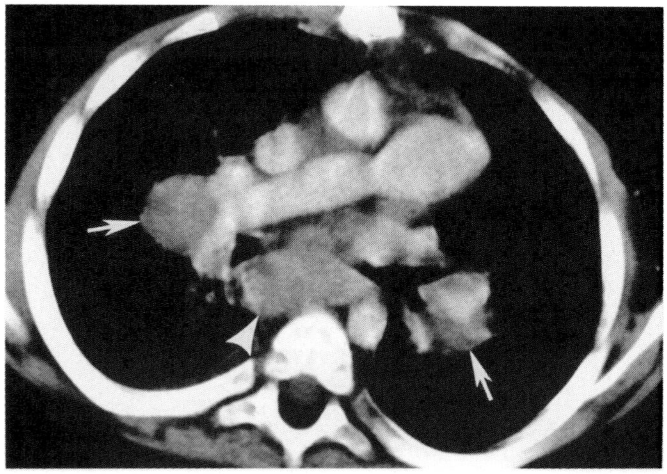

Figure 17-14. Lymphoproliferative disorder in a 6-year-old boy after a heart transplantation. A CT scan shows bilateral hilar (arrows) and mediastinal (arrowhead) lymphadenopathy.

liver, splenic masses appear as areas of low attenuation on CT scans and are hypoechoic on sonography.

Bowel involvement can be manifested as circumferential bowel wall thickening (Figure 17-13), an eccentric focal mass or masses, aneurysmal dilatation (Figure 17-13), or luminal narrowing. Additional findings include perforation and intussusception. Less common sites of abdominal disease include the abdominal wall, genitourinary tract, pancreas, and peritoneum.

In patients with lymphoproliferative disorder that involves the chest, the most common manifestation is mediastinal, hilar, or axillary lymphadenopathy (Figure 17-14). Lung nodules also are common. Other features of thoracic lymphoproliferative disorder include nonspecific lung consolidation, peribronchial thickening, and chest wall masses. The cervical region is another common site for lymphoproliferative disorder, manifested by involvement of lymph nodes (Figure 17-15) or oropharyngeal lymphatic tissues (Figure 17-16).

The initial therapy for a solid-organ recipient who develops lymphoproliferative disorder is a reduction in the degree of immunosuppression. Many cases of polyclonal lymphoprolifer-

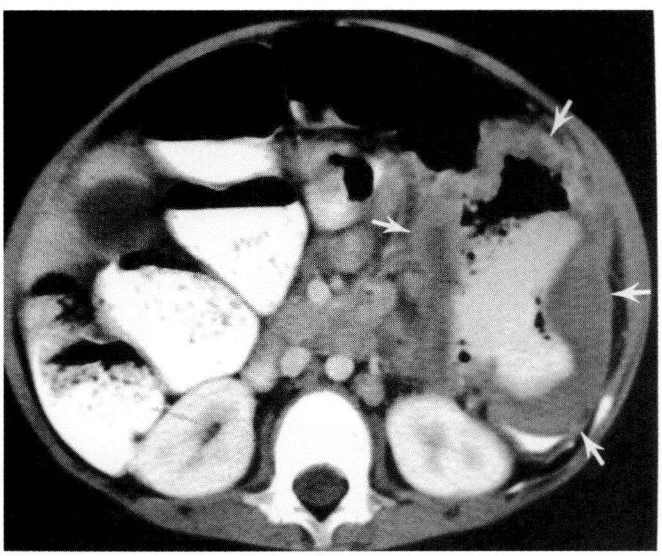

Figure 17-13. Lymphoproliferative disorder in an 8-year-old boy with Wiskott-Aldrich syndrome. A CT scan shows aneurysmal dilatation and marked bowel wall thickening (arrows) involving a segment of the jejunum.

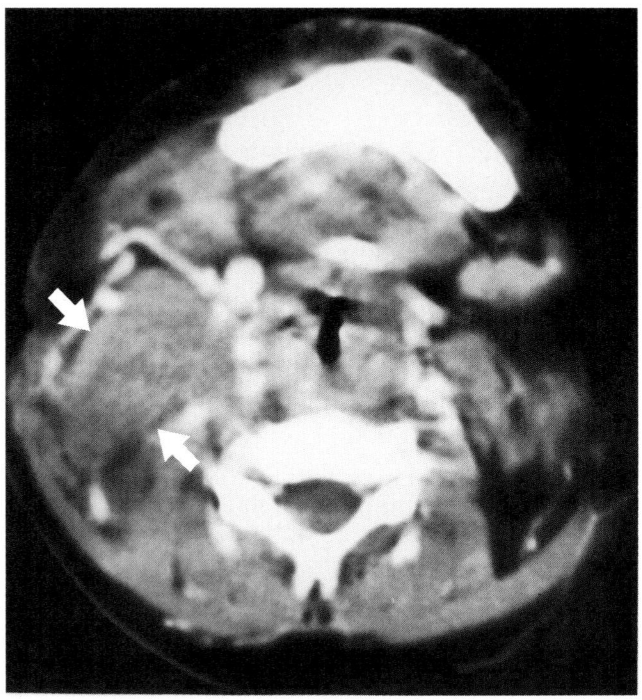

Figure 17-15. Lymphoproliferative disorder in a 5-year-old boy after heart transplantation. A CT scan shows a mass (arrows) in the right posterior cervical triangle.

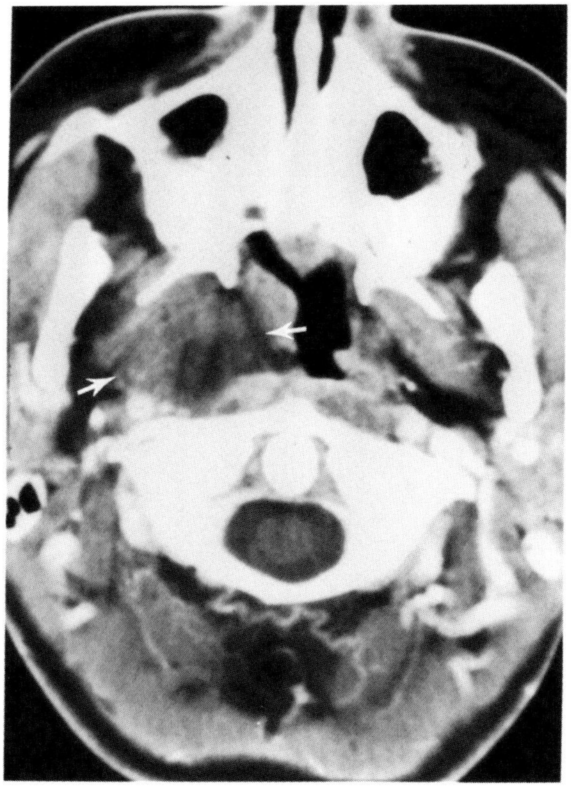

Figure 17-16. Lymphoproliferative disorder in a 14-year-old girl after heart transplantation. A CT scan shows a low-attenuation right parapharyngeal mass (arrows).

ative disorder and some cases of monoclonal lymphoproliferative disorder will resolve with a reduction in the degree of immunosuppression alone. Only when this measure fails is chemotherapy instituted (**Option (F) is false**). The prognosis of lymphoproliferative disorder after solid-organ transplantation is related to the extent of disease; widespread distribution is associated with a poorer prognosis than is localized disease. However, evaluation of patients with lymphoproliferative disorder of all causes has shown that the prognosis is much less closely related to the anatomic extent of disease than to the cause of the underlying immunodeficiency (**Option (B) is true**). Patients with fixed causes of immunosuppression, such as bone marrow transplant recipients and children with primary immunodeficiencies, have a much poorer prognosis than do patients with adjustable causes of immunodeficiency, such as immunosuppression to prevent rejection of a solid-organ transplant. Likewise, the degree of immunosuppression required to prevent rejection varies with the different solid-organ transplants; the prognosis of lymphoproliferative disorders in these patients is directly related to this factor. Heart transplants require higher degrees of immunosuppression than do many other solid-organ transplants, and heart transplant recipients who develop lymphoproliferative disorder have a worse prognosis than do liver transplant recipients with lymphoproliferative disorder.

Question 84

Concerning mesenteric adenitis,

(A) the diagnosis is usually made by biopsy of affected lymph nodes
(B) leukocytosis is rarely present
(C) CT typically shows lymph node enlargement in the large bowel mesentery
(D) the cause is usually bacterial
(E) nodal involvement is usually more diffusely distributed than the mesenteric adenopathy seen in patients with appendicitis

Mesenteric adenitis is a clinical entity related to benign inflammation of the lymph nodes in the mesentery and right lower quadrant of the abdomen, sometimes associated with enteritis. It is a diagnosis of exclusion based on a constellation of clinical symptoms, imaging findings, and clinical course. Therefore, diagnosis is not made on the basis of biopsy of affected lymph nodes (**Option (A) is false**). The cause of mesenteric adenitis is usually not identified. However, viruses and bacteria (*Yersinia* species and *Mycobacterium* species) have been implicated as causes. Most cases of mesenteric adenitis are thought to be related to a viral infection (**Option (D) is false**).

Since mesenteric adenitis is a benign, self-limited illness, the ideal treatment is conservative medical support. However, the true clinical relevance of mesenteric adenitis arises in differentiating this condition from appendicitis. The marked overlap in the symptoms of these two conditions makes this differentiation extremely difficult, if not impossible, on a clinical basis. Therefore, the diagnosis of mesenteric adenitis is often made during a laparotomy and nontherapeutic appendectomy. Clinically, patients with mesenteric adenitis present with nausea, vomiting, diarrhea, right lower quadrant abdominal pain and tenderness, fever, and leukocytosis (**Option (B) is false**). These are the same clinical symptoms as those of appendicitis. In a review of 651 children and adults who had an admission diagnosis of appendicitis, Rao et al. showed that 8% had a discharge diagnosis of mesenteric adenitis.

Differentiation between appendicitis and mesenteric adenitis on the basis of imaging is also difficult. CT images in mesenteric adenitis show enlarged and clustered lymph nodes (Figure 17-17) in the small bowel mesentery; a common site of involvement is just anterior to the right psoas muscle (**Option (C) is false**). Associated ileal wall thickening also can occur. Right lower quadrant lymphadenopathy alone is not helpful in differentiating appendicitis from mesenteric adenitis, since it is also present on CT images in about 80% of patients with documented appendicitis. The distribution and pattern of the lymphadenopathy can, however, be helpful in the differential diagnosis. In patients with appendicitis, lymphadenopathy is most commonly isolated to the region immediately anterior to the right psoas muscle, presumably in the mesentery of the appendix. In patients with mesenteric adenitis, the involved nodes

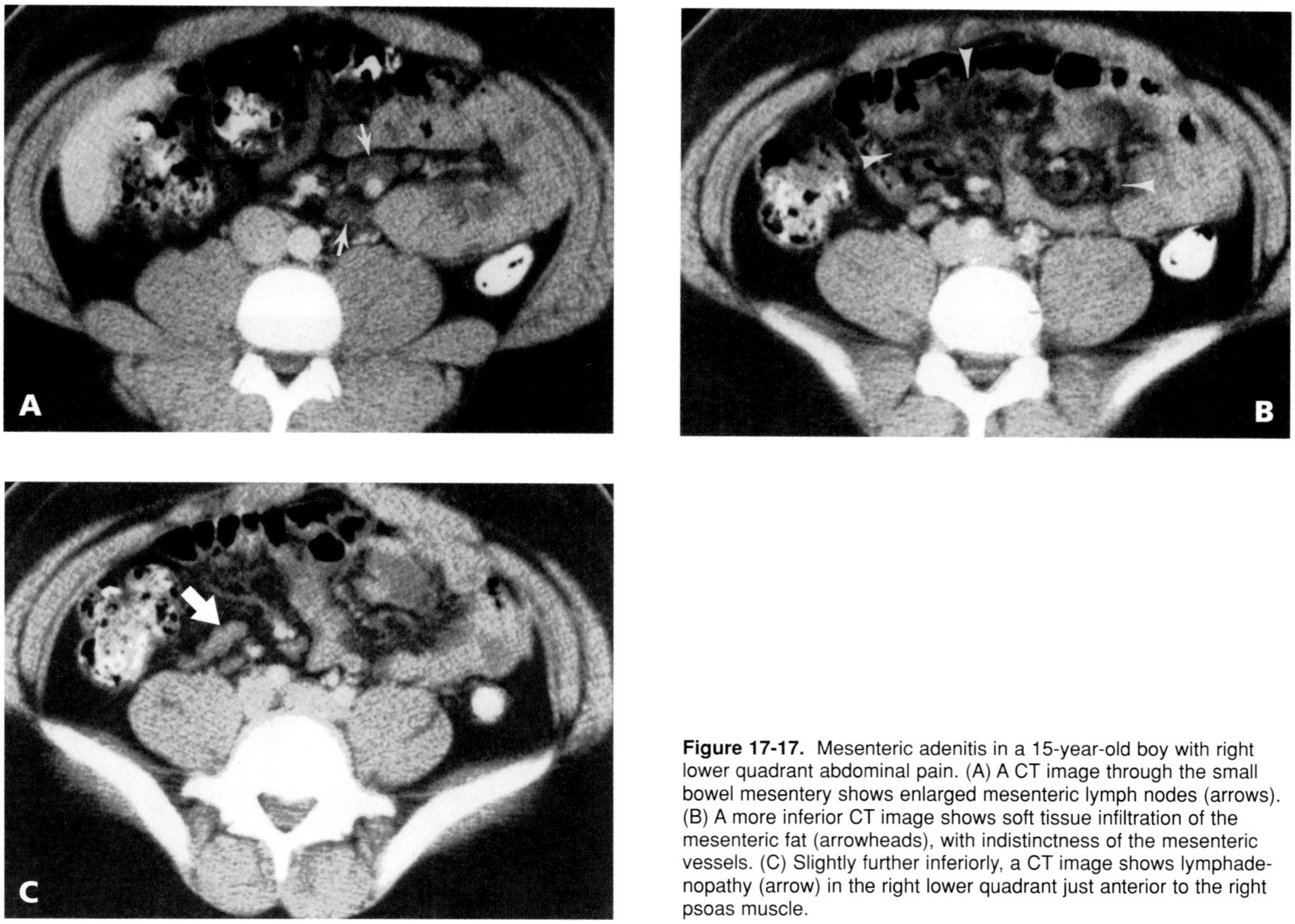

Figure 17-17. Mesenteric adenitis in a 15-year-old boy with right lower quadrant abdominal pain. (A) A CT image through the small bowel mesentery shows enlarged mesenteric lymph nodes (arrows). (B) A more inferior CT image shows soft tissue infiltration of the mesenteric fat (arrowheads), with indistinctness of the mesenteric vessels. (C) Slightly further inferiorly, a CT image shows lymphadenopathy (arrow) in the right lower quadrant just anterior to the right psoas muscle.

often involve more of the small bowel mesentery and are more numerous. This more diffuse distribution of lymphadenopathy can be used as supportive evidence of mesenteric adenitis (**Option (E) is true**). Probably the most important finding in support of a CT diagnosis of mesenteric adenitis is the absence of the findings of appendicitis. The CT criteria for the diagnosis of appendicitis include distension of the appendix (>6 mm in diameter) or the presence of one or more appendicoliths with associated adjacent inflammatory stranding of the periappendiceal fat. Secondary signs include right lower quadrant inflammatory changes, such as phlegmon, abscess, or extraluminal gas; evidence of small bowel obstruction; and cecal inflammatory changes.

Sonography also has been used to identify lymphadenopathy and ileal wall thickening as supportive findings of mesenteric adenitis. As with CT, the sonographic diagnosis of mesenteric adenitis is based on exclusion of the sonographic findings of appendicitis, such as a noncompressible, blind-ending tubular structure greater than 6 mm in diameter or an appendicolith.

Question 85

Concerning diseases that involve the mesentery in children,

(A) a mass near the root of the mesentery is more likely to be malignant than benign
(B) the mesentery is involved in more than 50% of children with non-Hodgkin's lymphoma
(C) cystic lymphangiomas tend to be unilocular
(D) on CT, mesenteric lymph nodes less than 5 mm in diameter are normal

Although a number of mesenteries exist, the most common reference is to the jejunoileal mesentery, a membrane composed of two folds of peritoneum suspending the jejunal and ileal bowel loops from the posterior abdominal wall. The mesentery is located in the midabdomen and contains a number of structures, including nerve plexuses, fat, lymph nodes, and blood vessels. The jejunoileal mesentery can be involved with a variety of disorders in children.

The mesentery does not have easily recognizable boundaries during imaging, so that localization of an abnormality to the mesentery can be difficult. In adults, the greater amount of fat aids in defining mesenteric processes. The relative paucity of mesenteric fat in the pediatric population can make detection and localization of processes in the mesentery more difficult. The following criteria are helpful in localizing a process to the mesentery in children: partial or complete envelopment of the superior mesenteric artery or vein, peripheral displacement of jejunal or ileal bowel loops, or extension of the process from superoposterior to inferoanterior.

To help limit the differential diagnosis for a mesenteric process, it is useful to characterize mesenteric processes into one of the following categories: diffuse involvement, solitary mass, or multifocal masses. Processes that can involve the mesentery diffusely include edema, hemorrhage, and inflammation. Features seen on cross-sectional imaging are generally nonspecific, and the diagnosis depends on associated findings as well as clinical information. The characteristic CT findings of a diffuse mesenteric process include replacement of mesenteric fat with soft tissue attenuation and loss of vascular definition (Figure 17-18). Mesenteric edema can have many causes, including hypoalbuminemia, heart failure, cirrhosis, and vascular thrombosis or obstruction. Inflammatory changes can occur in the mesentery secondary to severe bowel inflammation, e.g., attributable to Crohn's disease or graft-versus-host disease (Figure 17-18). Mesenteric inflammatory changes also can occur secondary to adjacent peritonitis, e.g., intraloop abscesses as a result of a perforated appendix, or from extension of inflammation in the anterior pararenal space associated with pancreatitis. Hemorrhage into the mesentery is usually the result of trauma or coagulopathy.

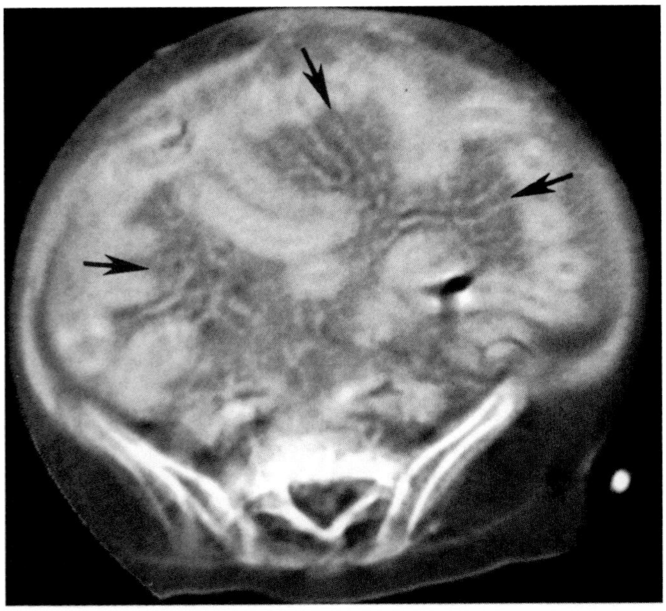

Figure 17-18. Diffuse abnormality of the mesentery secondary to graft-versus-host disease in a 9-month-old boy after bone marrow transplantation for Wiskott-Aldrich syndrome. A CT scan shows increased attenuation throughout the mesenteric fat (arrows), with associated indistinctness of the mesenteric vessels. Also note the diffuse mucosal enhancement of the small and large bowel loops associated with bowel wall thickening.

Focal masses within the mesentery in the pediatric population can be secondary to lymphoma, mesenteric cysts, desmoid tumors, teratomas, and lipomas. Mesenteric involvement in patients with lymphoma can be manifested as multifocal adenopathy or, less commonly, as a focal soft tissue mass. In general, masses located near the root of the mesentery are more likely to be of a malignant etiology than are lesions located more peripherally (**Option (A) is true**).

Mesenteric cysts, also known as cystic lymphangiomas, are believed to be developmental anomalies in which focal lymphatic channels fail to establish connections with the central lymphatic system. Most lymphangiomas are found in the neck and axilla. The less common intra-abdominal lymphangiomas are most likely to occur within the mesentery. Their appearance can vary, but the diagnosis can be suggested when a low-attenuation mass with no discernible wall is identified by CT. Lymphangiomas usually are multiseptate and quite large (Figure 17-19) (**Option (C) is false**).

Desmoid tumors are found in patients with prior abdominal surgery, trauma, or Gardner's syndrome. Lipomas are recognized by their low attenuation (typically lower than that of water) on CT scans or high signal intensity on T1-weighted MR images (Figure 17-20). Additional considerations for a focal mass include inflammatory pseudotumor, as well as nodes from neoplastic or inflammatory processes such as mesenteric adenitis.

Multifocal mesenteric masses most commonly represent lymphadenopathy. On CT, mesenteric lymph nodes are considered abnormal if they are greater than 5 mm in diameter (**Option (D) is true**). Mesenteric lymphadenopathy can be a manifestation of malignant processes, such as lymphoma (Figure 17-21), lymphoproliferative disorders (Figure 17-2), or metastatic disease, or of inflammatory processes. Lymphomatous involvement of the mesentery is usually attributable to non-Hodgkin's lymphoma and usually involves both the mesentery and the retroperitoneum (Figure 17-21). The mesentery is involved in the overwhelming majority of chil-

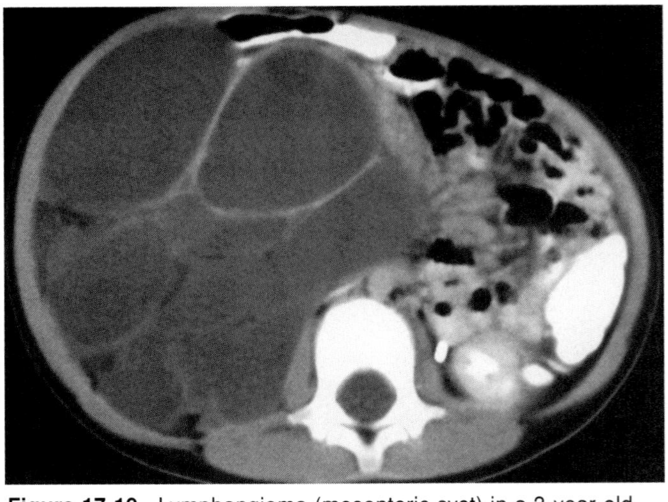

Figure 17-19. Lymphangioma (mesenteric cyst) in a 3-year-old girl. A CT scan shows a large multilocular cystic mass within the mesentery.

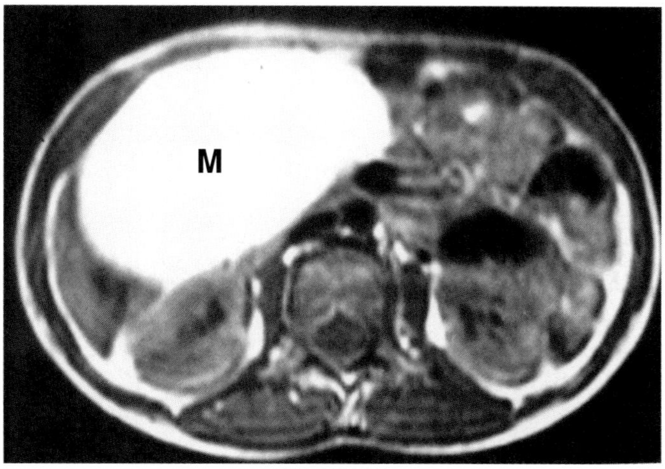

SE 800/20

Figure 17-20. Mesenteric lipoma in a 6-year-old girl. An axial T1-weighted spin-echo MR image shows a focal, well-defined mass (M) of homogeneous high signal intensity. The signal within the mass is isointense relative to the subcutaneous fat.

dren with abdominal involvement from non-Hodgkin's lymphoma (**Option (B) is true**). Lymphadenopathy also can be attributable to infections such as cat scratch disease, fungal infection, or tuberculosis (Figure 17-7). It has been suggested that in children with tuberculosis, the mesenteric adenopathy is often more pronounced than the retroperitoneal adenopathy. Central low attenuation and peripheral enhancement of mesenteric nodes have been described as highly suggestive of an inflammatory process, especially tuberculosis (Figure 17-7). However, this appearance can be associated with any neoplastic or inflammatory process associated with central necrosis. Other inflammatory causes of mesenteric lymphadenopathy in children include mesenteric adenitis (Figure 17-17) and sarcoidosis. Other causes of multifocal mesenteric processes include

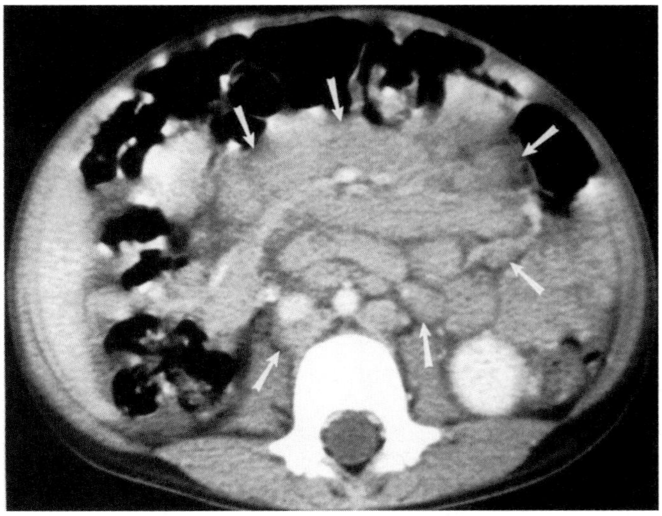

Figure 17-21. Non-Hodgkin's lymphoma in a 3-year-old boy. A CT scan shows extensive lymphadenopathy (arrows) within the mesentery and retroperitoneum. The density of the lymphadenopathy is homogeneous and similar to that of skeletal muscle.

lymphangiomas or plexiform neurofibromas in patients with von Recklinghausen's disease.

SUGGESTED READINGS

LYMPHOPROLIFERATIVE DISORDER

1. Bragg DG, Chor PJ, Murray KA, Kjeldsberg CR. Lymphoproliferative disorders of the lung: histopathology, clinical manifestations, and imaging features. AJR 1994; 163:273–281
2. Carignan S, Staples CA, Muller NL. Intrathoracic lymphoproliferative disorders in the immunocompromised patient: CT findings. Radiology 1995; 197:53–58
3. Day DL, Shapiro RS, Yueh N, McClain K, Allan BT, Filipovich AH. B-cell lymphoproliferative disorders in children after bone marrow transplantation: radiologic manifestations. Radiology 1987; 162:807–810
4. Dodd GD III, Ledesma-Medina J, Baron RL, Fuhrman CR. Posttransplant lymphoproliferative disorder: intrathoracic manifestations. Radiology 1992; 184:65–69
5. Donnelly LF, Frush DP, Marshall KW, White KS. Lymphoproliferative disorders: CT findings in immunocompromised children. AJR 1998; 171: 725–731
6. Harris KM, Schwartz ML, Slasky BS, Nalesnik M, Makowka L. Posttransplantation cyclosporine-induced lymphoproliferative disorders: clinical and radiologic manifestations. Radiology 1987; 162:697–700
7. McGuinness G, Scholes JV, Jagirdar JS, et al. Unusual lymphoproliferative disorders in nine adults with HIV or AIDS: CT and pathologic findings. Radiology 1995; 197:59–65
8. Mulvihill DM, Munden MM, Edell D. Lymphoproliferative disorder involving the liver following transplantation: CT appearance. J Comput Assist Tomogr 1994; 18:47–48
9. Nalesnik MA, Makowka L, Starzl TE. The diagnosis and treatment of posttransplant lymphoproliferative disorders. Curr Probl Surg 1988; 25: 367–472
10. Pickhardt PJ, Siegel MJ. Abdominal manifestations of posttransplantation lymphoproliferative disorders. AJR 1998; 171:1007–1013
11. Pickhardt PJ, Siegel MJ. Posttransplantation lymphoproliferative disorder of the abdomen: CT evaluation in 51 patients. Radiology 1999; 213:73–78
12. Pickhardt PJ, Siegel MJ, Anderson DC, Hayashi R, DeBaun MR. Chest radiography as a predictor of outcome in posttransplantation lymphoproliferative disorder in lung allograft recipients. AJR 1998; 171:375–382

KAWASAKI DISEASE

13. Bisset GS III, Strife JL, McCloskey J. MR imaging of coronary artery aneurysms in a child with Kawasaki disease. AJR 1989; 152:805–807
14. Chung CJ, Stein L. Kawasaki disease: a review. Radiology 1998; 208:25–33
15. Kato H, Sugimura T, Akagi T, et al. Long-term complications of Kawasaki disease. A 10- to 21-year follow-up study of 594 patients. Circulation 1996; 94:1379–1385
16. Kawasaki T. Acute febrile mucocutaneous syndrome with lymphoid involvement with specific desquamation of the fingers and toes in children. Arerugi 1967; 16:178–222

TUBERCULOSIS

17. Bloom BR, Murray CJ. Tuberculosis: commentary on a reemergent killer. Science 1992: 257:1055–1064
18. Cremin BJ. Tuberculosis: the resurgence of our most lethal infectious disease—a review. Pediatr Radiol 1995; 25:620–626
19. Gilinsky NH, Marks IN, Kotter RE, Price SK. Abdominal tuberculosis. A 10-year review. S Afr Med J 1983; 64:849–857
20. Hulnick DH, Megibow AJ, Naidich DP, Hilton S, Cho KC, Balthazar EJ. Abdominal tuberculosis: CT evaluation. Radiology 1985; 157:199–204
21. Johnson CA, Hill ID, Bowie MD. Abdominal tuberculosis in children. A

survey of cases at the Red Cross War Memorial Children's Hospital, 1976–1985. S Afr Med J 1987; 72:20–22

22. Leder RA, Low VH. Tuberculosis of the abdomen. Radiol Clin North Am 1995; 33:691–705
23. Rubin SA. Tuberculosis. Captain of all these men of death. Radiol Clin North Am 1995; 33:619–639

CHRONIC GRANULOMATOUS DISEASE OF CHILDHOOD

24. Barton LL, Moussa SL, Villar RG, Hulett RL. Gastrointestinal complications of chronic granulomatous disease: case report and literature review. Clin Pediatr (Phila) 1998; 37:231–236
25. Stiehm ER (ed). Immunologic disorders in infants and children. Philadelphia: WB Saunders; 1995:443–468

MESENTERIC ADENITIS

26. Puylaert JB. Mesenteric adenitis and acute terminal ileitis: US evaluation using graded compression. Radiology 1986; 161:691–695
27. Rao PM, Rhea JT, Novelline RA. CT diagnosis of mesenteric adenitis. Radiology 1997; 202:145–149
28. Rao PM, Rhea JT, Novelline RA, et al. Helical CT technique for the diagnosis of appendicitis: prospective evaluation of a focused appendix CT examination. Radiology 1997; 202:134–144
29. Sivit CJ, Newman KD, Chandra RS. Visualization of enlarged mesenteric lymph nodes at US examination: clinical significance. Pediatr Radiol 1993; 23:471–475

ABNORMALITIES OF THE MESENTERY

30. Casillas J, Sais GJ, Greve, JL, Iparraguirre MC, Morillo G. Imaging of intra- and extraabdominal desmoid tumors. RadioGraphics 1991; 11: 959–968
31. Donnelly LF, Morris CL. Acute graft-versus-host disease in children: abdominal CT findings. Radiology 1996; 199:265–268
32. Donnelly LF, Rencken IO, deLorimier AA, Gooding CA. Left paraduodenal hernia leading to ileal obstruction. Pediatr Radiol 1996; 26:534–536
33. Friedland JA, Siegel MJ. CT appearance of acute appendicitis in childhood. AJR 1997; 168:439–442
34. Hamrick-Turner JE, Chiechi MV, Abbitt PL, Ros PR. Neoplastic and inflammatory processes of the peritoneum, omentum, and mesentery: diagnosis with CT. RadioGraphics 1992; 12:1051–1068
35. Keesling CA, Frush DP, O'Hara SM, Fordham LA. Clinical and imaging manifestations of pediatric sarcoidosis. Acad Radiol 1998; 5:122–132
36. Ko SF, Ng SH, Shieh CS, Lin JW, Huang CC, Lee TY. Mesenteric cystic lymphangioma with myxoid degeneration: unusual CT and MR manifestations. Pediatr Radiol 1995; 25:525–527
37. Matsuki K, Kakitsubata Y, Watanabe K, Tsukino H, Nakajima K. Mesenteric plexiform neurofibroma associated with Recklinghausen's disease. Pediatr Radiol 1997; 27:255–256
38. Mindelzun RE, Jeffrey RB Jr, Lane MJ, Silverman PM. The misty mesentery on CT: differential diagnosis. AJR 1996; 167:61–65
39. Ruess L, Frazier AA, Sivit CJ. CT of the mesentery, omentum, and peritoneum in children. RadioGraphics 1995; 15:89–104
40. Siegel MJ, Glazer HS, St. Amour TE, Rosenthal DD. Lymphangiomas in children: MR imaging. Radiology 1989; 170:467–470
41. Silverman PM, Baker ME, Cooper C, Kelvin M. CT appearance of diffuse mesenteric edema. J Comput Assist Tomogr 1986; 10:67–70

CASE 18

Donald P. Frush, M.D.

Langerhans Cell Histiocytosis

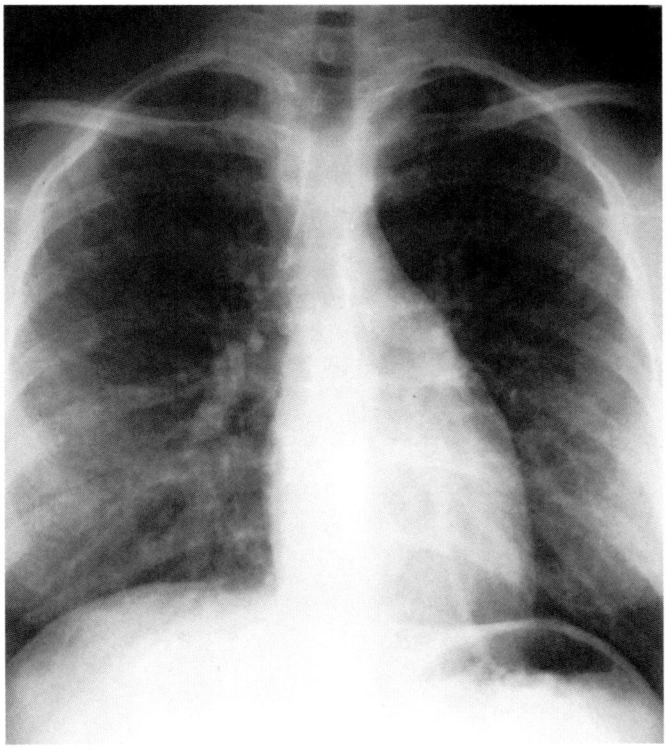

Figure 18-1

Question 86

This 17-year-old girl had a recent onset of mild exertional dyspnea. You are shown a posteroanterior chest radiograph (Figure 18-1) and two axial CT images (Figure 18-2).

Which *one* of the following is the MOST likely diagnosis?

(A) Prior *Pneumocystis carinii* infection
(B) Bronchiectasis
(C) Tuberculosis
(D) Papillomatosis
(E) Langerhans cell histiocytosis

The chest radiograph (Figure 18-1) demonstrates a reticulonodular interstitial disease that is more pronounced in the upper lungs. Lung volumes are normal. No hilar or mediastinal adenopathy and no pleural effusion are noted. The axial CT examination (Figure 18-2) confirms the presence of interstitial disease in the upper lung zones. There are several small (subcentimeter) solid nodules with scattered cavitation (Figure 18-3A). The CT appearance of the lower lungs is nearly normal (Figure 18-3B). These findings are most consistent with a diagnosis of Langerhans cell histiocytosis (LCH) (**Option (E) is correct**).

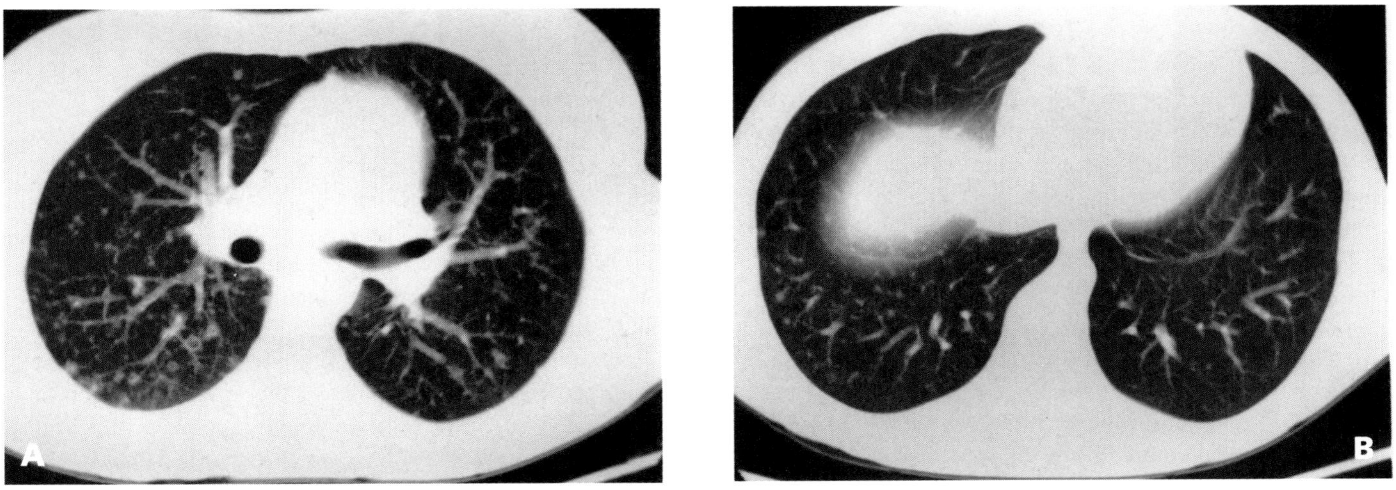

Figure 18-2

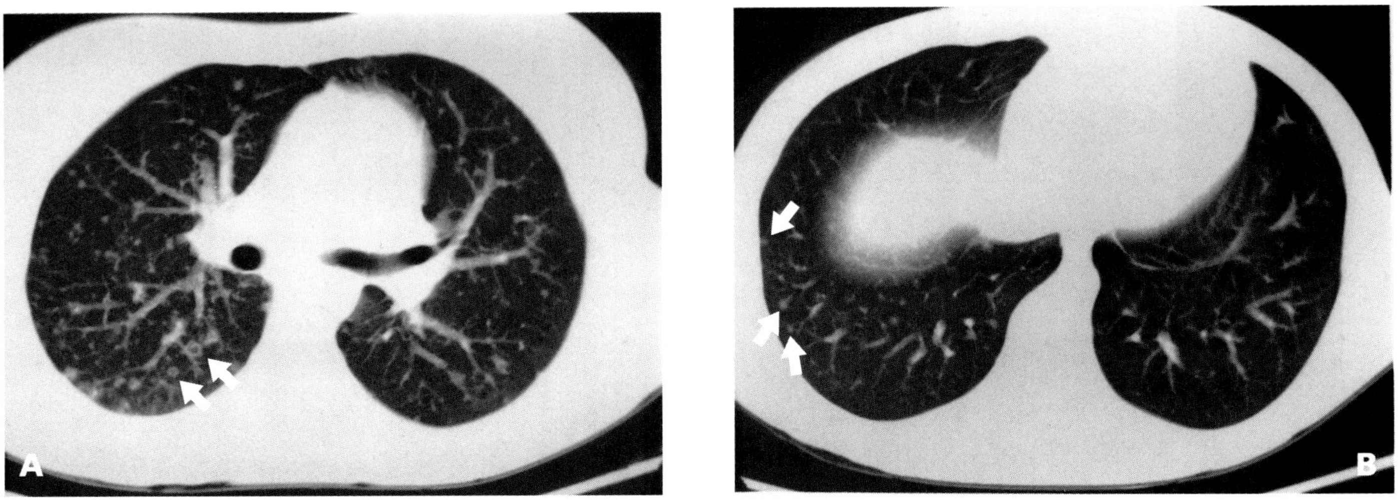

Figure 18-3 (Same as Figure 18-2). Langerhans cell histiocytosis. (A) An axial CT image obtained near the level of the origin of the upper lobe bronchi depicts the subcentimeter small nodular and cavitary nodular lesions (arrows) in both lungs. (B) A CT examination through the lung bases shows only a few scattered small nodules (arrows).

Pneumocystis carinii is a ubiquitous organism, but is rarely a respiratory pathogen in healthy individuals. However, in the setting of acquired immunodeficiency (e.g., human immunodeficiency virus [HIV] infection) or primary immunodeficiency (e.g., severe combined immunodeficiency), *P. carinii* can cause significant morbidity and mortality. Most infections are *P. carinii* pneumonia (PCP) and are a result of inhalation of the organism. The acute-phase radiographic and CT findings for PCP consist of interstitial or airspace disease (or a combination of both) with a continuum from focal to diffuse involvement. Subacute- or chronic-phase imaging features of PCP include those associated with fibrosis (either from the infection itself or secondary to adult respiratory distress syndrome) and cysts, likely representing pneumatoceles. These cysts are not associated with nodular interstitial disease and are typically subpleural in location. The exact frequency of cyst formation following PCP infection in children is unknown, but it is uncommon. Hence, prior *P. carinii* infection (Option (A)) is unlikely.

Bronchiectasis (Option (B)) is a feature of many pulmonary disorders. The term implies an irreversible dilatation of bronchi. Bronchiectasis is seen in a variety of disorders that are, in general, chronic in nature. The most familiar of these (and the most common cause overall of bronchiectasis) is cystic fibrosis. Bronchiectasis (unrelated to cystic fibrosis) occurs in about 1% of children evaluated for chronic suppurative pulmonary disease; in screening, bronchiectasis is found in fewer than 2 of 10,000 children. Excluding cystic fibrosis, just over 33% of children with bronchiectasis have no known underlying disorder, although the majority of these children have a past history of severe pulmonary infections. For the remaining two thirds of children, bronchiectasis is attributed to immunologic disorders in nearly half (either primary or acquired, such as following lung transplantation). Congenital malformations, including ciliary dysmotility, bronchial anomalies, such as Williams-Campbell syndrome (Figure 18-4), and foreign-body aspiration account for the remainder. Irrespective of the underlying disorder, bronchiectasis is associated with infection in about 70% of cases. In the past, tuberculosis, pertussis, and measles were the primary infectious causes of bronchiectasis.

Bronchiectasis usually occurs in medium-size bronchi, as larger airways have more cartilaginous support. The pathogenesis of bronchiectasis is not well understood, but likely involves a combination of changes attributable to infection, obstruction (with luminal expansion attributable to secretions), and traction (with enlargement attributable to fibrosis as a result of adjacent parenchymal disease). Bronchial pathologic changes include columnar epithelial damage and metaplasia, glandular hypertrophy, and fibrosis and destruction of elastic tissue. The typical categories of bronchiectasis are, from most mild to most severe, cylindrical (or fusiform), varicose, and cystic. These appearances represent a continuum of airway dilatation, and abnormalities representing the range of bronchiectasis often coexist (Figure 18-5). Most children present with bronchiectasis during preschool years. Symptoms include cough in over 95% of cases, followed in descending order of frequency by sputum production, wheezing, chest pain, and hemoptysis. Dyspnea is rare and is found in less than 10% of patients.

The appearance of bronchiectasis on chest radiographs includes bronchial dilatation (Figure 18-5), peribronchial thickening, and volume loss or air trapping. Mucoid impaction also may be evident. All of these changes are well seen with CT, including high-resolution CT; thus, CT has replaced conventional bronchography. The depiction and detection of bronchiectasis also have been improved by use of slab reconstructions of helical CT data. In general, bronchiectatic changes are most common in the middle and lower lobes. However, the distribution depends in part on the etiology. For example, in cases of bronchiectasis attributable to aspiration, the posterior segments of the upper lobes can be involved. Cystic fibrosis is also a distinct exception, as bronchiectasis in this condition is found more often in the upper lungs, particularly on the right. The predominantly nodular pulmonary parenchymal disease in the test pa-

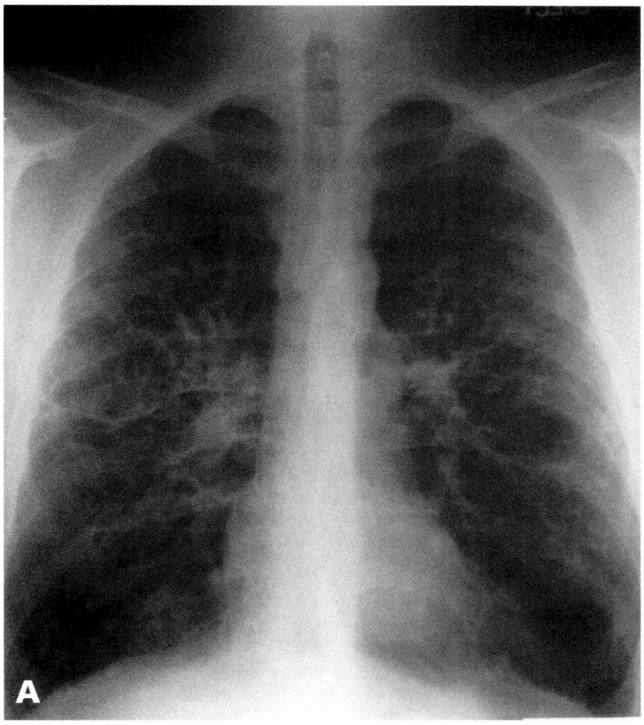

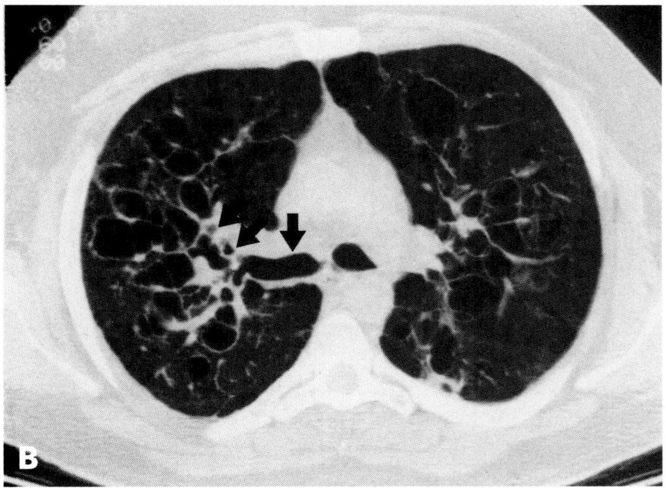

Figure 18-4. Williams-Campbell syndrome in a 24-year-old man. (A) Bronchiectasis attributable to the congenital cartilage deficiency in the fourth- to sixth-order bronchi is evident predominantly in the lower lungs on a posteroanterior radiograph. (B) A CT examination just below the carina shows the cystic bronchiectasis more clearly. The more proximal bronchi (arrows) are relatively normal in caliber. Note that bronchiectasis is also present in the upper lobes in this syndrome, unlike the majority of cases of bronchiectasis related to infection, which occur in the middle and lower lungs.

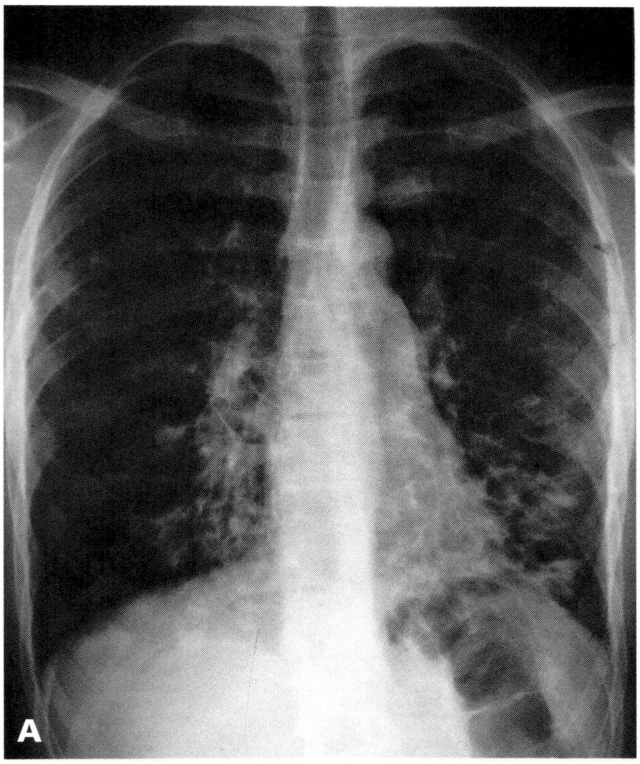

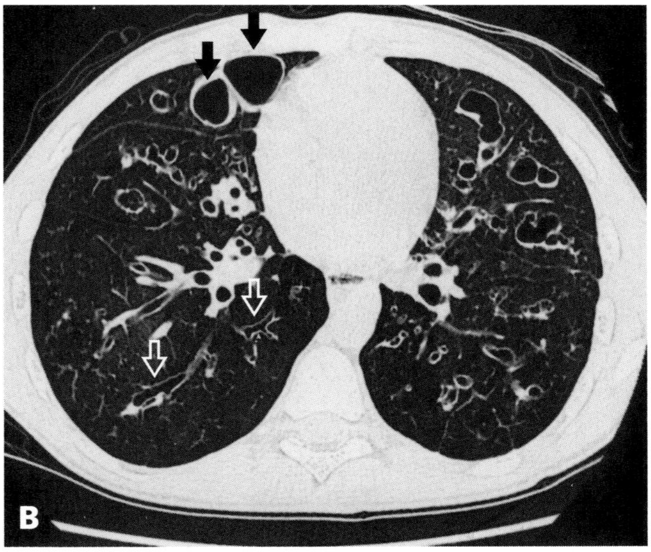

Figure 18-5. Bronchiectasis in a 15-year-old boy with ciliary dyskinesia. (A) Bronchiectasis is evident at both lung bases on a posteroanterior chest radiograph. Cystic bronchiectasis is most easily seen in the lower lungs. Scattered nodular opacities, particularly at the level of the right hemidiaphragm, are attributable to dilated bronchi filled with mucus. (B) A high-resolution CT image more clearly demonstrates the range of bronchiectatic changes. Cylindrical bronchiectasis is evident in the right lower lobe (open arrows). Larger, cystic bronchiectasis is particularly evident in the right middle lobe (solid arrows), as well as the lingula.

tient is not the radiographic appearance of bronchiectasis.

Therapy for bronchiectasis consists of medical and surgical options. Medical treatment is directed at preventing the progression of bronchiectatic changes and includes aggressive pulmonary toilet, antibiotics in the acute-phase setting (prophylaxis has been shown to be beneficial when there is a propensity for bronchiectasis, such as with cystic fibrosis or ciliary dysmotility), and aerosol therapy. Indications for surgery include localized bronchiectasis, failed medical therapy (including abscess formation), and recurrent hemoptysis.

Over 95% of primary tuberculosis (Option (C)) in children is pulmonary in origin. Pulmonary tuberculosis is an increasing public health issue in children as well as adults. In the

10 years prior to 1994, there was a 33% increase in the incidence of tuberculosis in children. Disease in children usually is attributable to primary infection; postprimary (i.e., reactivation of dormant disease) manifestations usually do not occur until adolescence and adulthood. Importantly, and in distinction from adults, children with tuberculosis may be asymptomatic.

The primary manifestations of tuberculosis in children are nonspecific and include cough, fever, and malaise. Airspace disease and regional adenopathy are typical. Enlarged lymph nodes can secondarily obstruct the airway, resulting in atelectasis (Figure 18-6). Air trapping is rare, as are cavitation, bronchiectasis, and pleural effusions. Diffuse pulmonary disease can be seen with miliary tuberculosis. Miliary disease is a complication of primary infection in which two or more organs (often the lungs) are involved, with hematogenous spread of tuberculosis. Miliary disease is most likely to develop in young children and infants, and the majority of these patients demonstrate significant signs of systemic infection, including meningitis, which is present in up to 50% of cases. Cavitation of pulmonary lesions is rare in miliary tuberculosis, and there is no upper lobe predilection. Cavitary changes are rarely associated with primary tuberculosis in children, as mentioned above. Cavitation is attributable to destruction as a reaction to infected parenchyma and to emphysematous changes following infection. The cystic regions can be isolated or confluent and can contain septations. Small cysts and cavitation of small nodules are not features of the cavitary lesions of tuberculosis, and this is not a likely diagnosis in the test patient.

The radiographic manifestations of primary pulmonary tuberculosis reflect involvement of the pulmonary parenchyma, the mediastinal and hilar lymph nodes, the tracheobronchial structures, and the pleura. When present, parenchymal involvement typically is identified as a region of homogeneous airspace consolidation with ill-defined margins. This consolidation can be subsegmental, segmental, or lobar. Superimposed atelectasis can be associated. Cavitation is uncommon and is seen in less than 3% of infants. When present, it is demonstrated as an air-filled or air-fluid-filled cavity in the region of the parenchymal consolidation. Hilar or paratracheal nodal enlargement is identified in most cases of primary pulmonary tuberculosis. Lymphadenopathy is usually unilateral. In some cases, contiguous pulmonary consolidation obscures hilar anatomy. Tracheobronchial involvement with tuberculosis is usually in the form of compression of the bronchi by moderately enlarged lymph nodes, often leading to atelectasis. Pleural effusions are not common with primary tuberculosis.

The classic radiographic feature of the sequelae of healed primary tuberculosis is termed Ranke's complex. This complex consists of a parenchymal scar and calcified hilar or paratracheal lymph nodes. The parenchymal scar, sometimes termed Ghon's lesion, may or may not be calcified. Parenchymal lung calcifications attributable to prior tuberculosis are usually less than 5 mm in diameter, whereas calcifications from prior histoplasmosis tend to be somewhat larger.

The radiographic features of tuberculosis in patients with acquired hypersensitivity and immunity often vary slightly from the features identified with primary tuberculosis. This condition is termed postprimary tuberculosis and includes instances of reinfection and cases of continuation of the primary disease. There seems to be a tendency for involvement of the

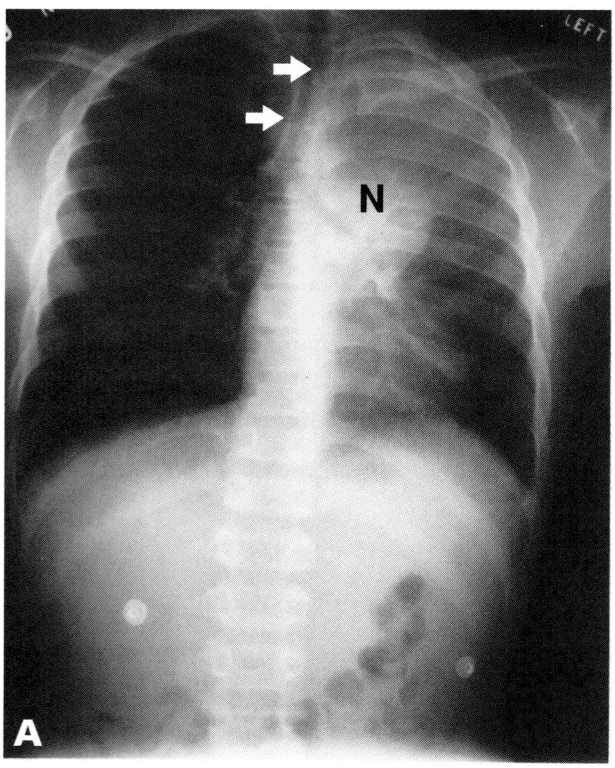

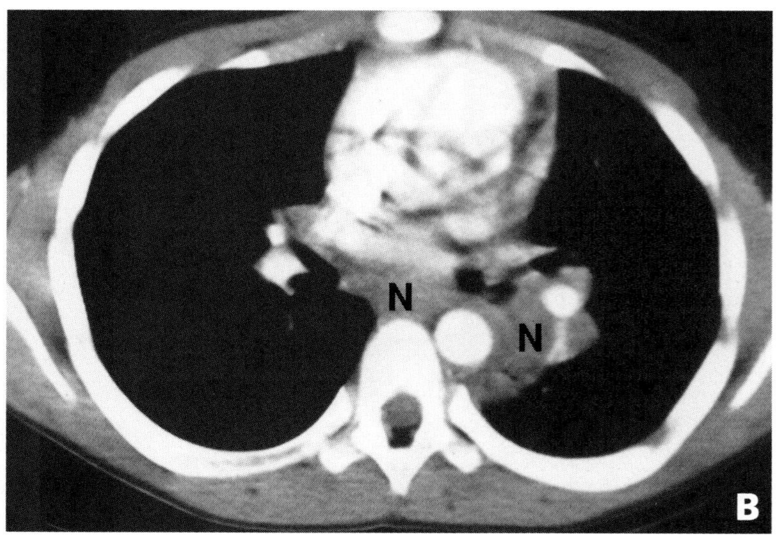

Figure 18-6. Tuberculosis in an 11-year-old boy. (A) Mediastinal left hilar adenopathy (N) results in partial left upper lobe collapse evident on a posteroanterior chest radiograph. Note the leftward shift of the trachea (arrows) attributable to atelectasis. (B) On a contrast-enhanced chest CT image (mediastinal window), the mediastinal adenopathy (N) is more evident.

apical and posterior segments of the upper lobes. The radiographic patterns in these patients vary. In some cases, there is a patchy or confluent airspace consolidation. Linear densities can be identified coursing toward the hilum; these are attributable to enlarged lymphatics. The poorly defined area of consolidation can be replaced by more sharply circumscribed densities. This area may show adjacent linear densities because of fibrosis.

Caseation is common in postprimary tuberculosis. Occasionally, the caseous material is expelled from the lesion into the bronchial tree. The resulting cavity usually has a fairly thick wall with a smooth inner surface. Dissemination of the material into the tracheobronchial tree can result in one or more areas of confluent airspace consolidation in adjacent or distant portions of the lung.

Hematogenous dissemination of tubercle bacilli can occur in either the primary or the postprimary form of the disease. Radiographic changes are more common, however, with postprimary disease. These cases of miliary tuberculosis are manifested radiographically by tiny, discrete foci distributed uniformly throughout the lung. Most often, the individual nodules are well defined and pinpoint in size. In untreated patients and in individuals with severe underlying illness, the nodules can reach 2 to 3 mm in size.

Papillomas are the most common laryngeal masses in children. These benign lesions are attributable to human papillomavirus infections. Papillomatosis (Option (D)) is most often localized to the larynx, but can involve the trachea and, more rarely, the lung parenchyma. Most patients present before 5 years of age with signs of airway compromise, cough, stridor, or dyspnea. Parenchymal lesions are invariably associated with airway papillomas, which appear as nodular soft tissue densities or focal thinking of the tracheal wall. Parenchymal lesions in papillomatosis tend to be central, basilar, and posterior in location. Upper lung involvement is seen with advanced cases, in which there is virtually always coexisting basilar disease. Isolated upper lung involvement is very rare. CT more clearly demonstrates the presence of airway and small parenchymal nodules than does radiography. Small nodules have a soft tissue attenuation. As they increase in size and outgrow their blood supply, they can cavitate. Although still histologically benign, pulmonary involvement by papillomatosis can result in significant morbidity. Infection and severe parenchymal destruction are notable complications. Squamous cell carcinoma is a rare, but significant, complication of recurrent papillomatosis in children. The older age of the test patient, recent rather than chronic history of dyspnea, the absence of tracheal nodules on CT, and the predominance of disease in the upper lung fields make papillomatosis an unlikely diagnosis.

LCH is a disorder in which single or multiple organ systems are affected by a mononuclear cellular infiltrate of histiocytes of the Langerhans cell type. The disease was formerly known as histiocytosis X. Historically, the term "eosinophilic granuloma" was applied to localized involvement of either lung or bone, and specific syndromes for systemic involvement of LCH were labeled Letterer-Siwe disease and Hand-Schüller-Christian disease.

In a recent multicenter review of 348 children with initial presentation of LCH, sites of involvement (in decreasing order of frequency) included bone (especially calvarium and skull base), skin, liver, central nervous system, lungs, marrow, lymph nodes, and spleen.

The median age at presentation for any manifestation of LCH is 30 months. Pulmonary LCH is more common in young adults (usually in the third or fourth decade), but about 13% of children have either imaging or clinical findings of lung involvement. Pulmonary LCH can be isolated or multifocal, with concomitant involvement of the skeleton (Figure 18-7). In general, multiorgan involvement or organ dysfunction is a poor prognostic factor. In addition to lung involvement, other independent factors indicating a poorer outcome include male gender; presentation in infancy; involvement of ear, nose, throat, or reticuloendothelial system; and poor response to therapy.

Clinical manifestations of pulmonary LCH are present in approximately 75% of individuals. These include dyspnea, cough, tachypnea, and systemic manifestations (fever and weight loss). LCH can cause spontaneous pneumothorax. The radiographic changes are typically worse than are the symptoms. Lung volumes are normal or slightly increased. Nodular interstitial disease located predominantly in the upper lungs (Figures 18-1 and 18-2) is typical. When more diffuse, LCH tends to spare the costophrenic angles. Nodules can cavitate. Larger bullae, linear densities, fibrosis (including a honeycomb pattern), and pneumothorax are rarer findings. Pleural effusion and adenopathy are uncommon. The pulmonary changes are more clearly demonstrated with CT. High-resolution CT findings are virtually diagnostic of LCH in up to 95% of early cases. The abnormalities include interstitial nodules that are peribronchiolar, usually less than 10 mm in size, and distributed in

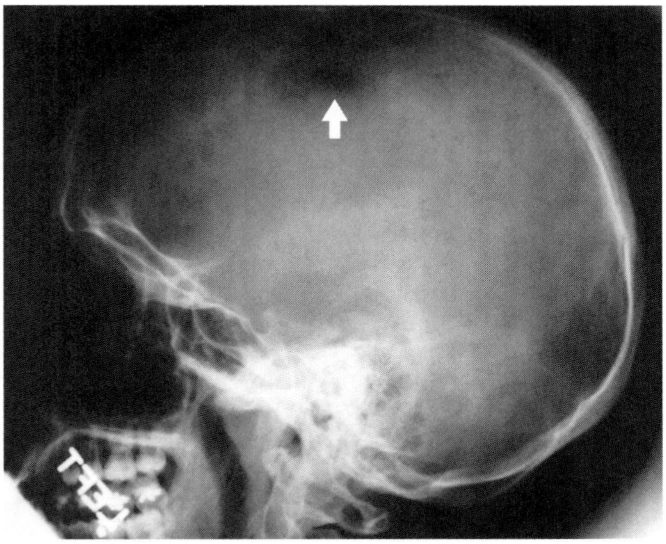

Figure 18-7. Same patient as in Figures 18-1 and 18-2. Langerhans cell histiocytosis. As part of a radiographic skeletal survey, a well-defined lytic lesion (arrow) was evident in the skull. This was the only skeletal involvement by LCH in this patient.

the upper lungs. Multiple cystic spaces (with variable wall thickness) (Figure 18-2) represent bronchiolar obstruction with a ball-valve effect. More extensive and emphysematous changes are occasionally present. In more advanced cases of LCH, with fibrosis and a honeycomb pattern, imaging features are not specific for LCH. Honeycomb lung can be present in LCH, interstitial pneumonia, sarcoidosis, rheumatoid lung, dermatomyositis, scleroderma, and bronchiectasis.

There is no standard treatment for LCH. The disease can spontaneously resolve, particularly if there is single-organ involvement and no organ dysfunction. However, when LCH persists or there is multiorgan involvement, especially with organ dysfunction, chemotherapy is indicated.

Question 87

Concerning *Pneumocystis carinii* pneumonia in children,

- (A) cystic changes are common in acute disease
- (B) it usually exhibits a reticulonodular pattern
- (C) hilar adenopathy is present in most patients
- (D) it is the most common pulmonary disease in children with AIDS
- (E) pleural effusions are common

P. carinii is a ubiquitous pathogen. Infection presumably occurs through inhalation of the organism, and the overwhelming majority of manifestations of *P. carinii* infection are pulmonary. PCP occurs almost exclusively in immunocompromised hosts and causes substantial morbidity and mortality in this population.

P. carinii is the leading cause of opportunistic pulmonary infections in children with HIV infection. In addition, *P. carinii* is a potential pathogen in any condition in which there is altered T-cell function. Such conditions include severe combined immunodeficiency, immunosuppression for transplants (i.e., bone marrow), and treatment of a variety of childhood malignancies. Despite the varied reasons for the underlying immunosuppression, the presentation, imaging features, and treatment of PCP are similar.

Up to 20% of HIV-infected children have been reported to have PCP at some time during the course of the disease. The frequency of PCP is probably decreasing because of earlier detection of HIV infection in children, chiefly as a result of maternal screening, PCP prophylaxis, and treatment with multidrug regimens that include protease inhibitors. For example, in one investigation, Simonds et al. reported that infants and children diagnosed with either PCP or cytomegalovirus infections had a significantly higher median survival rate (eight times) when born between 1993 and 1998 than when born before 1993.

Symptoms in pediatric PCP infections are usually acute and consist of tachypnea, cough, fever, and hypoxemia. The diagnosis can be established by bronchoalveolar lavage. Children with acute lung infections are often too sick to undergo open lung biopsy. Treatment options include trimethoprim-sulfamethoxazole and pentamidine. It is clear that the most effective means of reducing the morbidity of PCP is with sulfa drug prophylaxis. Of note is the fact that children with AIDS-related lymphocytic interstitial pneumonitis (LIP) (discussed below) are less likely to develop PCP than children without LIP. An explanation is that the lymphoid aggregates in LIP signify a better immune response and a lower rate of opportunistic infections.

Several different radiographic patterns are seen with PCP. The usual appearance (80% of cases) is fine, diffuse, granular, bilateral parenchymal opacities radiating from the hilar regions of the lung (**Option (B) is true**). Some degree of scattered alveolar consolidation is usually present, particularly later in the disease process (Figure 18-8). As the infection progresses, there is usually increasing opacification of the more peripheral aspects of the lung. The findings may represent pulmonary edema or may mimic acute cytomegalovirus pneumonia. Focal airspace disease and nodules are rare. Pleural effusions, which are rare, are usually small (**Option (E) is false**). Mediastinal and hilar lymphadenopathy attributable to PCP are rare (**Option (C) is false**). Cavitary or cystic areas, likely representing pneumatoceles (Figure 18-9), have been reported in both adults and children with PCP. However, the frequency is low, and pneumatoceles are even more rare with acute infections (**Option (A) is false**). As in adults, these pneumatoceles in children occur in the upper lobes and are transient. Proposed etiologies for these pneumatoceles include emphysema attributable to proximal bronchial obstruction, parenchymal necrosis, and acquired bronchopleural communication. High-resolution CT can be

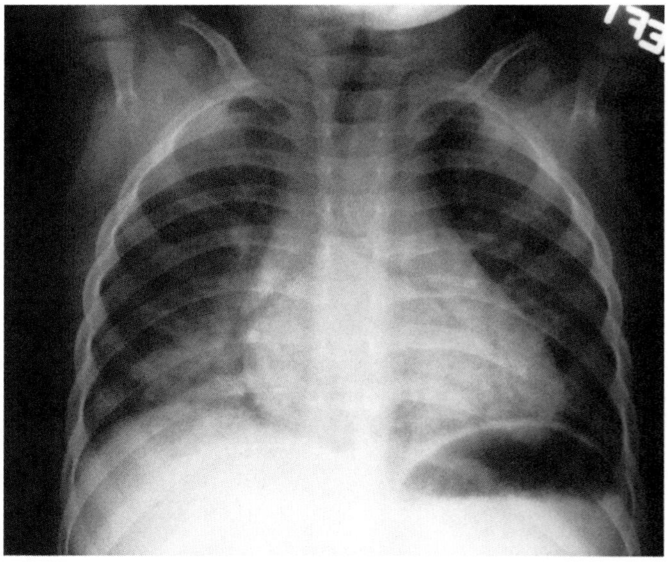

Figure 18-8. *Pneumocystis carinii* pneumonia in a 12-month-old boy with severe combined immunodeficiency syndrome. A posteroanterior chest radiograph demonstrates ill-defined opacities in a principally perihilar and lower lung distribution.

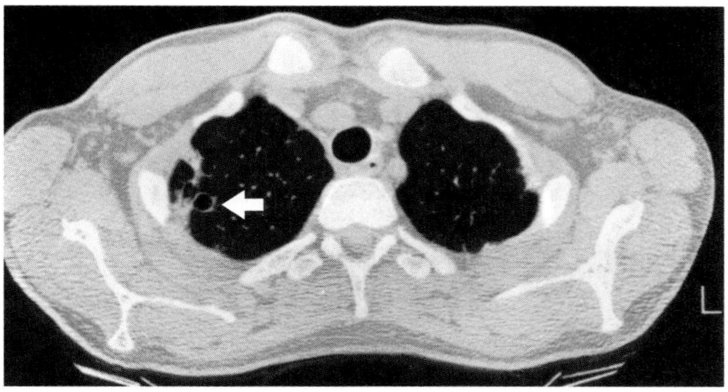

Figure 18-9. Pneumatocele associated with *Pneumocystis carinii* pneumonia in a 19-year-old man with HIV infection acquired through transfusion for hemophilia. A CT examination was performed several weeks following an episode of PCP. An axial CT image at the level of the upper lungs shows bilateral peripheral bandlike opacities. On the right, these changes are more evident, and there is a small, thin-walled cystic area (arrow) representing a postinfectious pneumatocele.

useful when chest radiographs are normal or equivocal. These early changes on CT include ground-glass opacities with inter- or intralobular septal thickening or extensive ground-glass opacities.

Overall, pulmonary disease is the most frequent clinical manifestation in children with AIDS. Although PCP is one cause of pulmonary disease, other pulmonary disease processes (e.g., bacterial pneumonia, cytomegalovirus pneumonia) are, together, more common in children infected with HIV (**Option (D) is false**). These processes include LIP, bronchiectasis, and infections attributable to viruses, bacteria, fungi, or mycobacteria. Viral infections, such as cytomegalovirus infection, can have a radiographic appearance identical to that of PCP. Although the appearances of infections attributable to other organisms are quite varied, focal consolidations are more typical of mycobacterial and bacterial infections.

LIP occurs in 30% to 40% of children with HIV infection. The cause is unknown. With LIP, lymphocytes and plasma cells infiltrate and proliferate in the lung interstitium. There is no consensus regarding the relationship between LIP and other types of lymphoid proliferation in children with AIDS. For example, the entity pulmonary lymphoid hyperplasia has been considered to include LIP or to be a distinct entity. In this entity, lymphoid aggregates are noted within the lung parenchyma or adjacent to bronchi.

Symptoms in children with LIP are generally mild initially and consist of tachypnea and cough. These features can slowly progress over months or years, with episodes of more acute exacerbations. The diagnosis of LIP used to be established by biopsy, but recently the combination of mild respiratory symptoms and radiographic appearance has been considered sufficient for diagnosis.

The primary radiographic finding of LIP is nodular interstitial disease that is symmetric and often diffuse (Figure 18-10). Adenopathy is not rare, but is seen in less than 50% of cases. Pleural effusions are rare. Focal consolidation and bronchiectasis are seen in a minority of cases. Cavitation does not occur in nodular interstitial disease. Corticosteroids have been the traditional form of treatment, although mild cases may not be treated.

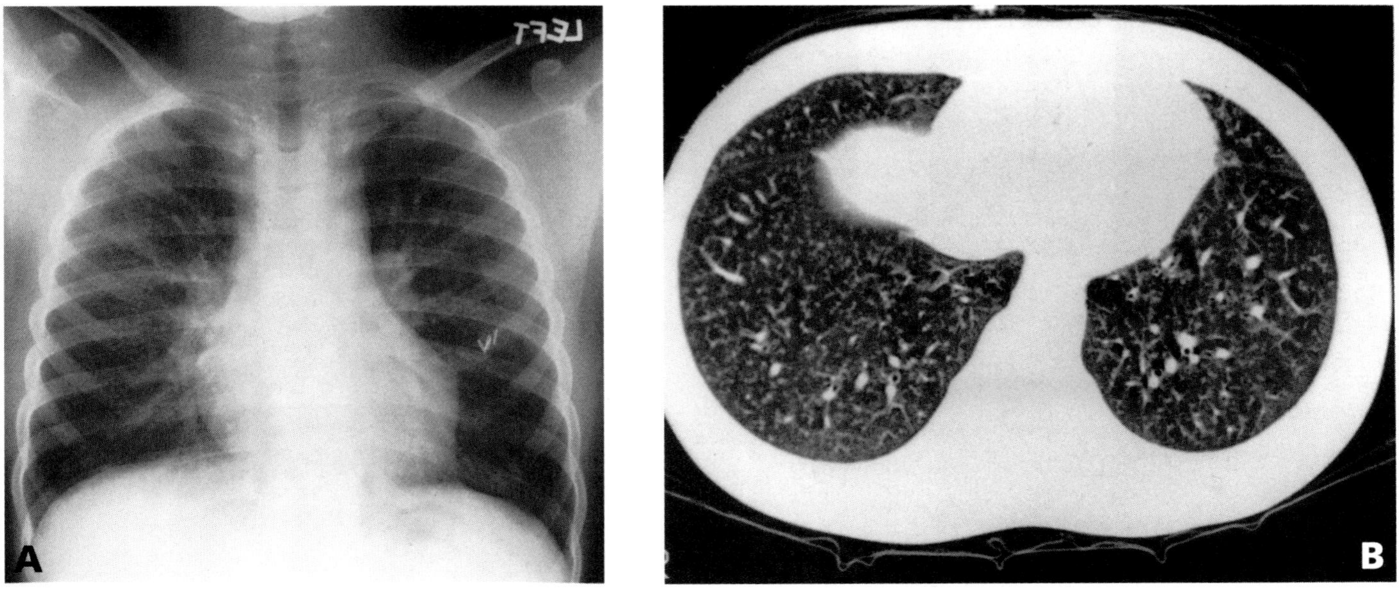

Figure 18-10. Lymphocytic interstitial pneumonitis in a 10-year-old girl with HIV infection. (A) Diffuse nodular interstitial disease is evident on a posteroanterior chest radiograph. Changes as a result of biopsy, by which the diagnosis was confirmed, are evident in the left lung. (B) A high-resolution chest CT image obtained 2 years later, when the symptoms of shortness of breath had improved, shows diffuse subtle reticulonodular changes.

Question 88

Concerning papillomatosis of the airway in children,

(A) it is usually diagnosed at birth
(B) it most often involves the laryngotracheal region
(C) pulmonary involvement occurs in about 5% of patients
(D) it is associated with an increased risk of squamous cell carcinoma
(E) it involutes spontaneously in most patients
(F) pulmonary involvement is characterized by subpleural nodules

Over 90% of laryngeal and tracheal neoplasms in children are benign. These can be either mesenchymal or epithelial in origin. The vast majority of mesenchymal tumors are hemangiomas occurring in infants and young children. Other reported mesenchymal tumors, including fibromas, neurofibromas, and schwannomas, are rare. Virtually all epithelial tumors of the larynx and trachea in childhood are papillomas. Moreover, papillomas are the most common laryngeal and tracheal neoplasms in children.

The descriptor "laryngeal papillomatosis" is used when involvement is limited to the larynx. The term "recurrent respiratory papillomatosis" (RRP) is another term to describe papillomatosis that is protracted, especially with lower respiratory tract involvement. Terms synonymous with RRP include respiratory papillomatosis and juvenile laryngeal papillomatosis.

The vast majority of papillomas are isolated to the laryngotracheal region (**Option (B) is true**). Lower respiratory tract involvement occurs only in a minority of patients; 5% to 17% of cases involve the distal trachea and proximal bronchi. Less than 1% of cases involve bronchoalveolar spread (**Option (C) is false**). Suggested mechanisms of spread include multicentric viral contamination, spontaneous direct spread throughout the respiratory tract, and aerosol spread by dissemination following intervention. Dissemination of disease is increased with tracheotomies (in particular with chronic cannulation), with subsequent development of peristomial and more distant sites of papillomatosis.

Papillomatosis is a virus-related disorder in which human papillomavirus (most often types 6 and 11; infrequently type 16) is implicated. Although there is a strong viral relationship, the etiology of papillomatosis is multifactorial and incompletely understood. The triad of first born, teenage mothers, and vaginal delivery is found in 70% to 75% of cases of pediatric papillomatosis. Although the explanation for the rarity of the entity in subsequent children is unclear, vertical transmission has been documented. This mode of spread is supported by the fact that in 50% of cases of pediatric papillomatosis, there is a history of maternal papillomavirus infection; 70% of mothers have human papillomavirus manifested as genital condyloma acuminatum. Host immunity probably also plays a role given the relative frequency of condylomata in mothers compared to the rarity of papillomatosis.

The majority of cases of papillomatosis occur before 5 years of age, and approximately 25% of cases occur during infancy. Given the slowly progressive symptoms, however, diagnosis at birth is rare (**Option (A) is false**). A second peak occurs during the third decade of life, with up to about 33% of all cases being diagnosed in patients between 16 and 50 years of age. Boys and girls are affected with equal frequency.

The papillomas are either sessile or pedunculated excrescences with squamous epithelium and a central core composed of fibrous and vascular tissues. The clinical manifestations of papillomas are related to either vocal cord involvement or airway compromise. Infants can have a weak or hoarse cry. Obstructive phenomena include cough, stridor, dyspnea or, when there is pulmonary involvement, recurrent respiratory infections or hemoptysis. With greater degrees of obstruction, respiratory difficulty, including tachypnea and retractions, also can be present. Overall, stridor and dyspnea are the most common symptoms, found in about 65% of children with papillomatosis. Because of both the slowly growing nature of the papillomas and their location in areas accessible only via endoscopy, symptoms often can be present for months before the diagnosis of papillomatosis is established. The physical examination can be normal, or papillomas can be found in the mouth and nose.

Chest radiography is used primarily for the evaluation and monitoring of lung involvement with papillomatosis. Radiography is insensitive for the detection of small nodules. When lung involvement is evident radiographically, nodular densities, cavitary lesions, or a combination of both can be present. The development of air-fluid levels within cavitary lesions suggests superimposed infection. Indications for CT include the evaluation of a rapidly growing soft tissue mass or adenopathy seen or suspected on chest radiography; evaluation of clinically suspected airway obstruction; and determination of the extent or depth of papillomatous involvement when endoscopy is not diagnostic. Although the advent of helical CT techniques and three-dimensional capabilities, including virtual endoscopy and bronchoscopy, has provided a noninvasive means for airway evaluation in settings including airway stenoses (e.g., following lung transplantation) and tracheal involvement by lung cancer, the benefit of helical CT for assessing papillomatosis has not been established.

Papillomas in the airway are evident as nodular soft tissue densities or regions of focal mural thickening (Figure 18-11). The nodules are usually multiple, variably sized, and well circumscribed (Figure 18-11). They tend to be located primarily in the central regions (**Option (F) is false**), lung bases, and posterior aspects of the lungs. When small, the nodules are solid and have the attenuation of soft tissue. As the nodules grow, they may cavitate. With cavitation, the walls are usually 3 mm or less in thickness (Figures 18-11 and 18-12). Coalescence of cavities occurs with more advanced lung disease, and these cystic areas can be several centimeters in size (Figure 18-12). Proposed mechanisms for cavitation with papillomatosis of the lung include postobstructive emphysema, pneumatocele formation, or necrosis with cyst formation. As with radiography, the

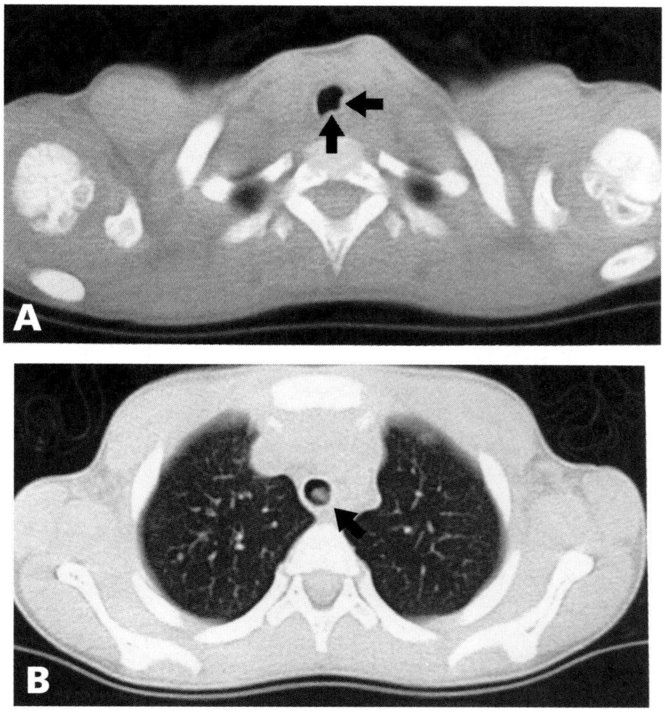

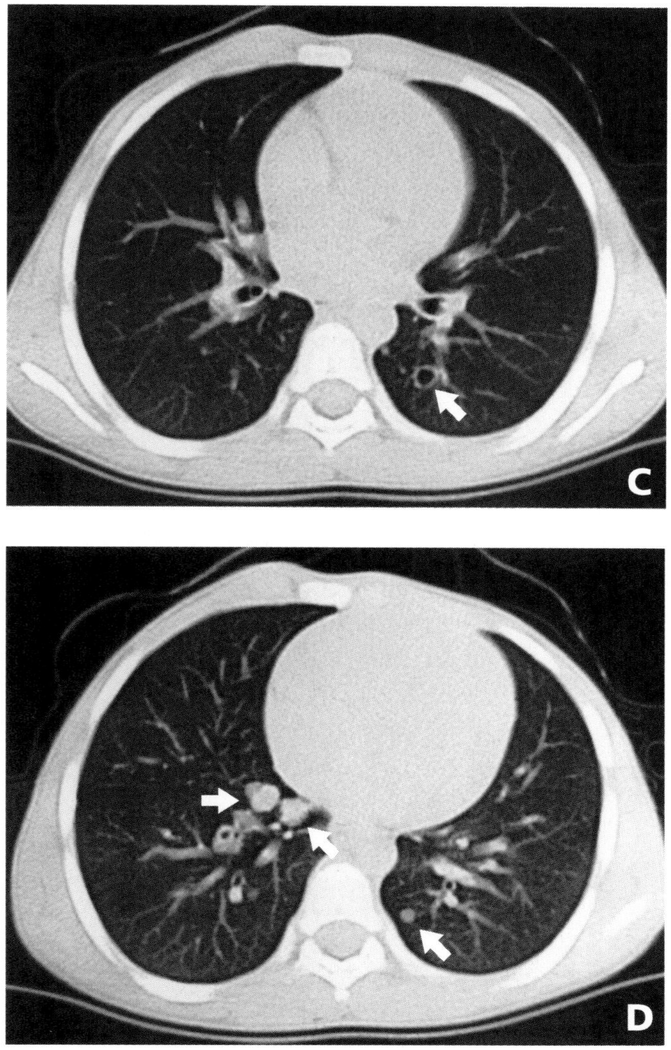

Figure 18-11. Chest CT examination of a 6-year-old boy with papillomatosis. (A) Nodular thickening of the left and posterior aspect of the trachea, attributable to papillomas (arrows), is evident near the level of the thoracic inlet on this axial CT image. (B) An axial CT image obtained just above the level of the aortic arch shows the intraluminal extent of a more polypoid tracheal papilloma (arrow). (C) On this CT image, a cavitary lesion is evident in the left lower lobe (arrow), along with smaller scattered lesions in the posterior aspects of both lungs. (D) On this CT image, obtained slightly more inferiorly than the image in panel C, pulmonary papillomatosis is more obvious. Note multiple, variably sized parenchymal papillomas principally in a central, basilar, and posterior distribution (arrows). (Case courtesy of Alan Brody, M.D., Children's Hospital Medical Center, Cincinnati, OH.)

development of air-fluid levels seen by CT suggests infection.

Malignancy (squamous cell carcinoma), although uncommon, develops with increased frequency (**Option (D) is true**), being found in 2% to 3% of cases of respiratory papillomatosis; malignancy tends to develop in the larynx in adults, but in the lungs in children. Rapid growth of solid nodules (Figure 18-12) suggests the development of squamous cell carcinoma and warrants transbronchial, percutaneous CT-guided, or open-lung biopsy. Other CT features of malignancy include the presence of new adenopathy and invasion of the medias-tinum, chest wall, or pericardium.

CT is also an excellent method for depicting the sequelae of papillomatosis, which are primarily attributable to central obstruction (from either papillomas or mucus plugging) or infection. These include collapse, bronchiectasis, consolidation, and empyema. Pneumothorax and pneumomediastinum are rare complications of lung involvement and are well seen by either CT or radiography. The role of MRI for detection and surveillance is limited. Papillomas have been noted to demonstrate intermediate signal intensity with T1-weighted sequences.

The course of papillomatosis in children is highly variable. Spontaneous remission has been reported but is unpredictable. Only about 25% of children younger than 16 years of age will have spontaneous remission (**Option (E) is false**). When remission occurs in children, it is usually at puberty, implicating a hormonal association. Remission can be found with laryngeal and tracheal diseases, but pulmonary disease virtually always progresses. Recurrence or exacerbation can occur after many years of remission or quiescence. In children with papillomatosis, many procedures, including routine bronchoscopy and laryngoscopy, may be necessary to monitor the disease. This requirement is in addition to the palliative ablations that also can be frequent.

Treatment for papillomatosis is ablation, and the best results have been obtained with lasers. Surgical intervention removes visible lesions, but recurrence is typical because of occult adjacent mucosal involvement. Complications of ablation include stenosis, laryngeal or tracheal perforation, pneumothorax, pneumomediastinum, and hemorrhage. Adjuvant therapy has not been successful, although several methods are under investigation, including interferon, antiviral chemotherapy,

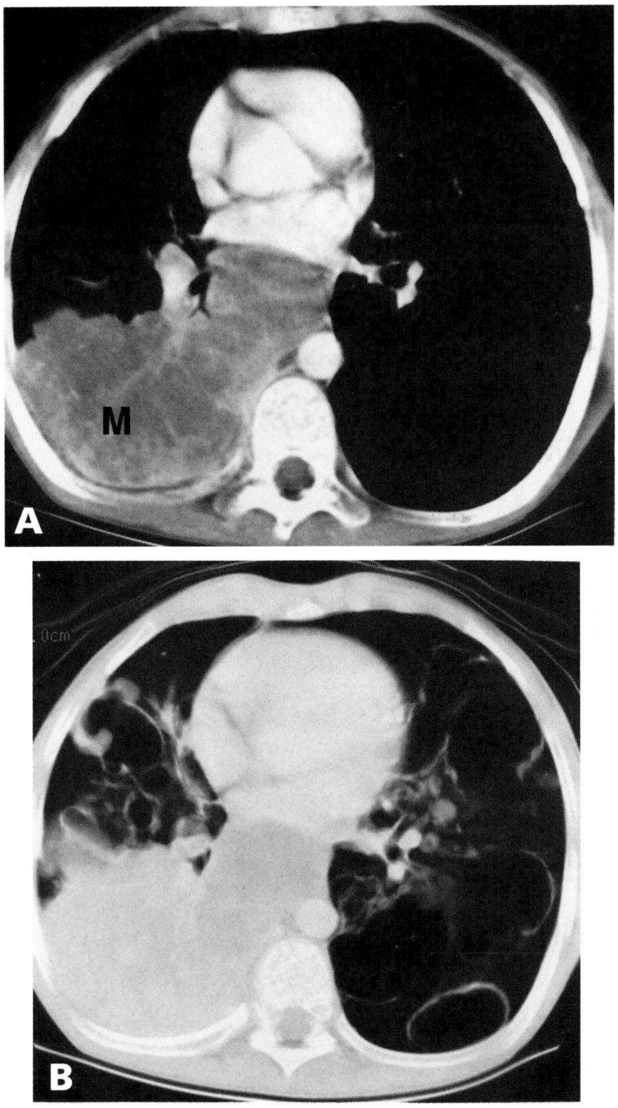

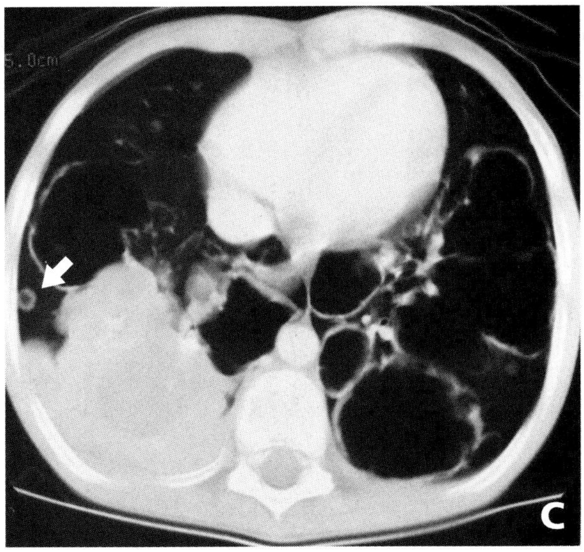

Figure 18-12. Papillomatosis with the development of squamous cell carcinoma in an 11-year-old boy. (A) On the soft tissue window of a chest CT examination, a heterogeneous, large soft tissue mass (M) attributable to carcinoma is present in the posterior aspect of the right lung and extending into the azygoesophageal recess. Note the anterior displacement of the heart. (B) On a CT image (lung window) obtained slightly lower in the chest, multiple large cavitary lesions with thin walls are evident in both lungs. Smaller, noncavitary papillomas are present in both lung bases as well. (C) The range of pulmonary parenchymal changes of RRP is well seen on this axial CT image through the lung bases. Thin-walled, variably sized cystic lesions, including a small cavitary lesion, are seen in addition to the smaller papillomas (arrow) in the right lower lung. (Case courtesy of Lane F. Donnelly, M.D., Children's Hospital Medical Center, Cincinnati, OH.)

indole-3-carbinol, retinoic acid, and photodynamic therapy. Death may be caused by progressive obstruction with respiratory failure, complications of superimposed infection or, very rarely, the development of malignancy.

Question 89

Disorders associated with cystic lung disease in children include:

(A) Niemann-Pick disease
(B) tuberous sclerosis
(C) von Hippel-Lindau disease
(D) Kawasaki's disease
(E) ciliary dyskinesia syndrome (Kartagener's syndrome)
(F) Ehlers-Danlos syndrome

Niemann-Pick disease is one of the group of genetic disorders characterized by enzymatic defects that result in abnormal accumulation of lipids within cells in a variety of organs in the body. Other disorders of lipid accumulation include Tay-Sachs disease, Gaucher's disease, GM1 gangliosidosis type I, Krabbe's disease, and metachromatic leukodystrophy. Niemann-Pick disease is actually a collection of biochemically heterogeneous disorders unified by an abnormal lysosomal accumulation of sphingomyelin and other lipids that results in foamy histiocytes

(Pick cells). Niemann-Pick disease can affect the brain, reticuloendothelial system (liver, spleen, lymph nodes, and bone marrow), and lungs. The diagnosis is established on the basis of clinical features and identification of the enzyme defect from blood samples (leukocytes) or skin biopsy specimens and culturing.

The classic type of Niemann-Pick disease is type A (infantile or neuronopathic type). The typical presentation is failure to thrive, deterioration of neurologic function, hepatomegaly, and macular cherry red spots (in about 50% of cases). Most children do not survive beyond young childhood. In type B, there is no central nervous system involvement and visceral manifestations predominate. The later-onset types (C, D, and E) have slower progression than type A and may not be evident until adulthood.

Lung involvement has been reported mostly for Niemann-Pick disease type B. Manifestations of respiratory tract involvement include cough, dyspnea, wheezing, and upper respiratory tract symptoms, including recurrent respiratory tract infections. Radiographic changes include interstitial disease (Figures 18-13 and 18-14), which can be chronic and can coalesce with areas of airspace disease. Pathologically, there is interstitial and intra-alveolar accumulation of foamy cells. The lower lungs are involved more often. The interstitial involvement is evident on CT as diffuse thickening of the secondary pulmonary lobule (Figure 18-14). High-resolution CT also has demonstrated centrilobular ground-glass opacities (possibly attributable to alveolar foamy cells) in the upper and middle lungs. There is no nodularity, and lung cysts are not found with Niemann-Pick involvement of the lungs (**Option (A) is false**).

Bone marrow transplantation has been successful in treating Niemann-Pick disease type A. The other types (B to E) do not require therapy if the disease is mild.

Tuberous sclerosis is one of a group of genetic neurocutaneous diseases that also includes neurofibromatosis, Sturge-Weber syndrome, ataxia telangiectasia, and von Hippel-Lindau disease. Tuberous sclerosis occurs in about 1 in 100,000 to 150,000 live births. The disease is inherited as an autosomal dominant trait, although about 50% of cases are caused by spontaneous mutations. The classic triad of tuberous sclerosis includes seizures, mental retardation, and sebaceous adenoma. Hamartomatous involvement can occur in virtually any organ. Typical sites of involvement include the brain (periventricular tubers and gliomas), skin, skeletal system (sclerotic lesions and cortical thickening), heart (rhabdomyomas), kidneys (renal

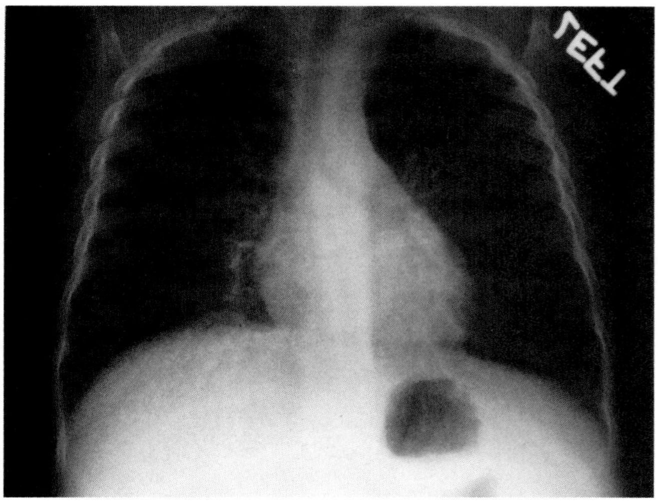

Figure 18-13. Niemann-Pick disease (type B) in a 2-year-old boy with splenomegaly and failure to thrive. A posteroanterior chest radiograph demonstrates subtle diffuse reticular interstitial lung disease.

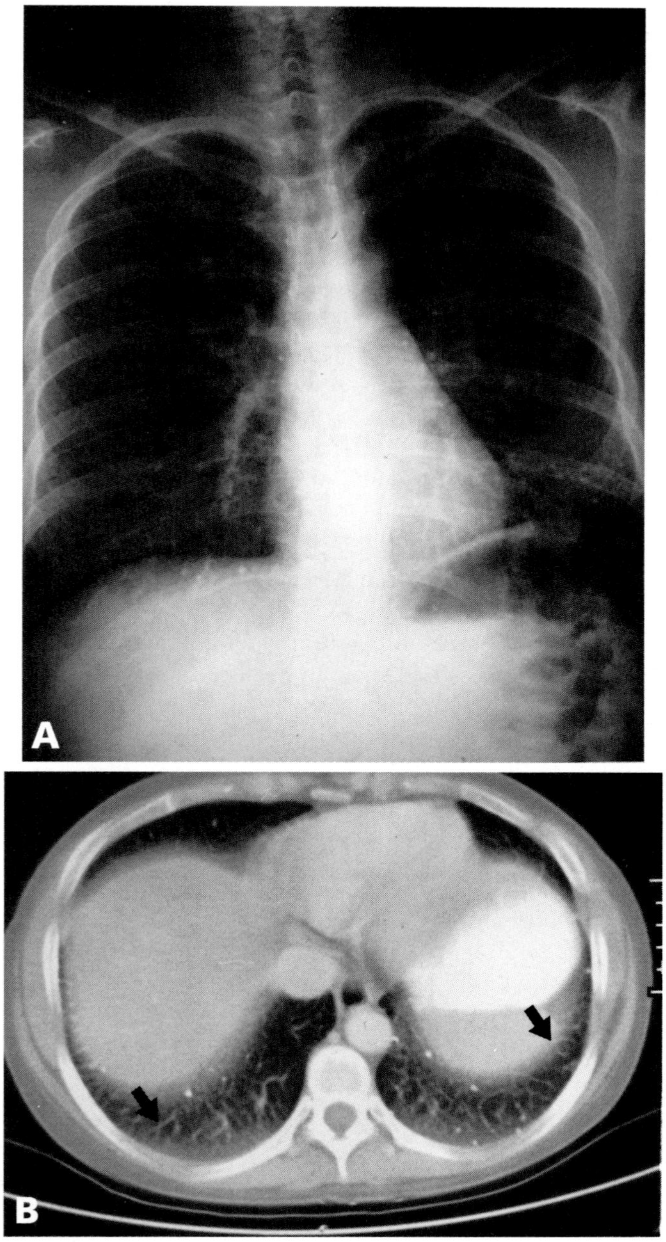

Figure 18-14. Niemann-Pick disease (type B) in a 31-year-old woman. (A) A frontal chest radiograph demonstrates basilar interstitial disease. Punctate densities scattered throughout both lungs are calcified granulomas attributable to childhood tuberculosis. (B) Basilar interstitial disease is demonstrated by a CT examination. Interstitial thickening is evident in the posterior aspects of both lung bases, with some regions more clearly involving the secondary pulmonary lobule (arrows). Calcified granulomas are present bilaterally.

cysts and hamartomas, including angiomyolipomas), liver, spleen, and lungs. Lung involvement is rare, however, occurring in only about 1% of children with tuberous sclerosis. Pulmonary lymphangioleiomyomatosis and tuberous sclerosis are pathologically identical (smooth muscle proliferation), but are distinguished on the basis of clinical features. Lymphangioleiomyomatosis, also known as lymphangiomatosis, is found almost exclusively in premenopausal women.

Lung involvement with tuberous sclerosis and lymphangioleiomyomatosis is characterized by interstitial thickening attributable to smooth muscle proliferation (Figure 18-15). Air trapping, with resultant formation of blebs and cysts (ranging from a few millimeters to several centimeters in size) **(Option (B) is true)** and complicated clinically by pneumothorax, is likely secondary to obstruction from the increase in smooth muscle around airways. Cyst walls contain smooth muscle and occasional columnar and cuboidal epithelia. The cystic and interstitial changes can be evident radiographically, but the extent and severity of abnormalities are best demonstrated by CT examination. Cysts are best characterized on high-resolution CT (Figure 18-16) and range in size from 0.5 to 5 cm, with walls that are typically less than 2.0 mm in thickness. They are distributed throughout all lobes. With severe pulmonary involvement, interstitial fibrosis can be seen. The diagnosis is established by open-lung or transbronchial biopsy.

Another disorder included in the constellation of neurocutaneous disorders is von Hippel-Lindau disease, in spite of the fact that there are no dermatologic manifestations of the syndrome. An autosomal dominant mode of inheritance is present in some cases. The constellation of features of von Hippel-Lindau disease includes retinal hemangiomas, posterior fossa hemangioblastomas, and renal and visceral neoplasms. Symptoms are related to ocular disease (visual loss) and cerebellar or spinal cord masses and are rarely present before adolescence. There are no pulmonary manifestations of von Hippel-Lindau disease **(Option (C) is false)**.

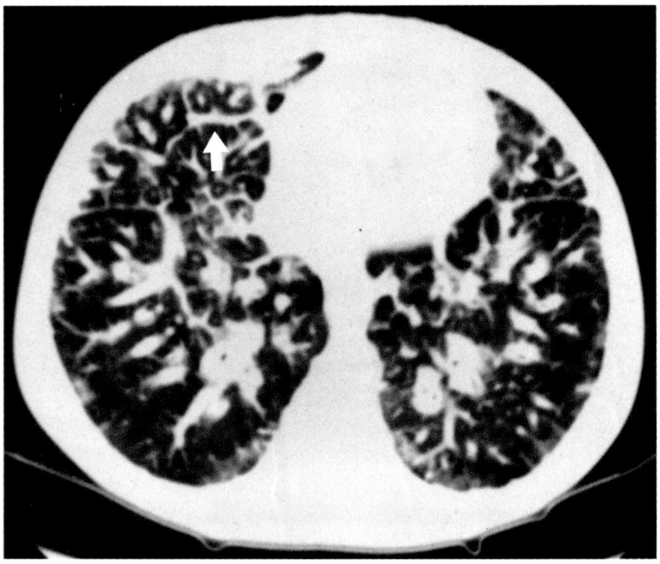

Figure 18-15. Biopsy-proven lymphangioleiomyomatosis in a 7-year-old boy with no other stigmata of tuberous sclerosis. A CT image of the lower lungs shows fairly symmetric and smooth septal thickening bilaterally. Note the secondary pulmonary lobule on the right (arrow). No cavitation is evident.

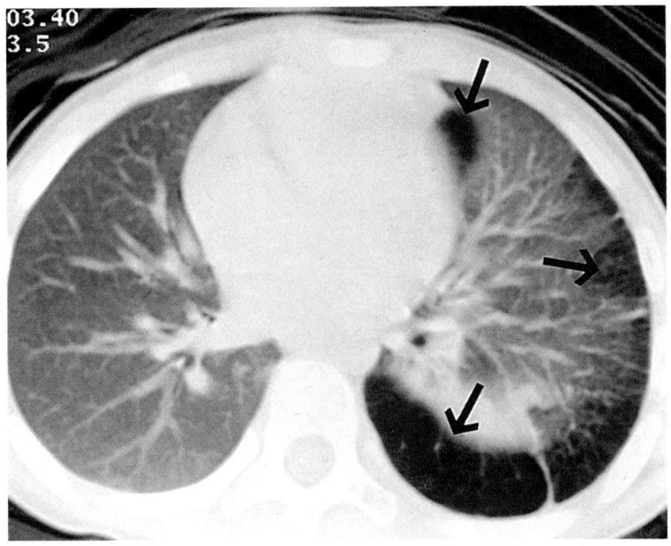

Figure 18-16. Tuberous sclerosis. A thin-section CT scan shows several areas of cystic emphysema (arrows) in the lower left lobe. (Case courtesy of Marilyn J. Siegel, M.D., Mallinckrodt Institute of Radiology, St. Louis, MO.)

Kawasaki's disease, also known as mucocutaneous lymph node syndrome, is a systemic vasculitic disorder of unknown etiology. An autoimmune response to infectious stimulation has been one predominant theory. Kawasaki's disease usually affects infants and young children, with 80% of cases occurring before the age of 5 years. The age of peak incidence in the United States for Kawasaki's disease is 1 to 2 years. The time course for Kawasaki's disease consists of acute (7 to 14 days), subacute (10 to 24 days), and convalescent (6 to 8 weeks) phases. The diagnosis is based on establishing a sufficient constellation of signs and symptoms. These include fever lasting several days and four or five of the following: bilateral conjunctivitis, mucosal abnormalities (strawberry tongue, pharyngeal erythema, and dry or cracked lips), erythema or edema of the distal extremities (including desquamation), rash, or cervical adenopathy. Other manifestations of organ involvement include arthralgias and arthritis, aseptic meningitis, inflammation of the genitourinary system (nephritis, epididymo-orchitis, cystitis, urethritis, and prostatitis), diarrhea, hepatopathy, and gallbladder hydrops. Thoracic manifestations are seen in the cardiovascular system and the lungs.

One of most significant sequelae of Kawasaki's disease is involvement of the cardiovascular system. Cardiac sequelae (including myocarditis, coronary aneurysms, and stenoses) are seen in about 10% of patients at the time of diagnosis. Up to 1% of children with Kawasaki's disease will succumb to cardiac complications. In the acute phase, the vasculitis results in phlebitis, myocarditis, pericarditis, endocarditis, or valvulitis. In both the acute and the convalescent phases, aneurysms of the coronary arteries and other medium-size arteries (e.g., axillary arteries) can occur. These aneurysms can persist, regress, or result in significant arterial stenosis.

Pulmonary involvement is rare and has been noted in less than 15% of children with Kawasaki's disease. In one series of 129 children, pulmonary findings were nonspecific and included a reticulonodular interstitial pattern (90%) and pleural effusion or peribronchial cuffing in less than 20%. Radiographic findings were present within 11 days from the onset of illness. Air trapping and atelectasis were rarely seen. On CT, parenchymal findings included diffuse interstitial disease or ill-defined nodules. Histopathologic changes were noted in 30% to 90% of autopsy cases and consisted of interstitial pneumonitis and arteritis. Lung cysts are not among the pulmonary manifestations of Kawasaki's disease **(Option (D) is false).**

The standard treatment for Kawasaki's disease is aspirin and intravenous gamma globulin. This combination is effective in reducing the duration and magnitude of acute-phase manifestations, in particular the development of coronary artery disease.

Kartagener's syndrome is an autosomal recessive syndrome; the classic triad consists of sinusitis, bronchiectasis, and situs inversus totalis (Figure 18-17). The frequency of Kartagener's syndrome varies and is reported to be from 1 in 15,000 to 1 in 130,000 individuals. Ciliary dyskinesia or dyskinetic cilia syndrome (also referred to as immotile cilia syndrome) encompasses Kartagener's syndrome and includes patients in whom cardiac situs and abdominal situs are normal. The aberration in ciliary dyskinesia is attributable to an abnormal ciliary structure or function. The characteristic abnormality is an alteration in the 9 + 2 configuration of microtubules or microtubular elements (dynein arms, radial spokes, and nexin links), resulting in ciliary dyskinesia. Other aberrations found in children with ciliary dyskinesia include ciliary aplasia and functional abnormalities despite normal ciliary structure. Clinical and imaging manifestations of ciliary dyskinesia are related to respiratory tract infections, reduced fertility in males, and situs inversus totalis.

The disorder rarely appears during infancy. In such cases, it is suspected only when recurrent respiratory tract infections

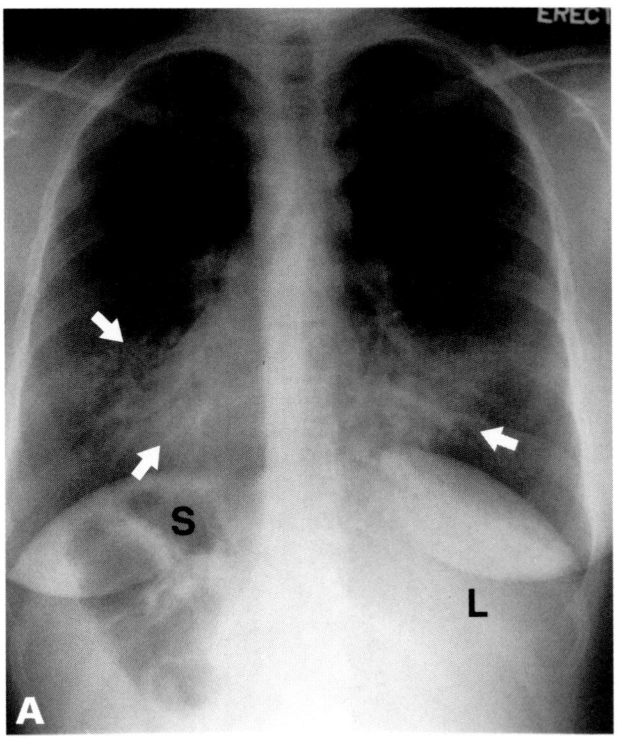

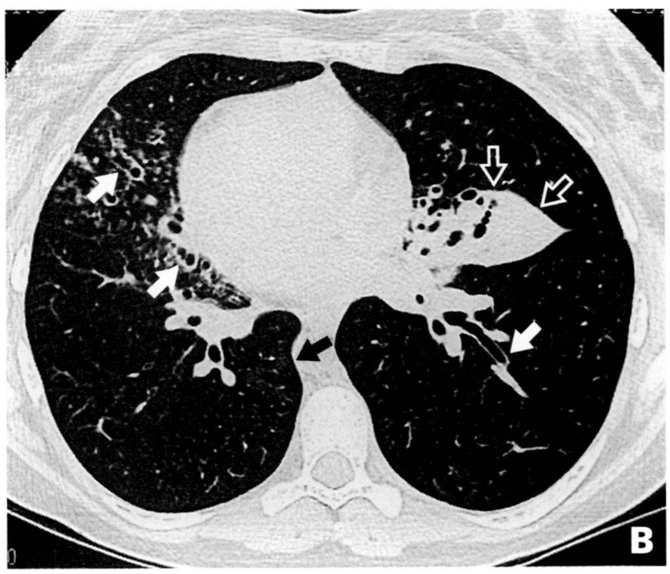

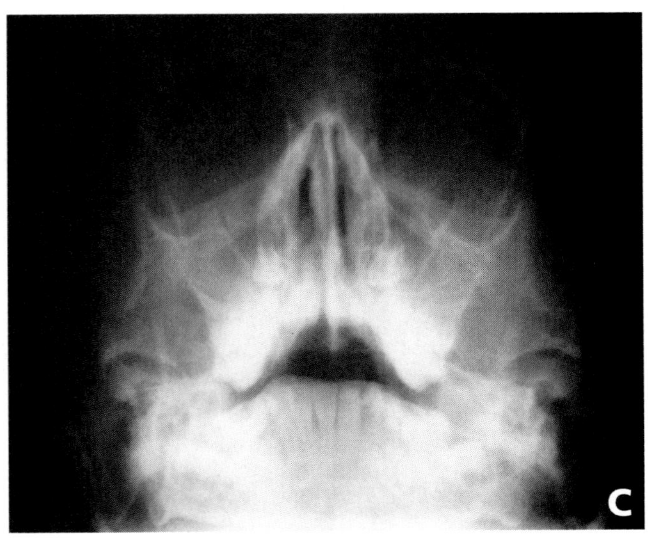

Figure 18-17. Kartagener's syndrome in a 14-year-old girl with recurrent sinus and pulmonary infections. (A) A posteroanterior chest radiograph demonstrates dextrocardia with abdominal situs inversus. The stomach bubble (S) is on the right, and the soft tissue density in the left upper quadrant corresponds to the liver (L). Streaky bibasilar opacities (arrows) are attributable to bronchiectasis. (B) A high-resolution CT image obtained at the level of the basilar bronchi more clearly demonstrates the areas of bronchiectasis (white arrows). There is reversal of bronchial anatomy, and the opacity on the left side (open arrows) is in the middle lobe. Note also the descending thoracic aorta, which is slightly to the right of midline (black arrow). (C) Nearly complete opacification of the left maxillary sinus and mucoperiosteal thickening of the right maxillary sinus are seen in this Water's view from a radiographic series.

are accompanied by situs inversus totalis. Otherwise, the diagnosis of ciliary dyskinesia usually is not established until childhood or adolescence. The most common clinical manifestation of ciliary dyskinesia is chronic cough, found in over 95% of individuals. Sinusitis is found in about 95%, otitis is found in 75%, and bronchiectasis is found in 60%.

Radiographic features include hyperinflation, peribronchial cuffing, consolidation or atelectasis, situs inversus totalis, and bronchiectasis, which can be cystic. However, parenchymal lung cysts are not a feature of this disease (**Option (E) is false**). The most frequent regions involved are the middle lobe and lingula and the lower lobes. Without situs inversus totalis, the radiographic features, in particular bronchiectasis, are nonspecific and can be found in a variety of pediatric disorders predisposing to recurrent pulmonary infections, including cystic fibrosis and primary immunodeficiency. These two entities are also the principal differential considerations of ciliary dyskinesia syndrome based on clinical features. Sinus CT features are those of sinus infection, including mucoperiosteal thickening, sinus opacification, and polyps.

It is interesting that 50% of children with ciliary dyskinesia have situs inversus totalis. This percentage implicates a contribution of normally functioning cilia in the early positioning of asymmetric body organs. In the absence of normal cilia, there is a random (50:50) distribution between normal and reversed configurations.

The diagnosis of ciliary dyskinesia is established with a combination of clinical and imaging features and biopsy of nasal cilia, with subsequent demonstration of abnormal ciliary function or structure.

With prompt recognition of ciliary dyskinesia and institution of therapy, which minimizes the progression of bronchiectasis, morbidity can be minimal and patients can have a normal life span. There is no cure, and treatment is directed at the prevention of respiratory tract infection (pulmonary toilet); management of complications, including antibiotics; and operative intervention, including tympanostomy tubes for otitis, nasal polypectomies, and partial lung resection for severe bronchiectasis or persistent consolidation.

There are nine subgroups of connective tissue disorders collectively known as Ehlers-Danlos syndrome. Most types have an autosomal dominant mode of inheritance, although a minority are either autosomal recessive or X-linked. The basis of these different types is a defect in collagen synthesis. The uniting feature of these types is a variable presence of hyperextensible skin and increased fragility predisposing to bruising and bleeding. Significant morbidity also can result from skeletal deformity, blindness, bowel rupture, aneurysms and dissection of the great vessels, and lung involvement. Patients having surgical procedures are also at increased risk for poor wound healing and dehiscence.

Lung involvement is uncommon and is most frequently reported with type IV Ehlers-Danlos syndrome. When present, pulmonary Ehlers-Danlos syndrome is manifested clinically by hemoptysis, pneumonia, respiratory distress, or pneumothorax. Structural features of pulmonary involvement include bronchiectasis, bulla formation, and tracheobronchomegaly. The frequency of pulmonary involvement is unknown, but it is very small. Findings of lung involvement on radiography and chest CT include variable numbers of solid pulmonary nodules, cysts that can contain fluid (**Option (F) is true**), and blebs (Figure 18-18). The cysts are believed to be secondary to blood vessel rupture and hemorrhage with subsequent cavitation. Changes of fibrosis attributable to defective healing include the formation of fibrous pseudotumors, which can be evident with radiography or CT.

SUGGESTED READINGS

LANGERHANS CELL HISTIOCYTOSIS

1. A multicentre retrospective survey of Langerhans' cell histiocytosis: 348 cases observed between 1983 and 1993. The French Langerhans' Cell Histiocytosis Study Group. Arch Dis Child 1996; 75:17–24
2. Brauner MW, Grenier P, Tijani K, Battesti JP, Valeyre D. Pulmonary Langerhans cell histiocytosis: evolution of lesions on CT scans. Radiology 1997; 204:497–502
3. Egeler RM, D'Angio GJ. Langerhans cell histiocytosis. J Pediatr 1995; 127:1–11
4. Meyer JS, Harty MP, Mahboubi S, et al. Langerhans cell histiocytosis: presentation and evolution of radiologic findings with clinical correlation. RadioGraphics 1995; 15:1135–1146

PNEUMOCYSTIS CARINII PNEUMONIA

5. Crans CA Jr, Boiselle PM. Imaging features of *Pneumocystis carinii* pneumonia. Crit Rev Diagn Imaging 1999; 40:251–284
6. Dollfus C. Pneumocystosis in infants and children with HIV: current concepts. Pediatr Pulmonol Suppl; 1997; 16:194–196
7. Markowitz RI, Ruchelli E. Pneumonia in infants and children: radiological-pathological correlation. Semin Roentgenol 1998; 33:151–162
8. Marks MJ, Haney PJ, McDermott MP, White CS, Vennos AD. Thoracic disease in children with AIDS. RadioGraphics 1996; 16:1349–1362

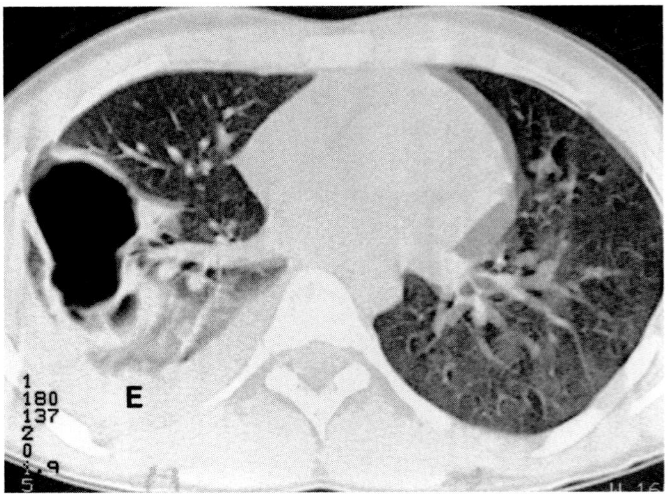

Figure 18-18. Ehlers-Danlos syndrome. A CT image shows a thick-walled cyst in the right lower lobe and a pleural effusion (E). The adjacent lung is compressed by both the cyst and the effusion. (Case courtesy of Marilyn J. Siegel, M.D.)

9. Miller CR. Pediatric aspects of AIDS. Radiol Clin North Am 1997; 35: 1191–1221
10. Simonds RJ, Lindegren ML, Thomas P, et al. Prophylaxis against *Pneumocystis carinii* pneumonia among children with perinatal acquired human immunodeficiency virus infection in the United States. *Pneumocystis carinii* Pneumonia Prophylaxis Evaluation Working Group. N Engl J Med 1995; 332:786–790
11. Uwyyed K, Bar-Ziv J, Kramer MR. Case report: *Pneumocystis carinii* pneumonia presenting as a solitary cavitating lung lesion in non-HIV immunosuppressed patients. Br J Radiol 1996; 69:472–475
12. Williams AJ, Duong T, McNally LM, et al. *Pneumocystis carinii* pneumonia and cytomegalovirus infection in children with vertically acquired HIV infection. AIDS 2001; 15:335–339

BRONCHIECTASIS

13. Agasthian T, Deschamps C, Trastek VF, Allen MS, Pairolero PC. Surgical management of bronchiectasis. Ann Thorac Surg 1996; 62:976–978
14. Case records of the Massachusetts General Hospital. Weekly clinicopathological exercises. Case 31-1998. An eight-year-old boy with bronchiectasis. N Engl J Med 1998; 339:1144–1151
15. Coleman LT, Kramer SS, Markowitz RI, Kravitz RM. Bronchiectasis in children. J Thorac Imaging 1995; 10:268–279
16. Hansell DM. Bronchiectasis. Radiol Clin North Am 1998; 36:107–128
17. Jones VF, Eid NS, Franco SM, Badgett JT, Buchino JJ. Familial congenital bronchiectasis: Williams-Campbell syndrome. Pediatr Pulmonol 1993; 16:263–267
18. Maffessanti M, Candusso M, Brizzi F, Piovesana F. Cystic fibrosis in children: HRCT findings and distribution of disease. J Thorac Imaging 1996; 11:27–38
19. McAdams HP, Erasmus J. Chest case of the day. Williams-Campbell syndrome. AJR 1995; 165:190–191

TUBERCULOSIS

20. Abernathy RS. Tuberculosis: an update. Pediatr Rev 1997; 18:50–58
21. Burroughs M, Beitel A, Kawamura A, et al. Clinical presentation of tuberculosis in culture-positive children. Pediatric Tuberculosis Consortium. Pediatr Infect Dis J 1999; 18:440–446
22. Correa AG. Unique aspects of tuberculosis in the pediatric population. Clin Chest Med 1997; 18:89–98
23. Vallejo JG, Starke JR. Intrathoracic tuberculosis in children. Semin Respir Infect 1996; 11:184–195

RESPIRATORY PAPILLOMATOSIS

24. Andrews SE. Laser ablation of recurrent laryngeal papillomas in children. AORN J 1995; 61:532–540, 543–544
25. Bauman NM, Smith RJ. Recurrent respiratory papillomatosis. Pediatr Clin North Am 1996; 43:1385–1401
26. Derkay CS. Recurrent respiratory papillomatosis. Laryngoscope 2001; 111:57–69
27. Lui D, Kumar A, Aggarwal S, Soto J. CT findings of malignant change in recurrent respiratory papillomatosis. J Comput Assist Tomogr 1995; 19:804–807
28. McCarthy MJ, Rosado-de-Christenson ML. Tumors of the trachea. J Thorac Imaging 1995; 10:180–198

NIEMANN-PICK DISEASE

29. Ferretti GR, Lantuejoul S, Brambilla E, Coulomb M. Case report. Pulmonary involvement in Niemann-Pick disease subtype B: CT findings. J Comput Assist Tomogr 1996; 20:990–992
30. Kovesi TA, Lee J, Shuckett B, Clarke JTR, Callahon JW, Phillips MJ. Pulmonary infiltration in Niemann-Pick disease type C. J Inherit Metab Dis 1996; 19:792–793
31. Weisz B, Spirer Z, Reif S. Niemann-Pick disease: newer classification based on genetic mutations of the disease. Adv Pediatr 1994; 41:415–426

TUBEROUS SCLEROSIS

32. Castro M, Shepherd CW, Gomez MR, Lie JT, Ryu JH. Pulmonary tuberous sclerosis. Chest 1995; 107:189–195
33. Collins J, Müller NL, Kazerooni EA, McAdams HP, Leung AN, Love RB. Lung transplantation for lymphangioleiomyomatosis: role of imaging in the assessment of complications related to the underlying disease. Radiology 1999; 210:325–332
34. Kalassian KG, Doyle R, Kao P, Ruoss S, Raffin TA. Lymphangioleiomyomatosis: new insights. Am J Respir Crit Care Med 1997; 155:1183–1186
35. Milledge RD, Gerald BE, Carter WJ. Pulmonary manifestations of tuberous sclerosis. AJR 1966; 98:734–738

KAWASAKI'S DISEASE

36. Chung CJ, Stein L. Kawasaki disease: a review. Radiology 1998; 208:25–33
37. Oki I, Tanihara S, Ojima T, Nakamura Y, Yanagawa H. A multicenter collaborative study on the risk factors of cardiac sequelae due to Kawasaki disease: a one-year follow-up study. Acta Paediatr 2000; 89:1435–1438
38. Umezawa T, Saji T, Matsuo N, Odagiri K. Chest x-ray findings in the acute phase of Kawasaki disease. Pediatr Radiol 1989; 20:48–51

CILIARY DYSKINESIA

39. Losa M, Ghelfi D, Hof E, Felix H, Fanconi S. Kartagener syndrome: an uncommon cause of neonatal respiratory distress? Eur J Pediatr 1995; 154:236–238
40. Teknos TN, Metson R, Chasse T, Balercia G, Dickersin GR. New developments in the diagnosis of Kartagener's syndrome. Otolaryngol Head Neck Surg 1997; 116:68–74
41. Tkebuchava T, Niederhauser U, Weder W, et al. Kartagener's syndrome: clinical presentation and cardiosurgical aspects. Ann Thorac Surg 1996; 62:1474–1479

EHLERS-DANLOS SYNDROME

42. Dowton SB, Pincott S, Demmer L. Respiratory complications of Ehlers-Danlos syndrome type IV. Clin Genet 1996; 50:510–514
43. Herman TE, McAlister WH. Cavitary pulmonary lesions in type IV Ehlers-Danlos syndrome. Pediatr Radiol 1994; 24:263–265
44. Murray RA, Poulton TB, Saltarelli MG, et al. Rare pulmonary manifestation of Ehlers-Danlos syndrome. J Thorac Imaging 1995; 10:138–141

PULMONARY DISEASE: GENERAL

45. Cherniak V, Boat TF (eds). Kendig's disorders of the respiratory tract in children. 6th ed. Philadelphia: WB Saunders; 1998
46. Siegel MJ. Pediatric body CT. Philadelphia: Lippincott Williams & Wilkins; 1999:101–140

CASE 19

Donald P. Frush, M.D.

Pulmonary Sling

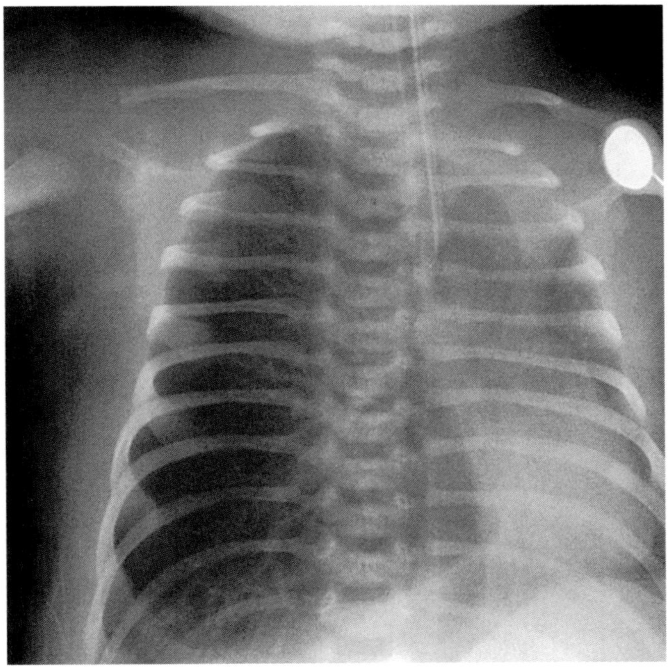

Figure 19-1

Question 90

This 11-day-old girl had respiratory distress requiring intubation. You are shown an anteroposterior chest radiograph (Figure 19-1).

Which *one* of the following is the MOST likely diagnosis?

(A) Pneumothorax
(B) Agenetic lung
(C) Pulmonary sling
(D) Diaphragmatic hernia
(E) Diaphragmatic paralysis

The test patient's chest radiograph (Figure 19-1) shows marked asymmetry in aeration. The right hemithorax is hyperlucent, with extension of the right lung across the midline. There is also a leftward shift of the heart and mediastinum, including the endotracheal tube.

A variety of conditions can result in asymmetric aeration in neonates and infants with respiratory distress. Such entities include developmental deficiencies of the airway and lung parenchyma (agenesis, aplasia, and hypoplasia), bronchopulmonary foregut malformations (congenital lobar emphysema) (Figure 19-2), congenital cystic adenomatoid malformations (CAM) (Figure 19-3), lung cysts, bronchial atresia, endobronchial abnormalities (most commonly mucus plugs) (Figure 19-4), exobronchial compression (Figure 19-5), and postinfectious pneumatoceles or bronchiolitis obliterans. Because the majority of these abnormalities have similar respiratory symptoms, imaging is an integral part of the evaluation when these conditions are suspected.

Exobronchial causes of obstructive hyperaeration include mediastinal masses, adenopathy, and anomalies of the cardiovascular system. Airway compression (and aeration disturbances) secondary to anomalies of the cardiovascular system can be attributable to chamber enlargement (e.g., left atrial enlargement) or enlargement or atypical course of the great vessels. One of these anomalies, the pulmonary sling, typically is seen in infants with signs of respiratory distress and a hyperaerated right lung. Of the options listed, pulmonary sling is the best explanation for the radiographic findings in the test patient (Figure 19-6) (**Option (C) is correct**). The pulmonary sling consists of an ectopic origin of the left pulmonary artery from the right pulmonary artery. The course of the aberrant artery is adjacent to the right bronchus and, subsequently, posterior to the trachea. Airway compromise can be attributable to a combination of factors, including direct compression by the vessel, resultant tracheomalacia and, occasionally, complete tracheal rings or stenosis. MRI is ideally suited for evaluation of the pulmonary sling because multiplanar depiction will clearly demonstrate the aberrant vessel (Figure 19-6B) and the extent and severity of the airway compromise.

Congenital unilateral deficiencies in pulmonary tissue include agenesis, aplasia, and hypoplasia. With pulmonary agenesis (Option (B)), there is a complete absence of lobes and bronchi on the affected side. The trachea continues into a single bronchus. Right- and left-sided involvement occur with equal frequency. In unilateral pulmonary aplasia, there is a rudimentary, blindly ending bronchus with no distal lung parenchyma. Clinically, agenesis and aplasia are identical. The radiographic appearance of either agenesis or aplasia is hyperin-

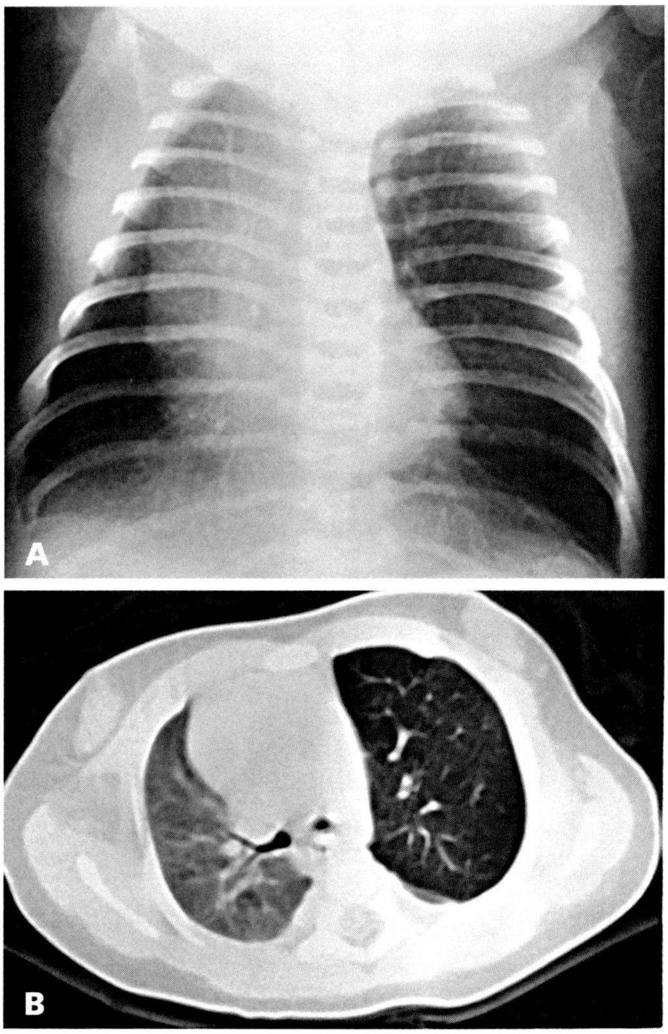

Figure 19-2. Left upper lobe congenital lobar emphysema in a 5-day-old boy with dyspnea. (A) A radiograph shows marked hyperinflation of the left lung and rightward shift of the mediastinum. (B) A CT examination at a level just below the carina confirms the presence of emphysematous lung parenchyma.

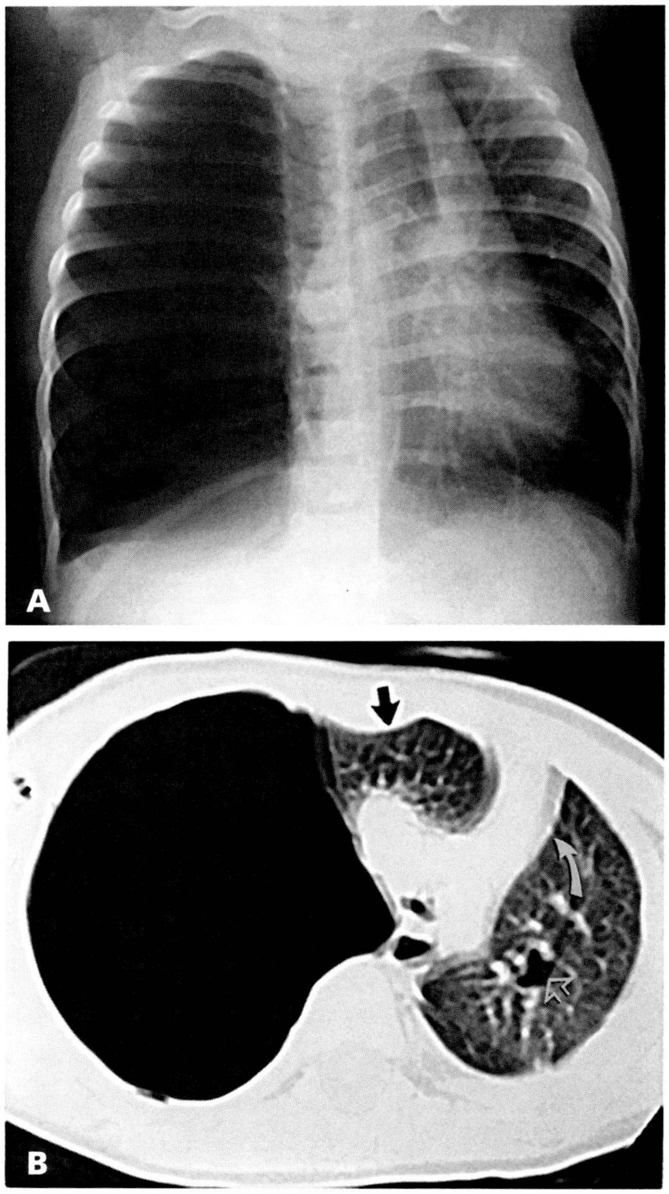

Figure 19-3. Large congenital cystic adenomatoid malformation (CAM) in a 16-month-old boy with respiratory distress. (A) An anteroposterior chest radiograph demonstrates hyperlucency and increased size of the right hemithorax. Note the leftward shift of the heart and mediastinum. (B) A subsequent CT examination of the chest at the level of the aortic arch demonstrates an enlarged, unilocular cystic area in the right lung. Note the mass effect, with both the right upper lobe (black arrow) and the thymus (curved arrow) being displaced toward the left. Note also a small focal lucency in the left upper lobe (open arrow). The etiology of this feature was uncertain, but it was believed also to be a CAM of the left lung. At surgery, the right-sided CAM was confined to the resected right middle lobe.

flation of one lung with marked cardiac and mediastinal shift, including posterior bowing of the trachea on lateral radiographs. CT examination can help to distinguish between the two entities (Figure 19-7). In aplasia, a rudimentary bronchus is demonstrated, whereas no bronchus is present with pulmonary agenesis. Lobar agenesis and aplasia are less common than these abnormalities in an entire lung. Pulmonary hypoplasia represents malformed pulmonary parenchyma and associated deficiency of the airway. Pulmonary hypoplasia is described in greater detail in the discussion of Question 91. Although the clinical findings for the test case could have been attributable to one of these congenital lung anomalies, the radiograph in Figure 19-6A demonstrates an anterior junction line separating the right and left lungs. Thus, agenesis of the left lung is not likely.

Congenital diaphragmatic hernia (Option (D)), also known as a Bochdalek's hernia, usually is manifested as respiratory distress in the first few hours of life. However, the radiographic features of congenital diaphragmatic hernia are quite different from those of the test case. Congenital diaphragmatic hernia occurs in the left hemithorax in 80% to 90% of cases. There is typically a multicystic radiographic appearance of the affected hemithorax attributable to stomach and intestine within the hemithorax. With the less common right-sided hernia, the right hemithorax is partially or completely opacified by the herniation of the liver into the hemithorax. The radiographic

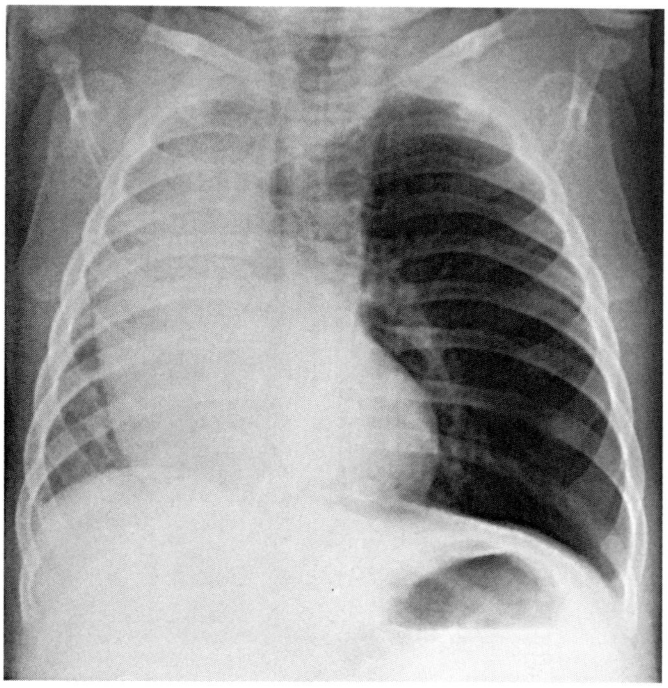

Figure 19-4. Asymmetric aeration attributable to right-lung atelectasis from a right bronchial mucus plug in a 3-month-old child with a lower respiratory tract viral infection. Note the compensatory hyperinflation of the left lung and the shift of the mediastinum and heart toward the right on the radiograph.

findings in the test patient do not suggest either a right or a left congenital diaphragmatic hernia.

Unilateral paralysis of the diaphragm (Option (E)) is usually a result of trauma, typically birth related or following surgery for congenital heart disease. Manifestations include respiratory distress and ventilator dependence. The radiographic features of diaphragmatic paralysis are asymmetric lung volumes, with the involved side being smaller. The ipsilateral diaphragm is elevated (Figure 19-8). Hyperinflation is not found with diaphragmatic paralysis.

On first inspection, a large right pneumothorax (Option

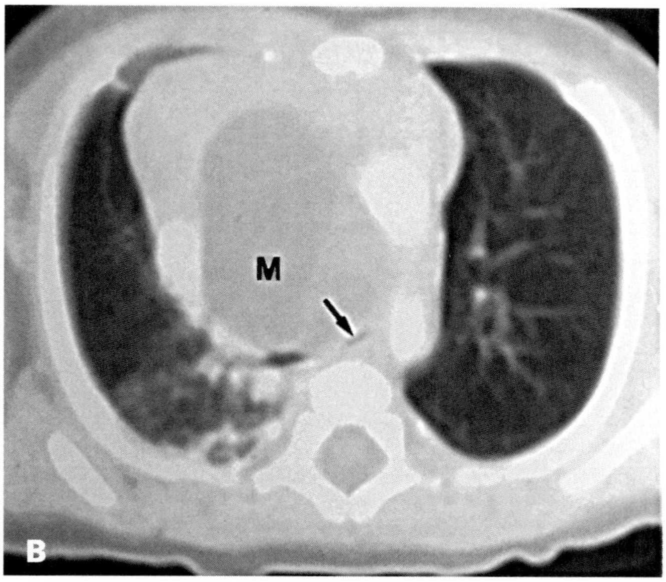

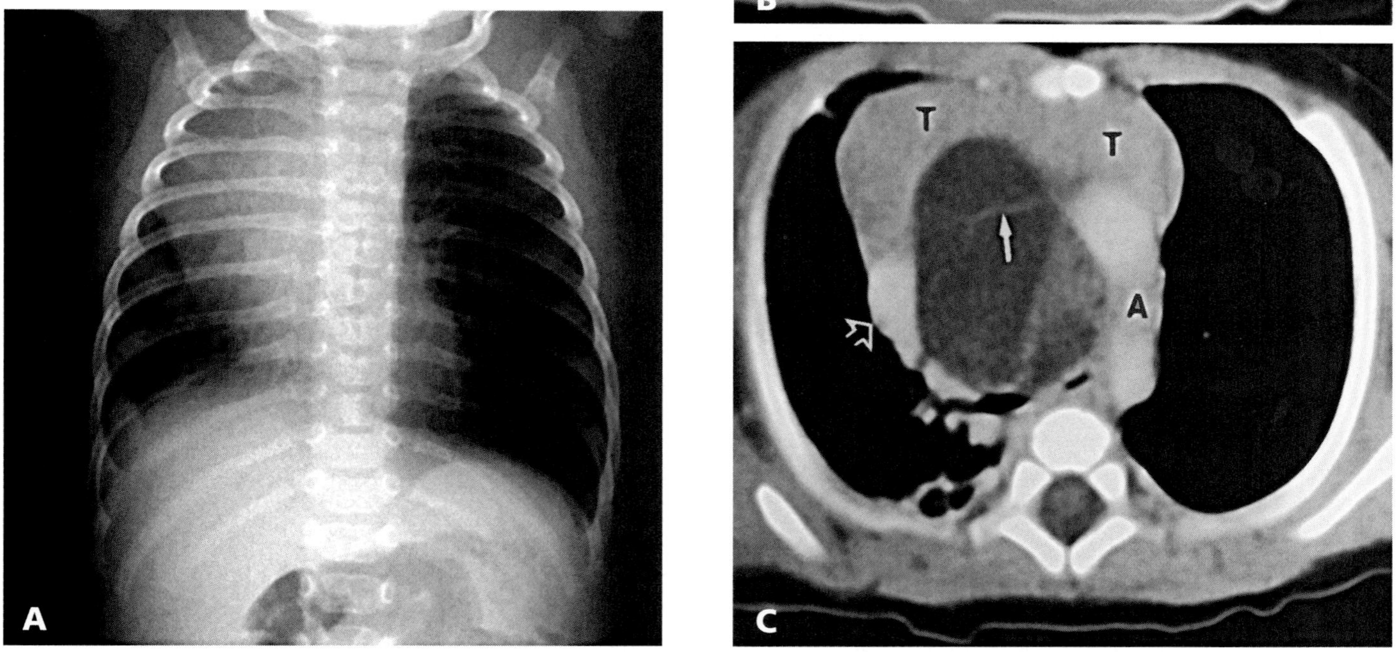

Figure 19-5. Mature teratoma in a 3-month-old boy. (A) An anteroposterior chest radiograph was obtained because of wheezing. Note the hyperlucent and hyperinflated left lung with evidence of flattening of the diaphragm and shifting of the cardiac and mediastinal silhouette to the right. (B) A CT examination confirms the asymmetry in aeration between the left and right lungs. There is posterior atelectasis. Note the narrowing of the left main bronchus (arrow) resulting in air trapping in the left lung because of an anterior mediastinal mass (M). (C) A CT image with mediastinal windows at the same level as in panel B better characterizes the large, predominantly low-attenuation mass in the anterior mediastinum, located dorsal to the thymus (T) and between the superior vena cava (open arrow) and the aortic arch (A). There was a thin septation within this cystic mass (solid arrow), and a higher-attenuation region was evident on the left.

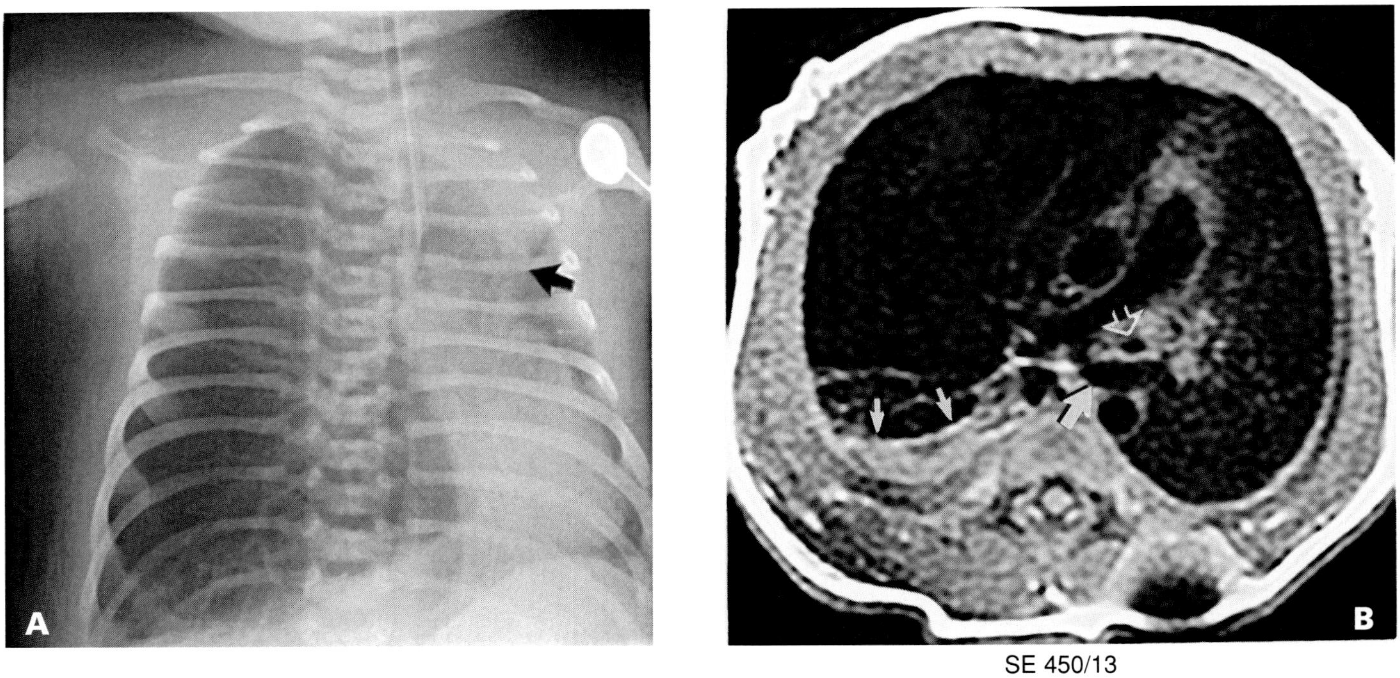

Figure 19-6. Same patient as in Figure 19-1. Asymmetric aeration attributable to air trapping in the right lung from pulmonary sling in an 11-day-old girl. (A) (Same as Figure 19-1) A pneumothorax was thought to be responsible for the respiratory distress and the large lucency on the right evident on the anteroposterior radiograph. Note tissue, likely thymic (arrow), at the anterior junction line separating the right and left lungs. A follow-up chest radiograph obtained after placement of a thoracostomy tube (not shown) showed no significant change. Because of the persistence of lucency, an MRI examination was obtained to evaluate for pulmonary sling. (B) An axial, cardiac-gated, T1-weighted MR image demonstrates that the origin of the slightly smaller left pulmonary artery (large solid arrow) is from the normally sized right pulmonary artery. The trachea (open arrow) is located between the right pulmonary and aberrant left pulmonary arteries. The larger size of the right lung is attributable to focal narrowing of the right main bronchus (not shown). Note the atelectasis of the right lower lobe (small solid arrows), which was a transient phenomenon. (Reprinted with permission from Frush [3].)

(A) might be considered in the test patient. However, the presence of vascular markings throughout the right lung and the absence of a well-defined interface between the pleural air collection and collapsed lung make this an unlikely explanation for the radiographic findings. Neonatal pneumothorax can be either spontaneous or associated with positive-pressure ventilation in the setting of reduced lung compliance. Pneumothoraces can be small and detected only by subtle signs, such as increased lucency of the hemithorax attributable to an anterior collection of air. An affected infant can be asymptomatic or

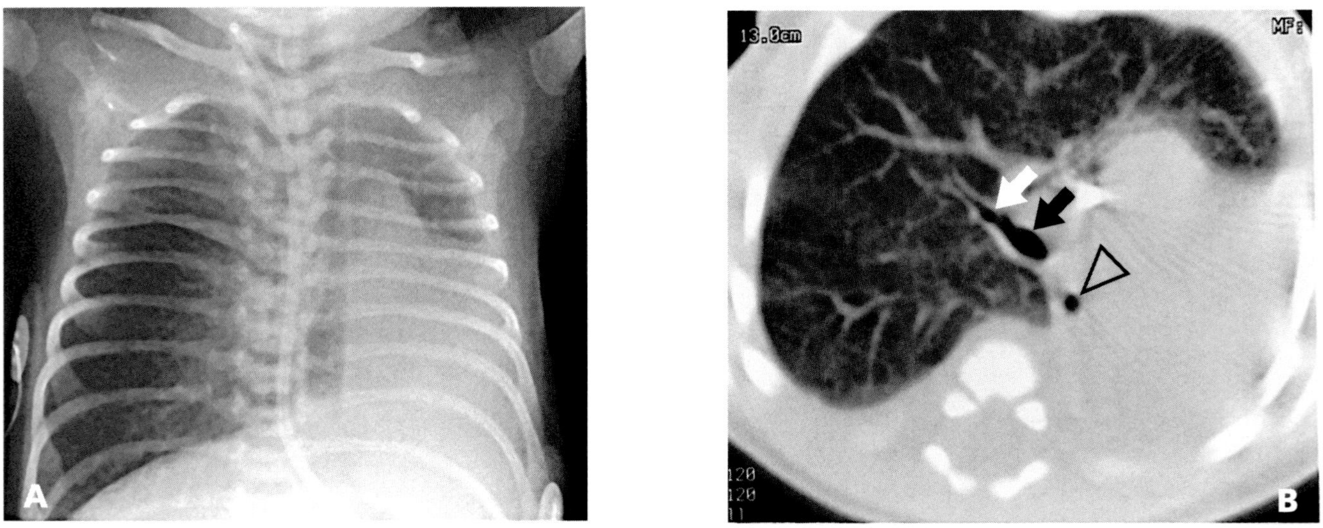

Figure 19-7. Newborn girl with severe respiratory stress attributable to left lung agenesis. (A) An anteroposterior chest radiograph shows marked asymmetry in the degree of aeration, with a hyperinflated right lung that extends well into the left hemithorax. (B) On CT evaluation (lung windows), the distal trachea (black arrow) and right bronchus (white arrow) are well demonstrated. There is no left bronchus. The air seen slightly more posterior (arrowhead) is in the esophagus. The heart and mediastinum constitute the soft tissue opacity in the left hemithorax. Note the extension of the right lung into the left hemithorax.

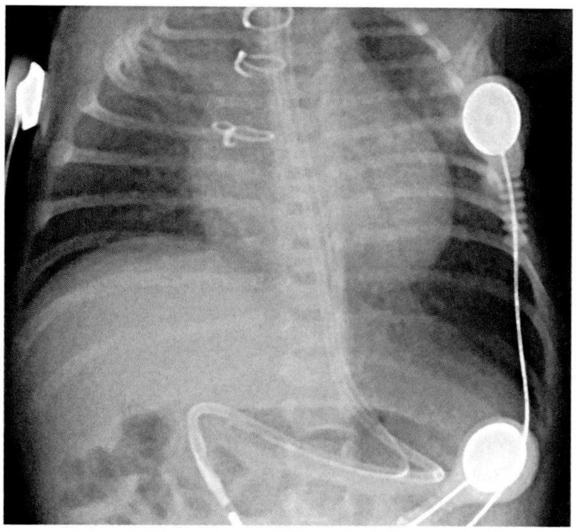

Figure 19-8. Diaphragmatic paralysis following repair of congenital heart disease in a 22-day-old girl. Paralysis of the right hemidiaphragm accounts for the large difference in the levels of the hemidiaphragms and the attendant asymmetric lung volumes on the radiograph.

can have mild respiratory distress. Alternatively, large pneumothoraces result in moderate or severe tachypnea, retractions, and hypoxemia. Large pneumothoraces can be detected clinically by auscultation, but usually are confirmed with radiography. When a large, tension pneumothorax is present, mediastinal and cardiac shift to the contralateral side and hyperlucency of the involved hemithorax are seen; an anterior junction line also may be evident.

Small spontaneous air collections will resorb by treatment with oxygen delivered via a hood for a period ranging from a few hours to a few days. Pneumothoraces attributable to positive-pressure ventilation are more problematic because they are under tension from the positive end-expiratory pressure and because the infant usually has underlying pulmonary or other organ failure compromising the respiratory status. Tube thoracostomies usually are necessary to treat these collections.

Question 91

Features associated with pulmonary hypoplasia include:

(A) systemic arterial supply
(B) accessory diaphragm
(C) pulmonary venous drainage to systemic vein
(D) oligohydramnios

The phrase "pulmonary hypoplasia" can refer to conditions in which the lung itself is unable to develop normally, such as with congenital diaphragmatic hernia, or to conditions in which thoracic development is restricted, such as with skeletal dysplasias or oligohydramnios (**Option (D) is true**). Pulmonary hypoplasia also can represent a developmental abnormality of the lung in which there are smaller airways and associated alveoli, as well as concomitant abnormalities in the pulmonary artery. Some authors consider hypoplasia a general term encompassing aplasia and agenesis. For the purposes of this discussion, the term "hypoplasia" will be used to refer to conditions in which the lung and pulmonary artery are present, but are small.

Pulmonary hypoplasia belongs to a broader group of entities referred to as congenital pulmonary venolobar syndrome. Components of this syndrome include lobar agenesis, aplasia, or hypoplasia (collectively referred to as hypogenetic lung); partial anomalous pulmonary venous return; absent pulmonary artery; pulmonary sequestration; systemic arterialization of the lung without airway sequestration; absence of the inferior vena cava; and duplication of the diaphragm (accessory diaphragm) (**Option (B) is true**).

One of the most widely recognized types of pulmonary hypoplasia is known as scimitar syndrome. Features of scimitar syndrome include lung and pulmonary artery hypoplasia, an anomalous draining pulmonary vein (radiographically, the widened course of this vessel distally resembles a scimitar), hyparterial bronchus, cardiac dextroposition, systemic drainage of the lower lobe pulmonary vein, systemic arterial supply to the lung (**Option (A) is true**), and accessory diaphragm or incomplete right hemidiaphragm (including eventration or Bochdalek's hernia).

The most constant findings in scimitar syndrome are the hypogenetic lung and partial anomalous venous return. The vein usually drains the entire lung, but drainage from a single lobe also is found. The anomalous vein most commonly drains into the inferior vena cava, near or at the junction with the right atrium, but drainage into the right atrium and subdiaphragmatic veins (portal veins, azygous veins, and hepatic veins) also has been reported (**Option (C) is true**).

The accessory diaphragm in scimitar syndrome is a membrane that fuses with the diaphragm anteriorly and the posterior chest wall. Because the subjacent lung (either middle or lower lobe) is "trapped," a band of opacity may be seen on lateral radiographs. When the subjacent lung is aerated, an oblique line (on lateral radiographs) that is indistinguishable from an accessory fissure is all that may be present.

Associated cardiac and spinal anomalies are common (25% to 50%). Atrial septal defect (secundum type) is the most common defect, seen in 25% of patients with scimitar syndrome and congenital heart defects. Other defects include tetralogy of Fallot, pulmonic stenosis, ventricular septal defect (VSD), and patent ductus arteriosus.

With scimitar syndrome, the anomalies are almost always on the right. The reason for this distribution is not known. The incidence is estimated to be 1 to 3 per 100,000 births. Most individuals are asymptomatic, and the anomaly is discovered incidentally.

When symptomatic, patients can be diagnosed in infancy.

In this setting, symptoms are attributable to associated cardiac defects that result in either congestive heart failure or cyanosis. In one series of 13 infants reported by Gao et al., 11 (85%) had severe symptoms, including congestive heart failure attributable to other cardiovascular abnormalities, respiratory symptoms (including wheezing or cough), and rhythm abnormalities. Symptoms related to the respiratory system also can be manifested in childhood. These include recurrent infections or shortness of breath. In adults, symptoms are most often attributable to recurrent pulmonary infections. Although the anomalous veinous drainage results in a left-to-right shunt, rarely is the ratio of pulmonary flow to systemic flow greater than 2:1. Patients are rarely symptomatic because of this small degree of shunting, and surgery is unnecessary.

The radiographic features of scimitar syndrome include a small and hyperlucent right hemithorax. The right hemidiaphragm may be elevated. The heart is dextroposed, and the right hilum is small. An anomalous draining vein may be evident in the right lower chest, paralleling the right heart border (Figure 19-9). On lateral radiographs, an increased band of soft tissue along the anterior thorax is attributable to the superimposition of the left and smaller right hemithoraces. If there have been recurrent pulmonary infections, bronchiectasis may be evident.

Either CT or MRI will demonstrate the findings evident on radiography. Features that are not evident radiographically can be demonstrated with these cross-sectional modalities. For example, the abnormal systemic arterial supply to the hypoplastic lung can be demonstrated by either contrast-enhanced CT or MRI. With CT, imaging during the arterial phase is best for identifying the systemic arterial supply. Because of the normally rapid pulmonary circulation, CT is sufficient for identifying the abnormal pulmonary venous return (Figure 19-9). CT is also helpful in depicting bronchiectasis and demonstrating an accessory diaphragm (Figure 19-10), a hypoplastic right bronchus, or associated lung anomalies.

With MRI, routine spin-echo sequences can demonstrate the position of the heart and the smaller right hemithorax. Either a cine evaluation or MR angiography can be used to obtain information on potential systemic arterial supply to the right lung as well as the anomalous drainage. These sequences take advantage of either intrinsic signal characteristic of flowing blood or intravenous contrast media to help distinguish the vessels from adjacent lung.

The differential diagnostic considerations for scimitar syndrome are limited. Given the dextroposition of the heart, other entities resulting in a smaller hemithorax are unlikely. Entities that should be considered include bronchiolitis obliterans (including Swyer-James syndrome) (Figure 19-11) and pulmonary hypoplasia without an anomalous draining vein (Figure 19-12). Identification of the anomalous venous drainage confirms the diagnosis of scimitar syndrome.

In patients who have scimitar syndrome and who are symptomatic because of the shunt, surgical correction is aimed at anastomosis of the anomalous vein into the left atrium. When present, congenital heart defects also are repaired. When bronchiectasis is present, lobectomy should be considered.

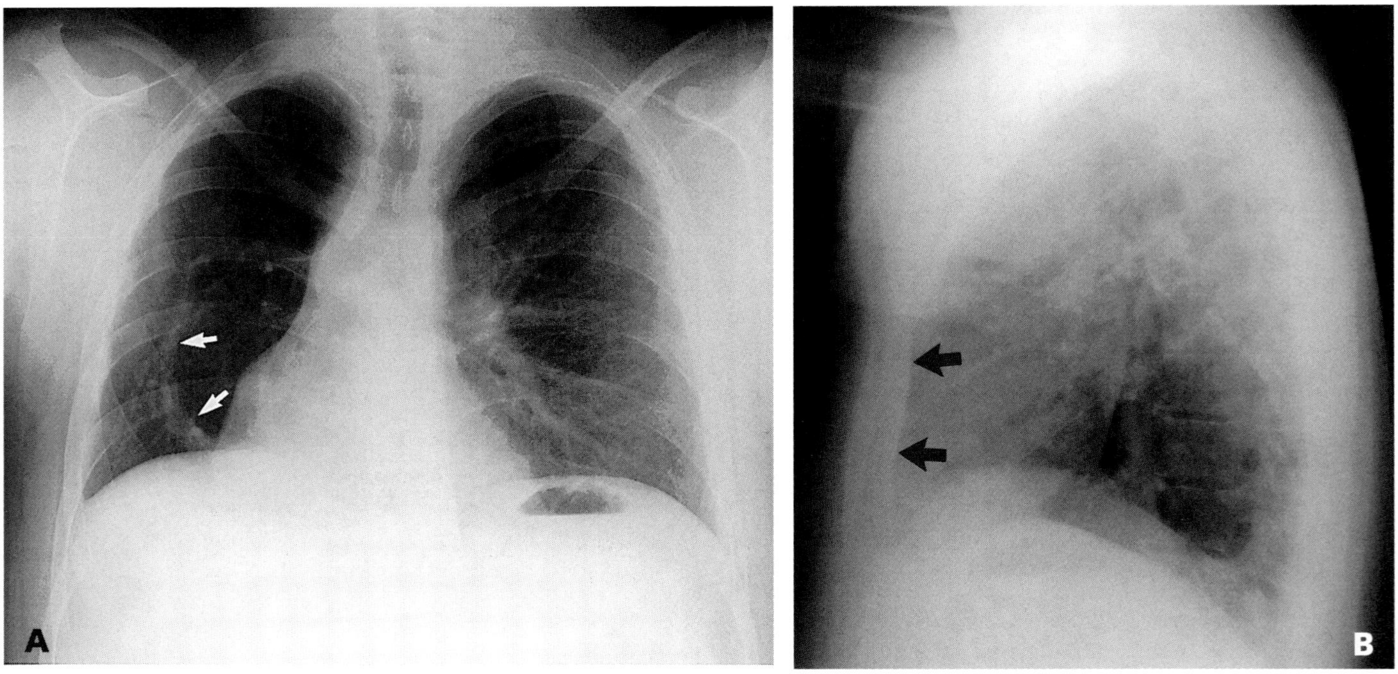

Figure 19-9. Scimitar syndrome in a 20-year-old man. (A) An anteroposterior chest radiograph shows pulmonary hypoplasia evident as a small right hemithorax as well as decreased pulmonary blood flow to the right lung. The anomalous pulmonary vein (arrows) is adjacent to the right heart border. (B) A bandlike opacity along the anterior hemithorax (arrows) on a lateral radiograph is attributable to superimposition of the smaller right hemithorax and the left hemithorax.

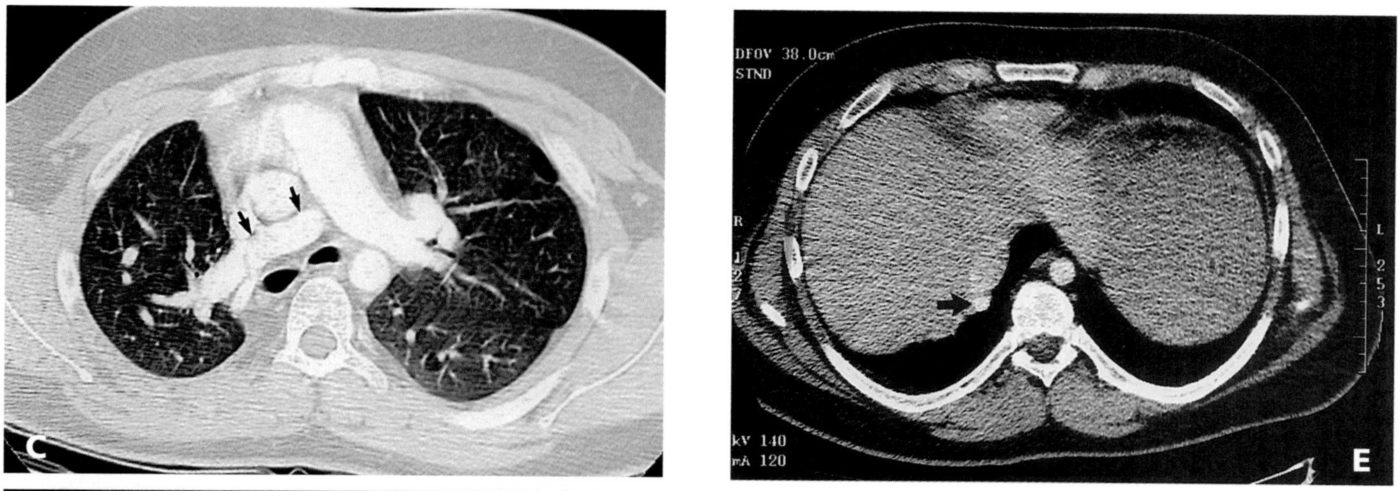

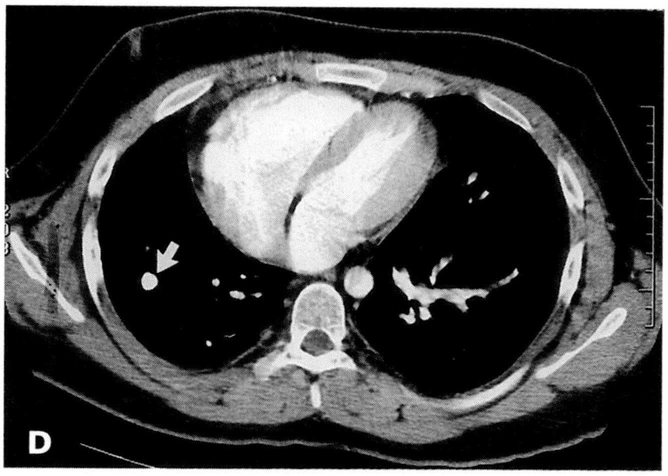

Figure 19-9 (Continued). Scimitar syndrome in a 20-year-old man. (C) An axial contrast-enhanced CT image (lung algorithm) just distal to the carina demonstrates the smaller right hemithorax. Note the smaller right pulmonary artery (arrows). In this example of scimitar syndrome, the right bronchus is not smaller than the left. (D) An axial contrast-enhanced CT image (soft tissue algorithm) at the level of the atrioventricular valves demonstrates the anomalous draining pulmonary vein (arrow) in the right lower lobe. Note the shift of the heart toward the right. (E) An axial contrast-enhanced CT image (soft tissue algorithm) at the level of the hemidiaphragms shows connection of this anomalous pulmonary vein (arrow) with the intrahepatic inferior vena cava.

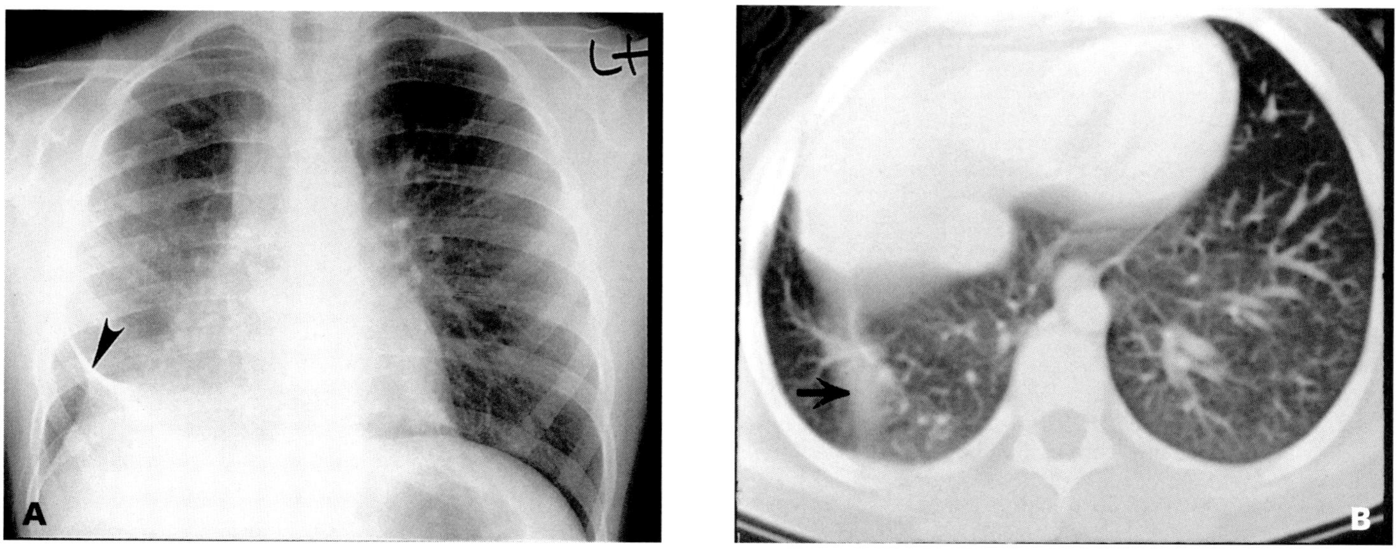

Figure 19-10. Hypogenetic lung syndrome (scimitar syndrome) with an accessory hemidiaphragm in a 7-month-old boy with recurrent pneumonia. (A) A frontal chest radiograph reveals a small right hemithorax and shift of the cardiac silhouette to the right. The pulmonary vasculature of the right lung is diminutive compared with that of the left lung. A large linear density (arrowhead) coursing caudally through the lung base represents an accessory right hemidiaphragm. (B) A CT scan through the right lower lobe also shows the accessory hemidiaphragm (arrow) and the mediastinal shift from left to right. The vessels in the right lung are smaller than those in the left and have a disorganized branching pattern. The anomalous vessel (not shown) entered the right atrium. (Case courtesy of Marilyn J. Siegel, M.D., Mallinckrodt Institute of Radiology, St. Louis, MO.)

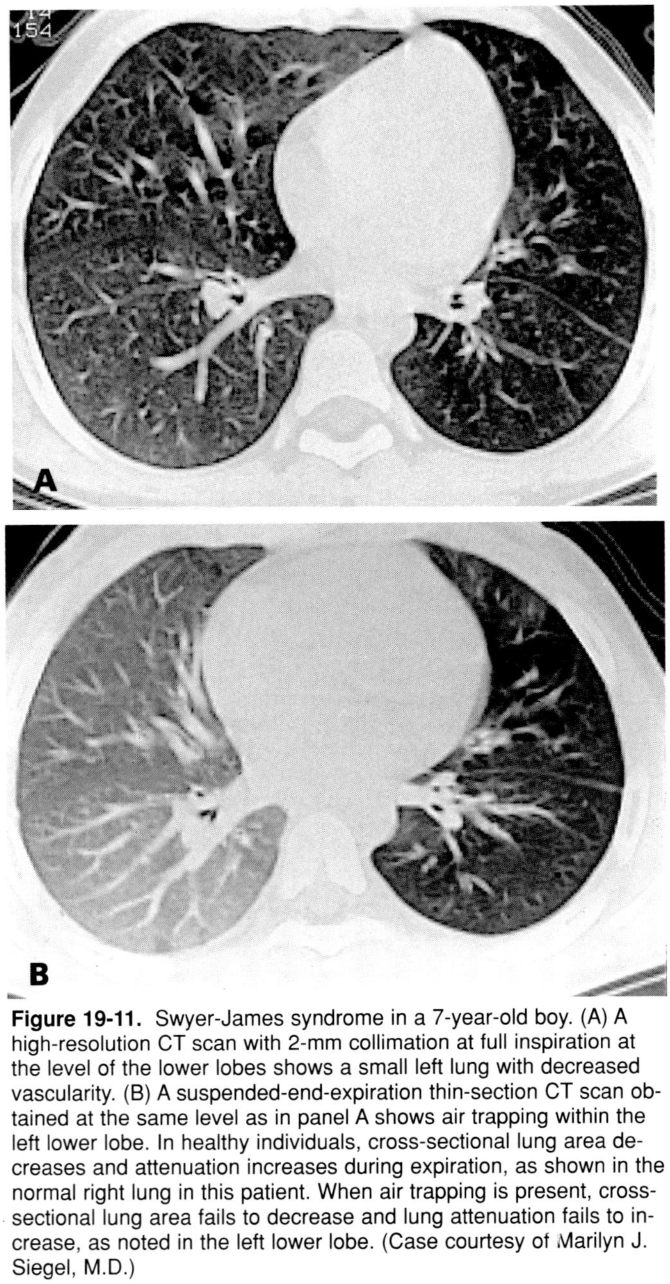

Figure 19-11. Swyer-James syndrome in a 7-year-old boy. (A) A high-resolution CT scan with 2-mm collimation at full inspiration at the level of the lower lobes shows a small left lung with decreased vascularity. (B) A suspended-end-expiration thin-section CT scan obtained at the same level as in panel A shows air trapping within the left lower lobe. In healthy individuals, cross-sectional lung area decreases and attenuation increases during expiration, as shown in the normal right lung in this patient. When air trapping is present, cross-sectional lung area fails to decrease and lung attenuation fails to increase, as noted in the left lower lobe. (Case courtesy of Marilyn J. Siegel, M.D.)

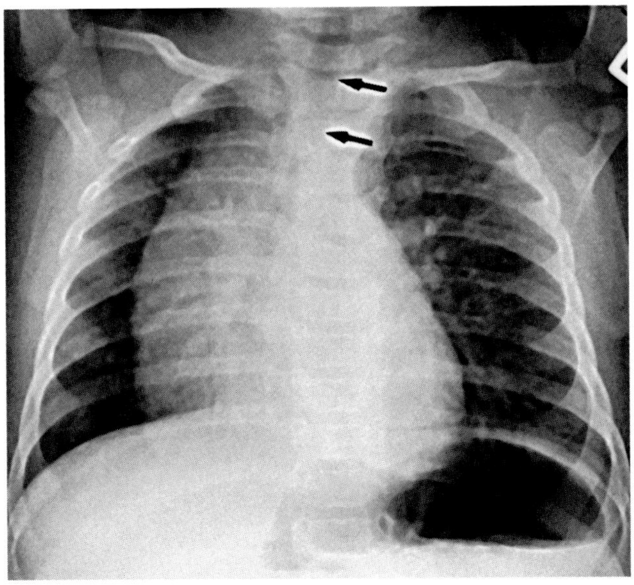

Figure 19-12. Hypoplastic right lung in a 16-month-old boy. A slight rightward shift of the trachea (arrows) and other portions of the mediastinum is evident on the posteroanterior chest radiograph. The diagnosis of hypoplastic right lung was established by CT (not shown).

Question 92

Concerning congenital diaphragmatic hernia,

(A) it occurs with equal frequency on both sides
(B) ultrasonography helps to distinguish a small one from an eventration
(C) associated malrotation is infrequent
(D) the contralateral lung is nearly always normal
(E) it is synonymous with Bochdalek's hernia

There are a number of abnormalities of the diaphragm. These include congenital abnormalities, such as Bochdalek's hernia (better known as congenital diaphragmatic hernia) (**Option (E) is true**) in the posterolateral region, Morgagni's hernia in the substernal space, herniation through the esophageal hiatus, and eventration. Of these, congenital diaphragmatic hernia is the most common.

Congenital diaphragmatic hernia occurs in 1 in 2,000 to 5,000 births. Congenital diaphragmatic hernia occurs on the left side in 80% to 90% of cases; the remaining 10% to 20% occur on the right side (bilateral occurrence is extremely rare) (**Option (A) is false**). There are two proposed mechanisms for this difference. The first is that the liver may serve a protective function, preventing herniation. Supporting this idea is the observation that delayed presentations of congenital diaphragmatic hernia are more common on the right. The second is based on evidence that the closure of diaphragmatic components occurs embryologically later on the left, exposing this side to a longer period during which abdominal contents may herniate into the chest.

The period during which the diaphragm normally completes the separation between chest and abdomen is from gestational weeks 5 to 10. Embryologically, congenital diaphragmatic hernia results from incomplete development of the components of the diaphragm. These components are the central tendon, the dorsolateral portions, the dorsal crura, and the pos terolateral muscles. The central tendon separates the thoracic from the abdominal contents and forms from the transverse septum. The dorsolateral portions are formed from the pleuroperitoneal membranes. Embryologically, these pleuroperitoneal membranes grow medially and inferiorly to fuse with both the central tendon and the dorsal crura. The posterolateral muscles are formed from the intercostal muscles.

The diaphragmatic defect in congenital diaphragmatic hernia arises when there is failure of closure of the pleuroperitoneal membranes. Because of their anatomic location posteriorly and laterally, this is the area where the hernia occurs. The actual defect is 2.0 to 4.0 cm in size, but can result in herniation of substantial amounts of abdominal viscera into the chest.

On the left, components of the gastrointestinal tract in addition to the left lobe of the liver, spleen, and kidney can herniate. On the right, the liver as well as the kidney and portions of the gastrointestinal tract can herniate. The herniated contents can be contained in a thin pleural or peritoneal membrane (10% to 20% of cases) or can be present without a sac.

Overall, 18% to 60% of infants with congenital diaphragmatic hernia have associated anomalies. These include anomalies of the cardiovascular, musculoskeletal, and gastrointestinal systems. With associated anomalies, survival decreases and can be as low as 6%. Among gastrointestinal abnormalities, virtually all neonates with congenital diaphragmatic hernia have malrotation (**Option (C) is false**). Although the gut herniates normally into the yolk sac, its return to the abdomen at about 10 weeks coincides with the presence of the diaphragmatic defect. At this point, viscera may ascend unimpeded into the chest. Further rotation and fixation are halted.

The abnormality can be detected during fetal ultrasonography as a mass in the chest with cardiac and mediastinal shift to the contralateral chest. With postnatal presentations, symptoms are invariably related to the degree of associated pulmonary hypoplasia.

Although the defect in congenital diaphragmatic hernia is attributable to a diaphragmatic anomaly and the predominant radiographic manifestations are attributable to herniation of the viscera, by far the greatest physiologic consequence is attributable to the effects on the lungs. Because the embryologic development of the lungs occurs at the same period of time (gestational weeks 14 to 16) during which the abdominal viscera are occupying the thorax, there is a decrease in bronchial branching. This decrease in branching results in pulmonary hypoplasia. There is concomitant vascular hypoplasia. Moreover, because of herniation of the mediastinum and heart to the contralateral side, there is hypoplasia of the contralateral lung (**Option (D) is false**) in about 30% of cases, although to a lesser degree than the ipsilateral lung.

The majority of patients with congenital diaphragmatic hernia (up to 94%) appear within the first 6 hours of life with severe respiratory distress, hypoxemia, and hypercapnia requiring ventilatory support. Because pulmonary arterial hypertension can coexist with failure of closure of the ductus arteriosus (from profound hypoxia), persistent fetal circulation can result. With persistent fetal circulation, systemic venous blood is shunted across the foramen ovale and from right to left across the patent ductus arteriosus, compounding the hypoxemia attributable to pulmonary hypoplasia. Additional physical examination findings include a scaphoid abdomen, asymmetric sizes of the hemithoraces, and asymmetric breath and cardiac sounds. A minority of children manifest symptoms of congenital dia-phragmatic hernia later (after 24 hours). Respiratory symptoms are milder in degree.

In addition to the pulmonary abnormalities attributable to congenital diaphragmatic hernia, gastrointestinal manifestations can occur. Although less frequent than pulmonary features, gastrointestinal findings include anatomic compression of the gastroesophageal junction because of distortion of the normal gastric position. Esophageal dilatation and abnormal peristalsis also can be present.

The diagnosis of congenital diaphragmatic hernia usually is confirmed radiographically. Within the first few hours of life, before the bowel becomes aerated, the herniated contents can mimic a solid mass. After aeration of the bowel, a more typical air-filled cystic appearance will be evident (Figures 19-13 and 19-14). The gastric tube tip extends into the hemithorax when the stomach is in the chest. With large hernias, there is a shift of the heart and mediastinum into the contralateral chest. In cases of severe pulmonary hypoplasia, pulmonary compliance is low and positive-pressure ventilation can cause a pneumothorax. The pneumothorax is usually on the contralateral side, as the lung is more compliant and, therefore, more susceptible to barotrauma.

Emergent management of congenital diaphragmatic hernia includes intubation and gastric tube placement and suction. This technique decompresses the space-occupying viscus, improving pulmonary compliance. Pharmacologic paralysis also can improve compliance by reducing bowel gas and relaxing thoracic musculature; however, increased chest wall edema can decrease compliance, diminishing or negating these effects. The selective pulmonary vasodilator nitric oxide also has been used, although this is not standard therapy.

Whereas previously congenital diaphragmatic hernia was

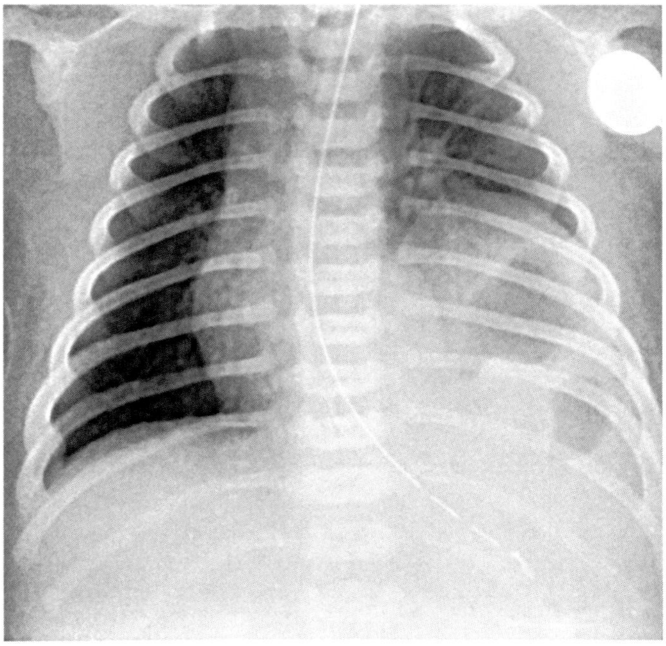

Figure 19-13. Left-sided congenital diaphragmatic hernia in a newborn girl. An anteroposterior chest radiograph demonstrates in the left lower lung a mixed lucent and soft tissue mass that displaces the heart, mediastinum, and orogastric and endotracheal tubes to the right. Small and large intestines are herniated into the thorax.

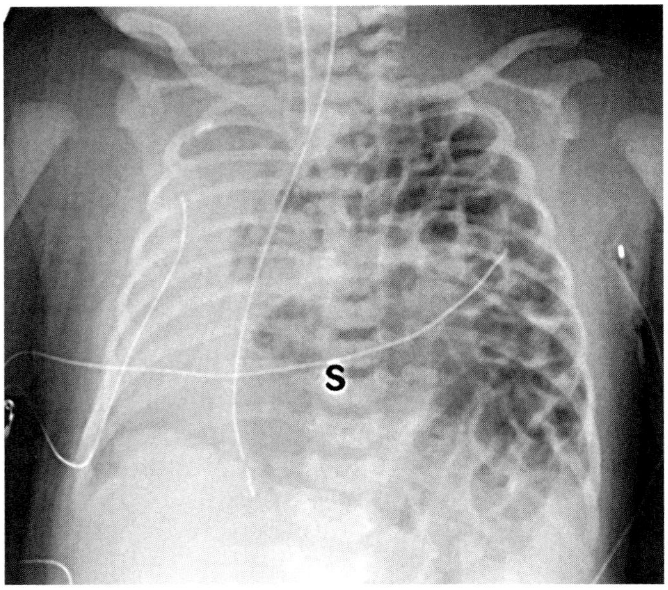

Figure 19-14. Congenital diaphragmatic hernia in a 1-day-old boy. An anteroposterior chest radiograph shows extensive multicystic lucencies in the left lung and marked shift of the heart and mediastinum toward the right, which is nearly completely opacified because of atelectasis. The large lucency in the lower midchest is the stomach (S).

considered an emergent surgical condition ("early" repair), the current trend is toward stabilization of the pulmonary status, if possible. During the first week or so after birth, there can be a decrease in the amount and lability of pulmonary hypertension and improvement in pulmonary compliance. This "delayed" surgical strategy has resulted in improved operative success. Survival rates in cases of early repair vary from 12% to 43%, whereas investigations reporting on delayed closure note survival rates ranging from 48% to 78%. Infants who are poor surgical candidates include those with other severe associated anomalies or those who remain consistently hypoxemic or hypercapnic because of persistent fetal circulation or pulmonary hypoplasia. The role of extracorporeal membrane oxygenation is controversial. There are reports of improved survival rates (up to about 65%), but there is still disagreement about the indications for the use of extracorporal oxygenation in congenital diaphragmatic hernia. Finally, congenital diaphragmatic hernia is one of the conditions for which fetal surgery has shown promise. Prognosis is dependent on factors such as the severity of associated abnormalities, hypoxemia, hypercapnia, and acidosis.

Surgical correction of congenital diaphragmatic hernia consists of primary closure of the defect. If the defect is large and there is insufficient tissue posteriorly, prosthetic material can be used. Late sequelae in children who have had repair of congenital diaphragmatic hernia include occasional mild restrictive lung disease, gastroesophageal reflux (up to 30% at 1 year of age), and gastrointestinal motility abnormalities.

The radiologic differential diagnosis of congenital diaphragmatic hernia includes other congenital anomalies of the diaphragm, including eventration and Morgagni's hernia. In addition, CAM can have a similar radiologic appearance.

Morgagni's hernia is rarer than congenital diaphragmatic hernia and accounts for only about 2% of all congenital hernias. Morgagni's hernia is attributable to anterior agenesis of the diaphragm, at the hiatus for the internal mammary artery, at about the level of the eighth rib. The hernia is more common on the right than on the left. Bilateral involvement (up to 30%) is more common than with congenital diaphragmatic hernia, as the embryologic basis of Morgagni's hernia is related to the failure of fusion of the transverse septum and the anterior thoracic wall centrally. The majority of Morgagni's hernias are asymptomatic. When symptoms are present, they are usually gastrointestinal in nature. The anterior location helps to distinguish congenital diaphragmatic hernia radiographically from the more anterior Morgagni's hernia when the latter is detected in a neonate. The role of CT and MRI in evaluation of the diaphragm itself is limited. However, multiplanar depictions can demonstrate that the nature of a basilar opacity is related to abdominal structures associated with either hernia or eventration.

Eventration represents muscular thinning of the diaphragm, but the diaphragm is continuous. Muscle fibers are thin but intact, and grossly, there is a membranous appearance. Some consider that true eventration is only congenital, whereas others also include acquired muscular atrophy attributable to conditions such as phrenic nerve injury or anomalies of the spinal cord. Eventration is seen in approximately 1 in 1,400 individuals and is up to nine times more common on the left. Small eventrations are asymptomatic, but larger abnormalities can result in respiratory symptoms, including dyspnea and recurrent pulmonary infections. Eventration (Figure 19-15) can be radiographically indistinguishable from a small congenital diaphragmatic hernia (the latter is rare). However, ultrasonography can help to distinguish the two conditions. The demon-

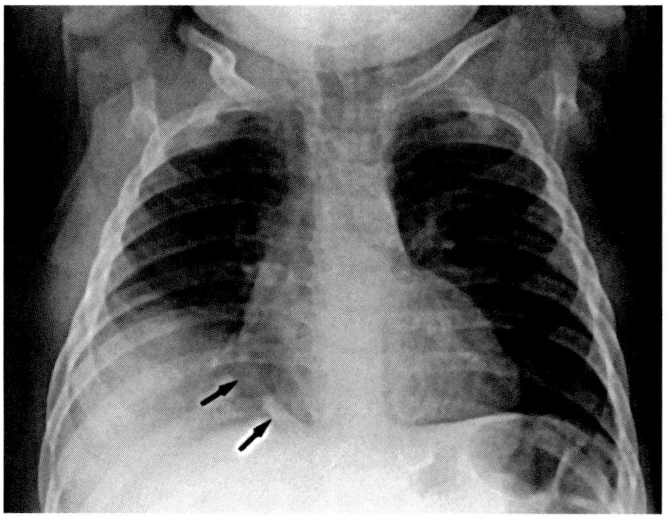

Figure 19-15. Right hemidiaphragmatic eventration in a 2-month-old boy with mild tachypnea. A radiograph shows that a soft tissue opacity in the right lower lung is not associated with mass effect. There is atelectasis (arrows) in the right lower lobe. A CT examination (not shown) was performed for unrelated reasons and demonstrated that the liver constituted the soft tissue opacity. Although these findings could represent hernia of the diaphragm, eventration was confirmed at surgery.

stration of clearly defined echoes in the area of the diaphragmatic bulge favors the diagnosis of eventration (**Option (B) is true**). Dynamic evaluation of the diaphragm with either ultrasonography or fluoroscopy yields similar findings. There is a paradoxic response of the subjacent viscera during the respiratory cycle; the viscera do not distend on inspiration.

CAM can have a radiographic appearance similar to that of congenital diaphragmatic hernia. CAM initially can appear solid, but can become progressively cystic in appearance as fluid is reabsorbed from hamartomatous cysts. If a cystic mass is not continuous with the diaphragm or is located on the right side and is associated with a normally positioned stomach and bowel, CAM should be considered.

Question 93

Congenital cardiovascular anomalies commonly associated with asymmetric pulmonary aeration include:

(A) atrioventricular septal defect
(B) Ebstein's anomaly
(C) aberrant right subclavian artery
(D) pulmonary sling
(E) tetralogy of Fallot with absence of the pulmonic valve

Aeration disturbances in the lungs can be secondary to cardiovascular causes. Three mechanisms are responsible for these aeration abnormalities: (1) bronchiolar compression from either edema or enlarged adjacent arterioles; (2) extrinsic compression of the airway by an anomalous vessel, an abnormal course or enlargement of vessels (i.e., pulmonary arteries), or an enlarged cardiac chamber (i.e., left atrium); or (3) structural airway abnormalities (e.g., complete cartilaginous rings, tracheomalacia, or bronchial stenosis). Airway abnormalities can be either secondary to impingement from adjacent cardiovascular structures or attributable to a primary airway deficiency associated with cardiovascular abnormalities. Diagnostic imaging plays a critical role in determining the presence, nature, and extent of cardiovascular and, when present, airway anomalies resulting in aeration disturbances in infants and children.

In structural heart disease with increased pulmonary blood flow, enlargement of pulmonary arterioles can result in narrowing of adjacent bronchioles and air trapping attributable to compression from the vessels themselves. Pulmonary venous hypertension attributable to increased left atrial pressure can cause bronchial edema and also can result in narrowing with air trapping. The most common situation in which these problems occur is with left-to-right shunts that result in increased pulmonary arterial flow and pressure, such as an atrioventricular septal defect (AVSD) or a VSD (Figure 19-16). The resultant disturbance in aeration is symmetric (**Option (A) is false**). Clinically, the manifestations of air trapping can be relatively silent, but there may be respiratory symptoms, such as cough, tachypnea, and wheezing.

The radiologic evaluation will demonstrate both air trapping and the cardiovascular abnormalities. With respect to the

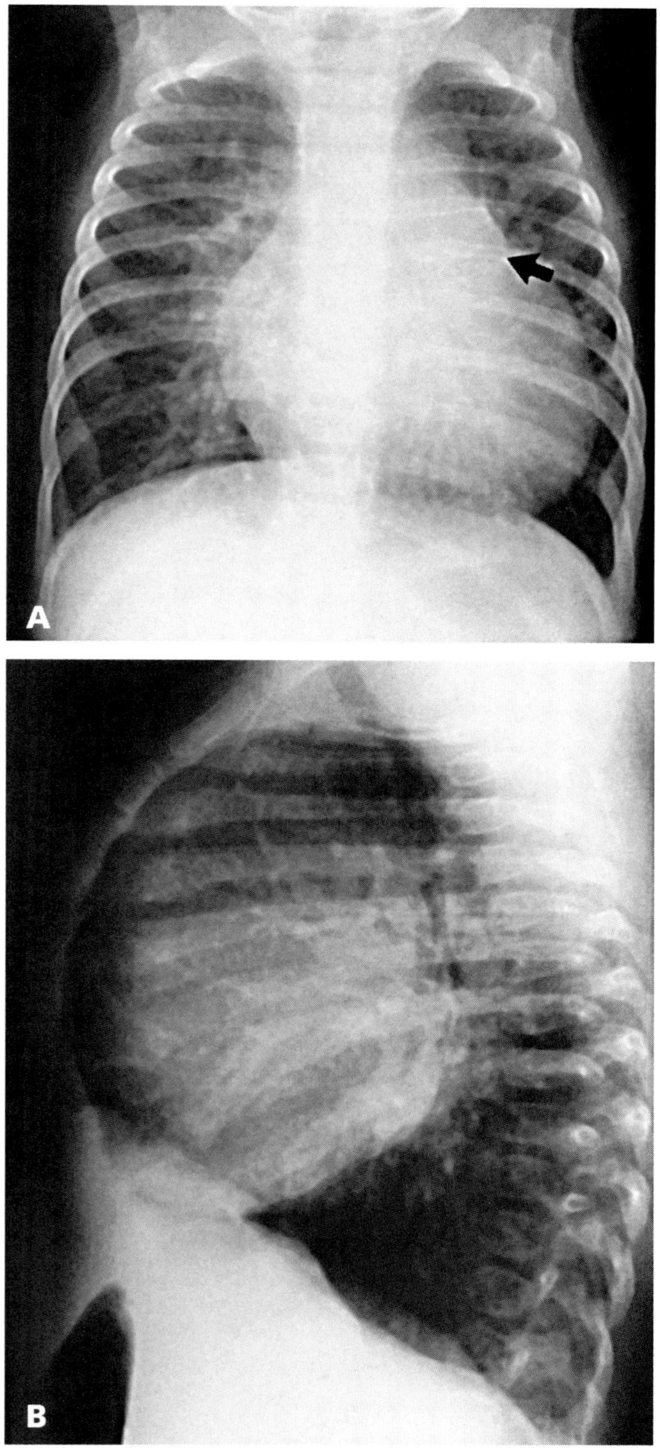

Figure 19-16. Air trapping associated with a left-to-right shunt from a ventricular septal defect in a 2-month-old girl. (A) A posteroanterior chest radiograph shows cardiomegaly and increased pulmonary vascularity. Note the prominent main pulmonary artery (arrow). (B) The hyperinflation is most evident on a lateral radiograph, with increased anteroposterior diameter and flattening of the hemidiaphragm.

cardiovascular findings, cardiomegaly is usually present with biventricular enlargement in the case of either an AVSD or a VSD. The right atrium is normal; the left may be enlarged in the setting of a VSD. Although MRI can depict the nature of the intracardiac defects, echocardiography is usually sufficient in determining the type and severity of these and other intracardiac lesions. Angiography usually is not required for the diagnosis and preoperative evaluation of these lesions, unless echocardiography is insufficient. With surgical correction of these left-to-right shunts, the symptoms and radiographic findings will resolve.

Aeration disturbances also can be attributable to cardiac chamber enlargement. Because of the intimate relationship of the left atrium and carina (Figure 19-17), the left main bronchus can be compressed between the enlarged left atrium inferiorly and the left pulmonary artery superiorly. This situation can result in either atelectasis or postobstructive air trapping. Because the right atrium and the right ventricle are located anteriorly, enlargement of these chambers usually does not result in airway compression, except when the heart is displaced posteriorly (e.g., Ebstein's anomaly), in which case airway compression is a secondary phenomenon.

In Ebstein's anomaly, there is abnormal formation of the tricuspid valve, with resultant abnormal inferior displacement of the tricuspid leaflets and "atrialization" of a large portion of the right ventricle. There is often obstruction of pulmonary blood flow. Radiologically, cardiomegaly is often marked, with decreased pulmonary blood flow seen bilaterally. Two other scenarios in which this degree of cardiomegaly can be present in infants are pulmonary atresia with an intact ventricular septum and tricuspid atresia. In each of these predominantly right heart lesions with obstruction of pulmonary blood flow, the right side of the heart is markedly dilated.

In Ebstein's anomaly, displacement of the heart because of right heart enlargement can cause left main bronchial compression and associated asymmetry of pulmonary aeration (**Option (B) is true**) (Figure 19-18). In infancy and childhood, Ebstein's anomaly usually is well seen by echocardiography. However, this modality will miss airway compression, which is well seen by conventional radiography.

Aeration disturbances also can be attributable to aberrant vessels. With an aberrant left pulmonary artery (also known as pulmonary artery sling), the left pulmonary artery arises from the posterior aspect of the right pulmonary artery, encircles the right main bronchus, and travels posterior to the trachea (and anterior to the esophagus) (Figure 19-19A) before reaching the left hilum. In particular, pulmonary artery sling can cause either air trapping (more commonly) or atelectasis because of the relationship with the adjacent airway.

With an aberrant left pulmonary artery, symptoms are usually evident within the first few months of life, and the vast majority of children are diagnosed before 1 year of age. Symptoms are related to the airway compression and include respiratory distress (which can be severe), consisting of tachypnea, retractions, and cyanosis. The etiology is likely attributable to failure of the development of the left pulmonary artery from the left sixth aortic arch.

The pulmonary sling is divided into two types. Type 1 has normal airway branching and a left pulmonary artery that encircles the trachea and the right main bronchus. In type 2 lesions, the course of the aberrant artery is lower, with more extensive tracheal abnormalities (i.e., stenosis) as well as abnormal branching of the right-sided airways. This type is associated with other airway anomalies, such as complete tracheal rings, tracheomalacia, and tracheal stenosis. The combination of tracheal rings and aberrant left pulmonary artery has been termed the "ring-sling" complex.

The radiographic features are most commonly attributable to hyperinflation of the right lung (seen in at least 33% of cases) (**Option (D) is true**). Other findings include atelectasis in the right lung, bilateral hyperinflation or left lung hyperinflation (the left bronchus can be affected as well), tracheal nar-

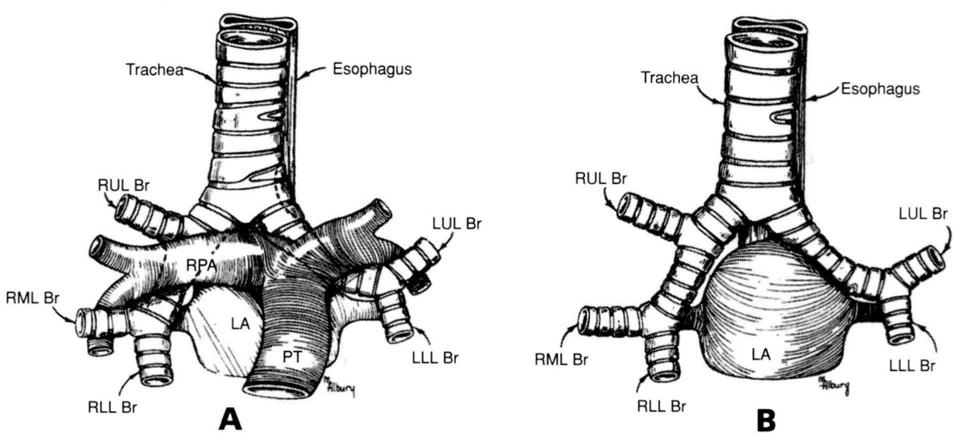

Figure 19-17. Schematic diagrams of the anatomic relationships among airways, pulmonary arteries, and left atrium, as viewed anteriorly with (A) and without (B) the pulmonary arteries. RUL = right upper lobe; RML = right middle lobe; RLL = right lower lobe; LUL = left upper lobe; LLL = left lower lobe; RPA = right pulmonary artery; PT = pulmonary outflow tract; LA = left atrium; Br = bronchus. (Reprinted with permission from Berlinger et al. [27].)

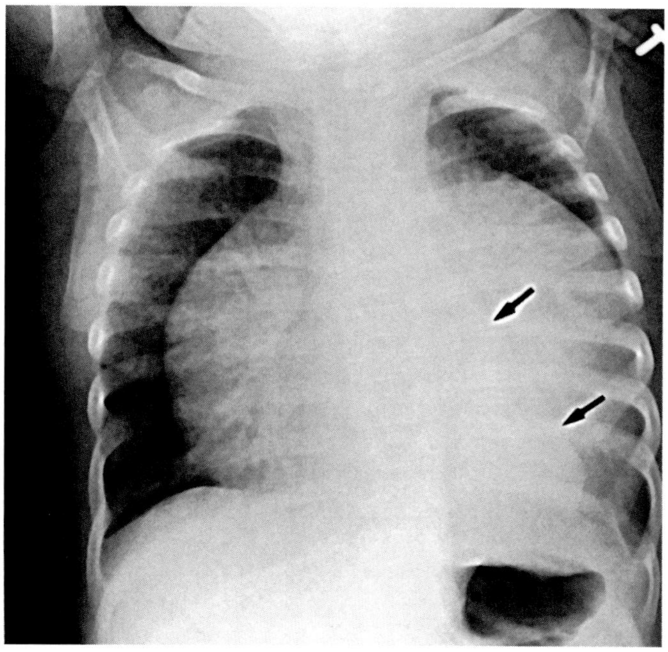

Figure 19-18. Massive cardiomegaly attributable to Ebstein's anomaly in a 1-year-old girl. A posteroanterior radiograph shows marked cardiomegaly. Note the collapse of the left lower lobe (arrows) attributable to compression of the left main bronchus.

rowing, or secondary features, such as pneumonia. The aberrant vessel is not seen radiographically.

A contrast esophagram may depict the anterior impression by the aberrant pulmonary artery, but this characteristic is present in only about one third of cases. If there is a strong suspicion of pulmonary sling, preoperative evaluation is best performed by MRI.

Although echocardiography can demonstrate the presence of an aberrant vessel, MRI best depicts the relationship of the vascular anomaly to the adjacent airway. In particular, the length of airway involvement, which is critical in operative planning, can be assessed. MRI is also excellent at demonstrating the course of the left pulmonary artery itself (Figure 19-6B). The left pulmonary artery is usually normal in size. Cine evaluation also has been used to illustrate the relative asymmetry in perfusion that can result from asymmetry in pulmonary artery size.

CT also has been advocated as a modality for evaluating pulmonary sling (Figure 19-20). With the advent of helical technology, there may be increasing use of this modality. In particular, CT angiography with three-dimensional reconstructions and virtual bronchoscopy may prove to be useful in the evaluation of infants with an aberrant left pulmonary artery.

Surgical correction is performed by a midline sternotomy with anastomosis of the left pulmonary artery to the left side of the main pulmonary artery (Figure 19-19B). Complications (postoperative stenosis) are rare.

Several other vascular abnormalities can affect the airway. These include the "rings" of a right-sided aortic arch with an aberrant left subclavian artery; a right-sided aortic arch with mirror-image branching; a left-sided aortic arch with an aberrant right subclavian artery (and right ductus ligament); circumflex and double aortic arch (Figure 19-21); and innominate artery compression of the trachea. In these situations, symptoms may not be present. When present, symptoms are usually respiratory in nature, consisting of cough or wheezing. However, because the trachea is involved, there is no aeration asymmetry (**Option (C) is false**).

Nevertheless, the chest radiograph is very useful in the evaluation of suspected rings. In one investigation, Pickhardt et al. evaluated 41 children with symptomatic vascular rings. On frontal radiographs, findings included right aortic arch (85%), distal tracheal indentation (73%), and right descending aorta (66%). All of these were present in 48% of patients. On lateral examinations, increased retrotracheal opacity was noted in 79% of children, anterior tracheal bowing was noted in 92%, and tracheal narrowing was noted in 77%. All of these findings

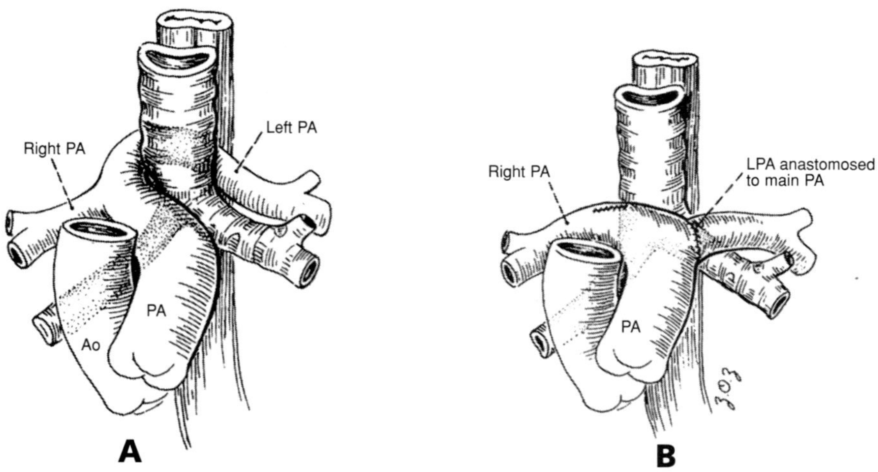

Figure 19-19. Schematic diagrams depicting pulmonary sling. (A) Origin of the left pulmonary artery (PA) from the right pulmonary artery, constituting pulmonary sling. (B) The airway compromise is corrected by anastomosing the left pulmonary artery (LPA) to the left side of the main pulmonary artery. Ao = aorta. (Reprinted with permission from Backer and Idriss [26].)

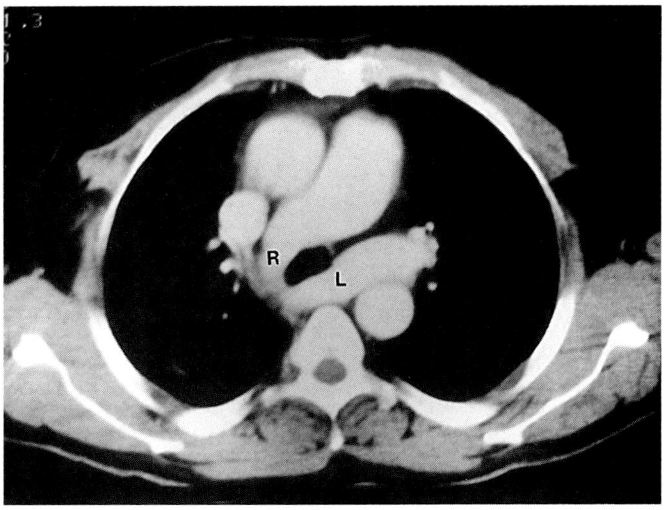

Figure 19-20. Pulmonary artery sling. A contrast-enhanced CT image demonstrates the left pulmonary artery (L) arising posteriorly from the right pulmonary artery (R), before crossing behind the trachea to reach the left lung. (Case courtesy of Marilyn J. Siegel, M.D.)

were present in 62% of lateral examinations. Altogether, there was at least one abnormality on either the frontal or the lateral chest radiograph for all patients. The authors concluded that in symptomatic children, a normal chest radiograph virtually excludes a vascular ring. However, these abnormalities are not related to aeration disturbances.

The benefits of barium esophagography versus MRI have been debated. Although contrast examination can depict vascular rings, contemporary practice usually calls for a more complete demonstration of the vascular anatomy for operative

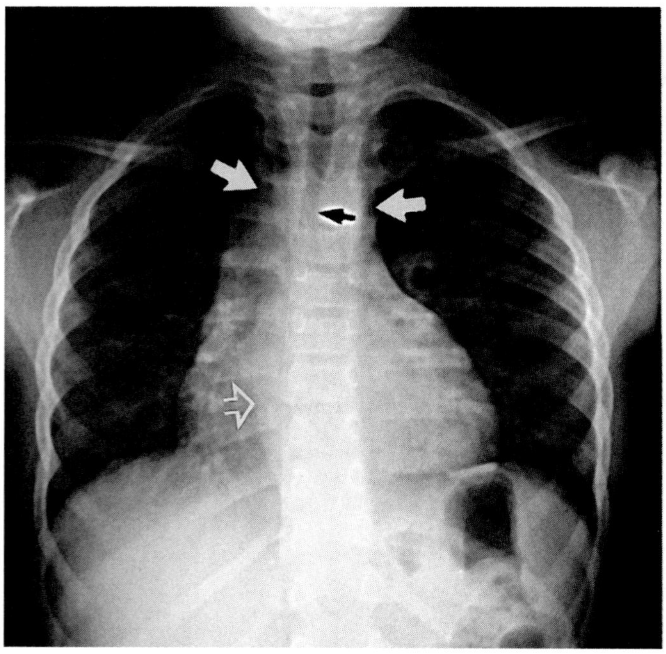

Figure 19-21. Double aortic arch in a 6-year-old boy with a history of wheezing. A posteroanterior chest radiograph demonstrates the left- and right-sided aortic arches (solid white arrows), which result in mild narrowing of the distal trachea (black arrow). The descending thoracic aorta is evident to the right of the spine (open arrow).

planning. If there is a high suspicion of a ring on the basis of radiography, an appropriate next step would be MRI. With MRI, the nature of the vascular abnormality and the severity of the airway compromise are well depicted. Echocardiography can demonstrate some vascular abnormalities but, as with pulmonary sling, the presence and extent of airway involvement are not appreciated. Although helical CT can depict vessels and airways and has advantages in terms of cost, examination time, and availability, its role in depicting vascular rings has not been established as has the role of MRI.

Surgical considerations depend on the lesion type. In general, procedures are aimed at releasing the compression of the airway (e.g., division of a ligamentum arteriosum or division of the smaller of the two aortic branches in double aortic arch). Between 70% and 92% of patients will have complete remission of symptoms, whereas up to 30% may have persistent upper- and lower-airway symptoms.

Extrinsic compression of airways occurs with enlargement of adjacent vessels, particularly the pulmonary arteries. This scenario is exemplified in the entity of tetralogy of Fallot with an absent pulmonic valve. Agenesis of the pulmonic valve can be an isolated finding. However, in about 10% of cases, there is an association with tetralogy of Fallot. All lesions that involve agenesis of the pulmonic valve can be referred to as absent pulmonic valve syndrome.

In classic tetralogy of Fallot, the constellation of findings is related to aberrant conotruncal development, which results in a VSD, overriding of the ventricular septum by the aorta, pulmonary outflow (infundibular and valvar) stenosis, and right ventricular hypertrophy. With agenesis of the pulmonic valve, seen in 2% to 6% of all cases of tetralogy, the valve is either absent or rudimentary, with malformed cusps. There is still infundibular stenosis. The etiology of the absent pulmonic valve syndrome in association with tetralogy is not clear. It may result either from dysplasia at the base of the pulmonary arteries or from the hemodynamic consequences of the VSD and pulmonic regurgitation. Frequently, there is an absent ductus arteriosus, and the lack of decompression also may be a factor. With absent pulmonic valve and tetralogy, the pulmonary trunk and proximal right and left pulmonary arteries dilate markedly and result in tracheobronchial compression. This compression can be severe and can be associated with significant tracheobronchial malacia, typically with bilateral air trapping (**Option (E) is false**).

There are two recognized patterns of presentation. The first is in the neonatal period, with marked respiratory symptoms. In this setting, morbidity and mortality are higher than at later times because of marked airway compromise. The second presentation is in older children, and the airway is not as severely affected. The VSD may result in left-to-right shunting if the infundibular stenosis is not severe. In this case, pulmonary edema can be the etiology of symptoms. If the stenosis is severe, then right-to-left shunting may predominate.

With chest radiography, the features of tetralogy of Fallot may be seen (normal to slightly enlarged heart, right ventricular hypertrophy, and right-sided aortic arch). However, the marked dilatation of the main and proximal right and left pulmonary arteries (Figures 19-22 and 19-23) separates tetralogy with absent pulmonic valve from classic tetralogy. This pulmonary artery enlargement results in posterior displacement and narrowing of the trachea, as appreciated in the lateral radiograph (Figure 19-22B).

Echocardiography can demonstrate the constellation of lesions, including pulmonic regurgitation from the pulmonic valve anomaly. The degree of airway involvement is better depicted by either CT or MRI. With these modalities, both the degree and the extent of airway anomalies are well displayed.

Surgical options depend on the severity of airway symptoms. Considerations include repair of the tetralogy of Fallot complex, including valve conduit placement, and aneurysmorrhaphy of the pulmonary arteries. The utility of the latter procedure is debatable, because there have been varied results. If airway symptoms are not substantial, then reduction of aneurysms generally is not performed.

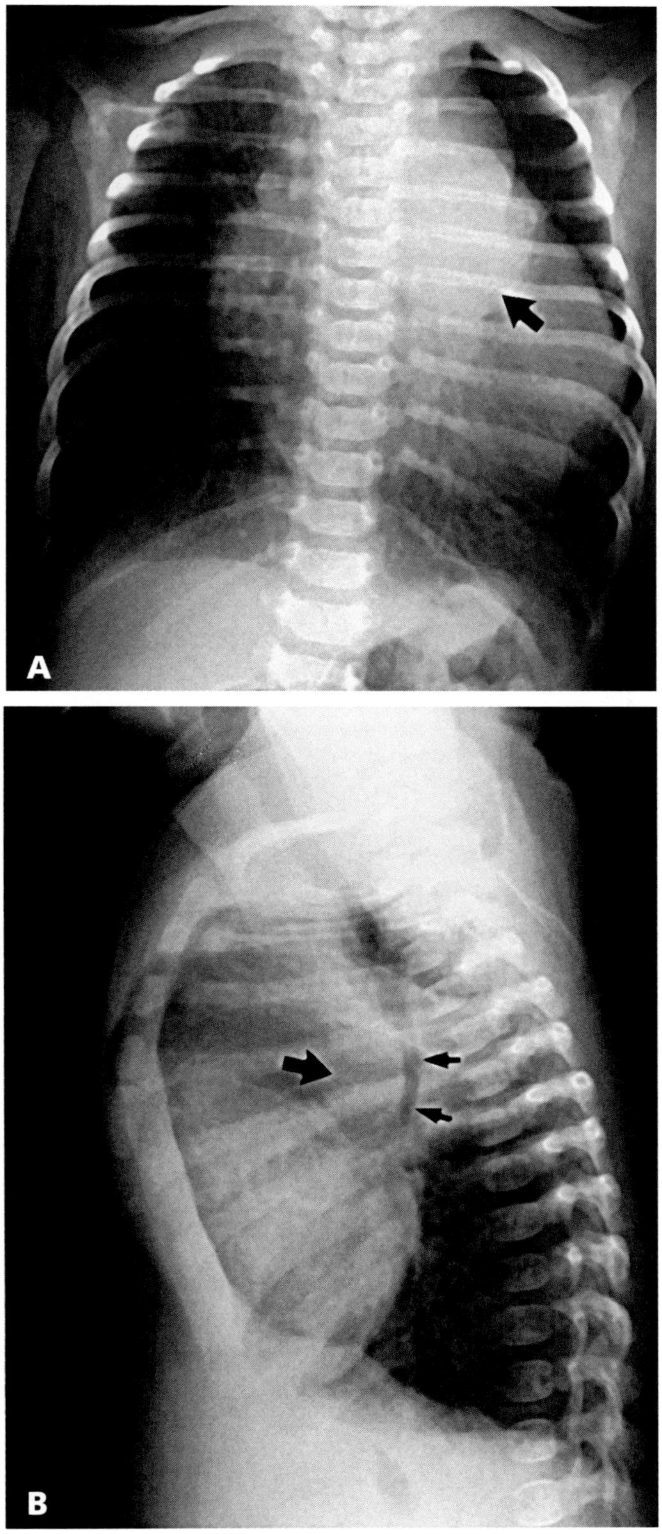

Figure 19-22. Tetralogy of Fallot with absent pulmonic valve in a 2-month-old boy. (A) A posteroanterior chest radiograph demonstrates cardiomegaly. The cardiac apex is uplifted, representing right ventricular hypertrophy. Note the prominent main pulmonary artery segment (arrow). There is hyperinflation attributable to compression of the carina and associated tracheomalacia with resultant bilateral air trapping. (B) A lateral radiograph more clearly demonstrates the relationship of the enlarged pulmonary artery (large arrow) with the distal trachea and bronchi, with narrowing and posterior displacement (small arrows).

SUGGESTED READINGS

PULMONARY SLING

1. Anand R, Dooley KJ, Williams WH, Vincent RN. Follow-up of surgical correction of vascular anomalies causing tracheobronchial compression. Pediatr Cardiol 1994; 15:58–61
2. Backer CL, Idriss FS, Holinger LD, Mavroudis C. Pulmonary artery sling. Results of surgical repair in infancy. J Thorac Cardiovasc Surg 1992; 103:683–691
3. Frush DP. Pediatric radiology. In: Provenzale JM, Nelson RC (eds). Duke radiology case review. Philadelphia: Lipincott-Raven Publishers; 1998: 412–467
4. Newman B, Meza MP, Towbin RB, Nido PD. Left pulmonary artery sling: diagnosis and delineation of associated tracheobronchial anomalies with MR. Pediatr Radiol 1996; 26:661–668
5. Siripornpitak S, Reddy GP, Schwitter J, Higgins CB. Pulmonary artery sling: anatomical and functional evaluation by MRI. J Comput Assist Tomogr 1997; 21:766–768

PULMONARY HYPOPLASIA

6. Canver CC. Isolated unilateral pulmonary artery agenesis. J Thorac Cardiovasc Surg 1993; 105:766
7. Cirillo RL. The scimitar sign. Radiology 1998; 206:623–624
8. Ferrari VA, Reilly MP, Axel L, Sutton MG. Images in cardiovascular medicine. Scimitar syndrome. Circulation 1998; 98:1583–1584
9. Foker J, Long C, Lucas RV. Tracheobronchial compression in acyanotic congenital heart disease. Ann Otol Rhinol Laryngol 1983:387–390
10. Gao YA, Burrows PE, Benson LN, Rabinovitch M, Freedom RM. Scimitar syndrome in infancy. J Am Coll Cardiol 1993; 22:873–882
11. Gilkeson RC, Basile V, Sands MJ, Hsu JT. Chest case of the day. Scimitar syndrome. AJR 1997; 169:267, 270
12. Krummel TM. Congenital malformation of the lower respiratory tract. In: Chernick V, Boat TF, Kendig EL Jr (eds), Kendig's disorders of the respiratory tract in children. 6th ed. Philadelphia: WB Saunders; 1998: 287–327
13. Mulligan ME. History of scimitar syndrome. Radiology 1999; 210:288–290
14. Najim HK, Williams WG, Coles JG, Rebeyka IM, Freedom RM. Scimitar syndrome: twenty years' experience and results of repair. J Thorac Cardiovasc Surg 1996; 112:1161–1169

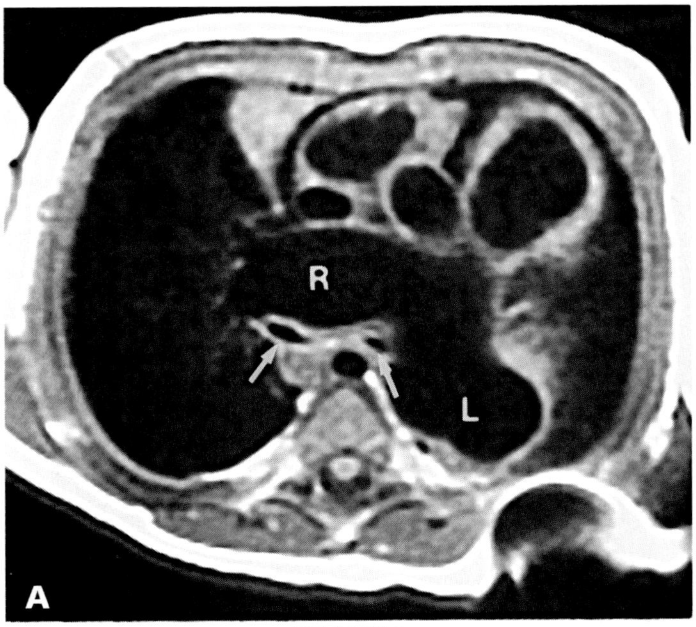

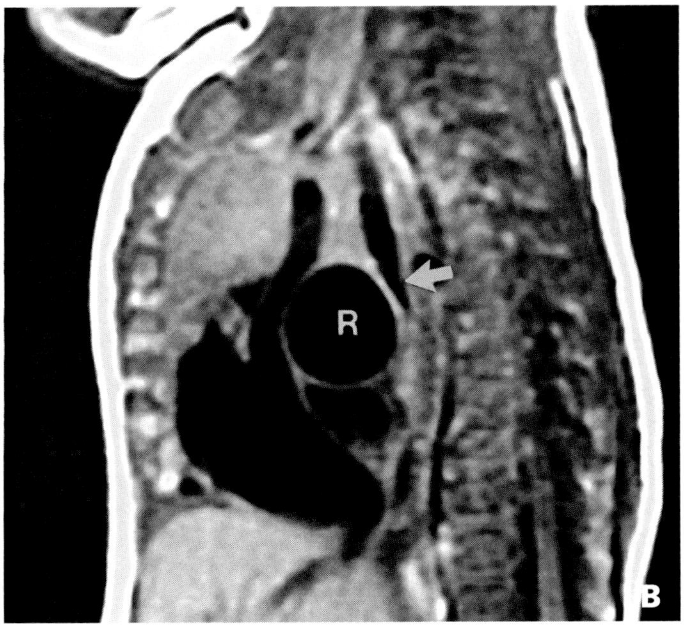

Figure 19-23. Tetralogy of Fallot with absent pulmonic valve in a 2-month old girl. (A) An axial, T1-weighted, cardiac-gated MR image just below the carina demonstrates the aneurysmal dilatation of the pulmonary outflow tract and right (R) and left (L) pulmonary arteries. Note the relationship to the right and left main bronchi (arrows); the left main bronchus is narrowed more than the right main bronchus. (B) A sagittal, T1-weighted, cardiac-gated MR image just to the right of the midline illustrates the relationship of the dilated right pulmonary artery (R) and distal trachea (arrow), which is narrowed and posteriorly displaced.

15. Newman B, Gondor M. MR evaluation of right pulmonary agenesis and vascular airway compression in pediatric patients. AJR 1997; 168:55–58
16. Vrachliotis TG, Bis KG, Shetty AN, Simonetti O, Madrazo B. Hypogenetic lung syndrome: functional and anatomic evaluation with magnetic resonance imaging and magnetic resonance angiography. J Magn Reson Imaging 1996; 6:798–800
17. Woodring JH, Howard TA, Kanga JF. Congenital pulmonary venolobar syndrome revisited. RadioGraphics 1994; 14:349–369

CONGENITAL DIAPHRAGMATIC HERNIA

18. Brink JA, Heiken JP, Semenkovich J, Teefey SA, McClennan BL, Sagel SS. Abnormalities of the diaphragm and adjacent structures: findings on multiplanar spiral CT scans. AJR 1994; 163:307–310
19. Deslauriers J. Eventration of the diaphragm. Chest Surg Clin North Am 1998; 8:315–330
20. Donnelly LF, Sakurai M, Klosterman LA, Delong DM, Strife JL. Correlation between findings in chest radiographs and survivial in neonates with congenital diaphragmatic hernia. AJR 1999; 73:1589–1593
21. Greenholz SK. Congenital diaphragmatic hernia: an overview. Semin Pediatr Surg 1996; 5:216–223
22. Sarihan H, Cay A, Akyazici R, Abes M, Imamoglu M. Congenital diaphragmatic eventration: treatment and postoperative evaluation. J Cardiovasc Surg (Torino) 1996; 37:173–176
23. Stolar CJH. Congenital diaphragmatic hernia. In: Oldham KT, Colombani PM, Foglia RP (eds), Surgery of infants and children: scientific principles and practice. Philadelphia: Lippincott-Raven Publishers; 1997: 883–895
24. Thibeault DW, Haney B. Lung volume, pulmonary vasculature, and factors affecting survival in congenital diaphragmatic hernia. Pediatrics 1998; 101:289–295
25. Vanamo K. A 45-year perspective of congenital diaphragmatic hernia. Br J Surg 1996; 83:1758–1762

CARDIOVASCULAR ABNORMALITIES AND AERATION DISTURBANCES

26. Backer CL, Idriss FS. Tracheoesophageal compressive syndromes of vascular origin. In: Baue AE, Geha AS, Hammond GL, Laks H, Naunheim KS (eds). Glenn's thoracic and cardiovascular surgery. 5th ed. Norwalk, CT: Appleton and Lange; 1991:963–970
27. Berlinger NT, Foker J. Long C, Lucas RV. Tracheobronchial compression in acyanotic congenital heart disease. Ann Otol Rhinol Laryngol 1983: 387–390
28. Corno A, Giamberti A, Giannico S, et al. Airway obstructions associated with congenital heart disease in infancy. J Thorac Cardiovasc Surg 1990; 99:1091–1098
29. Corr L, McCarthy PA, Lavender JP, Hallidie-Smith KA. Bronchial compression by an enlarged left atrium in infants; a cause of hypovascularity of the left lung. Pediatr Radiol 1988; 18:459–463
30. Donnelly LF, Strife JL, Bailey WW. Extrinsic airway compression secondary to pulmonary arterial conduits: MR findings. Pediatr Radiol 1997; 27:268–270
31. Hungate RG, Newman B, Meza MP. Left mainstem bronchial narrowing: a vascular compression syndrome? Evaluation by magnetic resonance imaging. Pediatr Radiol 1998; 28:527–532
32. Jekel L, Benatar A, Bennink GB, Woolley SR, van de Wal HJ. Tetralogy of Fallot with absent pulmonary valve. A continuing challenge. Scand Cardiovasc J 1998; 32:213–217
33. Pickhardt PJ, Siegel MJ, Gutierrez FR. Vascular rings in symptomatic children: frequency of chest radiographic findings. Radiology 1997; 203: 423–426
34. Subramanian V, Anstead M, Cottrill CM, Kanga J, Gurley J. Tetralogy of Fallot with absent pulmonary valve and bronchial compression: treatment with endobronchial stents. Pediatr Cardiol 1997; 18:237–239
35. van Son JA, Julsrud PR, Hagler DJ, et al. Imaging strategies for vascular rings. Ann Thorac Surg 1994; 57:604–610

Marta Hernanz-Schulman, M.D.

Ectopic Ureterocele

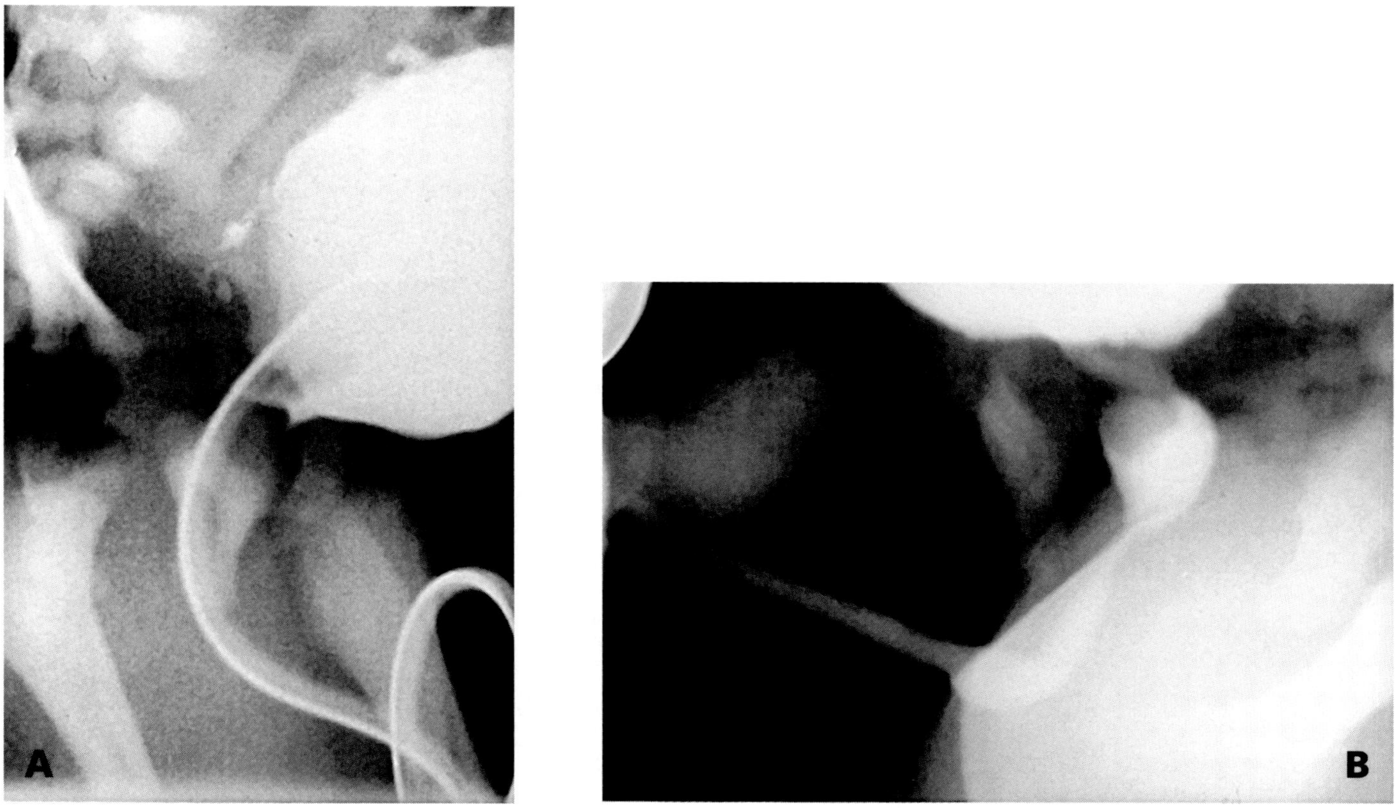

Figure 20-1

Question 94

This 1-week-old boy has a urinary tract infection. You are shown prevoiding (Figure 20-1A) and voiding (Figure 20-1B) images from a voiding cystourethrogram.

Which *one* of the following is the MOST likely diagnosis?

(A) Posterior urethral valves
(B) Neurogenic dysfunction of the bladder
(C) Urethral polyp
(D) Ectopic ureterocele
(E) Rhabdomyosarcoma

The prevoiding film (Figure 20-1A) demonstrates a large, smooth intravesical filling defect (Figure 20-2A) within a trabeculated bladder with multiple diverticula. The contrast material does not extend circumferentially around the filling defect, but rather outlines only its intravesical extension, suggesting that it arises from the bladder wall. On voiding (Figure 20-1B), there is prolapse of the filling defect into the posterior urethra (Figure 20-2B). These findings are characteristic of a prolapsing intravesical ureterocele **(Option (D) is correct)**. A sonogram performed on this child demonstrated the dynamic left-sided intravesical ureterocele (Figure 20-3A to C) and bilateral duplicated renal systems (Figure 20-3D and E). Hydronephrosis of all four moieties and obstruction at the bladder and bladder outlet can be seen.

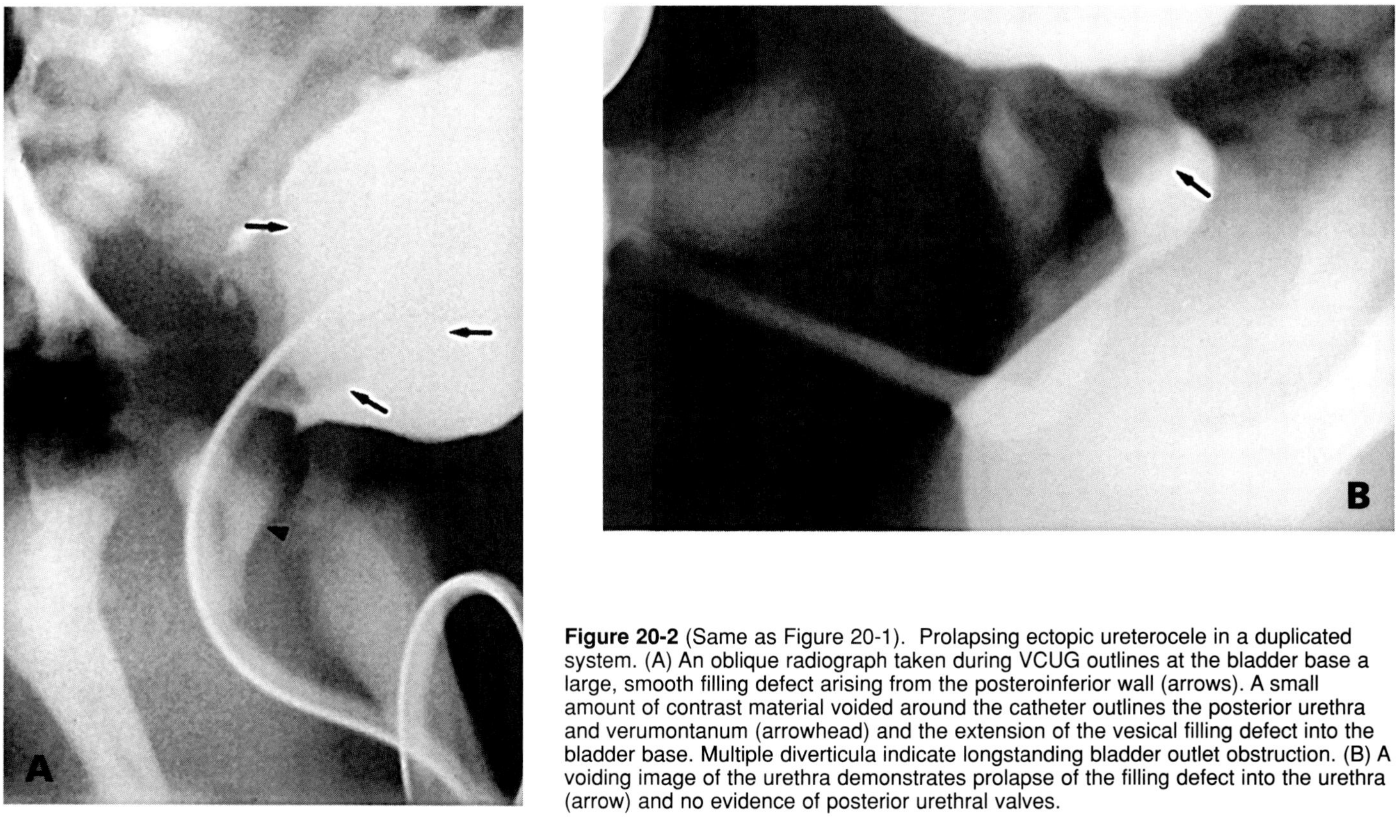

Figure 20-2 (Same as Figure 20-1). Prolapsing ectopic ureterocele in a duplicated system. (A) An oblique radiograph taken during VCUG outlines at the bladder base a large, smooth filling defect arising from the posteroinferior wall (arrows). A small amount of contrast material voided around the catheter outlines the posterior urethra and verumontanum (arrowhead) and the extension of the vesical filling defect into the bladder base. Multiple diverticula indicate longstanding bladder outlet obstruction. (B) A voiding image of the urethra demonstrates prolapse of the filling defect into the urethra (arrow) and no evidence of posterior urethral valves.

Posterior urethral valves (Option (A)) cause anatomic and functional obstruction to bladder emptying; they are situated in the posterior urethra at the base of the verumontanum. On voiding cystourethrography (VCUG), they have a characteristic appearance of dilatation of the prostatic urethra, which comes to a point at the site of the valves. The urinary stream continues along the aperture of the obstructing valves and becomes markedly thinned in caliber (Figure 20-4). A filling defect extending from the vesical lumen into the posterior urethra, as seen in the test patient, is not a feature of posterior urethral valves.

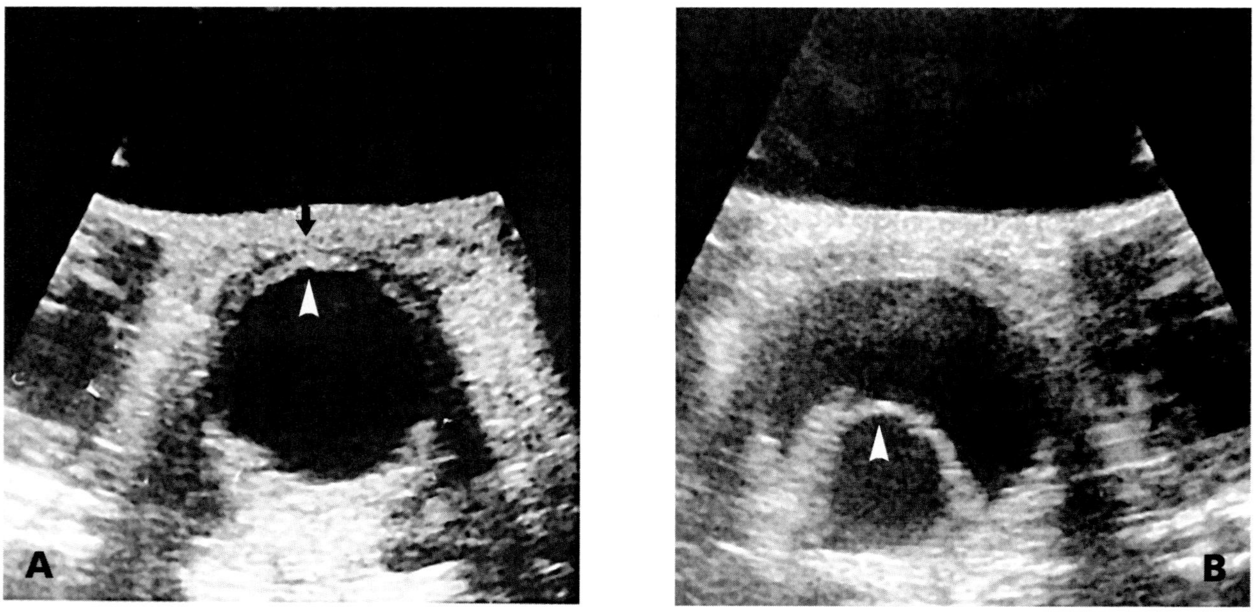

Figure 20-3. Same patient as in Figures 20-1 and 20-2. Prolapsing ectopic ureterocele in a duplicated system. (A) A transverse sonographic image of the bladder performed with a linear 5-MHz transducer through a stand-off device initially suggests a thick-walled bladder. However, on closer inspection, one can see the ureterocele (arrowhead) outlined by a thin layer of anechoic urine interposed between the ureterocele and the bladder wall (arrow). (B) A transverse sonographic image taken a few minutes after the image shown in panel A shows a change in the size of the left-sided ureterocele (arrowhead).

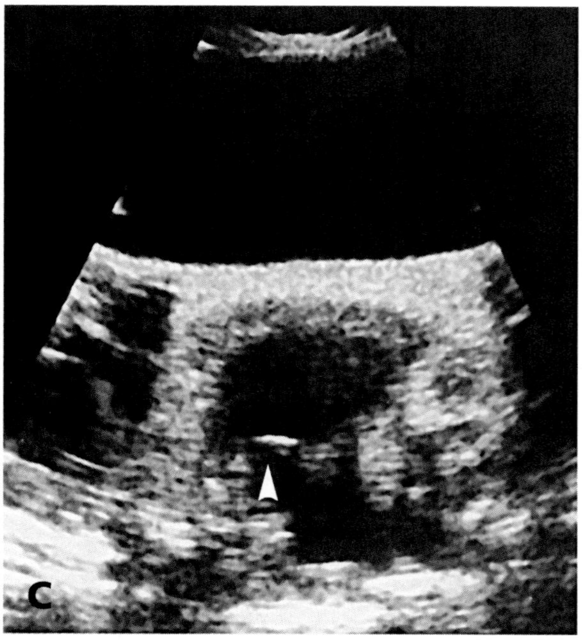

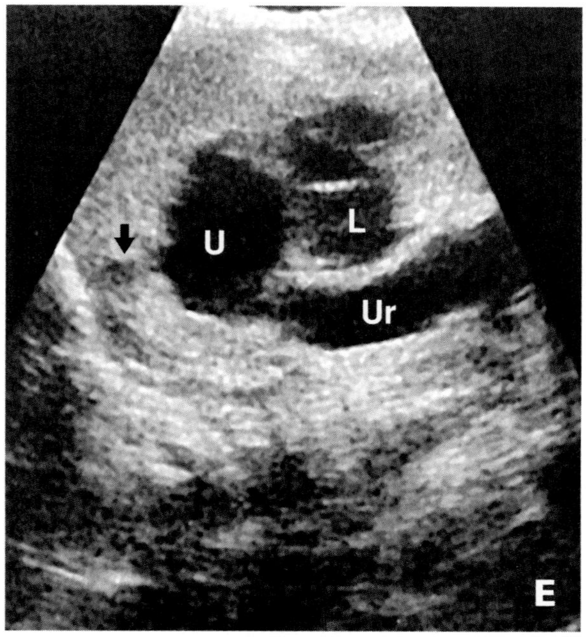

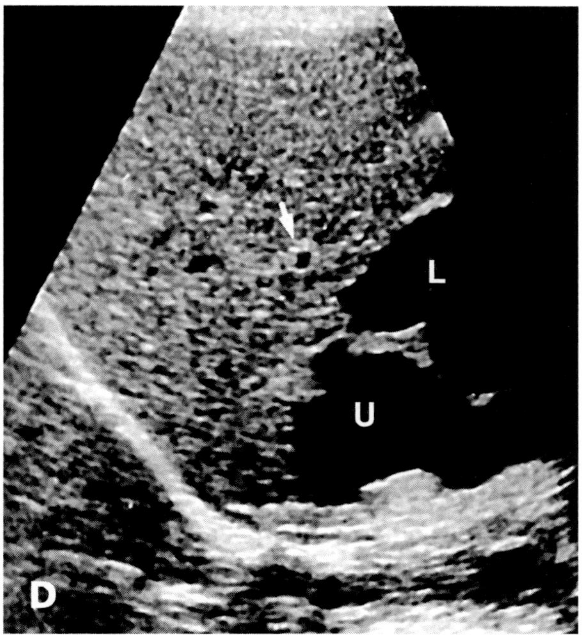

Figure 20-3 (Continued). Prolapsing ectopic ureterocele in a duplicated system. (C) A transverse sonographic image taken a few seconds after the image shown in panel B shows a further change in the size of the ureterocele (arrowhead). (D) A coronal image taken along the right flank with a curved 5-MHz transducer shows hydronephrosis of upper (U) and lower (L) renal pelves. Renal parenchyma is isoechoic relative to the liver and lacks corticomedullary differentiation. A small peripheral cortical cyst (arrow) is present. (E) A coronal image taken along the left flank with a curved 5-MHz transducer shows the dilated left upper pole pelvis (U) and dilated ureter (Ur), which courses medial to the hydronephrotic lower pole pelvis (L). The renal parenchyma is hyperechoic compared to adjacent spleen, lacks corticomedullary differentiation, and exhibits a cortical cyst (arrow).

Neurogenic dysfunction of the bladder (Option (B)) is a condition in which the coordinated neuromuscular and sphincteric responses to bladder filling and intravesical pressure are abnormal or lacking. The most common cause is disruption of the neurospinal axis in patients with myelodysplasia. The degree of urinary voiding dysfunction is variable. The level of the neurologic lesion usually is within three vertebral levels of the bony lesion. Patients in whom the lesion affects the reflex arc through segments S2 to S4 can have an atonic bladder and a lower motor neuron lesion; patients with a lesion at a higher level more often have upper motor neuron dysfunction and bladder spasticity. Urodynamic examination of patients with myelodysplasia allows classification of the condition into three broad categories: synergic; dyssynergic, with and without detrusor hypertonicity; and complete denervation. Synergy is characterized by relaxation of sphincteric activity during detrusor contraction, whereas dyssynergy occurs when sphincteric activity persists or increases with detrusor contraction or with an increase in intravesical pressure. Denervation is defined as failure of sphincteric activity during the micturition cycle or in response to Credé's maneuver (caudally directed manual pressure on the bladder dome) or sacral stimulation. Obstruction to bladder emptying, such as that present in infants with dyssynergic bladders, places the upper tracts at risk. These patients are managed with prophylactic, frequent, clean intermittent catheterization, with or without anticholinergic pharmacological intervention. Chronically elevated intravesical pressures are associated with obstruction, reflux, hyronephrosis, infection, and upper tract functional deterioration

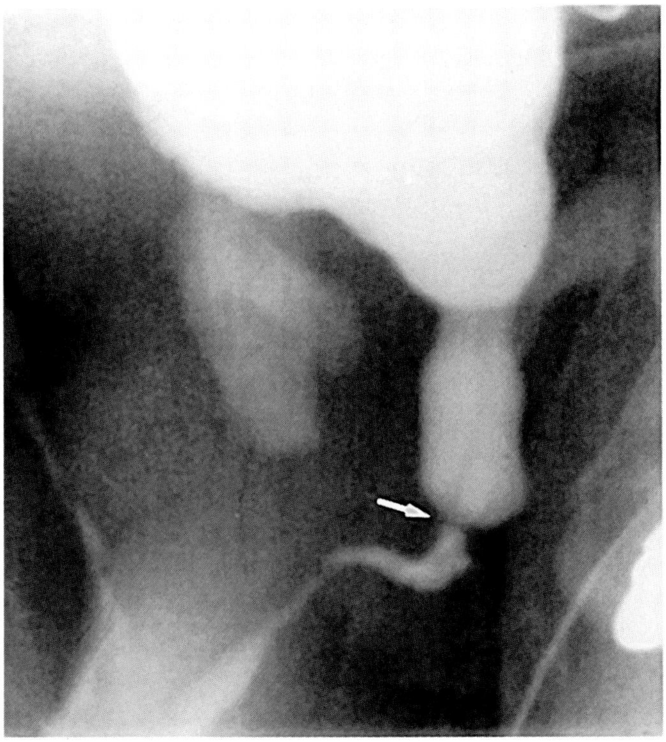

Figure 20-4. Posterior urethral valves. Voiding image of an infant during VCUG. Note the abrupt narrowing at the base of the posterior urethra (arrow) and the diminished caliber of the urethra distal to the obstruction.

in the majority of patients.

Other causes of neurogenic bladder dysfunction include central nervous system insults such as cerebral palsy, traumatic injuries to the spine, and repeated infections. As many as 80% of patients with cerebral palsy or another type of central lesion can exhibit a pattern of detrusor hyperreflexia, with or without sphincteric dyssynergia. Patients with spinal cord injury, such as trauma and transverse myelitis, can demonstrate transient or permanent voiding dysfunction with detrusor hyperreflexia. In children with recurrent urinary tract infections, symptoms of frequency, urgency, and dysuria can persist after the infection has cleared. It is postulated that cystitis may lead to increased irritability of the detrusor muscle, poor bladder compliance, and inappropriate sphincteric contractions. A vicious cycle of retained urine and repeated infections thus may be established. Treatment for these patients is geared to elimination of recurrent infections, psychosocial training, and antispasmodic agents.

Children who are otherwise neurologically normal can have a spectrum of functional voiding abnormalities, a situation that is believed to be an acquired problem, with persistence of the transitional phase of bladder functional control and inappropriate sphincteric contraction, rooted in overly severe toilet training for the particular child's maturation and ability. This condition is known as Hinman or Hinman-Allen syndrome, nonneurogenic neurogenic bladder, or psychological nonneuropathic bladder. The dyssynergy between detrusor contractions and sphincteric relaxation leads to ineffective detrusor contractions, bladder trabeculation, hydronephrosis, and secondary reflux. Some children can show evidence of constipation. Treatment is geared to reeducation and institution of appropriate voiding habits, with the addition of pharmacologic therapy and intermittent catheterization as needed.

The findings at VCUG in patients with neurogenic dysfunction of the bladder differ depending on the type of lesion that is present and associated findings. Patients with atonic bladder have a smooth-walled bladder and urinary dribbling. Patients with various forms of dyssynergic activity often have a trabeculated bladder with multiple diverticula and show failure of complete relaxation of the sphincter during voiding (Figure 20-5). These findings, however, are unassociated with an intravesical filling or prolapsing defect such as that present in the test case.

Urethral polyps (Option (C)) are pedunculated fibroepithelial lesions with a fibromuscular stroma invested by transitional epithelium. They are rare, benign lesions that occur most commonly in the posterior urethra. Because they are pedunculated, vesical dynamics allow them to migrate in and out of the bladder base (Figure 20-6), and they can cause intermittent bladder outlet obstruction. Unlike the findings in the test case, these lesions arise in the urethra and migrate into the bladder, not vice versa; they are usually pedunculated and are approximately 1.5 cm long, on average.

Rhabdomyosarcomas (Option (E)) are soft tissue tumors that originate from the mesenchyma, which normally develops into muscle. They account for approximately 50% of pediatric soft tissue sarcomas and approximately 15% of pediatric solid tumors. The peak incidence occurs between 2 and 5 years of age, with a second peak between 15 and 19 years. Embryonal and botryoid tumors occur in younger children, whereas the alveolar histologic subtype occurs in older patients. Twenty percent of these tumors arise in the genitourinary system: prostate, bladder, and vagina. Approximately 60% or more of genitourinary tumors are of the embryonal histologic subtype. A rhabdomyosarcoma growing into a hollow viscus, such as the bladder or vagina, often assumes a polypoid shape resembling a cluster of grapes, termed sarcoma botryoides. Such tumors occur more commonly in boys, in the trigone and bladder neck, and can cause bladder outlet obstruction (Figure 20-7). However, their irregular, botryoid appearance is unlike the smooth outline of the mass seen in the test patient. The age of the test patient is also inconsistent with this diagnosis. Rhabdomyosarcomas arising in the prostate present with mass effect and elevation of the bladder base. Both prostate and intravesical tumors may present with urinary retention and hydronephrosis. Prognosis is dependent on staging at the time of diagnosis and on histologic subtype.

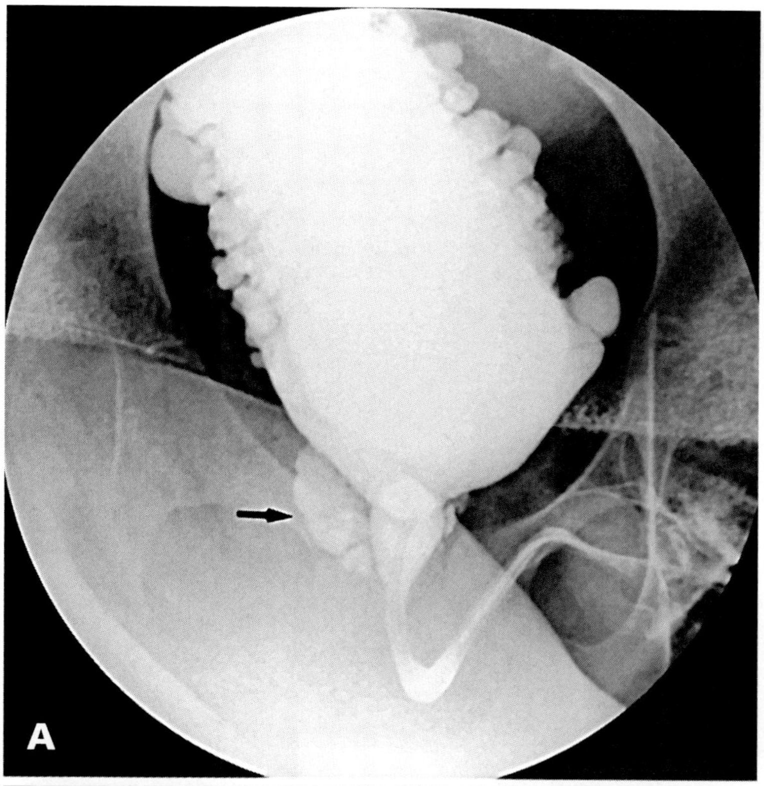

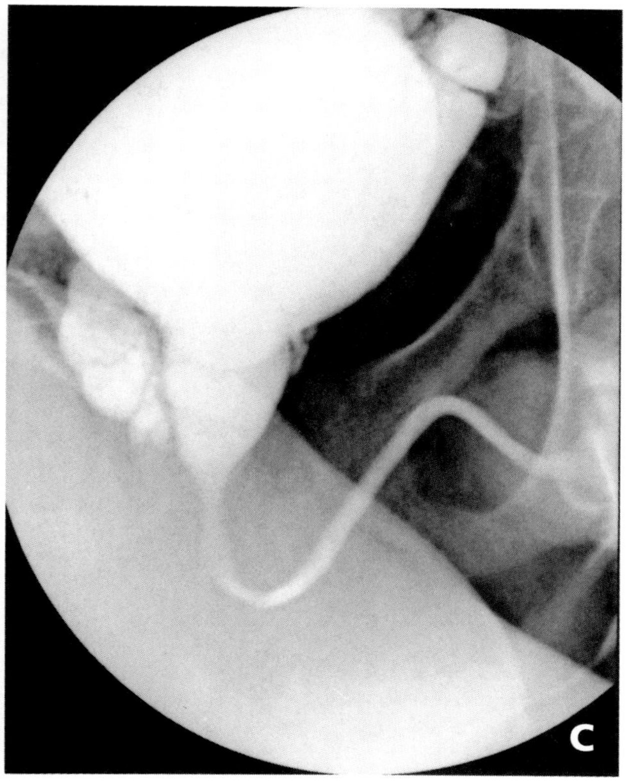

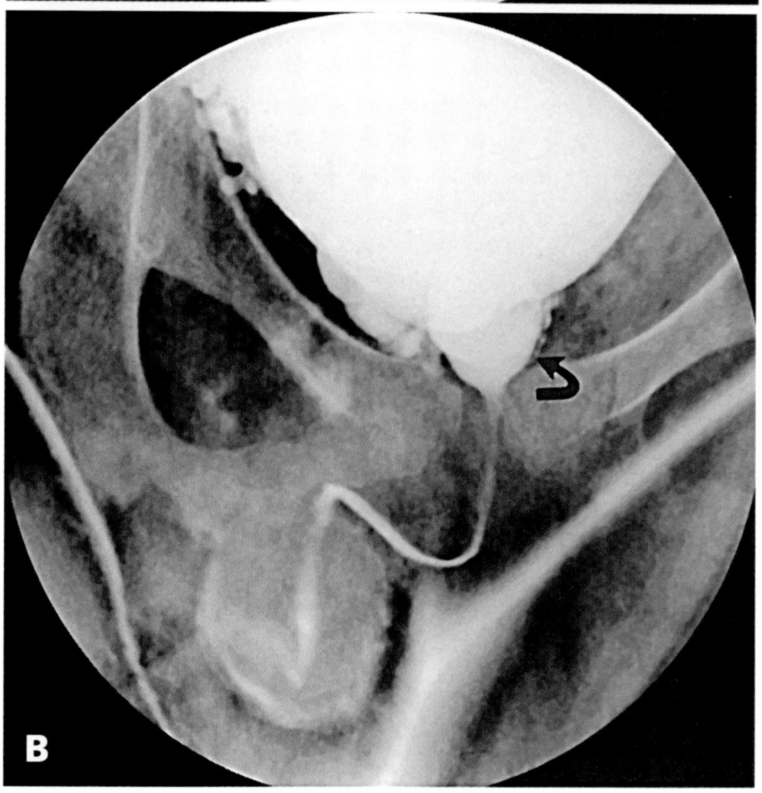

Figure 20-5. Neurogenic bladder dysfunction. (A) Radiograph taken during VCUG of an adolescent patient with myelomeningocele, with the catheter still in place. The urinary bladder is highly trabeculated, and there is extensive reflux into the prostatic ducts (arrow). (B) After removal of the catheter, there is failure of relaxation of the external sphincter, resulting in dilatation of the posterior urethra (curved arrow) and a markedly attenuated urinary stream. (C) Another image taken during momentary relaxation of the sphincter demonstrates the absence of an anatomic obstructing lesion, such as valves.

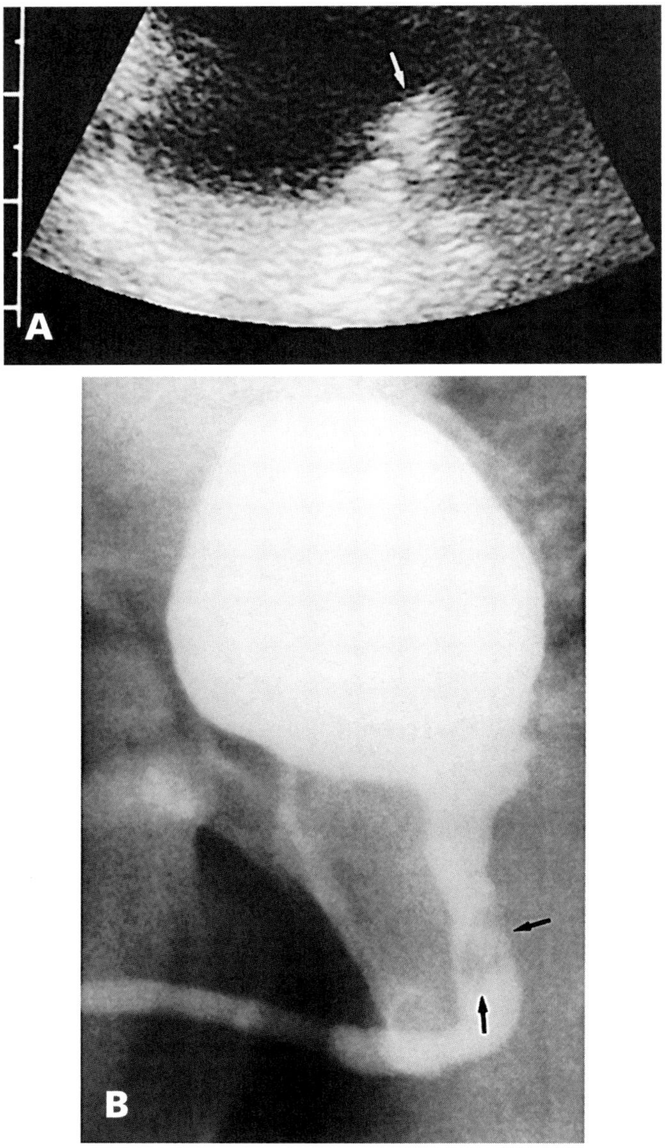

Figure 20-6. Urethral polyp. (A) A longitudinal sonographic image of the bladder base shows a solid 1-cm structure (arrow) protruding into the bladder base. (B) A voiding image from VCUG of the same patient illustrates the broad-based filling defect within the prostatic portion of the urethra (arrows). (Case courtesy of Lisa H. Lowe, M.D., Children's Mercy Hospital, University of Missouri—Kansas City, Kansas City, KS.)

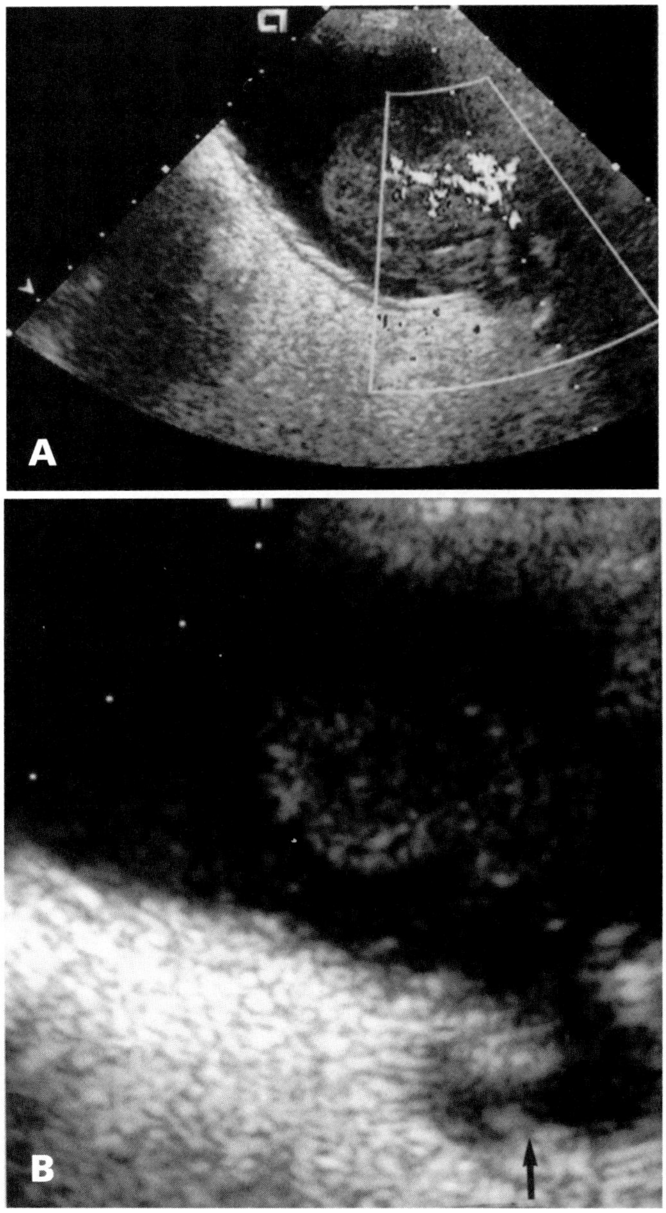

Figure 20-7. Rhabdomyosarcoma in a 2-year-old boy presenting with urinary retention. (A) A longitudinal sonographic image of the bladder angled to the left demonstrates a solid mass at the base of the bladder. Doppler interrogation demonstrates flow within the lesion, excluding the possibility of clot and indicating that it represents a neoplasm. (B) A magnified sonographic view of the left ureterovesical junction demonstrates a portion of the intravesical tumor and dilatation of the left ureter (arrow) outside the bladder.

Question 95

Concerning posterior urethral valves,

(A) they are the result of abnormal insertion of the mesonephric ducts
(B) they rarely occur in phenotypic girls
(C) nearly all patients have reflux
(D) they are the most common cause of urinary ascites in neonates
(E) on ultrasonography, a dilated prostatic urethra is a specific sign

Posterior urethral valves were classified in 1919 by Young, who described three types: I, II, and III. Type I valves were described as a membrane radiating caudally from the verumontanum, with a posterior aperture; type II valves were represented by folds also arising in the verumontanum, but radiating cranially to the posterolateral bladder neck; and type III valves were described as a membrane located immediately distal to the verumontanum, at the level of the membranous urethra, with the opening situated centrally.

Type II valves are now believed to represent enlarged superficial muscular bundles extending distally from the ureteral orifices to the verumontanum. These muscular bundles can undergo hypertrophy, notably in cases of bladder neck obstruction unrelated to the valves. However, type II valves are rarely obstructive and, therefore, in most cases do not represent a clinically significant entity.

Type I valves are the most common cause of urinary tract obstruction leading to renal failure in childhood and occur with an incidence variably reported at between 1 in 8,000 to 1 in 25,000 live births. End-stage renal disease occurs with a frequency ranging between 24% and 44%, depending on the length of follow-up of the patients. The valves are believed to result from an abnormal anterior insertion of the mesonephric ducts into the embryonic cloaca (**Option (A) is true).** This anomalous position prevents their normal lateral migration to form the plicae colliculi and results in persistence of the abnormal anterior insertion and anterolateral fusion of their distal ends. Thus, the obstruction takes the form of a membrane with a posterior aperture (Figure 20-8).

Type III valves constitute approximately 5% of posterior urethral valves. They consist of a membranous obstruction with a central rather than a posterior aperture. They are more commonly described as being located just distal to the verumontanum and are believed to represent failure of recanalization of the urogenital membrane (Figure 20-9). Their anatomy and elasticity permit them to "stretch," and in some cases they can have a wind sock appearance, prolapsing into the more distal urethra. Their clinical presentation, however, is similar to that of type I valves.

Posterior urethral valves occur exclusively in boys. Although rarely an obstructing valvelike lesion has been reported in girls, normal girls do not have a posterior urethra; therefore, such valves cannot occur in phenotypic girls (**Option (B) is false).** However, true posterior urethral valves have been encountered in masculinized female infants with the adrenogenital syndrome.

Valves have a wide spectrum of clinical findings, depending on the degree of obstruction, the presence of reflux, and the occurrence of spontaneous urinary decompression or "pop-off" mechanism. Thus, the clinical scenario includes prenatal presentation with oligohydramnios; neonatal presentation with pulmonary hypoplasia, bilateral hydroureteronephrosis (Figure 20-10A and B), urinoma or urinary ascites, or renal dysplasia; presentation in later childhood or even adulthood with enuresis, urinary tract infection or hematuria, or evidence of unrecognized renal damage, such as hypertension and elevated creatinine levels; or even presentation later in life with infertility.

Neonatal presentation usually is associated with a poorer outcome, likely because of a more significant degree of obstruction *in utero.* Prognosis correlates with the degree of reflux, hydroureteronephrosis, and renal dysplasia.

Reflux is present in approximately 50% of all patients with posterior urethral valves (**Option (C) is false).** Mortality rates are approximately 57% in patients with bilateral reflux,

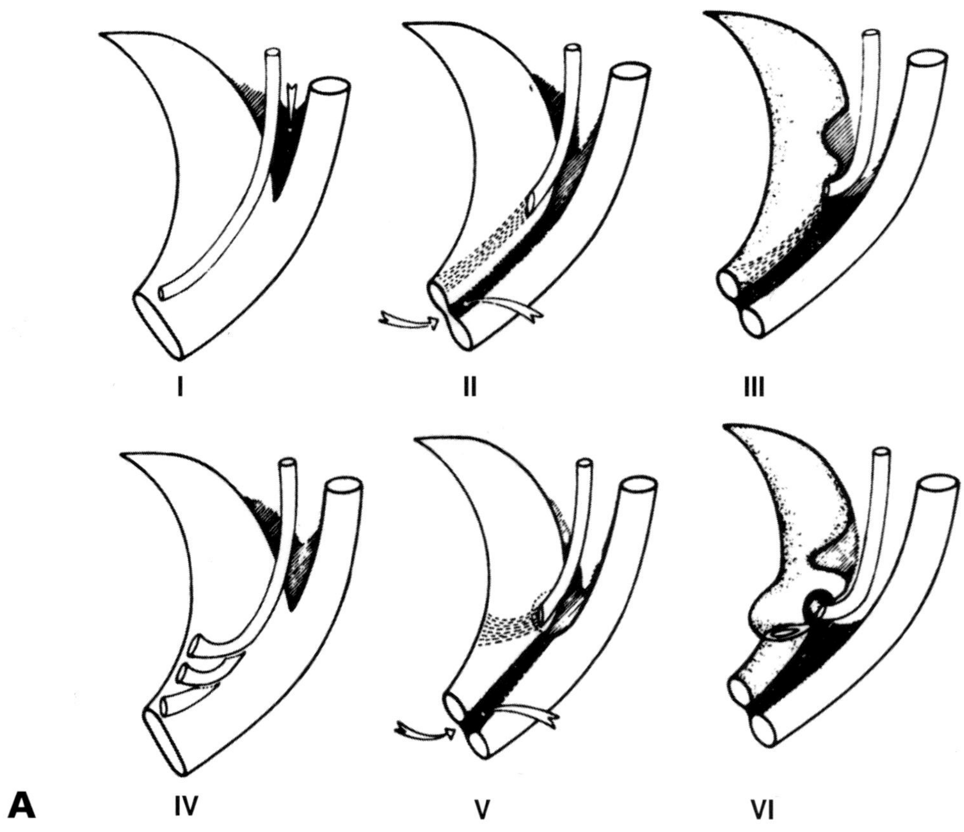

Figure 20-8. Posterior urethral valves. (A) Diagrammatic sketch of hypothetical etiology of type I posterior urethral valves. Diagrams I through III show the normal insertion and pathway of migration of the distal end of the mesonephric or Wolffian ducts. The dark band marks the urorectal septum, dividing the cloaca into the urogenital canal anteriorly and the anorectal canal posteriorly; the stippled band marks the path of the mesonephric ducts as the normal plicae colliculi. Diagrams IV through VI show an abnormal anterior insertion of the mesonephric ducts, leading to abnormal migration and circumferentially oriented ridges that fuse anteriorly in the midline, resulting in type I valves. (Adapted with permission from Kaplan and Scherz [25].)

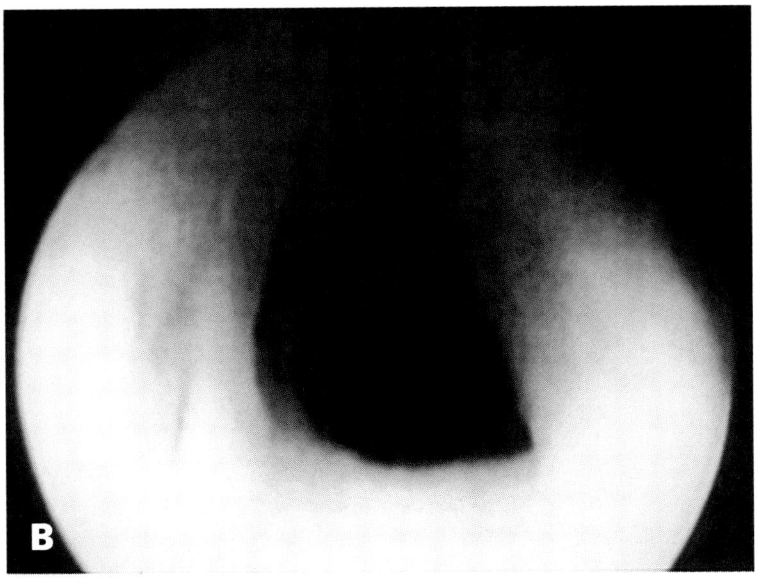

Figure 20-8 (Continued). Posterior urethral valves. (B) Photograph of posterior urethral valves taken through an endoscope. (Photograph courtesy of Mark Adams, M.D., Vanderbilt University Medical Center—Children's Hospital, Nashville, TN.)

approximately 17% in those with unilateral reflux, and about 9% in those with no reflux. The prognosis is also affected by the presence of a pop-off mechanism, which diverts the high pressure generated by the hypertrophied bladder from the upper tracts. Forniceal rupture can lead to the development of a urinoma or to urinary ascites, which results from tear of the renal capsule and Gerota's fascia, with transudation of urine across the peritoneal membrane. Although urinary ascites can occur from any type of urinary obstruction, urethral valves are the most common cause of urinary ascites in neonates **(Option (D) is true)**. Reflux into one kidney also can act as a protective mechanism for the contralateral kidney, and a patent urachus or large bladder diverticula also can exert a protective effect on the upper tracts.

Diminished renal function can be seen in as many as two

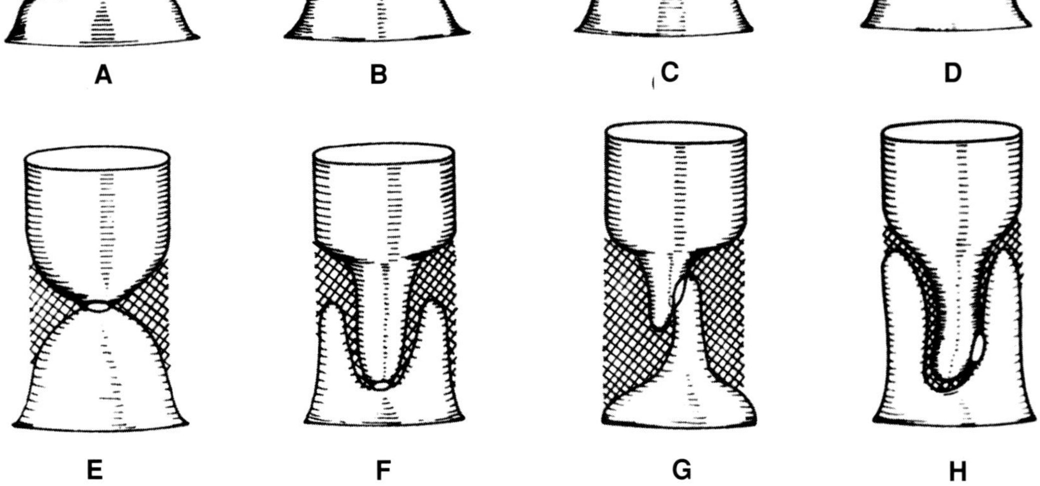

Figure 20-9. Diagrammatic sketch of hypothetical etiology of type III posterior urethral valves. Diagrams A to D outline the normal canalization of the urogenital membrane. Diagram E shows a narrow central opening of a persistent membrane. Diagram F shows stretching of the membrane resulting in a wind sock appearance. Diagrams G and H show an eccentric opening leading to a diverticulum-like wind sock appearance. (Reprinted with permission from Kaplan and Scherz [25].)

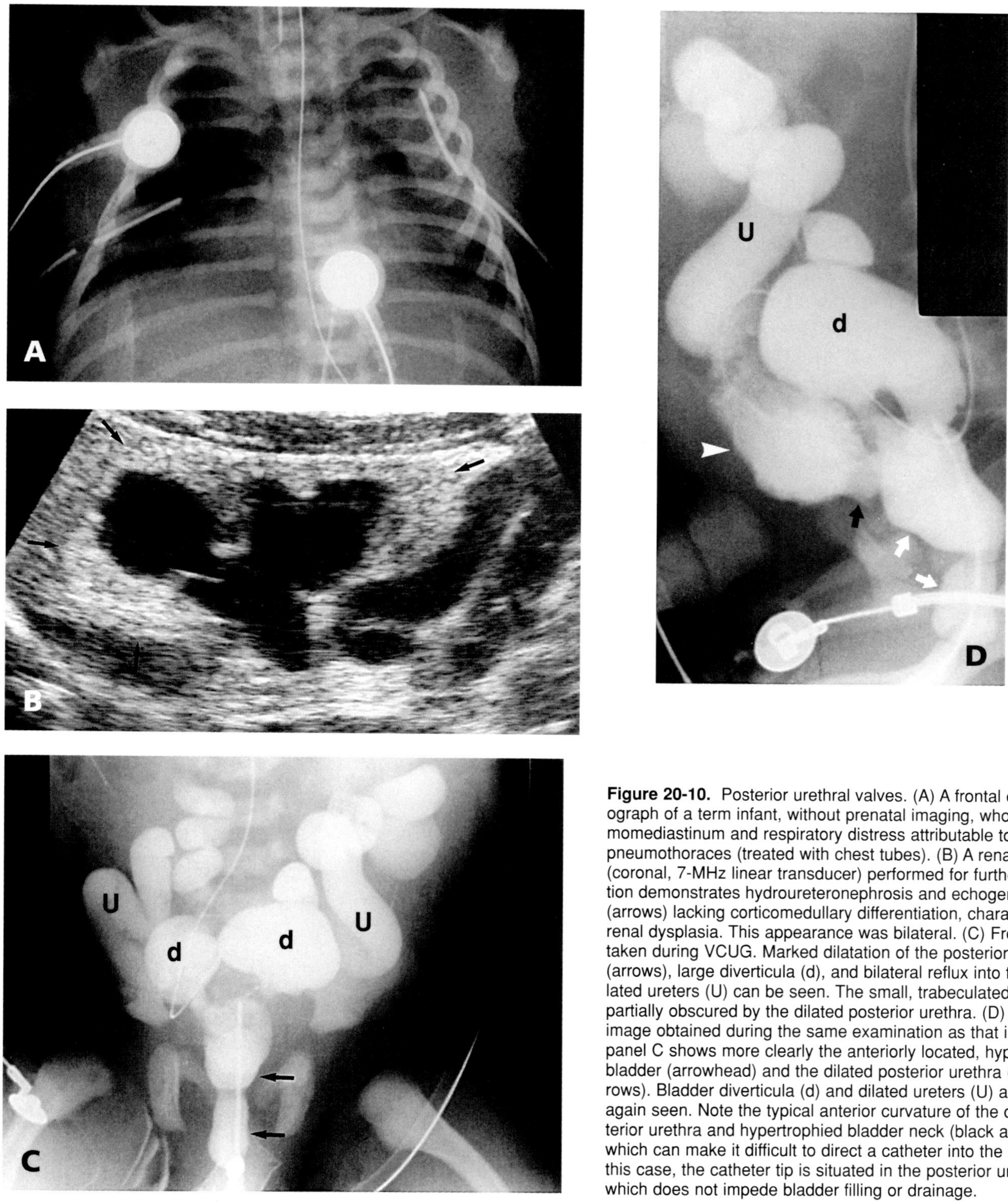

Figure 20-10. Posterior urethral valves. (A) A frontal chest radiograph of a term infant, without prenatal imaging, who had pneumomediastinum and respiratory distress attributable to bilateral pneumothoraces (treated with chest tubes). (B) A renal sonogram (coronal, 7-MHz linear transducer) performed for further evaluation demonstrates hydroureteronephrosis and echogenic kidneys (arrows) lacking corticomedullary differentiation, characteristic of renal dysplasia. This appearance was bilateral. (C) Frontal image taken during VCUG. Marked dilatation of the posterior urethra (arrows), large diverticula (d), and bilateral reflux into tortuous, dilated ureters (U) can be seen. The small, trabeculated bladder is partially obscured by the dilated posterior urethra. (D) An oblique image obtained during the same examination as that illustrated in panel C shows more clearly the anteriorly located, hypertrophied bladder (arrowhead) and the dilated posterior urethra (white arrows). Bladder diverticula (d) and dilated ureters (U) are once again seen. Note the typical anterior curvature of the dilated posterior urethra and hypertrophied bladder neck (black arrow), which can make it difficult to direct a catheter into the bladder. In this case, the catheter tip is situated in the posterior urethra, which does not impede bladder filling or drainage.

thirds of patients at presentation. Decreased urinary concentrating capacity is common. Deterioration in renal function may continue inexorably after repair of the valves, and as many as 26% of patients with initially normal renal function may develop chronic renal failure after 18 years of age. The reasons for this situation are postulated to be multifactorial and related to nephron damage secondary to hyperfiltration, repeated urinary tract infections and scarring, and persistent bladder dysfunction. The hypertrophied bladders of these children have a measurable increase in smooth muscle mass and may exhibit persistent dysfunction and diminished compliance. In addition, the hypertrophied muscle itself can obstruct the ureteral orifices.

The basis for the diagnosis of posterior urethral valves is VCUG. This technique permits visualization of the valves at the base of the verumontanum and passage of contrast material across the aperture (Figure 20-4). Obstructing valves have a highly variable appearance, with variable dilatation of the posterior urethra that is dependent on volume flow. Thus, imaging early or late during micturition can lead to failure to detect this dilatation. The bladder typically is hypertrophied, with multiple sacculations; large diverticula, often larger than the hypertrophied bladder, also can be present (Figure 20-10C and D). Reflux into one or both kidneys can be present, and pyelotubular backflow also may be visible during cystography (Figure 20-11).

Sonography is an important adjunct in the imaging evaluation of patients, and the diagnosis often is suspected during this examination. In typical cases, the bladder is hypertrophied and, when drained via a catheter, can resemble a solid pelvic mass (Figure 20-12). The degree of hydroureteronephrosis should be assessed, and the thickness of the renal parenchyma and presence or absence of cortical dysplasia also should be evaluated. Pathologically, renal dysplasia is characterized by variable numbers of functioning glomeruli, primitive ducts surrounded by fibromuscular tissue, cortical and medullary cysts, and metaplastic cartilage. Sonography typically demonstrates loss of normal corticomedullary differentiation and, in more severe cases, small peripheral cysts. Evaluation of the urethra with high-frequency transducers (7 to 10 MHz) may reveal dilatation of the posterior urethra. However, the absence of this finding in no way excludes the diagnosis, as dilatation of the posterior urethra may not be present in the absence of voiding. In addition, dilatation of the posterior urethra can be seen in other obstructive conditions, such as the presence of a urethral polyp, and in nonobstructive conditions with hypoplasia or absence of the verumontanum, such as the prune belly syndrome **(Option (E) is false).**

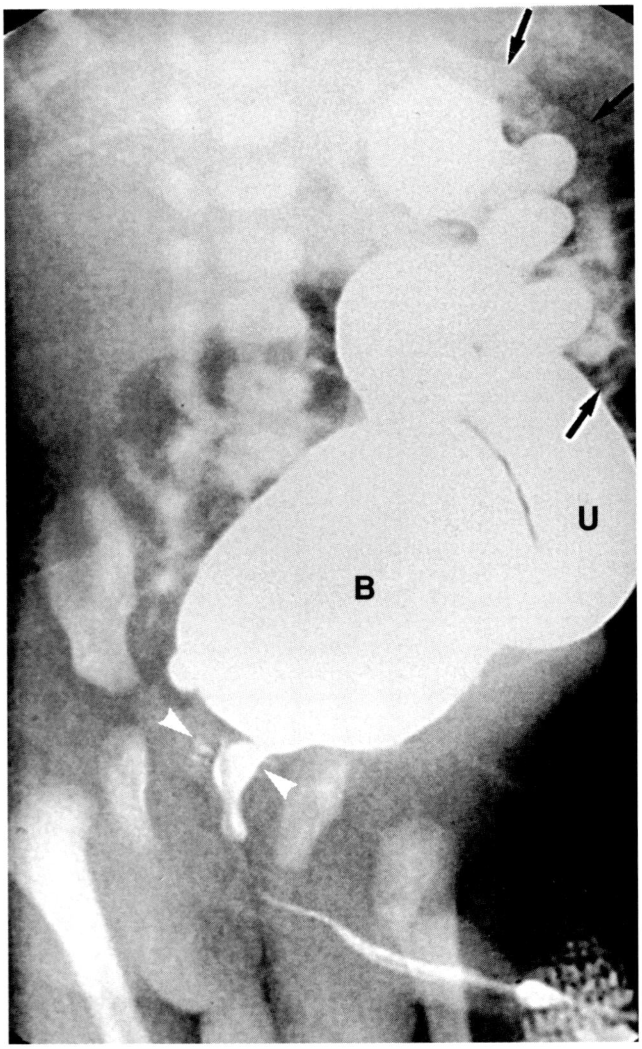

Figure 20-11. Posterior urethral valves. An oblique image from VCUG of an infant with posterior urethral valves shows less dilatation of the posterior urethra than in the infant whose imaging results are shown in Figure 20-10, but typical narrowing at the base of the verumontanum is evident. The bladder (B) of this infant lacks the large diverticula present in the infant whose imaging results are shown in Figure 20-10. However, reflux into the prostatic ducts (arrowheads) and marked unilateral reflux into the left kidney, with prominent pyelotubular backflow (arrows), can be seen. U = left ureter.

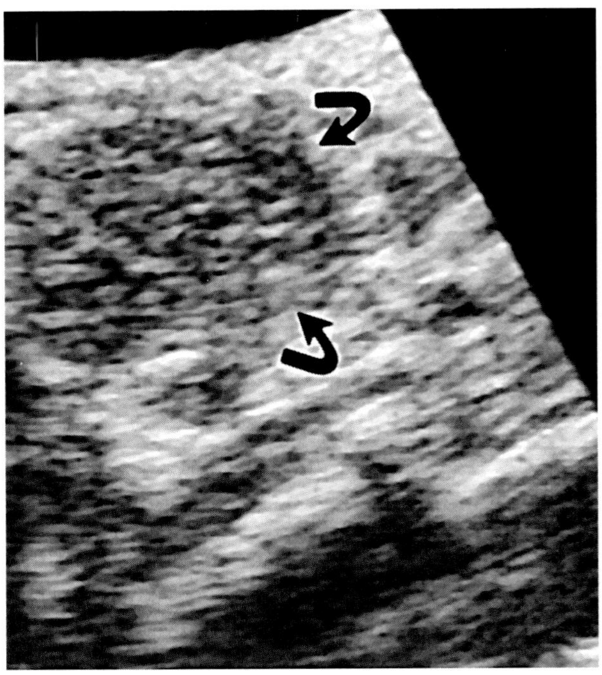

Figure 20-12. Posterior urethral valves. On a sonogram of the pelvis, obtained following catheter drainage of the bladder in an infant with posterior urethral valves, a thick-walled, empty bladder (arrows) resembles a solid pelvic mass.

Question 96

Concerning urethral polyps,

(A) they undergo malignant degeneration
(B) they often occur in the posterior urethra
(C) most are pedunculated
(D) they are a cause of prenatally detected hydronephrosis
(E) they mimic urethral diverticula on voiding cystourethrography

Genitourinary polyps, or benign fibroepithelial polyps, are tumors of mesodermal origin that consist of smooth muscle and connective tissue invested in transitional epithelium. These lesions are presumed to be of congenital origin, although some have been reported in older patients, indicating that some can be acquired or subclinical. They are uniformly benign and do not undergo malignant degeneration (**Option (A) is false**).

Genitourinary polyps occur most often in the posterior urethra in boys, at the level of the verumontanum (**Option (B) is true**). However, they have been reported in girls and in other areas of the urinary tract, from the renal pelvis to the anterior urethra. Extraurethral lesions typically are found in the ureter, where they occur more commonly on the left side. The lesions are rare, with only 16 cases identified in Mayo Clinic records between 1957 and 1992. Genitourinary polyps are typically pedunculated (**Option (C) is true**); urethral polyps often extend into the base of the bladder during bladder filling and can be reextruded into the urethra during voiding (Figure 20-6), leading to bladder neck obstruction of variable severity. Hydronephrosis or reflux can be seen in 20% to 50% of cases; these conditions can resolve spontaneously after ablation of the lesion.

The typical age at presentation of a patient with a urethral polyp is approximately 9 years, with symptoms of intermittent obstruction, urinary retention, hematuria, and dysuria. Thus, presentation in the neonatal period is rare, but polyps have been identified in neonates during postnatal investigation of hydronephrosis incidentally detected *in utero* (**Option (D) is true**). As noted above, urethral polyps occur almost exclusively in boys, but they have been reported in girls, in whom a prolapsing polyp can appear as an interlabial mass. Urethral polyps present as intermittent flank pain and hematuria, which occurs in approximately two thirds of patients.

The diagnosis of urethral polyp is made on VCUG (Figure 20-6B) by identification within the posterior urethra of a pedunculated lesion that is mobile during fluoroscopic observation. The polyp differs from the prolapsing ureterocele in its location, as the ureterocele arises in the bladder and protrudes into the urethra, whereas the polyp arises in the urethra and can extend into the bladder but, on voiding, usually is noted as a filling defect located exclusively within the urethra and extending distally along the urinary stream. The prolapsing ureterocele originates in an ectopically inserting ureter and is most often associated with an obstructed upper pole collecting system in girls, whereas the urethral polyp is not associated with this upper tract lesion and occurs almost exclusively in boys.

Congenital urethral diverticula can occur anywhere along the anterior urethra, most commonly in the bulbous urethra or at its junction with the penile urethra (70%); the rest are located along the course of the penile urethra. These diverticula, in various forms, are thought to encompass nearly all cases of so-called anterior urethral valves. The diverticula can arise from an incomplete urethral duplication or congenital cystic dilatation of a periurethral gland. During voiding, the diverticulum fills with urine, and as it distends, it encroaches upon the urethral lumen, obstructing urinary flow (Figure 20-13). The appearance of the diverticulum as a sessile contrast material-filled mass compressing the anterior urethra and separated from it by a ventral lip is thus quite different from that of the urethral polyp, which is seen as a mobile, pedunculated filling defect within the posterior urethra (**Option (E) is false**). Anterior urethral diverticula have a broad spectrum of findings, from marked bladder outlet obstruction and upper tract changes similar to those seen in severe cases of posterior urethral valves to small, narrow-necked lesions that are not obstructive.

Question 97

Concerning ureteroceles,

(A) they are a cause of enuresis
(B) ectopic ones usually are associated with the upper pole ureter of a duplicated system
(C) in boys, ectopic ones are most often associated with nonduplicated systems
(D) they are best demonstrated on cystography when the bladder is maximally distended

The term "ureterocele" refers to dilatation of the intramural portion of the distal ureter, which protrudes into the vesical cavity. Therefore, the ureterocele is a fluid-filled structure, containing urine derived from its ureter, with a bilayered wall (Figure 20-14). Viewed from the bladder, the wall of the ureterocele is vesical epithelium, whereas viewed from within the ureter, its wall is ureteral epithelium. Ureteroceles may or may not be associated with ureteral ectopia; conversely, an ectopic ureter may or may not terminate in a ureterocele.

In order for a discussion of the various types and complications of ureteroceles to be meaningful, an understanding of the embryology and pathophysiology of the ureteral bud is a prerequisite. The mesonephros and mesonephric duct are the templates from which the mature anatomy develops. The ureteric bud "buds" from the mesonephric duct at the site where the duct bends prior to insertion into the ventral portion of the cloaca. At this site, the ureteric bud encounters the metanephric blastema, and a normal kidney develops from

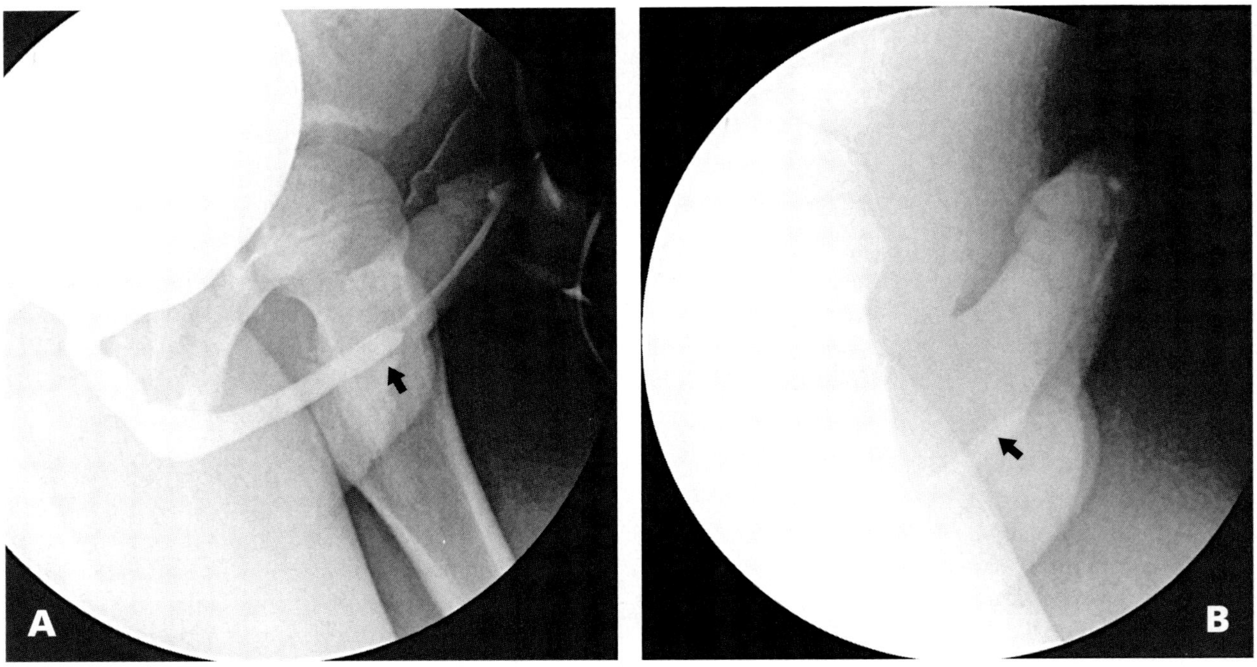

Figure 20-13. Congenital urethral diverticulum (anterior urethral valve). (A) A voiding image from a VCUG in a young boy with a congenital urethral diverticulum shows the contrast material-filled diverticulum (arrow) and the change in caliber of the urinary stream distal to the diverticulum. (B) An image taken at the end of voiding better outlines the linear filling defect (arrow) indicating the site of a membrane between the urethra dorsally and the diverticulum ventrally.

their interaction by a process of mutual induction. That portion of the mesonephric duct caudal to the origin of the ureteric bud becomes incorporated into the urogenital sinus to form the bladder trigone, such that the future normal or orthotropic ureter will drain at the corner of the trigone. That portion of the mesonephric duct cranial to the origin of the ureteric bud, on the other hand, migrates caudally and medially, crossing over the ureter to form the vas deferens in males and Gartner's duct in females; the latter duct lies along the lateral vaginal wall from the cervix to the hymen. It is thus clear that an abnormal cranial origin of the ureteric bud or, more commonly, the development of a duplicated bud cranial to the normal origin will result in insertion of that ureter medial and caudal to the orthotopic orifice at the trigone and that that ureter may open into any of the derivatives of the mesonephric duct (Figure 20-15). It is this embryologic origin that underlies the Weigert-Meyer rule, which states that the upper pole ureter lies medial and caudal to the lower pole orthotopic orifice, a direction that can extend beyond the confines of the bladder to the derivatives of the mesonephric duct in males and females. For this reason, an ectopic ureter in a male never inserts below the insertion of the ejaculatory duct, always lying above the external sphincter, and thus never leads to urinary incontinence. In females, on the other hand, the ectopic ureter can terminate anywhere along the wall of the vagina to the level of the perineum, below the external sphincter, and can cause dribbling (but not enuresis), alternating with periods of complete dryness. Urinary dribbling, therefore, would be the result of ureteral ectopia and would not be secondary to the presence of the ureterocele (**Option (A) is false**).

Although ureteral ectopia obeys the simple Weigert-Meyer rule based on the embryologic principles outlined above, dilatation of the intramural portion (ureterocele) of either an orthotopic or an ectopic ureter is an independent process, and its etiology is not known. It is hypothesized that this dilatation occurs as a result of stenosis of the ureteral orifice or that it occurs as a result of abnormal supporting structures, such as abnormal collagen and musculature in the wall of the distal ureter.

Various terms are used, sometimes interchangeably, to describe ureteroceles, and these can be confusing if not initially defined. "Simple" ureterocele is a term traditionally applied to dilatation of the orthotopically located ureter of a single system, associated with a normally functioning unit and showing a typical "cobra-head" appearance on the excretory urogram. This type of ureterocele is more common in adults than in children. "Ectopic" ureterocele, on the other hand, is associated with an abnormally positioned ureteral orifice, displaced caudally and medially with respect to the trigonal orifice; it is most often identified in children, typically, but not always, in association with the upper pole of a duplicated system. The orifice of the ureterocele can be small or stenotic, normal in size or patulous; reflux into the ureterocele and its ureter may or may not occur.

Recently, the Committee on Terminology, Nomenclature, and Classification of the American Academy of Pediatrics Section on Urology defined the terms as follows: a ureterocele located entirely within the bladder is identified as intravesical and corresponds to the simple ureterocele seen typically in adult patients, whereas one located entirely or partly at the

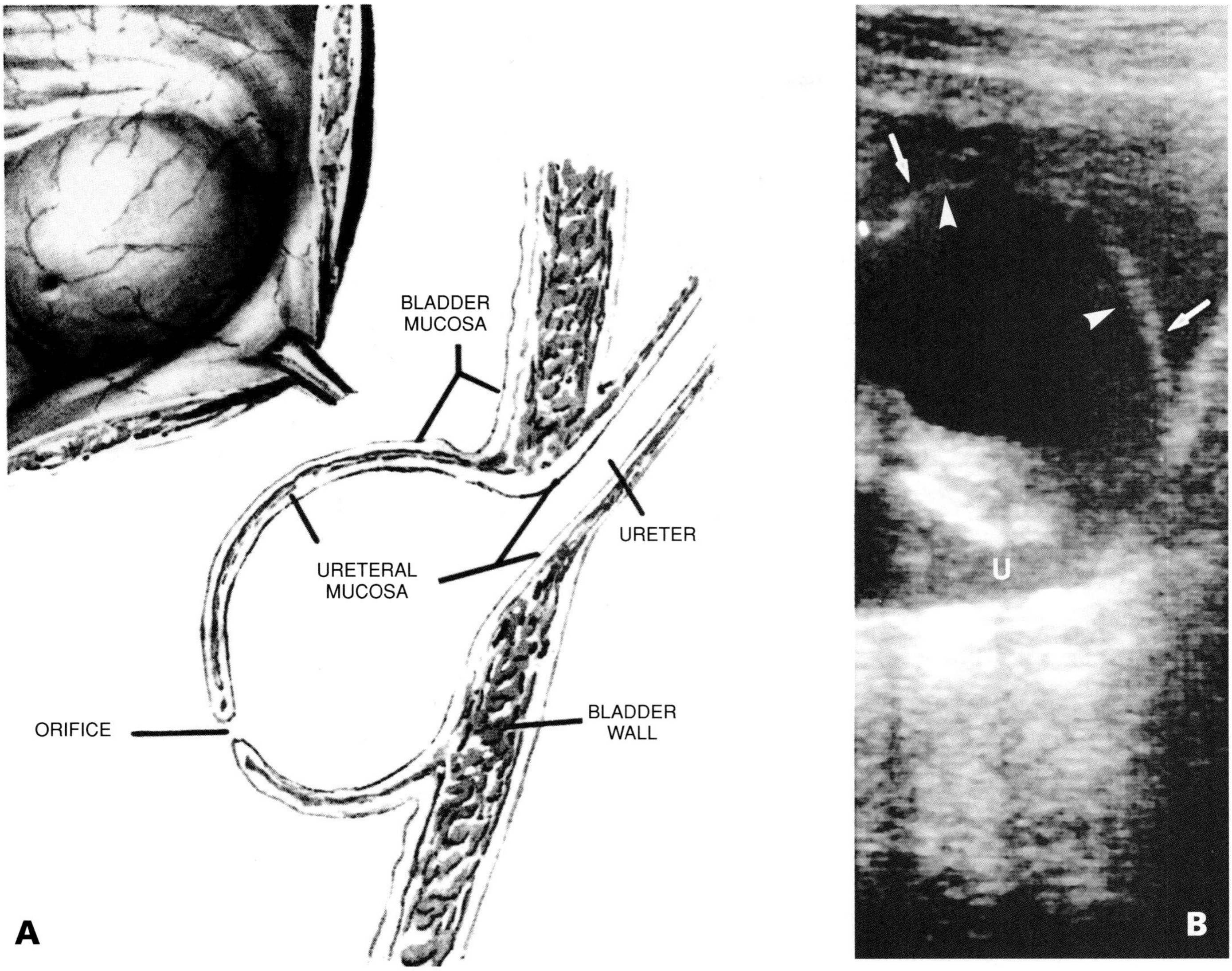

Figure 20-14. Intravesical ureterocele. (A) Pictorial representation of an intravesical ureterocele, outlining the appearance of the ureterocele protruding into the bladder and the relationship of its components to the bladder and ureteral walls. (Reprinted with permission from Netter et al. [9].) (B) Parasagittal sonogram demonstrating the urine-filled ureterocele and its continuity with the ureter (U); compare to illustration in panel A. The internal wall of the ureterocele is the continuation of ureteral mucosa (arrowheads), whereas the outer wall is the continuation of bladder mucosa (arrows), both stretched by the dilated distal ureter, or ureterocele.

bladder base or urethra is defined as ectopic and is related to an ectopically inserting ureter. Duplicated systems are defined as either incomplete (bifid pelvis or bifid ureter) or complete, in which two ureters drain separately. Ureteral orifices within this context are identified by the position of the subtended system: i.e., upper pole or lower pole orifices. Although a ureter can be ectopically located lateral to its normal insertion, a situation typically associated with reflux, the term "ectopic ureter" usually is reserved for ureters that insert abnormally caudally and medially. A single-system ureterocele, as the term implies, is associated with the ureter of a single-system kidney and can be intravesical, simple, or ectopic; a duplicated-system ureterocele is associated with a duplicated system, usually is ectopic and, in accordance with the Weigert-Meyer rule, subtends the upper pole ureter.

There are many variations in the presentation and symptoms caused by ureteroceles. Ureteroceles can be tense or relatively flaccid and can be compressed by a fully distended bladder; they can evert into their own ureter (Figure 20-16) or between the bladder musculature to resemble a paraureteral diverticulum at sonography or at radiography if filled with contrast material. Within the bladder, they can obstruct the orifice of the ipsilateral lower pole ureter (if from a duplicated system), the contralateral orifice(s), or the bladder outlet (if ectopic and prolapsing into the urethra, as in the test case). The most common abnormality in patients evaluated for urinary tract infections and who have complete ureteral duplication is reflux into the lower pole moiety. This reflux can occur if an adjacent ureterocele distorts the tunnel mechanism of the lower pole ureter. In the absence of such an effect, the cause of re-

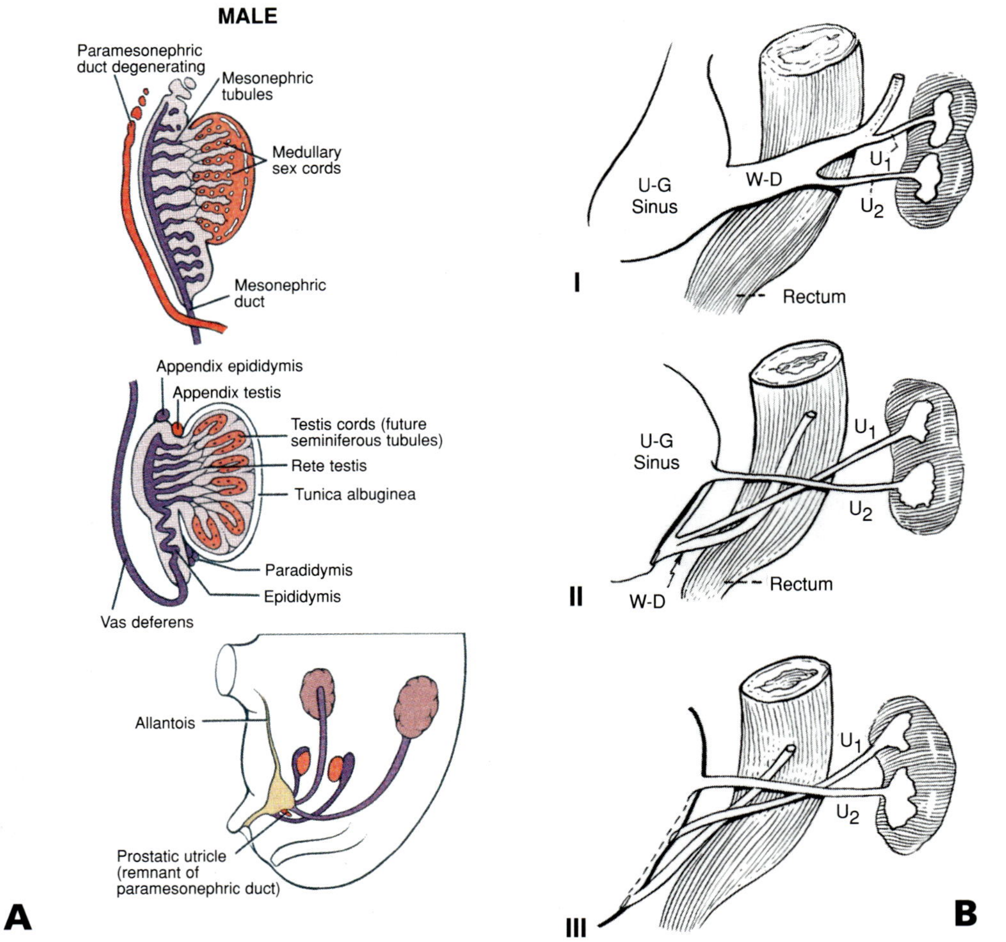

Figure 20-15. Ureteral development. (A) Diagrammatic representation of the developing anatomic relationships of the mesonephric duct and ureteral bud. The paramesonephric duct degenerates, although a small remnant can persist as the prostatic utricle. The portion of the mesonephric duct cranial to the ureteral bud is related to the developing gonad and migrates caudally, becoming the vas deferens and inserting in the prostatic urethra. (Reprinted with permission from Larsen [38].) (B) Diagrammatic representation of the development of orthotopic and ectopic ureters from a mesonephric duct or Wolffian duct. Diagram I shows that the lower pole or orthotopic ureter (U^2) originates from the Wolffian duct (W-D). The upper pole ureter (U^1) originates from an abnormal cranial location. Diagrams II and III show that as normal development of the Wolffian duct progresses, the upper pole ureter is carried caudally and medially. The caudal distance to which it is carried is dependent upon the distance cephalad to the orthotopic orifice from which it initially originates. U-G = urogenital. (Reprinted with permission from Gonzalez [3].)

flux into the lower pole of a duplicated system is thought to be an abnormal angle of insertion, similar to that occurring in a single system. In these cases, spontaneous resolution is usual if the reflux is mild to moderate (grades I to III); reimplantation may be needed if the reflux is severe (grades IV and V).

Approximately 80% of ectopic ureters subtend the upper pole of a duplicated system **(Option (B) is true)**; this proportion appears to be lower in Asians. Approximately 80% of ectopic ureters in girls drain the upper pole of a duplicated system, but in boys, the majority of ectopic ureters drain a single system **(Option (C) is true).** Interestingly, bilateral single-system ureteral ectopia is encountered more often in girls. The renal moiety drained by an ectopic ureter may be normal; in many patients, complete duplication is not associated with obstruction or reflux, and the resulting, uncomplicated duplication is of no clinical significance. However, there is often a variable degree of hydronephrosis and hydroureter, caused by obstruction, reflux, or a combination of the two, especially if present in combination with a ureterocele or severe degrees of ectopia. The parenchyma subtended by such a drainage system usually is dysplastic to a variable degree (Figure 20-17). These dysplastic changes can be the consequence of several mechanisms singly or in combination. Abnormally increased back pressure during renal development, such as that seen in some kidneys in patients with urethral valves, is one proposed mechanism. Another provocative theory advanced by Mackie and Stephens in 1975 suggests that a more distal location of the ureteral orifice from the trigone reflects a proportionally more cranial origin of the ectopic ureteral bud from the mesonephros and proportionally inadequate priming of the metanephric blastema that it encounters; the lack of response to the inductive mechanism leads to the development of a dysplastic and poorly functioning unit. The degree of dysplasia can be assessed at sonography by observing the lack of corticomedullary differentiation of the renal parenchyma, and the function can be further qualitatively or quantitatively evaluated via excretory urography or scintigraphy. At sonography, the degree of hydronephrosis of both upper and lower renal moieties, the characteristic course of the upper pole ureter medial to the lower pole pelvis, and the difference between the juxtaposed normal parenchyma of a lower pole and the dysplastic upper pole parenchyma can be demonstrated (Figure 20-17). Any of the renal units in duplicated systems can be affected by any other anomaly that can affect a single system, such as reflux, ureteropelvic junction obstruction, multicystic renal dysplasia, and neoplasms, such as nephrogenic rests (nephroblastomatosis) or frank Wilms' tumor. However, the majority of patients have symptoms of urinary tract infection.

In girls, urinary dribbling less frequently is an initial symptom and is distinguished from enuresis by the history of constant dampness, in contradistinction to episodes of incontinent urination with intermittent dryness. Purulent vaginal discharge is a less frequent sign of ureteral ectopia. In boys, insertion of the ureter along the course of the vas deferens, seminal vesicle, and ejaculatory duct can lead to recurrent epididymitis. Patients with large ureteroceles can have symptoms of infravesical obstruction or frank perineal prolapse of the ureterocele in girls. Patients diagnosed incidentally through routine prenatal sonography benefit by institution of prompt prophylaxis and treatment.

The imaging evaluation usually involves the typical examinations requested for patients with urinary tract infections. At

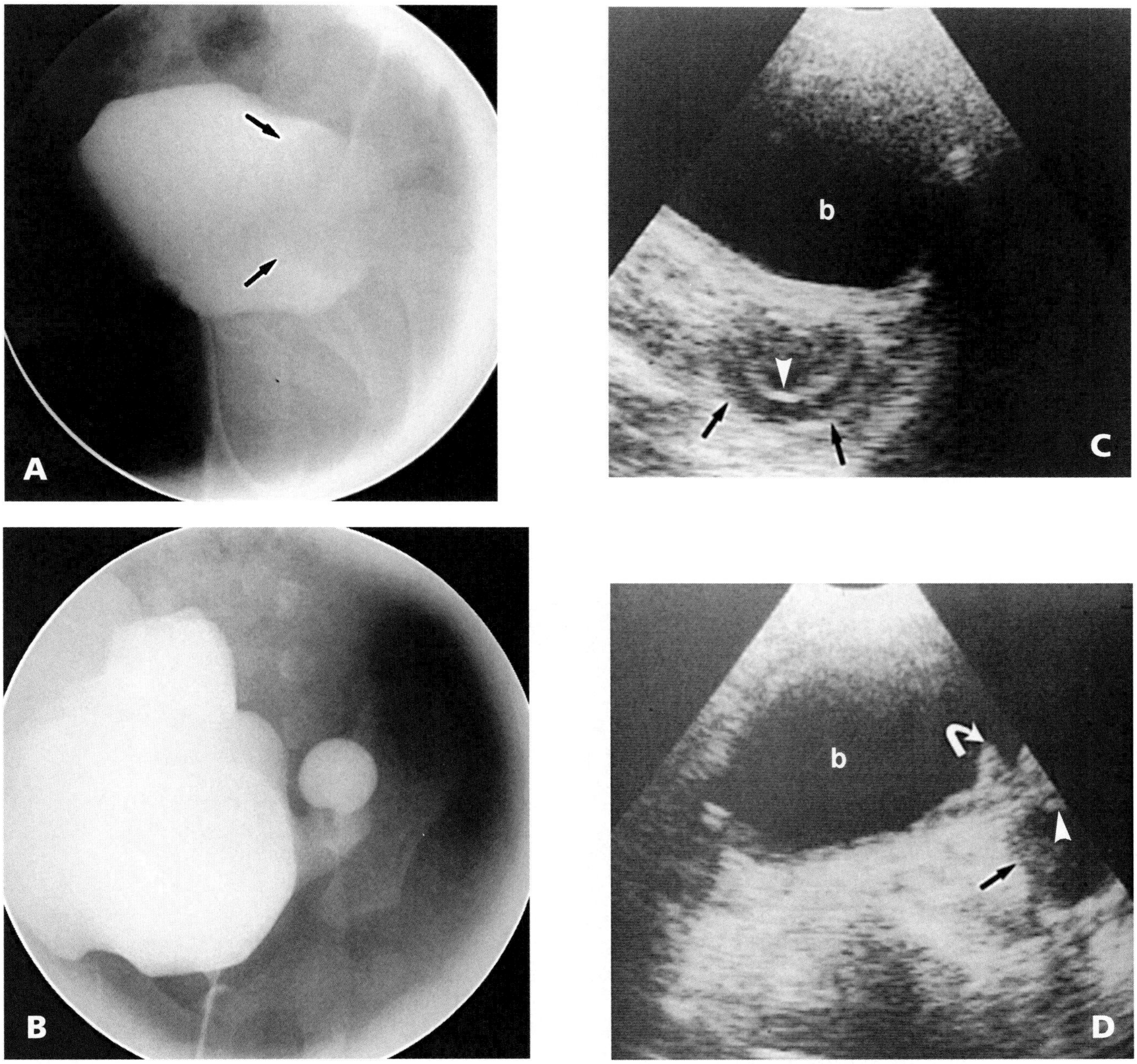

Figure 20-16. Everting ureterocele. (A and B) VCUG. (A) Oblique image in a neonate with a duplicated system and an upper pole ureterocele. The characteristic, smooth filling defect of the ureterocele is visible (arrows). (B) Anteroposterior image taken a few minutes subsequent to the image shown in panel A. The ureterocele has everted into its own ureter, resembling a diverticulum. (C and D) Sonography. (C) A sonogram of the bladder after VCUG demonstrates an everted ureterocele (arrowhead) within the dilated ureter (arrows). There is no ureterocele within the bladder (b). (D) A few seconds later, marked irregularity of the bladder (b) wall (curved arrow) was visible adjacent to the ureter (arrow)-ureterocele (arrowhead) complex.

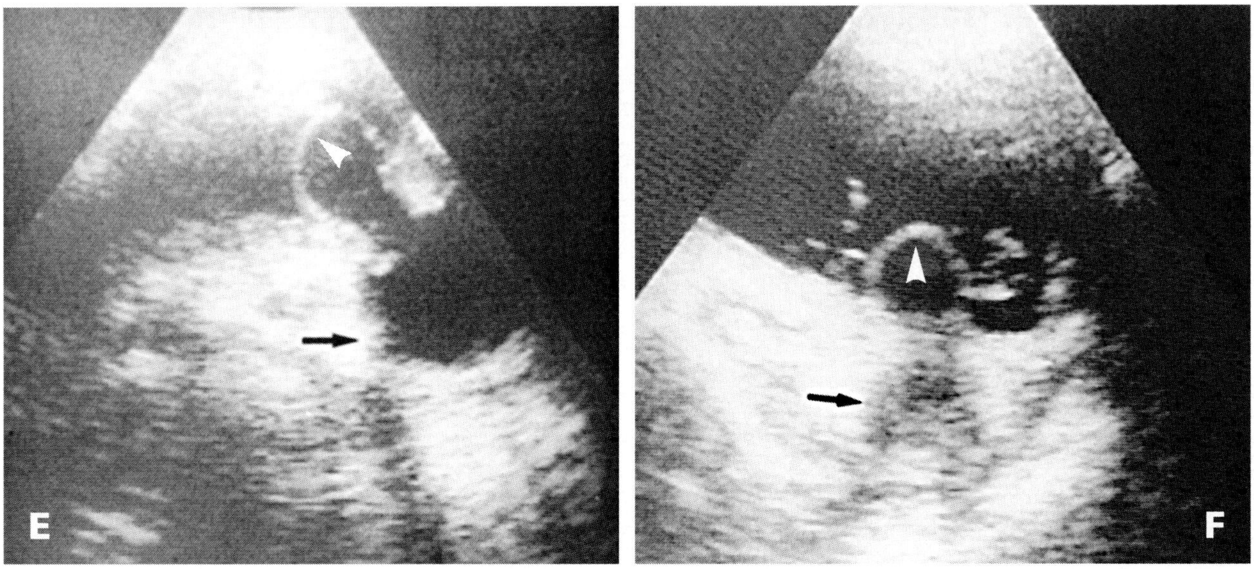

Figure 20-16 (Continued). Everting ureterocele. (E and F) Sonography. (E) A few seconds later, the ureterocele (arrowhead) protruded into the bladder base from the ureter (arrow). (F) A few seconds later, ureteral jets identified the intravesical intrusion of the ureterocele (arrowhead). The arrow indicates the ureter.

VCUG, a ureterocele is seen as a filling defect that can be mobile and that can be obscured by full bladder dissension or by the density of the contrast material; therefore, it is best demonstrated early in the course of the examination (**Option (D) is false**). If reflux occurs into the ureterocele, it will fill with contrast material, which can extend cephalad to outline the ureter and its pelvicalyceal system. Eversion of the ureterocele into its ureter can cause an initially confusing situation (Figure 20-16); paraureteral inversion through a weakness in the detrusor mechanism can simulate a Hutch diverticulum. For this reason, early fluoroscopic observation and correlation with other imaging results are essential. An ectopic infravesical ureter can be visible during voiding or may be demonstrated only after repeated episodes of voiding during cyclic VCUG (Figure 20-18).

At sonography, the dysplastic renal unit drained by an ectopic ureter, with or without ureterocele, can be large, hydronephrotic, and obvious. The ureterocele can be easily shown as an intravesical dilatation of the distal ureter and further identified by discovery of the urinary jet (Figure 20-16). However, not all cases demonstrate obvious findings; there may be little

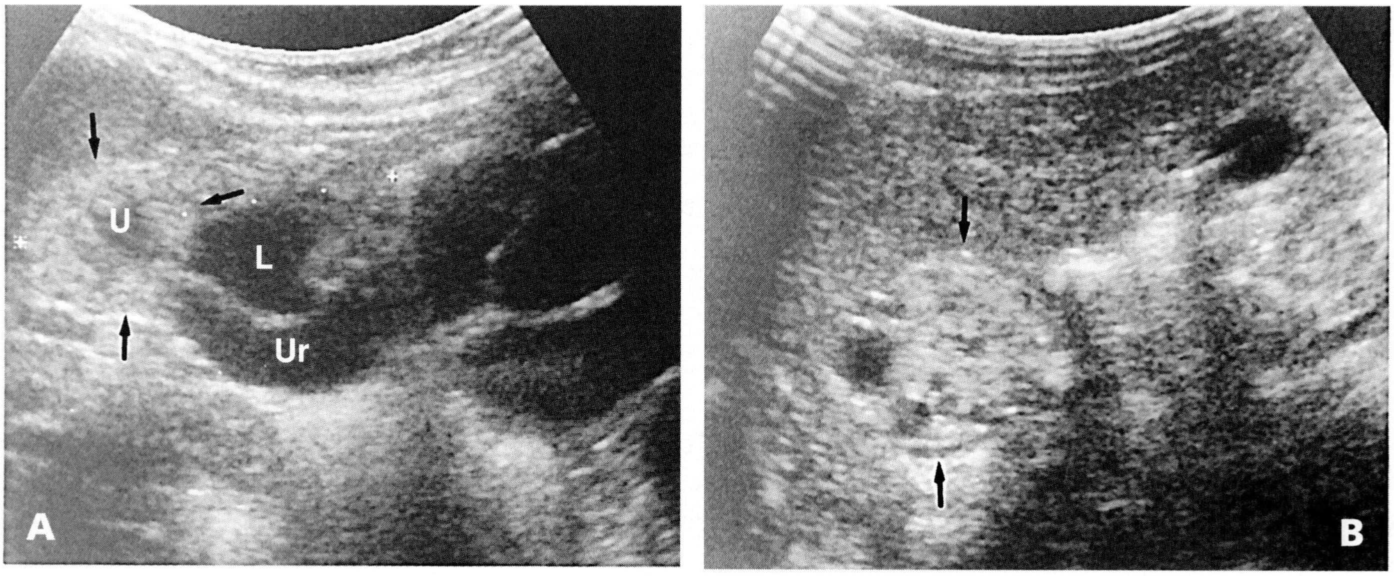

Figure 20-17. Duplicated system. (A) Longitudinal sonographic image of a right kidney (between the calipers) in a patient with a duplicated system and hydronephrosis of both moieties. Note the upper pole pelvis (U) and the typical course of the upper pole ureter (Ur) medial to the lower pole pelvis (L). Despite the marked dilatation and tortuosity of the upper pole ureter, hydronephrosis of the upper moiety is minimal. The parenchyma of the upper pole (arrows) is markedly abnormal, hyperechoic, and lacking in corticomedullary differentiation. (B) Transverse sonographic image of the upper pole (arrows) showing multiple peripheral cysts within hyperechoic parenchyma lacking corticomedullary differentiation; these are the sonographic characteristics of renal dysplasia.

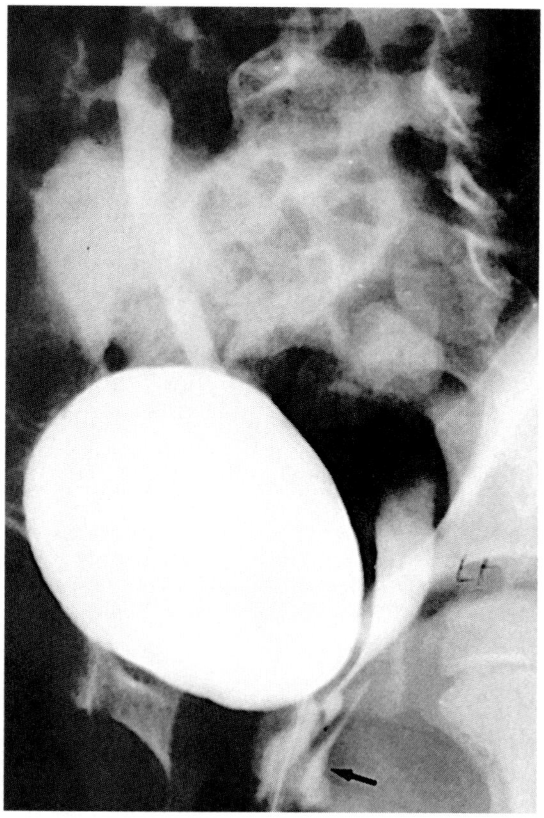

Figure 20-18. Reflux into ectopic infravesical ureter. An oblique radiograph taking during voiding in cyclic VCUG shows reflux into an ectopic ureter inserting at the urethral sphincter. A small amount of contrast material outlines the vaginal lumen (arrow). Reflux into the contralateral, orthotopic ureter is incidentally noted.

or no hydroureteronephrosis, a ureterocele may not be present, and the renal moiety may be severely dysplastic, very small, or atretic. At sonography, the adrenal gland should be identified, and the underlying parenchyma should be carefully inspected for any signs of a small, dysplastic upper renal unit in all patients with urinary tract infections or other symptoms suggestive of ureteral ectopia (Figure 20-19). Multicystic dilatation of the seminal vesicle(s) can be a clue to ectopic ureteral insertion in boys (Figure 20-20).

Excretory urography may demonstrate the following findings: (1) delayed function of the upper moiety when obstructed; (2) mass effect on the lower pole ureter by the dilated upper pole ureter, which displaces the ureter laterally from its normal position overlying the transverse processes of the lumbar vertebrae; and (3) abnormal axis of the lower pole calcyes, which point to the contralateral hip and ipsilateral shoulder, the result of displacement by the dilated upper pole moiety (Figure 20-21). Excretory urography is no longer used routinely to evaluate patients in most centers, because anatomic and functional information can be fully delineated with a combination of sonography and scintigraphy.

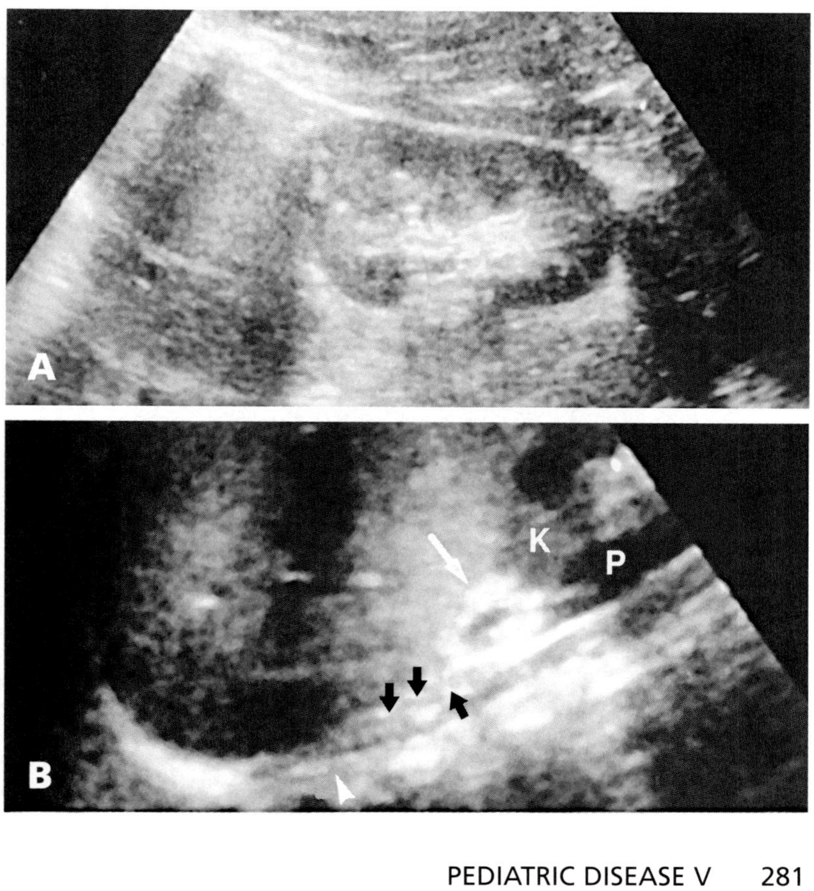

Figure 20-19. Small, dysplastic upper moiety. (A) A posterior sonogram of the left kidney in a 5-year-old girl with a urinary tract infection appears normal. (B) A coronal sonogram along the left flank outlines the diminutive upper pole (white arrow) lying below the ipsilateral adrenal gland (black arrows), medial to the diaphragmatic crus (arrowhead). K = normal lower pole of left kidney; P = psoas.

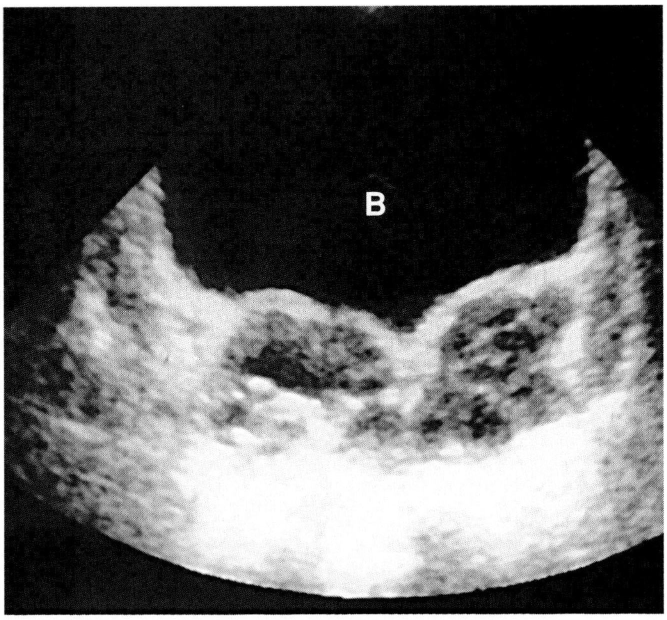

Figure 20-20. Ectopic ureteral insertion into seminal vesicles. A transverse sonogram through the bladder (B) in an adolescent boy with epididymitis shows bilateral enlargement of the seminal vesicles and multiple cysts. (Reprinted with permission from Hernanz-Schulman et al. [4].)

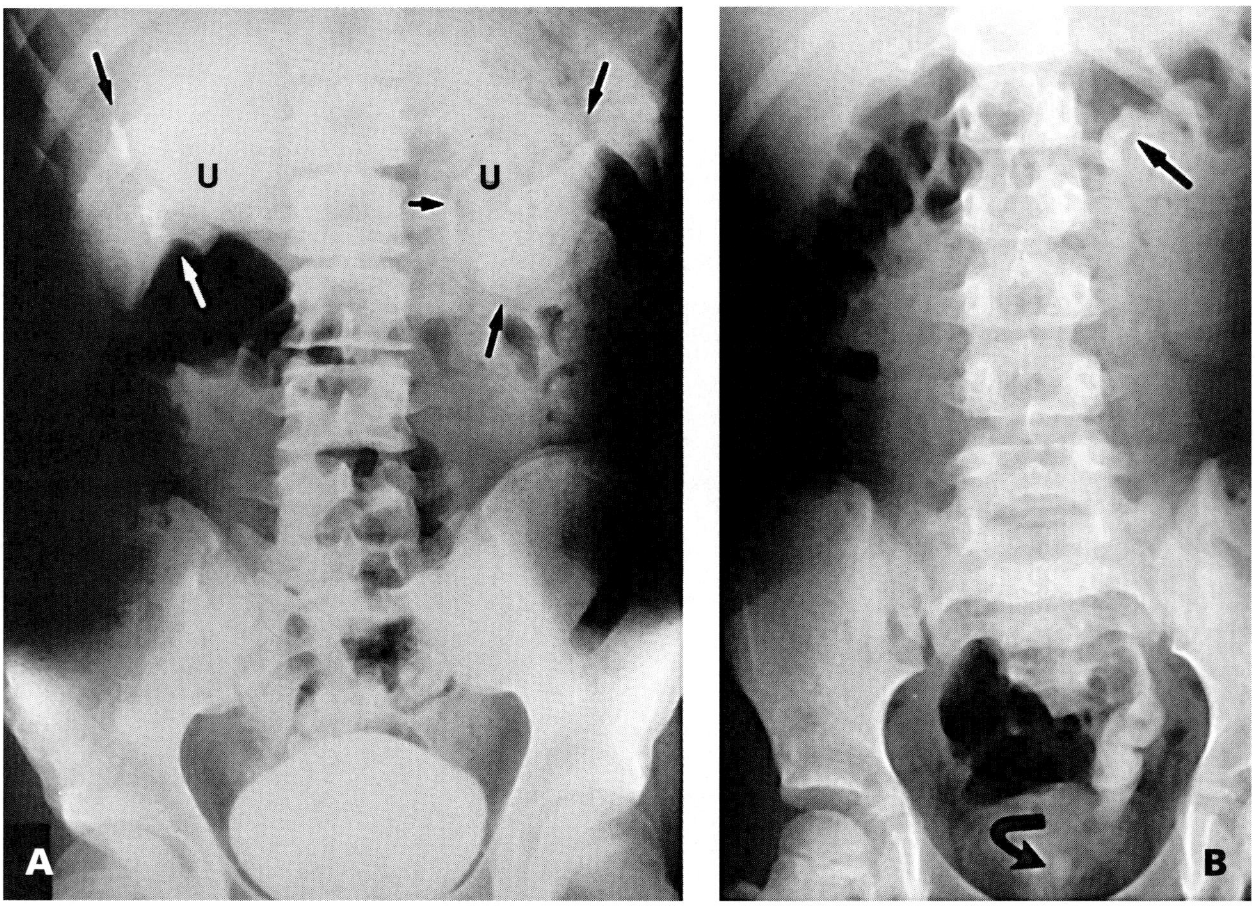

Figure 20-21. Excretory urography findings in patients with an obstructed upper pole. (A) Same patient as in Figure 20-20. A 4-hour radiograph shows an abnormal axis of the lower pole moieties (long arrows), a result of the "missing" upper pole calyces. The lower pole ureter is visible on the left (short arrow) and shows typical displacement lateral to the transverse processes, a result of the mass effect of the dilated upper pole ureter. At 4 hours, there is contrast material in the markedly dilated right upper pole pelvis (U) but none in the left upper pole pelvis (U). (Reprinted with permission from Hernanz-Schulman et al. [4].) (B) Same patient as in Figure 20-19. A 4-hour radiograph shows that contrast material has been excreted from the normal right kidney and left lower pole. However, the obstructed left upper pole is visible (straight arrow), as is the entire, obstructed upper pole ureter, terminating in a diminutive ureterocele at the bladder base (curved arrow). These findings could easily have been missed without delayed films.

SUGGESTED READINGS

URETERAL ECTOPIA AND URETEROCELE

1. Ben-Ami T, Gayer G, Hertz M, Lotan D, Boichis H. The natural history of reflux into the lower pole of duplicated collecting systems: a controlled study. Pediatr Radiol 1989; 19:308–310
2. Brown T, Mandell J, Lebowitz RL. Neonatal hydronephrosis in the era of sonography. AJR 1987; 148:959–963
3. Gonzalez ET Jr. Anomalies of the renal pelvis and ureter. In: Kelalis PP, King L, Belman A (eds). Clinical pediatric urology. 3rd ed. Vol. 1. St. Louis: WB Saunders; 1992:530–579
4. Hernanz-Schulman M, Genieser N, Ambrosino M, Hanna M. Bilateral duplex ectopic ureters terminating in the seminal vesicles: sonographic and CT diagnosis. Urol Radiol 1989; 11:49–52
5. Lubat E, Hernanz-Schulman M, Genieser NB, Ambrosino MM, Teele RL. Sonography of the simple and complicated ipsilateral fused kidney. J Ultrasound Med 1989; 8:109–114
6. Mackie GG, Stephens FD. Duplex kidneys: a correlation of renal dysplasia with position of the ureteral orifice. J Urol 1975; 114:274–280
7. Mandell J, Bauer SB, Colodny AH, Lebowitz RL, Retik AB. Ureteral ectopia in infants and children. J Urol 1981; 126:219–222
8. Mandell J, Colodny AH, Lebowitz R, Bauer SB, Retik AB. Ureteroceles in infants and children. J Urol 1980; 123:921–926
9. Netter FH, Shapter RK, Yonkman FF. Ciba collection of medical illustrations: kidneys, ureters and urinary bladder. Vol. 6. East Hanover, NJ: Novartis Medical Education; 1979:221–249
10. Share JC, Lebowitz RL. The unsuspected double collecting system on imaging studies and at cystoscopy. AJR 1990; 155:561–564
11. Share JC, Lebowitz RL. Ectopic ureterocele without ureteral and calyceal dilatation (ureterocele disproportion): findings on urography and sonography. AJR 1989; 152:567–571
12. Winters D, Lebowitz R. Importance of prenatal detection of hydronephrosis of the upper pole. AJR 1990; 155:125–129

URETHRAL VALVES

13. Bloom DA, Lebowitz RL, Bauer SB. Correlation of cystographic bladder morphology and neuroanatomy in boys with posterior urethral valves. Pediatr Radiol 1997; 27:553–556
14 Cherrie RJ, Leach GE, Raz S. Obstructing urethral valve in a woman: a case report. J Urol 1983; 129:1051–1052
15. Cuckow PM, Dinneen MD, Risdon RA, Ransley PG, Duffy PG. Long-term renal function in the posterior urethral valves, unilateral reflux and renal dysplasia syndrome. J Urol 1997; 158:1004–1007
16. Dinneen MD, Duffy PG. Posterior urethral valves. Br J Urol 1996; 78: 275–281
17. Donnelly LF, Gylys-Morin VM, Wacksman J, Gelfand MJ. Unilateral vesicoureteral reflux: association with protected renal function in patients with posterior urethral valves. AJR 1997; 168:823–826
18. Good CD, Vinnicombe SJ, Minty IL, King AD, Mather SJ, Dicks-Mireaux C. Posterior urethral valves in male infants and newborns: detection with US of the urethra before and during voiding. Radiology 1996; 198:387–391
19. Hendren W. Urinary undiversion—refunctionalizaton of the previously diverted urinary tract. In: Ashcraft K (ed). Pediatric urology. Philadelphia: WB Saunders; 1990:211–255
20. Holmdahl G. Bladder dysfunction in boys with posterior urethral valves. Scand J Urol Nephrol Suppl 1997; 188:1–36
21. Holmdahl G, Sillen U, Bachelard M, Hansson E, Hermansson G, Hjalmas K. The changing urodynamic pattern in valve bladders during infancy. J Urol 1995; 153:463–467
22. Holmdahl G, Sillen U, Bertilsson M, Hermansson G, Hjalmas K. Natural filling cystometry in small boys with posterior urethral valves: unstable valve bladders become stable during sleep. J Urol 1997; 158:1017–1021
23. Johnston JH, Kulatilake AE. The sequelae of posterior urethral valves. Br J Urol 1971; 43:743–748
24. Kaefer M, Keating MA, Adams MC, Rink RC. Posterior urethral valves, pressure pop-offs and bladder function. J Urol 1995; 154:708–711
25. Kaplan GW, Scherz HC. Infravesical obstruction. In: Kelalis PP, King L, Belman AP (eds). Clinical pediatric urology. 3rd ed. Vol 2. St. Louis: Harcourt; 1993:821–864
26. Pfister C, Wagner L, Dacher JN, Liard A, Boillot B, Mitrofanoff P. Long-term bladder dysfunction in boys with posterior urethral valves. Eur J Pediatr Surg 1996; 6:222–224
27. Pompino HJ, Bodecker RH, Trammer UA. Urethral valves during the first year of life—a retrospective, multicenter study. Eur J Pediatr Surg 1995; 5:3–8

NEUROGENIC DYSFUNCTION OF THE BLADDER

28. Bauer S. Anamolies of the upper urinary tract. In: Walsh P, Retik A, Stamey T, Vaughan EJ (eds). Campbell's urology. Philadelphia: WB Saunders; 1992:1357–1442
29. Bauer S. Neurogenic vesical dysfunction in children. In: Walsh P, Retik A, Stamey T, Vaughan EJ (eds). Campbell's urology. Philadelphia: WB Saunders; 1992:1634–1668
30. Bellinger M. Myelomeningocele and neuropathic bladder. In: Gillenwater J, Grayhack J, Howards S, Duckett J (eds). Adult and pediatric urology. St. Louis: CV Mosby; 1996:2489–2528

URETHRAL POLYPS

31. Arteaga J, Tran-Minh VA, Pracros JP, Mollard P. Sonographic diagnosis of polyp of the prostatic urethra in children. J Clin Ultrasound 1993; 21:188–193
32. Barzilai M, Shinawi M, Ish-Shalom N, Mecz Y, Peled N, Lurie A. A fibroepithelial urethral polyp protruding into the base of the bladder: sonographic diagnosis. Urol Int 1996; 57:129–131
33. Caro PA, Rosenberg HK, Snyder HM. Congenital urethral polyp. AJR 1986; 147:1041–1042
34. De Castro R, Campobasso P, Belloli G, Pavanello P. Solitary polyp of posterior urethra in children: report on seventeen cases. Eur J Pediatr Surg 1993; 3:92–96
35. Gleason PE, Kramer SA. Genitourinary polyps in children. Urology 1994; 44:106–109
36. Herman TE, Siegel MJ. Special imaging casebook. Congenital polyps of prostatic urethra. J Perinatol 1997; 17:500–502
37. Klee LW, Rink RC, Gleason PE, Ganesan GS, Mitchell ME, Heifetz SA. Urethral polyp presenting as interlabial mass in young girls. Urology 1993; 41:132–133
38. Larsen WJ. Human embryology. New York: Churchill Livingston; 1993: 261–310
39. Raviv G, Leibovitch I, Hanani J, Hertz M, Goldwasser B, Jonas P. Hematuria and voiding disorders in children caused by congenital urethral polyps. Principles of diagnosis and management. Eur Urol 1993; 23:382–385
40. Walsh IK, Keane PF, Herron B. Benign urethral polyps. Br J Urol 1993; 72:937–938

BLADDER RHABDOMYOSARCOMA

41. Newton WA Jr, Soule EH, Hamoudi AB, et al. Histopathology of childhood sarcomas, Intergroup Rhabdomyosarcoma Studies I and II: clinicopathologic correlation. J Clin Oncol 1988; 6:67–75

Lisa H. Lowe, M.D.
Marta Hernanz-Schulman, M.D.

Cat Scratch Disease

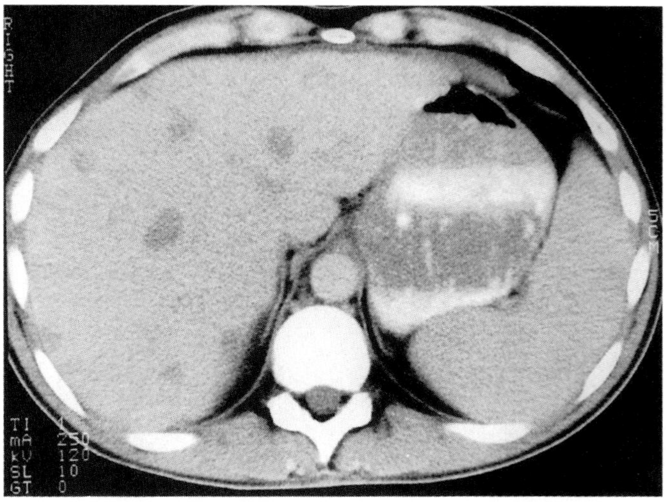

Figure 21-1

Question 98

This 12-year-old boy had persistent abdominal pain and low-grade fever for 1 week. A contrast-enhanced abdominal CT image was obtained; you are shown an axial image of the liver (Figure 21-1).

Likely explanations for the CT findings include:

(A) primary hepatic tumor
(B) metastases
(C) infection
(D) ductal dilatation
(E) unopacified veins

The CT image in the test case (Figure 21-1) shows multiple, round, hypodense areas throughout the liver (Figure 21-2). Because the lesions vary in size and are multiple, infection and metastatic disease are the most likely disease processes.

Hepatic metastases in children are most often attributable to neuroblastoma, Wilms' tumor, lymphoma, and leukemia. The imaging appearance of metastatic disease is variable, although most metastases are multiple, predominantly hypoechoic on sonography (Figure 21-3), and of a low density and

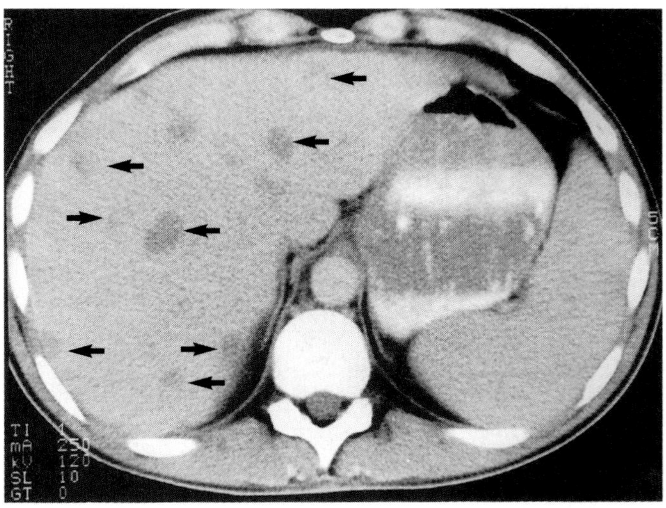

Figure 21-2 (Same as Figure 21-1). Cat scratch disease. An axial CT image of the liver after administration of contrast material reveals multiple, small, well-defined, low-density lesions (arrows) scattered throughout the liver.

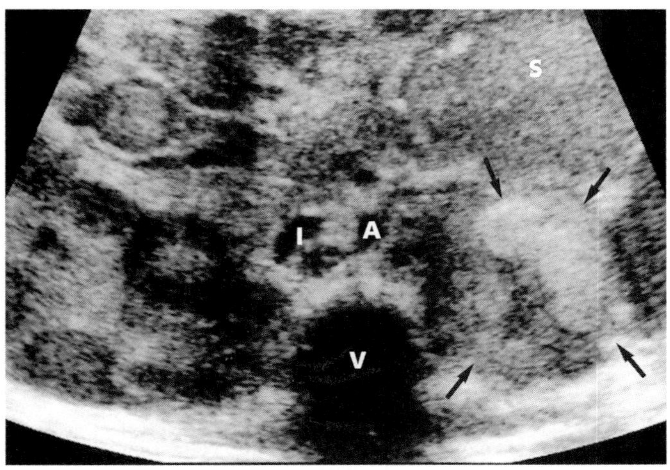

Figure 21-3. Metastatic neuroblastoma. A transverse abdominal sonogram reveals numerous heterogeneous hepatic lesions. The primary lesion (arrows) in the left adrenal gland is of mixed echogenicity. A = aorta; I = inferior vena cava; S = spleen; V = vertebra.

often peripherally enhancing on CT (**Option (B) is true**) (Figures 21-4). Involvement of both the liver and the spleen is distinctly unusual, except in leukemia and lymphoma. Sonography is most useful in the follow-up of patients with previously normal CT or MRI. CT usually is considered more sensitive than sonography and is the most common imaging modality used to detect metastatic disease. MRI is at least as sensitive as CT, with lesions most often having a low signal intensity on T1-weighted images and a high signal intensity on T2-weighted images. MRI and sonography have the advantage of demonstrating a pathologic process in multiple planes, a feature that is often helpful in assessing adjacent organ invasion by large masses. The choice between CT and MRI may be more a matter of availability and convenience than a difference in lesion detection capability. Although most hepatic metastases are discrete, leukemia, lymphoma, and neuroblastoma may diffusely infiltrate the liver (Figure 21-5). Diffuse hepatic metastases are difficult to detect; findings include architectural distortion and heterogeneous enhancement after intravenous contrast agent administration.

A variety of hepatic infections, ranging from viral to parasitic, occur in children. The imaging appearance varies with the specific infection. Cat scratch disease and fungal infections are most often seen as multiple, small, hypoechoic and hypodense lesions with peripheral enhancement after intravenous contrast material administration (**Option (C) is true**). The diagnosis of cat scratch disease was made in the test patient by liver biopsy and a positive skin test. The patient recovered with antibiotic treatment.

Although primary hepatic tumors are the third most common abdominal malignancy in children, they account for only 5% to 6% of solid abdominal neoplasms. The most common primary hepatic neoplasms are hepatoblastoma and hepatocellular carcinoma. Both are usually large at presentation, are twice as common in the right lobe, and are solitary in about 80% of children. The lesions in the test case are multiple and small (**Option (A) is false**).

Hepatoblastoma presents with a palpable upper abdominal mass, weight loss, and nausea or vomiting. Precocious puberty occasionally is observed. A persistently and markedly elevated

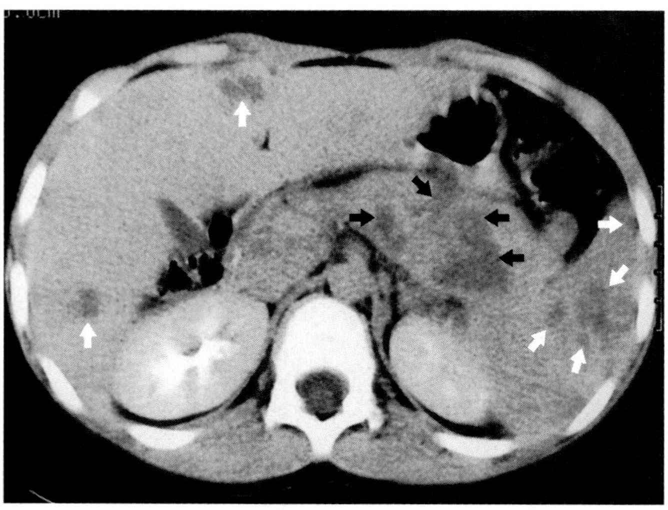

Figure 21-4. Lymphoma. An axial CT image of the liver during the late portal venous phase reveals multiple low-attenuation lesions (white arrows) throughout the liver and spleen. Necrotic peripancreatic nodes (black arrows) can be seen as well.

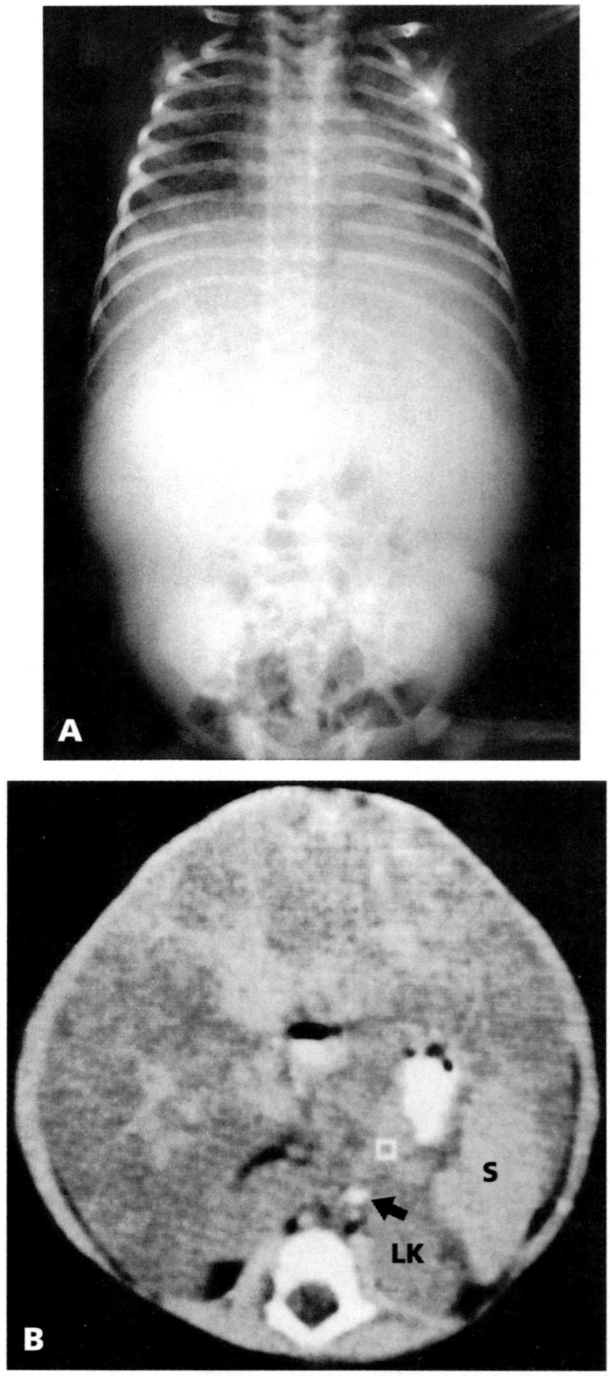

Figure 21-5. Neuroblastoma. (A) A radiograph of the chest and abdomen falsely suggests hepatosplenomegaly displacing bowel into the lower abdomen and pelvis. (B) A noncontrast CT image shows marked hepatic enlargement and architectural distortion consistent with diffuse involvement of the liver by metastatic disease. Calcification (arrow) in the left adrenal gland denotes the primary site of disease. The spleen (S) and the left kidney (LK) appear normal. The image was filmed with an inadvertent cursor over the left abdomen.

alpha-fetoprotein level is seen in over 70% of cases. Coarse calcifications or an osseous matrix is encountered in approximately 20% of cases. Sonography shows a large, heterogeneous echogenic mass (Figure 21-6); occasionally, cystic areas attributable to tissue necrosis are observed. CT demonstrates a hypointense tumor with peripheral rim enhancement. T1-weighted MRI most frequently shows a heterogeneous hypointense mass with hyperintense foci (hemorrhage). Likewise, T2-weighted MRI demonstrates a heterogeneous hyperintense mass with hypointense bands attributable to fibrous septae.

Hepatocellular carcinomas in children usually occur after the age of 4 years. They can be associated with paraneoplastic syndromes, such as sexual precocity, hypoglycemia, hypercalcemia, and carcinoid syndrome. These tumors can be associated with inborn errors of metabolism, such as tyrosinosis, galactosemia, type I glycogen storage disease (von Gierke's disease), and biliary atresia. These tumors invade the portal vein, hepatic vein, and occasionally the bile ducts. The liver frequently is very large, and there can be associated ascites. Sonographically, these tumors frequently appear as large hyperechoic tumors. CT demonstrates a hypodense mass or, rarely, an isodense mass. Enhancement during the arterial phase occurs in more than 80% of tumors. MRI shows a variable appearance. The tumors can appear isointense or hyperintense on T1-weighted images. Fre-

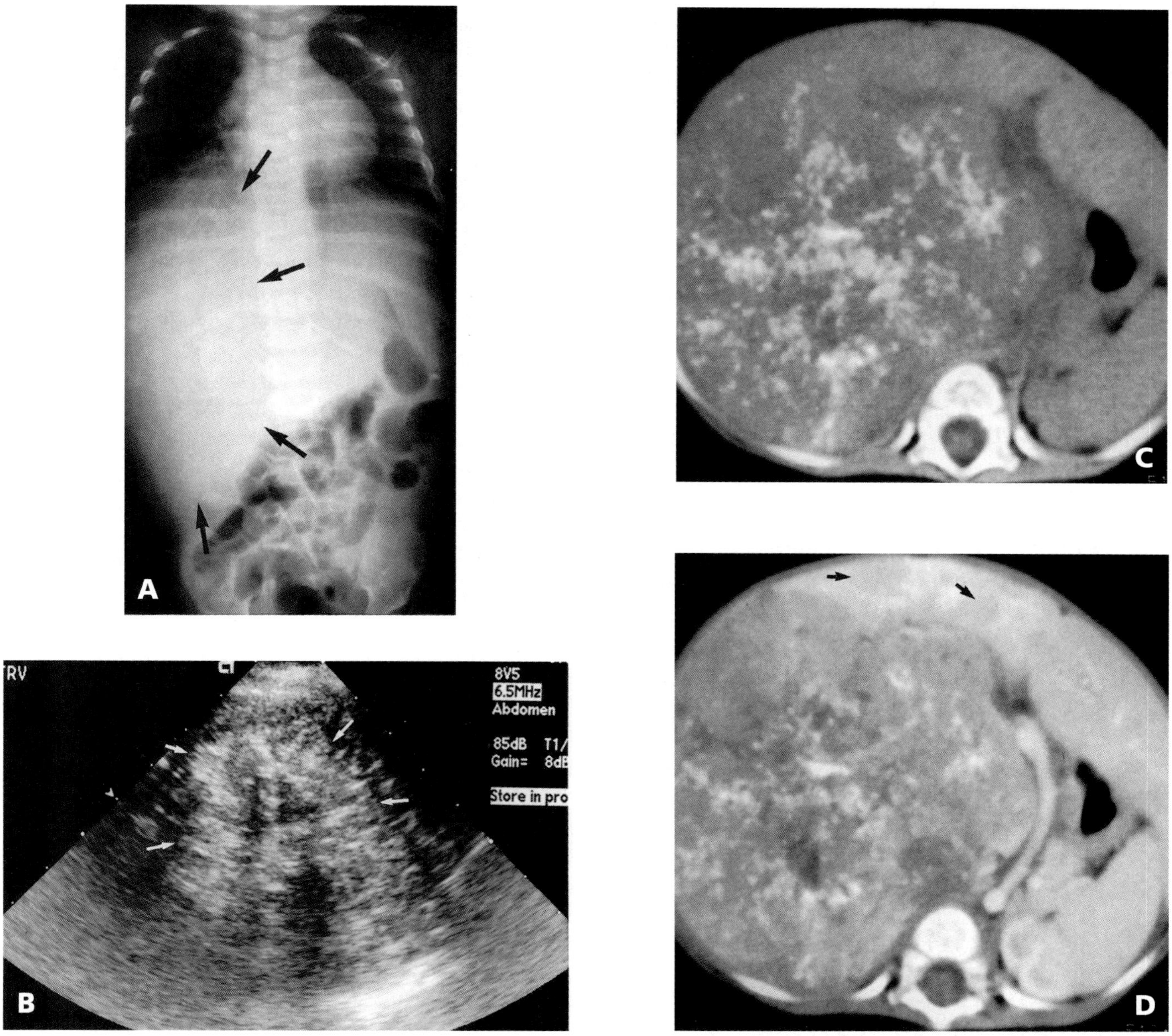

Figure 21-6. Hepatoblastoma. (A) An abdominal radiograph shows marked enlargement of the liver displacing bowel gas caudally and elevating the right hemidiaphragm. Extensive subtle calcifications (arrows) are present throughout the liver. (B) A transverse sonogram of the right hepatic lobe shows a large, heterogeneous mass (arrows) with central hypoechogenicity. (C and D) Axial CT images before (C) and after (D) intravenous administration of contrast material show a calcified, heterogeneously enhancing mass with areas of necrosis replacing the right lobe of the liver. Two subtle daughter nodules (arrows) can be seen in the medial segment of the left lobe of the liver.

quently, there is a well-defined capsule, which appears hypointense on T1-weighted images. Occasionally, an inner hypointense layer attributable to fibrous tissue and an outer hyperintense layer attributable to compressed blood vessels and bile ducts are demonstrated on T2-weighted images. Most lesions are hyperintense on T2-weighted images. Gadolinium chelate administration causes peripheral enhancement in less than 35%, central enhancement in less than 15%, mixed enhancement in 30%, and no enhancement in 20% of cases.

Biliary ductal dilatation can cause low-density areas in the liver. Enlarged ducts are seen as multiple, branching, tubular, or round structures that follow the portal triads and are not enhanced after contrast agent administration (Figure 21-7). These features are not seen in the test case **(Option (D) is false)**.

Ductal dilatation during childhood can be associated with a congenital abnormality or can occur secondary to acquired obstruction. The congenital abnormalities associated with bile duct dilatation are choledochal cyst and Caroli's disease. Caroli's disease involves nonobstructive saccular dilatation of the first- and second-order branches of the intrahepatic bile ducts. This condition also has been termed congenital biliary tract ectasia or congenital cystic dilatation of the biliary tree. The saccular dilatation of the bile ducts predisposes affected individuals to recurrent cholangitis, biliary lithiasis, liver abscess, and sepsis. This condition may or may not be associated with hepatic fibrosis. A definitive diagnosis of congenital biliary tract ectasia usually is established with noninvasive imaging modalities. These techniques demonstrate dilated intrahepatic bile ducts that communicate with large cystic areas. The common bile duct usually is normal in position and caliber. A choledochal cyst involves fusiform or diverticular dilatation of the common bile duct. In contradistinction to other cystic malformations of the biliary tract, a choledochal cyst typically is not associated with significant hepatic fibrosis and is only rarely associated with cystic renal disease. The diagnosis can be established readily with noninvasive cross-sectional imaging by demonstrating a disproportionately enlarged common bile duct with proximal dilatation and rapid peripheral tapering of the intrahepatic biliary ducts.

The etiologies of acquired biliary tract obstruction include tumors adjacent to the head of the pancreas, such as neuroblastomas in young children and lymphomas in older children. With these conditions, cross-sectional imaging will identify the extrahepatic mass and proportionate dilatation of the entire biliary tree. The higher the grade of obstruction, the more dilatation is identified. When biliary calculi are lodged in the distal common bile duct, cross-sectional imaging will show the same findings as those demonstrated for the adult population.

Unopacified veins are seen as tubular, branching structures that have a low attenuation during the arterial phase (Figure 21-8). However, the hepatic veins are enhanced during the portal venous phase of contrast enhancement. The lesions in the test case do not branch and are not enhanced with contrast agent administration **(Option (E) is false)**.

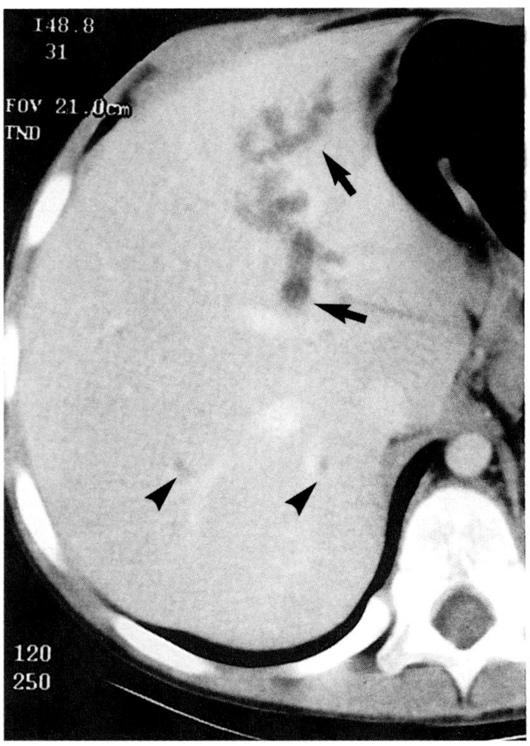

Figure 21-7. Dilated bile ducts. An axial CT image demonstrates a branching pattern of dilated bile ducts in the left lobe of the liver (arrows). Ducts in the right lobe also were slightly distended (arrowheads). Obstruction of ducts was attributable to choledocholithiasis.

Question 99

In children, features associated more often with the conventional than with the fibrolamellar form of hepatocellular carcinoma include:

(A) elevated serum alpha-fetoprotein levels
(B) association with type I glycogen storage disease
(C) younger mean patient age at diagnosis
(D) central calcifications
(E) portal vein invasion

Hepatocellular carcinoma is the second most common childhood hepatic malignancy, after hepatoblastoma, and represents about 25% of pediatric liver masses. There are two types of hepatocellular carcinoma, conventional and fibrolamellar, each distinct in presentation, imaging features, and prognosis. Conventional hepatocellular carcinoma is the most common primary liver tumor in children older than 4 years. It is more common in boys, involves the right lobe twice as often as the left, and has two peak ages of presentation, 4 to 5 years and 12 to 14 years. Serum alpha-fetoprotein levels are elevated in 55% to 80% of patients with conventional hepatocellular carcinoma and are normal in those with fibrolamellar hepatocellular carcinoma **(Option (A) is true)**. However, this finding is not a specific one, as about 90% of children with hepato-

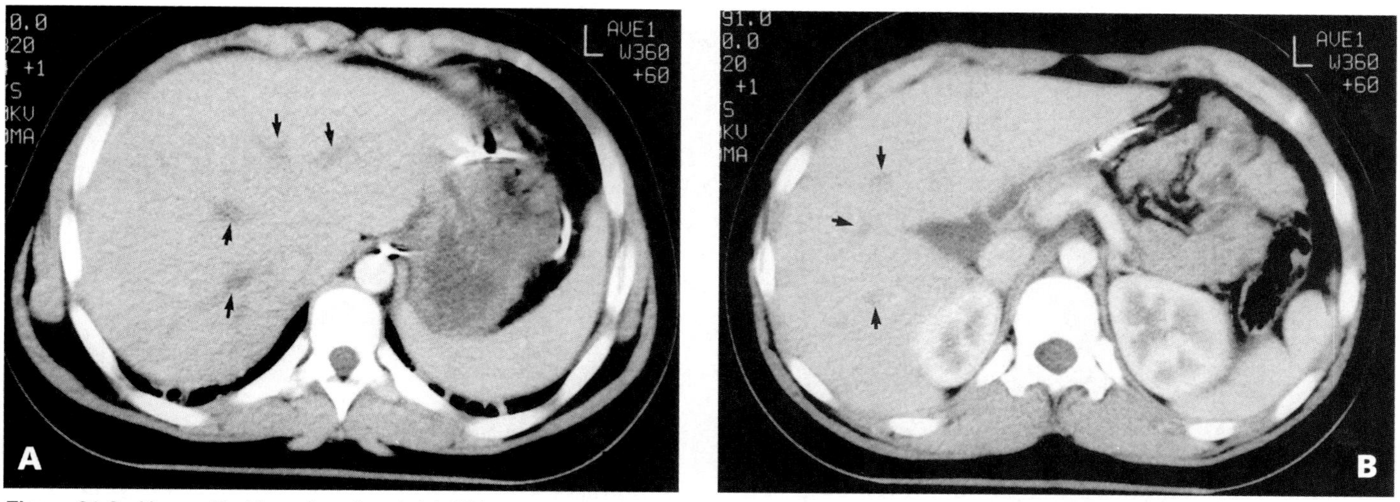

Figure 21-8. Unopacified hepatic veins. Axial CT images were obtained during the arterial phase after administration of the contrast agent bolus, through the superior liver (A) and at the level of the kidneys (B). Multiple branching, low-attenuation areas (arrows) converge toward the inferior vena cava on sequential images and should not be confused with a pathologic process. Other signs of arterial-phase imaging, including dense aortic opacification, enhancement of the renal cortex, and lack of opacification of the renal medulla, are demonstrated.

blastoma have elevated alpha-fetoprotein levels as well. Preexisting chronic liver diseases, such as type I glycogen storage disease, tyrosinemia, cystinosis, Wilson's disease, extrahepatic biliary atresia, alpha-1-antitrypsin deficiency, and giant cell hepatitis, are risk factors found in about 50% of patients with conventional hepatocellular carcinoma. These risk factors are not associated with the fibrolamellar form (**Option (B) is true**). Children with preexisting liver disease make up the majority of cases that occur during the second incidence peak.

Fibrolamellar hepatocellular carcinoma is distinct pathologically from conventional hepatocellular carcinoma. Histologic analysis demonstrates characteristic abundant fibrous bands arranged in a laminar fashion around hepatocytes with a deeply eosinophilic cytoplasm. It is most common in young adults, with the average age at presentation being 25 years (range, 5 to 69 years) (**Option (C) is true**). It typically occurs in otherwise normal livers and rarely is associated with necrosis or hemorrhage. Calcification occurs infrequently in conventional hepatocellular carcinomas and in 15% to 25% of fibrolamellar hepatocellular carcinomas (**Option (D) is false**). The most frequent pattern of calcification in fibrolamellar hepatocellular carcinoma is calcification within a stellate central scar.

The imaging appearance of conventional hepatocellular carcinomas is variable, although they are most often solitary and necrotic, may have daughter nodules, and invade the portal or hepatic veins in about 6% of cases (Figure 21-9). At sonography, they are most often hyperechoic, although they can be hypo- or isoechoic. On CT, the attenuation value of the tumor is typically lower than that of the adjacent liver (Figure 21-10), and most lesions enhance after contrast agent administration. Punctate calcifications are rarely seen on CT. Fifty percent of hepatocellular carcinomas are iso- or hyperintense on T1-weighted MRI sequences because of internal hemorrhage, hyperplasia, and steatosis. On T2-weighted sequences, more than 90% of lesions are hyperintense. Fibrolamellar hepatocellular carcinomas are usually solitary, more often involve the left lobe, and are hypervascular and well demarcated. They have satellite nodules in about 20% of cases and rarely invade the hepatic vasculature (**Option (E) is true**). Pathologically, most of these carcinomas are well circumscribed and are strikingly desmoplastic tumors, with calcifications and a fibrous central scar. The calcifications usually are central and stellate or have a trabecular formation. T1-weighted MRI frequently shows heterogeneous hypointensity; T2-weighted imaging shows a hyperintense character. The central scar appears hypointense on both T1- and T2-weighted images. The central scar that is seen with focal nodular hyperplasia frequently is hyperintense on T2-weighted images.

The prognosis of conventional hepatocellular carcinomas is poor; about 50% of patients have metastatic disease at presentation. Surgical resection is possible in only 30% of cases. The prognosis of fibrolamellar hepatocellular carcinomas is significantly better, with median survival averaging 45 to 60 months, compared with 6 months for patients diagnosed with conventional hepatocellular carcinomas.

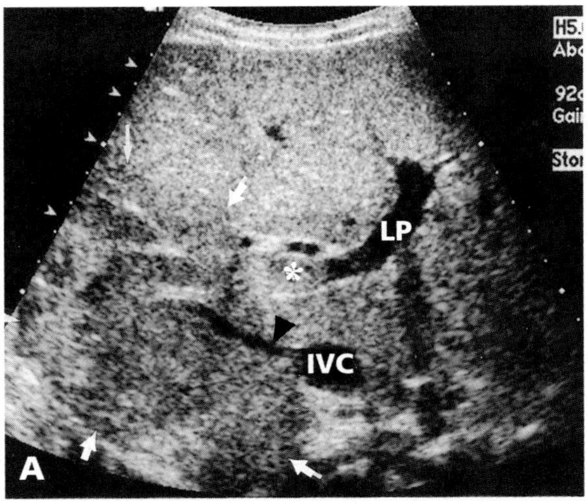

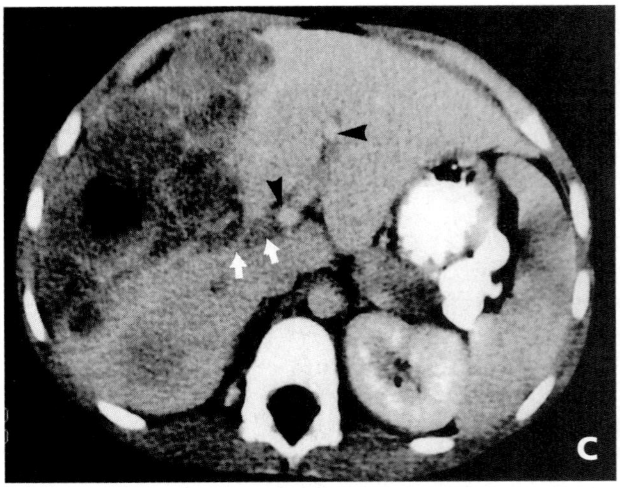

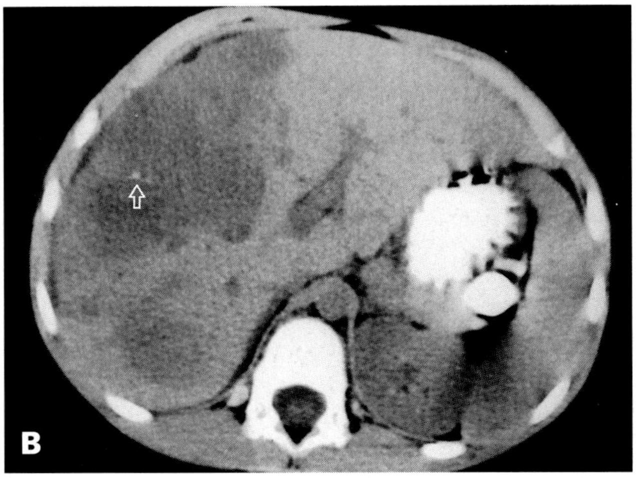

Figure 21-9. Conventional hepatocellular carcinoma. (A) A transverse sonogram of the liver at the main portal vein bifurcation demonstrates a heterogeneous, poorly defined mass (arrows) replacing the right lobe. A tumor thrombus is seen obliterating the lumen of the right portal vein (asterisk). The right hepatic vein (arrowhead) courses through the mass into the inferior vena cava (IVC). LP = left portal vein. (B and C) Axial CT images before (B) and after (C) intravenous contrast agent administration demonstrate a large, heterogeneously enhancing mass with focal calcification (open arrow). Vascular invasion is confirmed by the lack of enhancement in the expected location of the right portal vein (arrows) compared with the normal left portal vein (arrowheads).

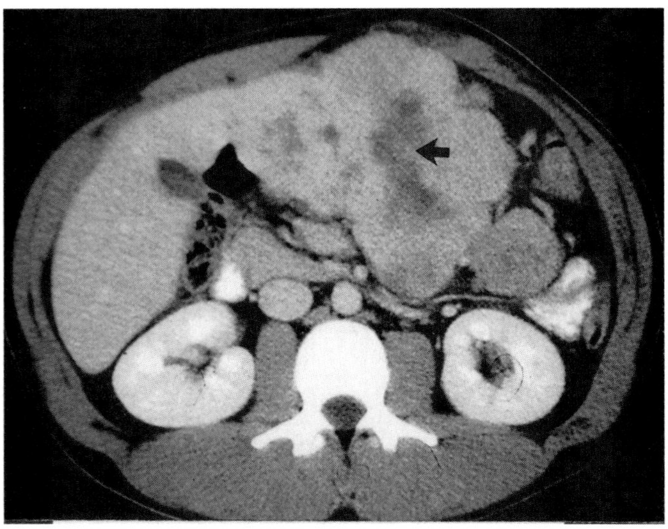

Figure 21-10. Fibrolamellar hepatocellular carcinoma. A contrast-enhanced CT image shows a large lobulated mass involving the left lobe of the liver. A central low-density area (arrow) proved to be scar at pathologic analysis.

Question 100

Which *one* of the following contrast enhancement phases is BEST for detecting hepatic metastatic disease?

(A) Arterial phase
(B) Early portal venous phase
(C) Late portal venous phase
(D) Equilibrium
(E) Late delayed phase

CT is the most common imaging modality used to detect hepatic metastases. Understanding the success of CT relates to two important pathophysiologic facts. First, the liver is unique relative to other abdominal organs in that it has a dual vascular supply, receiving 75% to 80% of its blood flow from the portal vein and 20% to 25% from the hepatic artery. Second, hepatic neoplasms are supplied almost exclusively by the hepatic arterial system. Prior to the intravenous administration of contrast agent, many hepatic lesions are not visualized because there is an insufficient difference in the attenuation values of the lesions and the normal liver parenchyma. This difference is increased by intravenous contrast agent administration, allowing many more lesions to be detected.

The phases of hepatic contrast enhancement include the arterial, early portal venous, late portal venous, equilibrium, and late delayed phases (Figure 21-11). Imaging during more than one of these phases recently has become possible with the advent of fast scanning techniques, specifically helical CT. The arterial phase occurs 20 to 30 seconds after the injection of the contrast agent bolus in children. In neonates, the arterial phase may occur as early as 10 to 15 seconds after contrast agent injection. During this phase, the aorta and its branches, including the hepatic artery, are opacified by the contrast agent. The hepatic parenchyma and hepatic veins are not significantly enhanced, as little contrast agent has passed through the portal venous system. Hypervascular neoplasms, such as hemangioendotheliomas, hemangiomas (Figure 21-12), and some metastases, are best detected during the arterial phase, as they enhance via contrast agent delivered by the hepatic artery and are set against a background of relatively unenhanced hepatic parenchyma. During the arterial phase, the hepatic veins may be seen as low-density areas within the liver and therefore can be confused with pathologic processes. However, normal hepatic veins are tubular, branching structures that converge toward the inferior vena cava on sequential images and are enhanced during the portal venous phase.

The hepatic arterial phase is followed by the early portal venous phase, which occurs 40 to 70 seconds after intravenous contrast agent injection. During this phase, the portal and hepatic veins become opacified. Contrast within the sinusoids of the normal hepatic parenchyma causes hypervascular lesions, which enhance during the arterial phase, to become isodense relative to the liver (Figure 21-12). Set against a background of normal hepatic parenchymal enhancement, hypovascular lesions, including most primary hepatic neoplasms and metastases, have low attenuation. The late portal venous phase occurs approximately 80 to 110 seconds after intravenous contrast agent administration. During this phase, most hypovasc accumulated enough contrast agent from the p become isodense relative to the liver and therefore less obvious.

Equilibrium follows the late portal venous phase and occurs when recirculation of the contrast agent causes nearly all hepatic lesions to be similar in density to hepatic parenchyma. Therefore, delayed-phase positivity is attributable to the slower uptake of hepatic lesions relative to normal liver. The late delayed phase occurs several minutes to hours later, after much of the intravenous contrast agent has been excreted by the kidneys. During this phase, lesions that are slow to accumulate contrast agent are occasionally detected as enhanced foci. Delayed-phase imaging is rarely performed, as it does not significantly increase the number of lesions detected and requires a significant increase in CT scanning time, a limiting factor in children.

The single most sensitive phase for the detection of metastases is the early portal venous phase **(Option (B) is correct).** However, multiphase imaging allows detection of the largest total number of metastatic lesions. The portal venous phase is always included in the evaluation of metastatic disease; other phases are included on a case-by-case basis. The performance of arterial-phase imaging has not proven practical and efficacious for every patient, although the consensus is that it should be performed in the setting of suspected hypervascular lesions. Precontrast images are useful when hemorrhage or calcification is possible.

The appropriate time delay between contrast agent injection and the beginning of the imaging sequence is influenced by many factors, including patient weight and the rate, volume, and type of contrast agent injected. In general, maximum hepatic enhancement is reached more quickly the faster the contrast agent is injected, the larger the volume (milliliters per kilogram) of the contrast agent, and with nonionic than with ionic contrast agents.

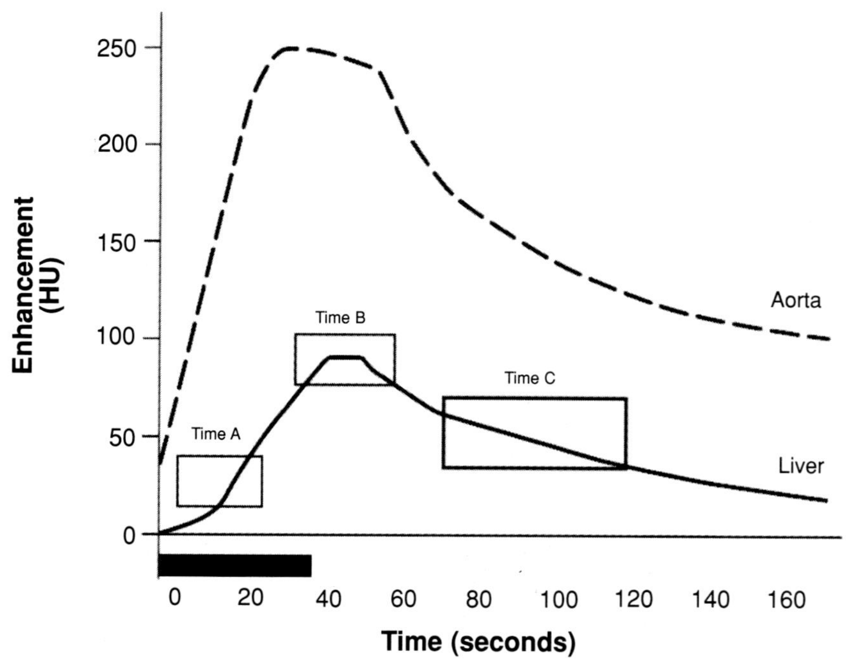

Figure 21-11. Graphic representation of the phases of hepatic intravenous contrast enhancement. Time-density enhancement curve for a typical patient after intravenous infusion of contrast agent in a dose of 2 mL/kg and at a rate of 2 to 3 mL/second. A sample infusion time for a 40-kg child is shown as a dark bar along the *x* axis. The aorta shows rapid enhancement until infusion is stopped. Then, a rapid but short decrease in aortic attenuation occurs, representing distribution of contrast material into extravascular spaces. The rapid decrease becomes a gradual decrease approximately 20 seconds after the contrast bolus injection is completed, representing the equilibrium phase of contrast agent delivery. The hepatic enhancement curve is similar in shape to the aortic curve, but has lower intensity and a later peak because of the delay required to deliver the contrast agent by portal venous flow and for the contrast material to diffuse into the extravascular spaces of hepatic parenchyma. The best time for detecting hypervascular tumors is during the arterial phase of contrast ehancement (Time A). The optimal time for detecting hypovascular tumors is during the portal venous phase (Time B), when there is peak hepatic enhancement. During the equilibrium phase (Time C), gradual excretion of contrast material through the kidneys and a gradual decrease in aortic attenuation occur. The late delayed phase occurs after 200 seconds and is beyond the limits of this graph.

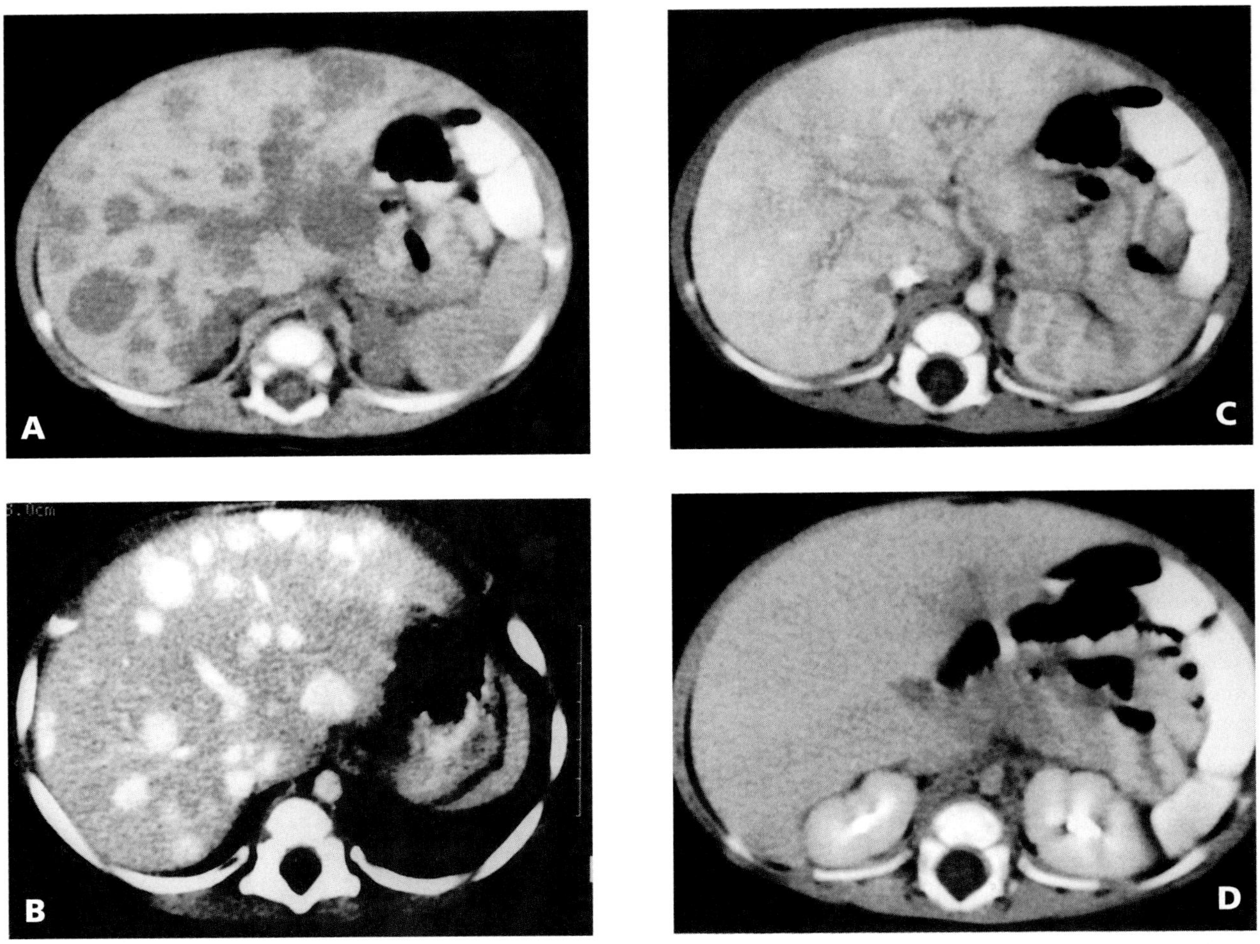

Figure 21-12. Hypervascular liver masses in a child with multiple hemangiomas. A multiphase CT scan shows the difference in lesion visualization that can occur during various phases of contrast enhancement. (A) An axial CT image obtained before the administration of intravenous contrast agent shows multiple, round, discrete, hypodense hepatic lesions. (B) These hypervascular lesions demonstrate bright enhancement during the arterial phase of the contrast bolus. (C and D) Early (C) and late (D) portal venous phase images show less enhancement of the lesions, which became nearly isodense relative to the hepatic parenchyma during the early portal venous phase and could not be visualized during the late portal venous phase.

Question 101

Concerning pyogenic hepatic abscesses in children,

(A) most are secondary to a source of infection elsewhere in the abdomen
(B) they are usually solitary
(C) an air-fluid level is present in most cases
(D) percutaneous drainage is successful therapy in greater than 80% of cases
(E) the most common complication of percutaneous drainage is peritonitis

In the past, the most common source of pyogenic hepatic abscesses in children was appendicitis, with the liver being seeded via the portal vein. Hepatic abscesses rarely complicate appendicitis today because of improved detection and earlier treatment. Instead, hepatic abscesses are now most often attributable to staphylococcal sepsis, with hematogenous spread to the liver (**Option (A) is false**). In infants, they may arise as a complication of umbilical artery catheterization. Pyogenic hepatic abscesses, both solitary and multiple, are more common in children with predisposing conditions, such as chronic granulomatous disease, immunodeficiency, and malignancy. Solitary abscesses are often discovered in children with persistent fever after an episode of sepsis. Although these abscesses occur most commonly after staphylococcal sepsis, cultures demonstrate multiple microorganisms in more than 50% of cases. Blood culture results are frequently normal or positive for microorganisms different from those aspirated from the abscess. Multiple pyogenic hepatic abscesses are most often the result of biliary disease, underlying malignancy with biliary obstruction, or hepatic trauma; they also may occur as a postsurgical complication.

Sonography and CT are both more than 90% sensitive for the detection of hepatic pyogenic abscesses. The imaging appearance is extremely variable, ranging from a single, round, homogeneous, well-marginated lesion to a multilocular, heterogeneous, poorly defined mass. About half of pyogenic abscesses in children are solitary (**Option (B) is true**). Gas produced by microorganisms within the abscess and air-fluid levels are specific findings, but occur in only about 20% of cases. A large amount of air resulting in a large air-fluid level is uncommon and should raise concern for a connection to the gut (**Option (C) is false**). Sonography demonstrates a round, sonolucent lesion with irregular margins, low-level echogenic internal debris that may form a fluid-debris level, enhanced through transmission, and no flow on Doppler imaging of the liquid necrotic center. CT is best performed with intravenous contrast agent administration and reveals a hypodense, unilocular lesion with internal septation, rim enhancement, and possibly internal gas (Figure 21-13).

Pyogenic abscesses are treated with antibiotics, percutaneous aspiration, and catheter drainage. Aspiration and antibiotics are often adequate treatment for discrete, unilocular lesions smaller than 5 cm. Larger abscesses, those that are multilocular, ill-defined, or chronic, or those that contain extremely viscous fluid often require percutaneous catheter drainage. A single catheter is often adequate despite septation and multiloculation, as there are often small connections between cavities. However, any areas that are not adequately drained by a single catheter may be treated successfully by aspiration or additional catheter placement.

Because the clinical presentation of hepatic abscesses is frequently insidious, delay in diagnosis is not uncommon, with mortality for solitary and multiple abscesses being 15% and 41%, respectively. With modern cross-sectional imaging techniques, early detection and percutaneous treatment have helped to dramatically decrease mortality from 32% to 2%. The rate of success of percutaneous drainage is 85% to 90% (**Option (D) is true**). Care should be taken to rule out amebic abscess, as it usually is treated with antimicrobial agents alone and rarely requires percutaneous intervention.

Complications related to percutaneous drainage are unusual, with bleeding being the most common. Peritonitis is very uncommon (**Option (E) is false**). Other uncommon, but potential, complications include septicemia, pneumothorax, empyema, and catheter dislodgment. Surgery, previously the mainstay of therapy, now is reserved for patients for whom catheter drainage has failed, who have a recurrence of abscess, or who require surgery to treat an underlying condition, such as malignancy.

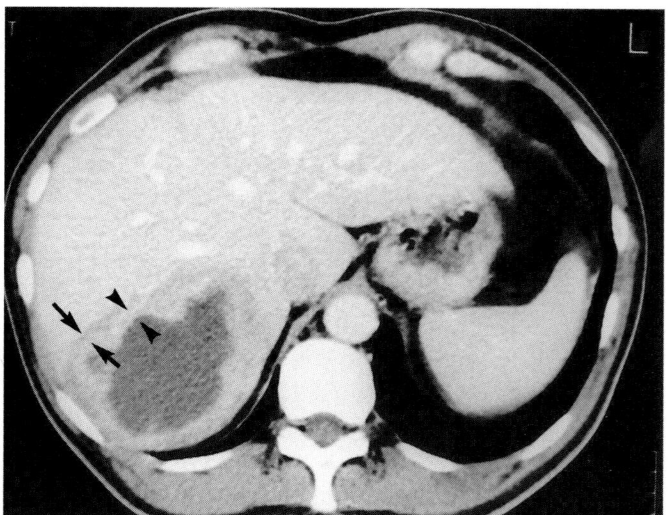

Figure 21-13. Pyogenic liver abscess. An axial CT image demonstrates, within the right lobe of the liver, a large, hypodense lesion with a thick enhancing wall (arrowheads) and a margin of low-attenuation edema (arrows).

Question 102

Concerning cat scratch disease,

(A) the causative agent is unknown
(B) painful adenopathy is the most common presenting sign
(C) hepatic involvement is present in most patients
(D) biopsy usually is necessary for diagnosis
(E) on sonography, hepatic lesions typically are echogenic
(F) hepatic lesions typically appear as target lesions on postcontrast CT

Cat scratch disease recently has been attributed to *Bartonella henselae*, a gram-negative bacillus that enters the host lymphatic system via a scratch from a cat (**Option (A) is false**). It usually is self-limiting, involving only the lymph nodes. The most common presenting complaint is painful adenopathy of one or more nodes proximal to the site of inoculation (**Option (B) is true**). The bacterium may access the venous system through the thoracic duct, and systemic infection may ensue. Disseminated disease occurs in 5% to 10% of patients and most often involves the liver and spleen (**Option (C) is false**). In such cases, it is not uncommon for children to have low-grade fever and abdominal pain, as in the test patient. The potential involvement of any organ system allows a variety of presenting complaints. Therefore, historical data and clinical information, such as recent acquisition of or exposure to a cat, are important in suspecting the diagnosis of cat scratch disease. The natural course of disease is the formation of granulomas that spontaneously resolve or occasionally calcify. A newly developed indirect serum fluorescent-antibody assay of blood or tissue is 85% to 100% sensitive and specific for detection of antibodies to *B. henselae*. A definitive diagnosis is possible with biopsy by detecting specific DNA in the organ(s) involved. However, because serum assays are now available, biopsy is not usually necessary (**Option (D) is false**).

The sonographic appearance of hepatosplenic disease includes typically hypoechoic, well-defined, round, homogeneous lesions (Figure 21-14) (**Option (E) is false**). The noncontrast CT appearance of hepatic cat scratch disease most often includes hypodense lesions smaller than 3 cm, as in the test patient. After the intravenous administration of contrast material, these granulomas can remain hypodense, become isodense, or demonstrate marginal enhancement (Figure 21-15). However, a target appearance is not typical (**Option (F) is false**).

Systemic involvement of the skeleton and less often of the brain can occur. Bone lesions appear as areas of increased tracer uptake on bone scintigraphy (Figure 21-15) and, if detectable, as lytic lesions on radiographs. Cerebral disease is very uncommon, with most reported cases having multiple, nonspecific, small lesions that involve the white matter and that are best detected on T2-weighted MR images. They are not usually seen on CT or T1-weighted MR images.

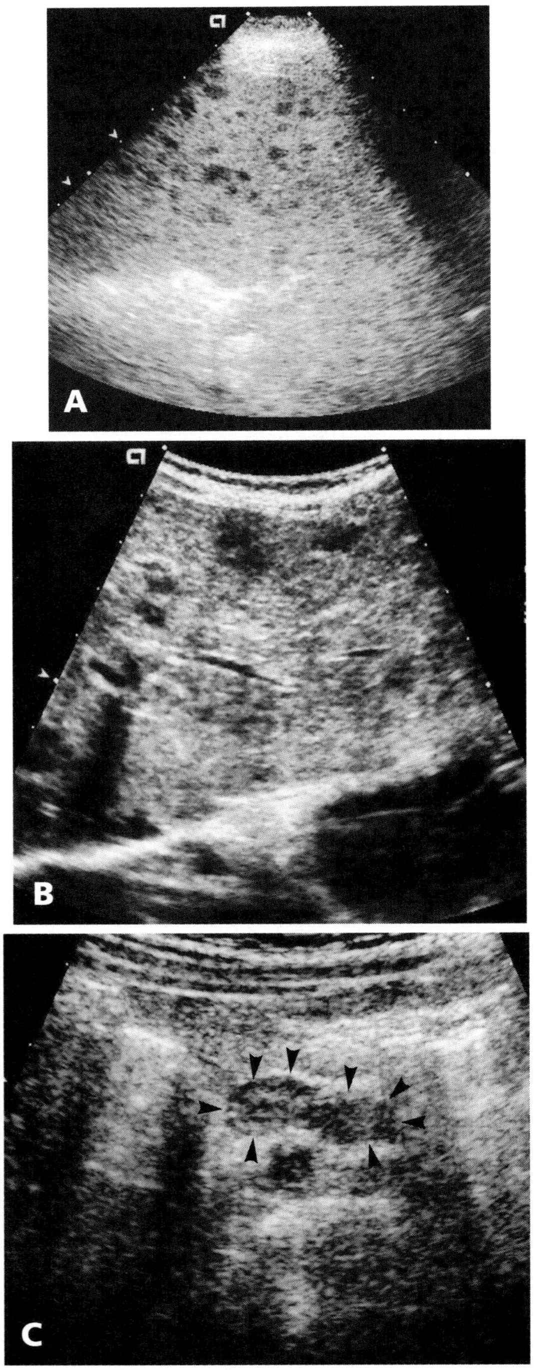

Figure 21-14. Cat scratch disease. Sonographic images of the spleen (A) and liver (B) show multiple, small, hypoechoic lesions scattered throughout both organs. (C) A transverse sonographic image of the retroperitoneum demonstrates enlarged periaortic lymph nodes (arrowheads).

Questions 103 through 106

For each of the numbered infections listed below (Questions 103 through 106), select the *one* lettered feature (A, B, C, D, or E) that is MOST closely associated with it. Each feature may be used once, more than once, or not at all.

103. Amebiasis
104. Candidiasis
105. Echinococcosis
106. Schistosomiasis

(A) diaphragmatic invasion
(B) target lesion on sonography
(C) peripheral hepatic calcification
(D) biliary ductal dilatation
(E) uniformly enhancing lesions on CT

Amebiasis, caused by the protozoan *Entamoeba histolytica*, is considered endemic between the 40° north and 30° south parallels. It colonizes the colon of 10% of the world's population, causes symptoms in 50 million people per year, and causes death in as many as 100,000. The highest rates of infestation are found in developing countries, such as Mexico, India, South Africa, East Africa, and parts of Central America and South America. Approximately 1,200 cases occur in the United States each year. They most often involve homosexual males, for reasons that are not clear.

Humans are the reservoir and principal host for *E. histolytica*. Infested persons excrete in their feces mature cysts that are subsequently ingested through contaminated water or food. The cyst wall is digested by trypsin in the small bowel, and four trophozoites per cyst are released to colonize and multiply in the colon, especially the cecum. The trophozoites can become invasive, causing ulceration of the gastrointestinal wall and penetrating the mesenteric or portal venous systems. Less than 10% of infested persons become symptomatic, usually with diarrhea and dysentery. A sufficient number of trophozoites in the small venules of the portal venous system can cause thrombosis and infarction of the hepatic parenchyma, allowing the development of an abscess. Hepatic abscess occurs in 3% to 8.5% of clinically symptomatic individuals. It is the second most common presentation and the most common extraintestinal manifestation. Rarely, the brain, skin, or genitals are affected.

Amebic abscesses of the liver can occur at any age, but are more common in adults over 20 years of age. These abscesses are usually solitary (about 85% of cases), involve the right lobe (nearly 75% of cases), and are easily detected by cross-sectional imaging. Presentation of hepatic disease is most often attributa-

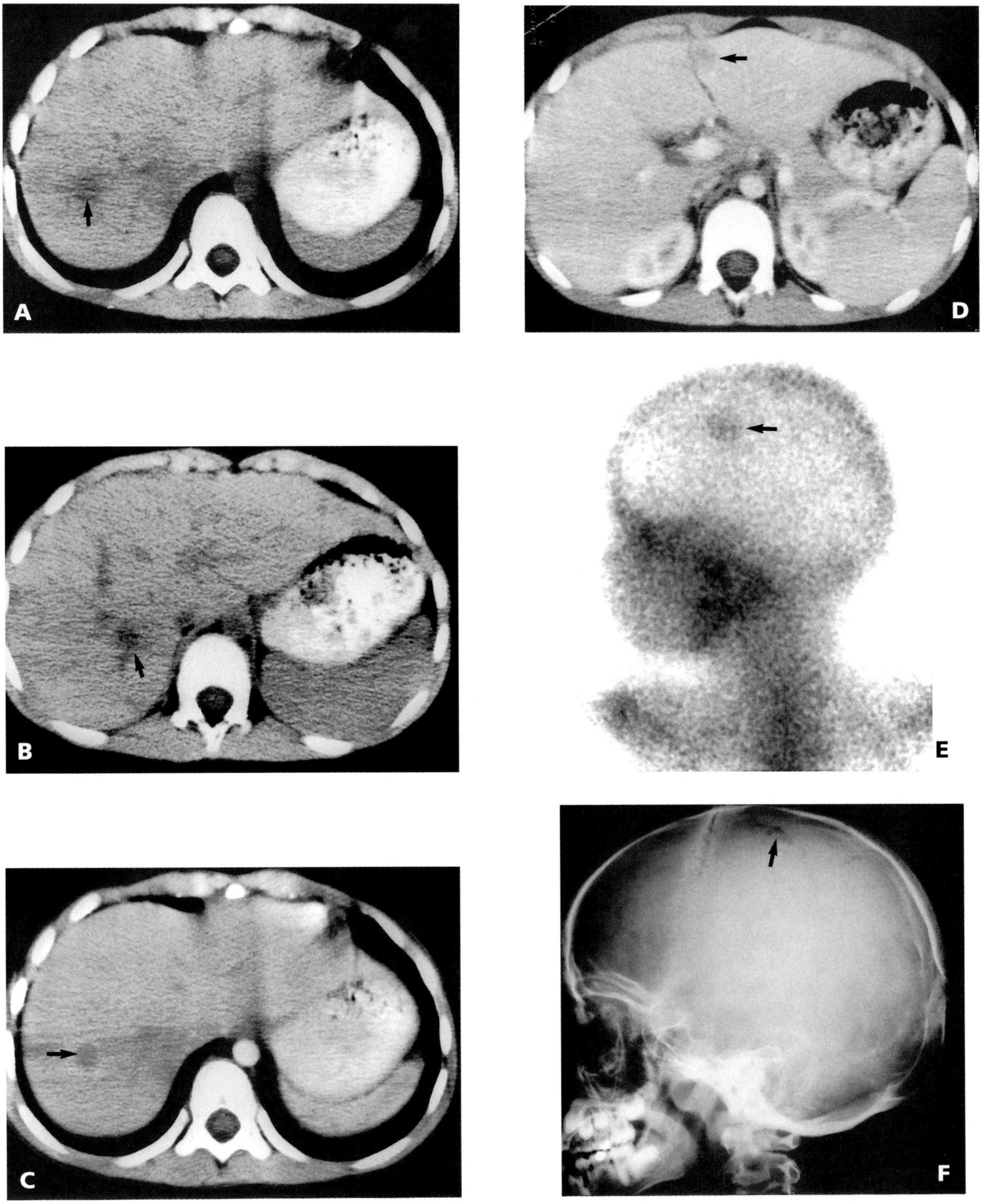

Figure 21-15. Cat scratch disease. Axial CT images before (A and B) and after (C and D) intravenous contrast agent administration show hypodense lesions with ill-defined margins before contrast agent administration and slight peripheral enhancement after contrast agent administration (arrows). (E and F) Bone scintigraphy (E) shows focally increased uptake in the parietal bone (arrow) that correlates with a lucent lesion (arrow) seen on a radiograph (F).

ble to mass effect or cyst rupture, causing abrupt right upper quadrant pain. Children with amebic abscesses are usually more acutely ill than are those with pyogenic abscesses. Distinction between amebic and pyogenic abscesses is important, as the treatment for amebic abscesses is most often medical, whereas pyogenic abscesses almost always require aspiration and drainage. The diagnosis of amebic abscess is made by a positive hemagglutination test in over 90% of cases. Positive amebic titers may be found, although there is a 2% to 18% false-negativity rate. Stool examination results are usually nonspecific or negative. When an amebic abscess is suspected on the basis of clinical or imaging findings, empiric treatment with antibiotics is initiated while laboratory results are pending.

The imaging appearance is nonspecific and depends on the stage of the lesion. Sonography is the imaging modality of choice, with features including the absence of significant wall echoes, an oval or round shape, decreased echogenicity, homogeneous low-level internal debris, peripheral location adjacent to or contacting the hepatic capsule, and enhanced through transmission. Amebic abscesses undergo a temporal progression in appearance on sonography, being hyperechoic early, at which time they can mimic a solid mass in about 5% of cases. Later, they become hypoechoic, with enhanced through transmission. On CT scans, amebic abscesses are round, well defined, and typically peripheral in location and have low attenuation values indicative of fluid. Postcontrast CT images show internal septation and marginal enhancement, with a more peripheral rim of surrounding low-attenuation edema (Figure 21-16). Target lesions, calcifications, ductal dilatation, and uniform contrast enhancement do not occur. MRI reveals decreased signal intensity on T1-weighted images and increased signal intensity on T2-weighted images, with a gadolinium chelate enhancement pattern similar to that seen on CT. Extension beyond the margin of the liver occurs in more than one third of patients. Thoracic involvement in amebiasis occurs in as many as 35% of patients and usually is attributable to rupture of an hepatic abscess across the diaphragm (**Option (A) is the correct answer to Question 103**). Chest radiographs are abnormal in up to 75% of all patients either because of direct extension of infection across the diaphragm or because of diaphragmatic irritation by an adjacent intrahepatic lesion. Findings on chest radiographs range from right hemidiaphragmatic elevation, pleural effusion, and atelectasis to empyema, lung abscess, or pericardial effusion.

Treatment with appropriate antimicrobial agents (most often metronidazole) is successful in more than 90% of patients, although therapy may be prolonged. Response to therapy usually is rapid, and failure to respond within 24 to 72 hours should raise concern for superimposed bacterial infection, which occurs in nearly 15% of patients. Although aspiration is not usually required in uncomplicated amebic abscesses, it is beneficial in certain situations, such as to differentiate amebic abscess from pyogenic abscess when there is no response to therapy and laboratory test results are negative; in the setting of strong clinical suspicion for impending rupture; to treat pyogenic superinfection of an amebic abscess; or when antimicrobial agents are inappropriate (pregnancy). Because of the threat of rupture into the pericardium, left lobe involvement adjacent to the diaphragm may be initially treated more aggressively with percutaneous aspiration or surgery. Although some

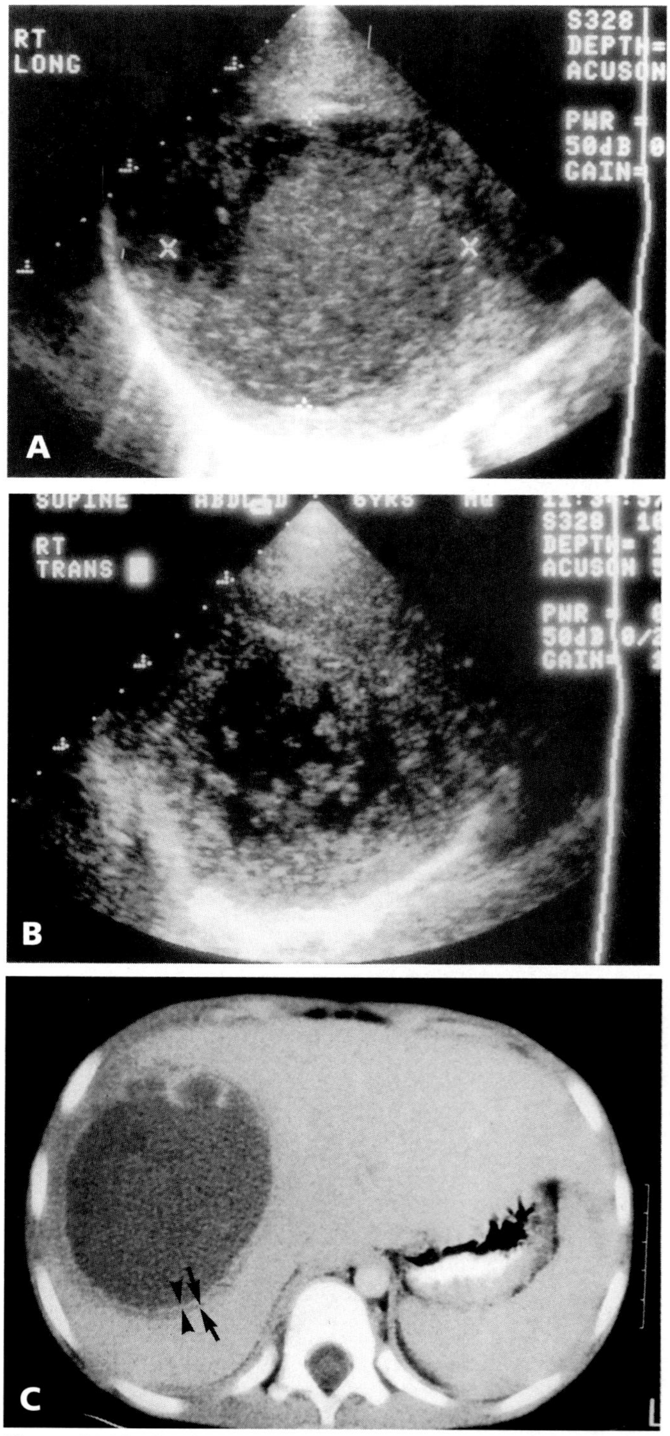

Figure 21-16. Amebiasis. (A and B) Longitudinal (A) and transverse (B) sonographic images show a round, hypoechoic lesion with internal debris in the right lobe of the liver (calipers). (C) An axial CT image shows a large, smoothly marginated, low-attenuation lesion with peripheral enhancement (arrowheads) and a more peripheral rim of hypodense edema (arrows) in the right lobe. Some septations are seen in the anterior aspect of the lesion.

investigators have advocated abscess aspiration to speed recovery, no study has proven this strategy beneficial, and most do not advocate routine aspiration of amebic abscesses unless there is an extenuating circumstance. Surgery is reserved for complicated cases in which other measures do not suffice.

Untreated amebic liver abscesses have a high mortality rate because of complications related to rupture, such as anaphylaxis and superimposed bacterial infection. The overall mortality rate increases from 1% to 6% with thoracic involvement. Rupture into the pericardium occurs in less than 1% of left lobe amebic abscesses, but it usually is fatal.

Candida albicans, a ubiquitous fungus and a normal part of the human flora, may spread hematogenously in immunocompromised patients. Candidiasis is particularly common in patients with AIDS, leukemia, lymphoma, lymphoproliferative disorders requiring high-dose chemotherapy, and bone marrow transplant patients. Nearly any organ can be affected, including the lungs, esophagus, liver, spleen, and kidneys but rarely the stomach, bile ducts, brain, bone, or lower gastrointestinal tract. The imaging appearance of hepatic candidiasis depends on the host immune response. During acute infection in a neutropenic patient, the lesions are microscopic and are usually not visible. When the patient recovers from neutropenia and mounts an immune response, microabscesses that can be detected by imaging form.

Four patterns of hepatic candidiasis on sonography have been described; all have in common multiple small (<4 mm) lesions throughout the liver. First, in the early stages of disease, a hyperechoic nidus of necrotic fungal elements is surrounded by echogenic inflammatory cells that are in turn surrounded by a peripheral zone of fibrosis, giving rise to a "wheel within a wheel" appearance. Second, when the host mounts a neutrophil response, the "bull's-eye" or "target" appearance is seen (Figure 21-17) (**Option (B) is the correct answer to Question 104**). This appearance represents a <4-mm lesion with a hyperechoic center and a hypoechoic rim. The third, and most common, appearance at sonography is "uniformly hypoechoic" lesions reflecting microabscesses and developing fibrosis (Figure 21-18). Finally, 1- to 4-mm "echogenic" lesions with or without acoustic shadowing are seen because of calcification or scarring (Figure 21-19). CT shows multiple, 2- to 20-mm, round, hypodense lesions that are scattered throughout the liver or spleen and that may be seen before or after intravenous contrast material administration (Figure 21-20). Slight hyperattenuation on noncontrast CT may indicate diffuse, homogeneous calcification; postcontrast-enhanced images often show peripheral microabscess enhancement. However, diaphragmatic invasion, peripheral hepatic calcification, biliary ductal dilatation, and uniform contrast enhancement do not occur. MRI can show small hepatosplenic lesions that may be missed on CT. Although a bull's-eye or target lesion seen at sonography can strongly suggest candidiasis, the appearance is not specific with any imaging modality. The differential diagnosis includes several infections not usually distinguished radiographically, including aspergillosis, cryptococcosis, histoplasmosis, mucormycosis, and atypical tuberculosis.

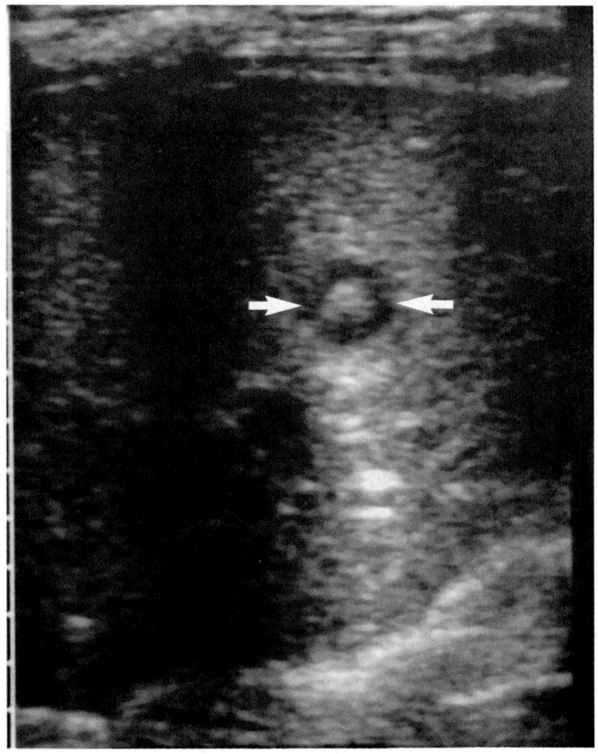

Figure 21-17. Hepatic candidiasis. A longitudinal sonogram of the liver in a 4-year-old boy with chronic granulomatous disease of childhood demonstrates a hypoechoic lesion (arrows) with a central echogenic focus ("bull's-eye lesion"). The adjacent bands of shadowing are attributable to ribs. (Case courtesy of Marilyn J. Siegel, M.D., Mallinckrodt Institute of Radiology, St. Louis, MO.)

Echinococcosis (hydatid disease) is caused by two main forms of tapeworms, *Echinococcus granulosus* and *Echinococcus multilocularis* (*E. alveolaris*). The disease usually is caused by the larval form of the parasite. It is most common in the Mid-

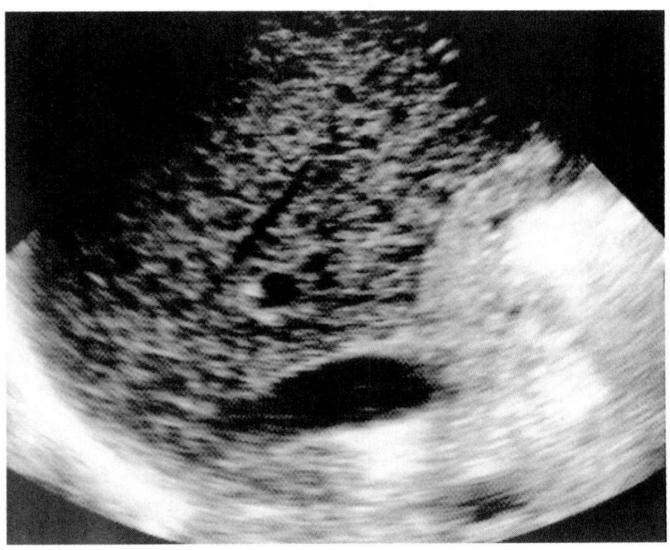

Figure 21-18. Candidiasis. A longitudinal sonogram shows numerous small, hypoechoic lesions of a similar size throughout the hepatic parenchyma.

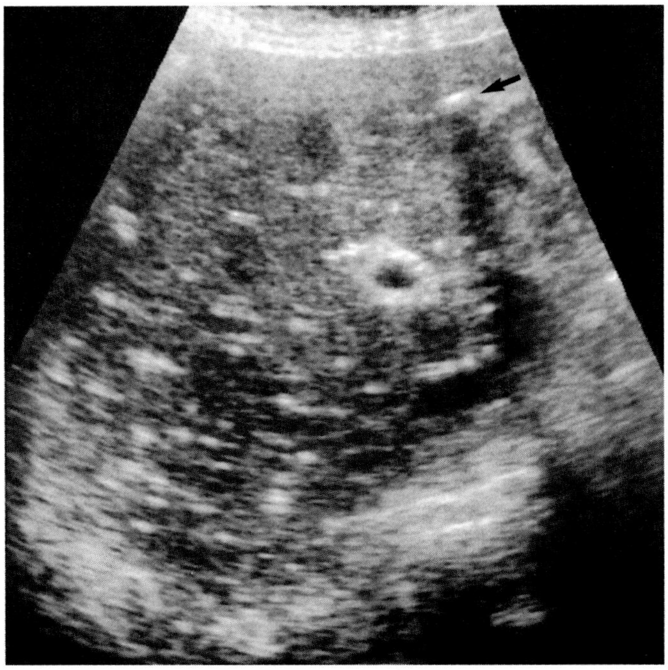

Figure 21-19. Healed candidiasis. A sonographic image shows heterogeneous echogenicity and multiple, tiny, hyperechoic foci scattered throughout the liver. Some demonstrate shadowing (arrow) consistent with punctate calcifications.

dle East, in the Mediterranean basin, and in all sheep-grazing countries. The definitive host of *E. granulosus* (dog, fox, or hyena) harbors adult worms that secrete eggs into host feces. Humans become infected as intermediate hosts by ingesting feces contaminated with the echinococcal eggs, most often through the ingestion of contaminated water or vegetables. The eggshell is digested in the duodenum, and a freed embryo can penetrate the intestinal mucosa. The embryos access the vascular system and are trapped within capillaries anywhere in

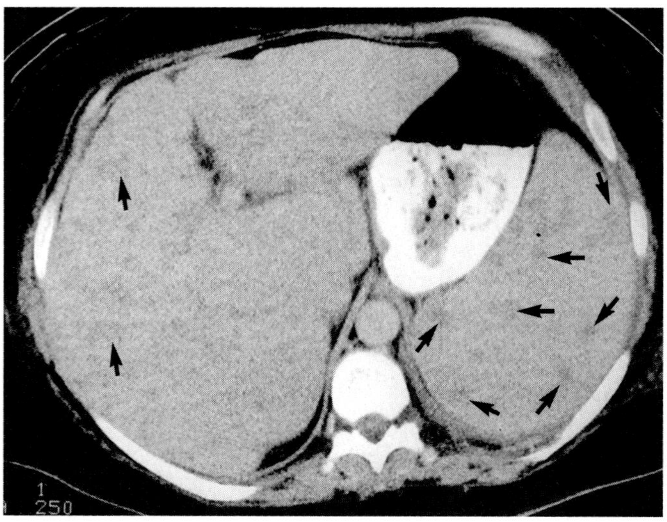

Figure 21-20. Candidiasis. A noncontrast axial CT image shows hepatosplenomegaly in addition to numerous small, hypodense foci (arrows) throughout the liver and spleen. The patient did not receive intravenous contrast agent because of renal dysfunction.

the body, most often the liver. Most embryos are destroyed, but those that survive form a cyst of 5 mm within the liver by 3 months. The cyst continues to slowly grow at a rate of 1 cm per year. The life cycle is completed when the intermediate host (most often a sheep and less often a human) dies and the larva-containing viscera are consumed by the definitive host (most often a dog). The life cycle of *E. multilocularis* is the same, with the exception that the definitive hosts are usually rodents and cats.

Echinococcosis is contracted during childhood, but presents 5 to 15 years later because of the slow growth of the cyst. The liver is the most common organ involved, although hematogenous dissemination in less than 5% of cases can allow the lungs and, less often, the spleen, kidneys, adrenal glands, bone, or central nervous system to be affected. Symptoms are most often the result of mass effect or complications related to rupture. The diagnosis is made by enzyme-linked immunosorbent assay detecting elevated serum echinococcal antibody titers, which are positive in more than 80% of cases.

Hepatic *E. granulosus* and *E. multilocularis* infestations have imaging features distinct from one another. *E. granulosus* infestation is more common and causes a unilocular form of hydatid disease in which the cyst has two main layers. The endocyst is a fragile, 2-mm-thick inner layer, and the pericyst is a tough, collagenous outer layer produced by the host in response to the parasite. The endocyst is filled with fluid under pressure (20 to 80 cm of water), and from its walls, brood capsules and scolices are secreted, forming hydatid sand. Daughter cysts, produced by the brood capsules, occur within the endocyst.

E. granulosus cysts are classified into three types reflecting changes in content and appearance during stages of development. Type 1 cysts contain no daughter cysts or matrix and have a "simple cyst" imaging appearance. Later, the walls of the endocyst grow out of proportion to the pericyst, becoming enfolded and redundant. Portions of the endocyst remote from nourishing cyst fluid degenerate, forming a gelatinous matrix. Type 2 cysts contain either internal daughter cysts or matrix (Figure 21-21). Calcified cysts are classified as type 3 (Figure 21-22). Calcification, seen on conventional radiographs in 20% to 30% of cases, occurs within the pericyst, the walls of the daughter cysts, clotted hepatic vessels, or the dead parasite. Parasite calcification is unrelated to viability, except in the setting of dense calcification, which usually indicates parasite death.

The pericyst layer of the hydatid cyst can be perforated by bile ducts that are often obstructed because of mass effect. Initially, high pressure within the intact endocyst prevents bile from leaking into the lesion. However, as the parasite outgrows the confined space of the pericyst, endocyst rupture can occur, allowing free exchange of fluid between the bile ducts and the hydatid cyst.

Cyst rupture can occur at any stage of development and is classified into three types: contained, communicating, and direct. Contained rupture is diagnosed at imaging when the delaminated endocyst membrane is seen floating as a wavy band within the hydatid fluid, termed the "water lily sign." In com-

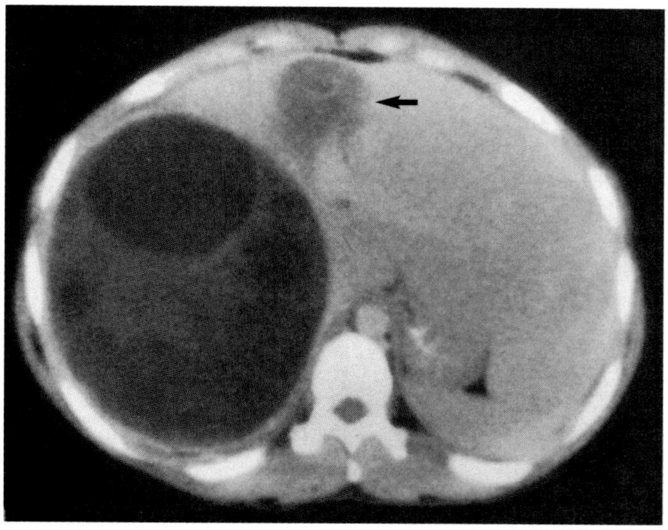

Figure 21-21. *E. granulosus* cyst. An axial CT image of the liver shows a round, smoothly marginated, low-attenuation lesion with internal septation in the right hepatic lobe. A second, smaller lesion is seen anteriorly (arrow).

municating rupture, the integrity of the endocyst is lost and hydatid fluid is forced into bile ducts that perforate the walls of the pericyst. As pressure between the bile ducts and the cyst equalizes, some bile flows into the cyst, often killing the parasite. Cyst contents spilled into the biliary tree may result in obstruction, ductal dilatation, bile stasis, or superimposed cholangitis. Bile duct enlargement can be caused by mass effect from an intact cyst or in the setting of cyst rupture (**Option (D) is the correct answer to Question 105**). Direct rupture into the substance of the liver can occur. Although it does not lead to anaphylaxis, it does allow the development of satellite lesions adjacent to the site of rupture. Rupture of both the endocyst and the pericyst allows spillage of cyst contents into the peritoneal cavity, often leading to life-threatening anaphylaxis.

The cross-sectional imaging appearance varies on the basis

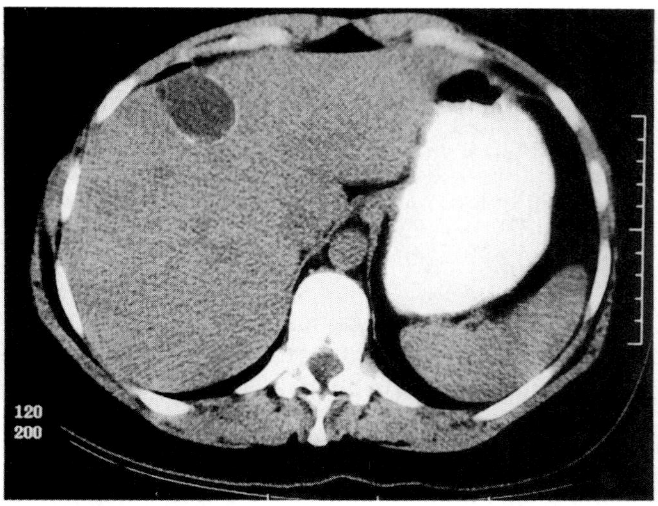

Figure 21-22. *E. granulosus* cyst. An axial CT image demonstrates a round, smoothly marginated lesion that is of fluid density centrally and has peripheral calcification.

of the stage of disease. Sonographic appearances include a sharply defined anechoic cyst, a cyst with layering debris (hydatid sand), a multiseptate cyst with daughter cysts and echogenic material between cysts, a cyst with a detached undulating membrane (the water lily sign), or a densely calcified mass. When superinfected, cysts become more hyperechoic and filled with debris. On CT, single or multilocular, well-defined cysts are seen. They can have daughter cysts, hydatid sand, or a central detached endocyst. Peripheral curvilinear cyst calcification is nearly pathognomonic. However, peripheral hepatic calcification does not occur. Similar anatomic changes are seen on MR images. The signal of hydatid cysts is similar to that of other cysts, hypointense on T1-weighted images and hyperintense on T2-weighted images. The fibrous pericyst has a low signal intensity on T1- and T2-weighted sequences.

E. multilocularis causes a less common, but more aggressive, form of hepatic echinococcosis. In contrast to those caused by *E. granulosus*, the cysts are poorly defined, more heterogeneous, infiltrative, nodular, and necrotic centrally. They are characterized by amorphous calcification, and their appearance simulates neoplastic disease on all imaging modalities. Therefore, a high index of suspicion may be required to make this diagnosis. Diaphragmatic invasion and target lesions are not seen with *Echinococcus* disease.

Treatment of echinococcosis includes removal of the cyst and its contents. Although believed dangerous in the past, percutaneous aspiration and drainage are now considered the treatments of choice. The cyst may not be amenable to percutaneous drainage if it is exophytic or if there is bile duct dilatation. Exophytic cysts have insufficient liver along their free margin to allow adequate pericyst development and maintenance of the cyst wall during catheter drainage. Exophytic cysts are usually drained surgically without delay, as they are unstable and more prone to intraperitoneal rupture. Hydatid cysts with adjacent bile duct dilatation should also be drained surgically because of an increased risk for communicating rupture, biliary infection, and biliary obstruction. Percutaneous drainage in the setting of bile duct dilatation causes inevitable development of a cyst into a biliary tree fistula. Because this communication can lead to additional problems, some authors have recommended that cyst fluid be aspirated for bile pigment testing before placement of a percutaneous drain is attempted. Some authors consider the presence of bile pigment in aspirated cyst fluid a contraindication to percutaneous catheter drainage and an indication for surgical drainage. Finally, the diagnosis of an echinococcal cyst must be determined to be certain by serologic analysis or percutaneous aspiration prior to catheter drainage because uncomplicated amebic and small pyogenic abscesses respond well to medical therapy alone. If a drain is placed, a large-bore 14-French catheter usually is required to drain the viscous cyst contents.

Schistosomiasis, a rare disease in North America, affects 200 million people worldwide, with about 10% of those in areas of endemicity developing hepatosplenic involvement. Three main forms of *Schistosoma* organisms affect humans: *S.*

japonicum, S. mansoni, and *S. haematobium. S. japonicum* is found in coastal China, Japan, Taiwan, and the Philippines. *S. mansoni* occurs in regions of Africa, the Middle East, the West Indies, and northern South America. *S. haematobium* is found in North Africa, southwestern Asia, and the Mediterranean basin. Infection occurs through bathing in contaminated water; schistosomal larvae released from snails (intermediate host) penetrate intact skin or mucous membranes of humans (definitive host). They migrate via the lymphatics through the heart and lungs to the mesenteric circulation, where they pass through capillaries into the portal venous system and mature into ova. Schistosomes that do not reach the mesenteric circulation die. The male and female organisms remain in the portal system for 10 to 15 years. The life cycle is completed when the mature female worm swims against blood flow to the venules of the urinary bladder (*S. haematobium*) or gut (*S. mansoni* and *S. japonicum*) and deposits eggs. The eggs can embolize to almost any organ, where they die, inciting a granulomatous response and causing most of the problems seen in humans. Schistosomes secrete more than 300 eggs per day, some of which hatch into motile miracidia. In warm static water, the miracidia infect a snail and undergo asexual reproduction into cercariae, the form of schistosome that can infect humans. Schistosomes may live for up to 30 years within the definitive host.

At the time of initial infection, a minority of patients experience significant clinical manifestations of schistosomiasis, termed Katayama fever. Most patients have no initial fever, and in those who do, the symptoms are usually mild and self-limiting enough that medical attention is not sought. Although little information is available on the acute-phase imaging features of schistosomiasis, sonography has shown multiple scattered hypoechoic areas within the liver and spleen as well as periportal lymphadenopathy. These lesions can persist for more than 4 weeks on CT, even after adequate treatment. The infestation is most commonly insidious in nature, with the liver being associated with the most morbidity. Chronic hepatic involvement is characterized by periportal fibrosis leading to presinusoidal portal hypertension, cirrhosis, and varices. Patients often have variceal bleeding or hematuria. The periportal fibrosis of schistosomiasis is seen at sonography as hyperechoic bands replacing the portal triads. Transverse images of portal triads near the bifurcations show echogenic rings with hypoechoic rims resembling a bird's claw. Changes of portal hypertension and cirrhosis, including surface lobulation, splenomegaly, and collateral vessels, also can be seen. *S. mansoni* and *S. haematobium* do not usually cause hepatic calcifications. However, periportal and pericapsular calcifications of *S. japonicum* ova have a classic CT appearance known as "tortoiseshell" or "turtleback" calcifications (Figure 21-23) (**Option (C) is the correct answer to Question 106**). Diaphragmatic invasion, biliary ductal dilatation, target lesions, and uniformly enhancing lesions do not occur. After intravenous contrast agent administration, there is often periportal enhancement on CT. MRI findings for *S. mansoni* infestation include isointense periportal bands on T1-weighted images that are hyperintense on T2-weighted images and enhance intensely after injection of gadolinium chelate. Enhancement after gadolinium chelate injection can be seen in the early and late stages of periportal fibrosis. Some authors have suggested that an advantage of MRI over sonography and CT is that it may be able to detect active inflammation by demonstrating a periportal bright signal on T2-weighted images. However, the role of MRI in schistosomiasis is still under investigation.

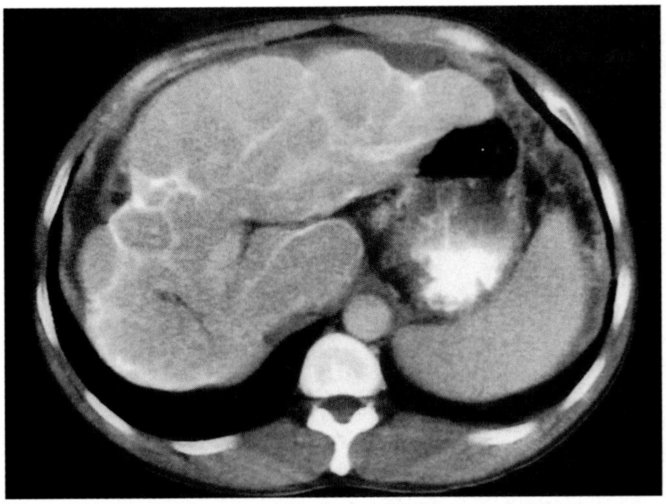

Figure 21-23. Schistosomiasis. An axial CT image demonstrates a "tortoiseshell" pattern of linear surface and peripheral parenchymal hepatic calcifications. Changes of cirrhosis, including lobulation of the liver margin and ascites, also can be seen.

SUGGESTED READINGS

CAT SCRATCH DISEASE

1. Bergmans AMC, Groothedde JW, Schellekens JFP, van Embden JDA, Ossewaarde JM, Schouls LM. Etiology of cat scratch disease: comparison of polymerase chain reaction detection of *Bartonella* (formerly *Rochalimaea*) and *Afipia felis* DNA with serology and skin tests. J Infect Dis 1995; 171:916–923
2. Hopkins KL, Simoneaux SF, Patrick LE, Wyly JB, Dalton MJ, Snitzer JA. Imaging manifestations of cat-scratch disease. AJR 1996; 166:435–438
3. Jackson LA, Perkins BA, Wenger JD. Cat scratch disease in the United States: an analysis of three national databases. Am J Public Health 1993; 83:1707–1711
4. Larsen CE, Patrick LE. Abdominal (liver, spleen) and bone manifestations of cat scratch disease. Pediatr Radiol 1992; 22:353–355
5. Margileth AM. Cat scratch disease. Adv Pediatr Infect Dis 1993; 8:1–21

HEPATOCELLULAR CARCINOMA

6. Brandt DJ, Johnson CD, Stephens DH, Weiland LH. Imaging of fibrolamellar hepatocellular carcinoma. AJR 1988; 151:295–299
7. Donnelly LF, Bisset GS III. Pediatric hepatic imaging. Radiol Clin North Am 1998; 36:413–427
8. Soyer P, Roche A, Levesque M, Legmann P. CT of fibrolamellar hepatocellular carcinoma. J Comput Assist Tomogr 1991; 15:533–538

LIVER METASTASIS

9. Mergo PJ, Ros PR. Imaging of diffuse liver disease. Radiol Clin North Am 1998; 36:365–375
10. Miller JH, Greenspan BS. Integrated imaging of hepatic tumors in childhood. Part I: malignant lesions (primary and metastatic). Radiology 1985; 154:83–90
11. Platt JF, Francis IR, Ellis JH, Reige KA. Liver metastases: early detection based on abnormal contrast material enhancement at dual-phase helical CT. Radiology 1997; 205:49–53

CONTRAST ENHANCEMENT OF THE LIVER

12. Baron RL. Understanding and optimizing use of contrast material for CT of the liver. AJR 1994; 163:323–331
13. Garcia PA, Bonaldi VM, Bret PM, Liang L, Reinhold C, Atri M. Effect of rate of contrast medium injection on hepatic enhancement at CT. Radiology 1996; 199:185–189
14. Halavaara JT, Hamberg LM, Leong FS, Hunter GJ, Gazelle GS, Wolf GL. Functional CT with an experimental intravascular contrast agent in the assessment of liver vascular physiology. Acad Radiol 1996; 3:946–952
15. Kopka L, Rodenwaldt J, Fischer U, Mueller DW, Oestmann JW, Grabbe E. Dual-phase helical CT of the liver: effects of bolus tracking and different volumes of contrast material. Radiology 1996; 201:321–326
16. Oliver JH III, Baron RL. Helical biphasic contrast-enhanced CT of the liver: technique, indications, interpretation, and pitfalls. Radiology 1996; 201:1–14
17. Silverman PM, O'Malley J, Tefft MC, Cooper C, Zeman RK. Conspicuity of hepatic metastases on helical CT: effect of different time delays between contrast administration and scanning. AJR 1995; 164:619–623

HEPATIC PYOGENIC ABSCESS

18. Do H, Lambiase RE, Deyoe L, Cronan JJ, Dorfman GS. Percutaneous drainage of hepatic abscesses: comparison of results in abscesses with and without intrahepatic biliary communication. AJR 1991; 157:1209–1212
19. Miller JH, Greenspan BS. Integrated imaging of hepatic tumors in childhood. Part II: benign lesions (congenital, reparative, and inflammatory). Radiology 1985; 154:91–100
20. Newlin N, Silver TM, Stuck KJ, Sandler MA. Ultrasonic features of pyogenic liver abscesses. Radiology 1981; 139:155–159
21. Robert JH, Mirescu D, Ambrosetti P, Khoury G, Greenstein AJ, Robner A. Critical review of the treatment of pyogenic hepatic abscess. Surg Gynecol Obstet 1992; 174:97–102
22. Stain SC, Yellin AE, Donovan AJ, Brien HW. Pyogenic liver abscess: modern treatment. Arch Surg 1991; 126:991–996

AMEBIASIS

23. Kimura K, Stoopen M, Reeder MM, Moncada R. Amebiasis: modern diagnostic imaging with pathological and clinical correlation. Semin Roentgenol 1997; 32:250–275
24. Kline MJ, Miller FH, Hoff F, Nemcek AA Jr, Abecassis MM. Case of the season. Amebic abscess (*Entamoeba histolytica*) of the liver. Semin Roentgenol 1998; 33:98–100
25. McDermott VG. What is the role of percutaneous drainage for treatment of amebic abscesses of the liver? AJR 1995; 165:1005–1006
26. Ralls PW. Focal inflammatory disease of the liver. Radiol Clin North Am 1998; 36:377–389

CANDIDIASIS

27. Lai PH, Lin SM, Pan HB, Yang CF. Disseminated miliary cerebral candidiasis. AJNR 1997; 18:1303–1306
28. Lenders C, Buonomo C, Jonas MM. Image of the month. Disseminated infections, especially candidiasis in immunocompromised individuals, cat-scratch fever, and infiltrative diseases such as leukemia or lymphoma. Gastroenterology 1997; 113:1432, 1815
29. Samuels BI, Bodey GP, Libshitz HI. Imaging in candidiasis. Semin Roentgenol 1996; 31:76–82
30. Semelka RC, Kelekis NL, Sallah S, Worawattanakul S, Ascher SM. Hepatosplenic fungal disease: diagnostic accuracy and spectrum of appearances on MR imaging. AJR 1997; 169:1311–1316

ECHINOCOCCOSIS

31. Khuroo MS, Wani NA, Javid G, et al. Percutaneous drainage compared with surgery for hepatic hydatid cysts. N Engl J Med 1997; 337:881–887
32. Lewall DB, Nyak P. Hydatid cysts of the liver: two cautionary signs. Br J Radiol 1998; 71:37–41
33. Reittner P, Szolar DH, Schmid M. Case report. Systemic manifestation of *Echinococcus alveolaris* infection. J Comput Assist Tomogr 1996; 20: 1030–1032
34. Stoupis C, Taylor HM, Paley MR, et al. The Rocky liver: radiologic-pathologic correlation of calcified hepatic masses. RadioGraphics 1998; 18:675–685

SCHISTOSOMIASIS

35. Cesmeli E, Vogelaers D, Voet D, et al. Ultrasound and CT changes of liver parenchyma in acute schistosomiasis. Br J Radiol 1997; 70:758–760
36. Palmer PE. Schistosomiasis. Semin Roentgenol 1998; 33:6–25
37. Willemsen UF, Pfluger T, Zoller WG, Kueffer G, Hahn K. MRI of hepatic schistosomiasis mansoni. J Comput Assist Tomogr 1995; 19:811–813

Michele H. Johnson, M.D.

Hypothalamic-Chiasmatic Glioma

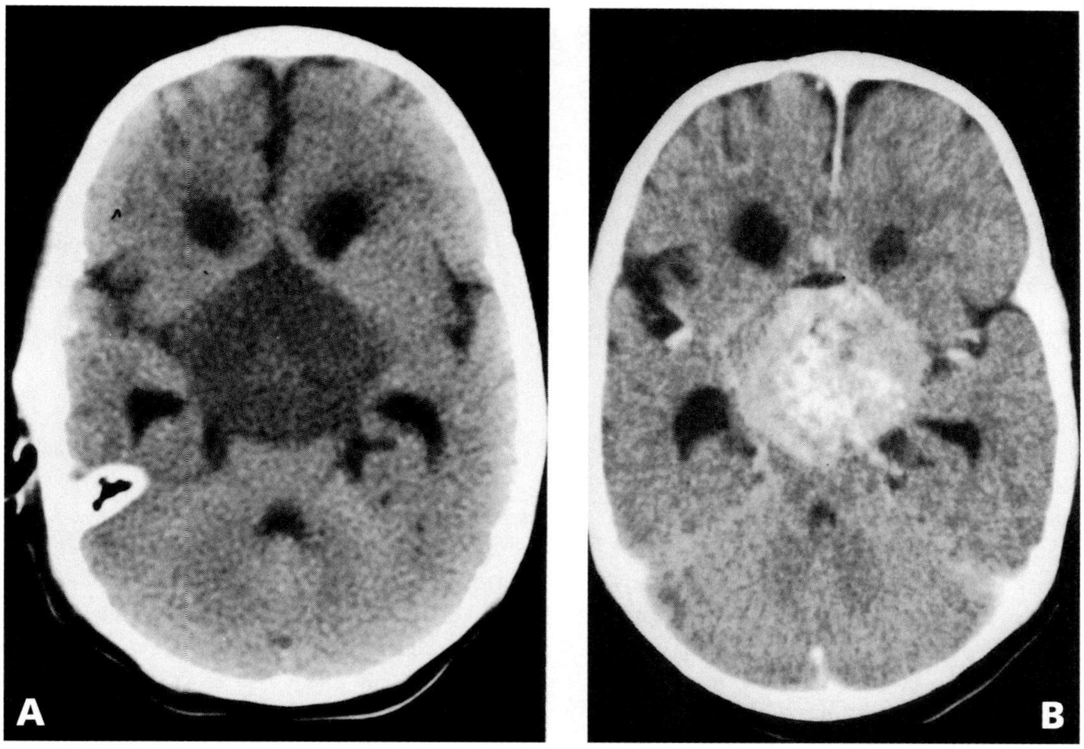

Figure 22-1

Question 107

This 7-month-old child has abnormal eye movements and hyperphagia. You are shown axial precontrast (A) and postcontrast (B) CT scans, as well as axial proton-density-weighted (C) and sagittal postcontrast T1-weighted (D) MR images (Figure 22-1).

Which *one* of the following is the MOST likely diagnosis?

(A) Langerhans cell histiocytosis
(B) Hypothalamic hamartoma
(C) Craniopharyngioma
(D) Suprasellar germinoma
(E) Hypothalamic-chiasmatic glioma

The axial noncontrast CT image (Figure 22-1A) demonstrates a large, hypodense, suprasellar mass expanding the suprasellar cistern. The mass is obstructing the drainage of the lateral ventricles, as evidenced by the enlargement of the frontal and temporal horns. No calcifications are present. Following the intravenous administration of contrast material, a heterogeneous pattern of enhancement is seen (Figure 22-1B). The mass obliterates the suprasellar cistern. An axial proton-density-weighted MR image confirms the location of the mass in the suprasellar cistern (Figure 22-1C). A sagittal postcontrast T1-weighted MR image demonstrates a bulky, homogeneously enhancing, predominantly suprasellar mass with extension into the sella (Figure 22-1D). The optic chiasm is not visible separate from the mass.

The sellar-parasellar region is composed of a variety of tis-

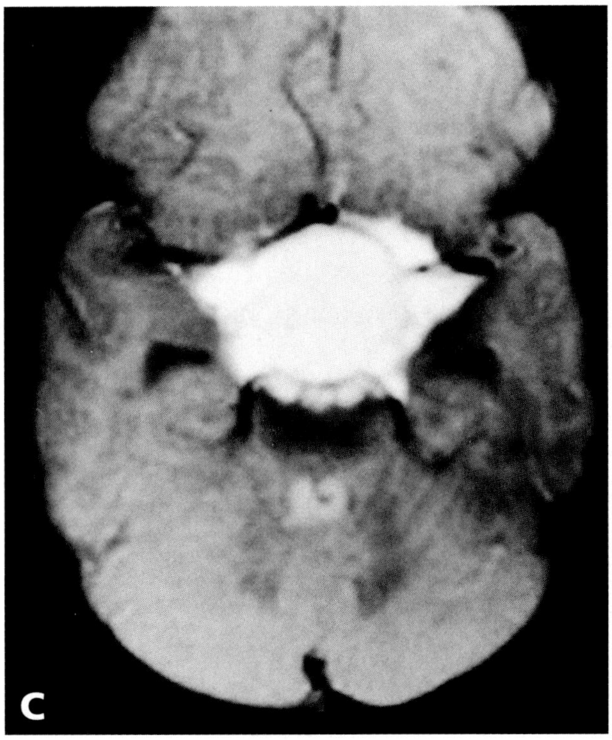

SE 3,000/45

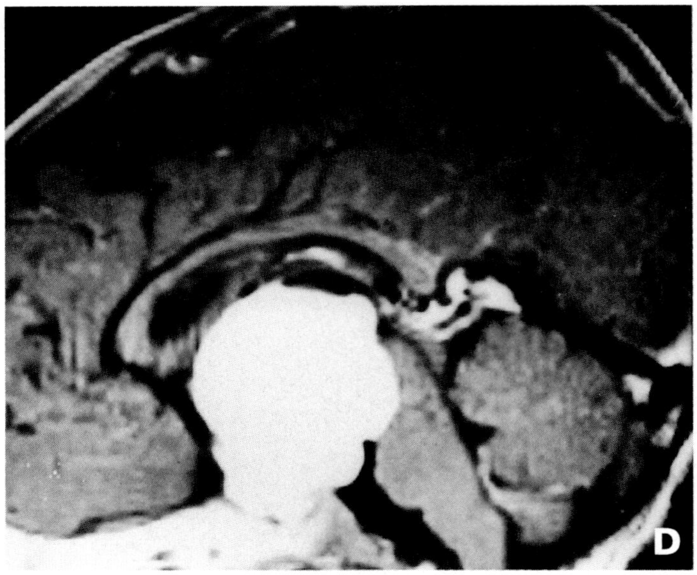

SE 700/20

Figure 22-1 (Continued)

sues, and each demonstrates complex embryologic development. This region of the brain is affected by a wide range of histologically different neoplasms and neoplasm-like diseases. Sellar and suprasellar tumors represent approximately 25% of all pediatric brain tumors. Both primary central nervous system tumors and developmental lesions can arise from embryonic cellular inclusions, neuroepithelial elements, the adenohypophysis, and surrounding bone, vessels, or meninges. Also, different hormonal and neural functions centered in this region of the brain lead to characteristic symptoms.

Hypothalamic-chiasmatic gliomas and craniopharyngiomas are the two most common lesions that arise in the suprasellar location in children and cause symptoms related to mass effect. The enlarging mass compresses the optic chiasm and the third ventricle, leading to visual impairment and ventricular obstruction. Hypothalamic-pituitary axis dysfunction is a later manifestation of the enlarging mass. Although their clinical features can be similar, these two lesions have imaging appearances that permit distinction in most cases. In the test patient, the presence of a bulky, homogeneous mass with moderate enhancement and the absence of calcifications or cyst formation strongly favor the diagnosis of hypothalamic-chiasmatic glioma (**Option (E) is correct**).

Craniopharyngiomas in children (Option (C)) typically are cystic and have calcifications within the lesion. Prior to the development of CT, calcification was identified on standard skull radiographs in over 70% of cases; it is seen on CT in over 90% of cases. The calcification can occur in the cyst wall or within the solid component of the tumor. Most often, the calcification will be irregular and can be dense or bone-like. The solid component of the lesion is frequently isodense with the surrounding normal brain. Over 90% of craniopharyngiomas enhance with intravenous contrast agent administration. Dominant cysts are demonstrated in more than 80% of cases. The cyst content is generally of low attenuation compared with the solid component of the tumor, but higher in attenuation than cerebrospinal fluid. The absence of calcifications and prominent cystic components makes craniopharyngioma an unlikely diagnosis in the test patient.

Langerhans cell histiocytosis (LCH) (Option (A)) and hypothalamic hamartoma (Option (B)) usually are smaller, more discrete lesions at the time of diagnosis than the tumor seen in the test patient. Each is often associated with a characteristic clinical syndrome, diabetes insipidus and diencephalic syndrome, respectively. LCH in the suprasellar region usually presents as a thickened infundibulum that is isodense on noncontrast CT or isointense on T1-weighted MR images. It is frequently associated with absence of the pituitary "bright spot," representing the neurohypophysis. There also may be a minimal decrease in the normal enhancement of the pituitary stalk. Occasionally, LCH appears on CT as a solitary mass in the region of the median eminence of the pituitary stalk. Hypothalamic hamartomas are lesions that are typically isodense relative to brain on CT. They typically exhibit no calcification or contrast enhancement. The size of the mass and the absence of classic symptoms in the test patient make both LCH and hypothalamic hamartoma unlikely diagnoses.

Germinomas (Option (D)) of the suprasellar region can

be hormonally active or can interrupt normal pituitary function by mass effect (Figure 22-2). The most common clinical manifestation is diabetes insipidus, followed by visual field defects and various syndromes of hypothalamic-pituitary dysfunction. Large lesions cause hydrocephalous either by obstructing the third ventricle or by interrupting the flow of cerebrospinal fluid through the suprasellar cistern. Small germinomas may first involve the pituitary stalk and region of the median eminence; rarely, they may extend to fill the sella turcica. Germinomas are isodense to hyperdense on CT and have a well-marginated appearance. Germinomas are hypointense on T1-weighted images and variable in appearance—from hypointense to mildly hyperintense—on T2-weighted images. The variability seems to be attributable to the level of cellularity of the tumor. Intense, homogeneous contrast enhancement is characteristic on both CT and MRI. In the test case, the hypodensity on noncontrast CT and the marked hyperintensity on T2-weighted MRI make germinoma an unlikely diagnosis.

Other solid lesions in the differential diagnosis of pediatric suprasellar masses include pituitary adenoma (Figure 22-3) and meningioma.

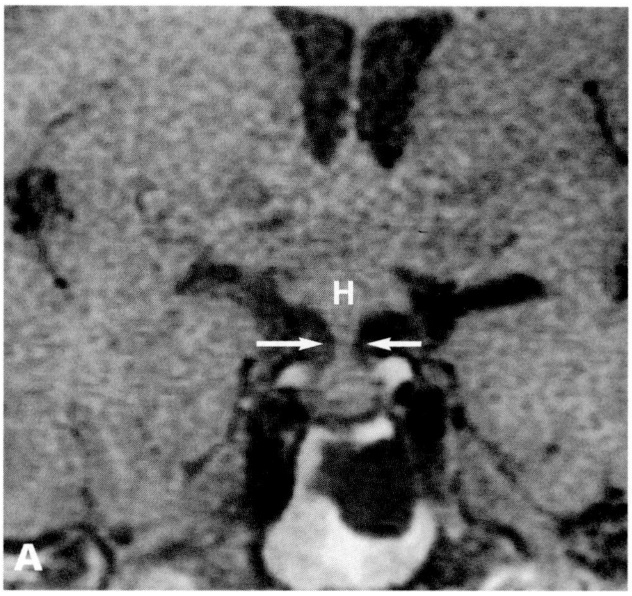

SE 500/20

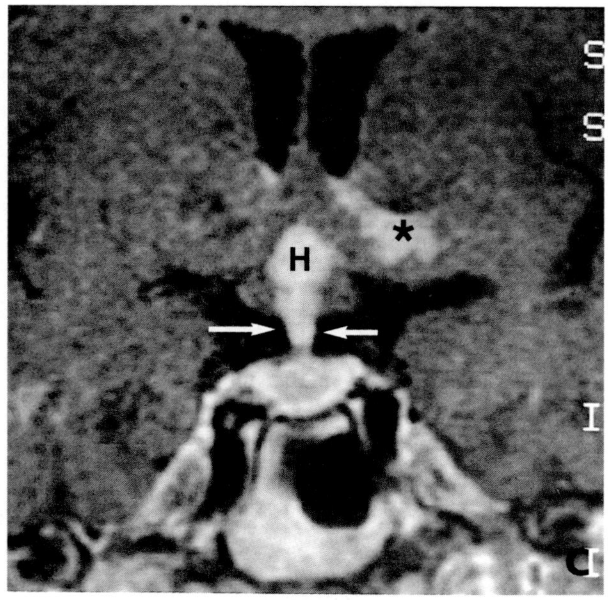

SE 500/25

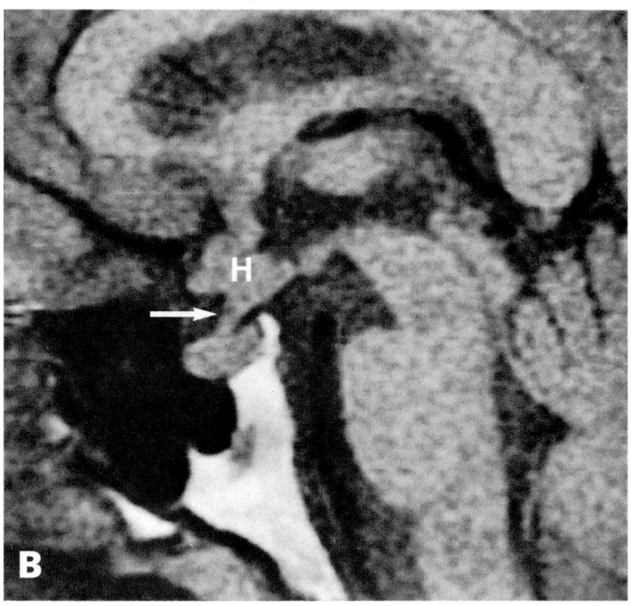

SE 500/20

Figure 22-2. Germinoma in a 19-year-old man with diabetes insipidus. Coronal (A) and sagittal (B) noncontrast T1-weighted MR images demonstrate thickening of the infundibulum (arrows) associated with enlargement of the hypothalamus (H). There is no posterior pituitary bright spot, a finding frequently identified in patients with diabetes insipidus. (C) A coronal T1-weighted MR image following gadolinium chelate administration reveals enhancement of the hypothalamus (H) and infundibulum (arrows). Note the parenchymal enhancement (*), indicative of extension of this suprasellar germinoma via the Virchow-Robin spaces.

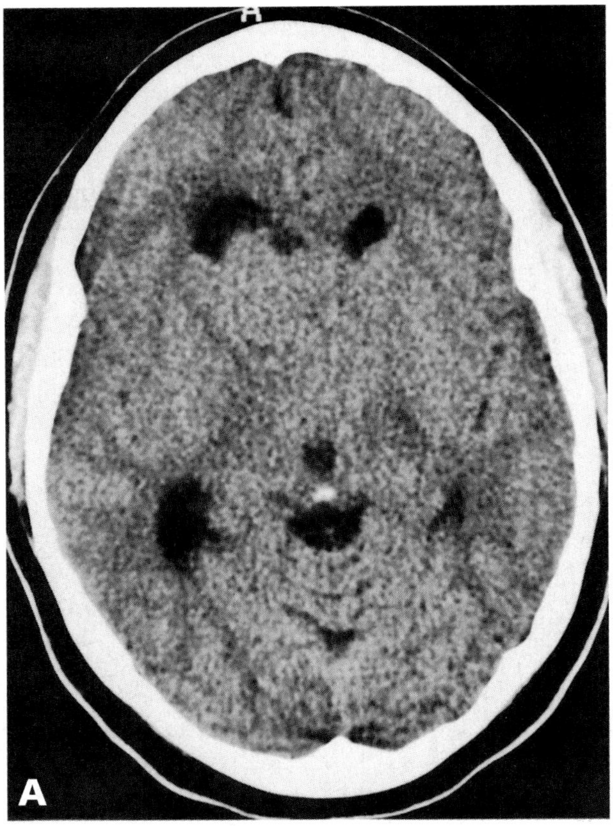

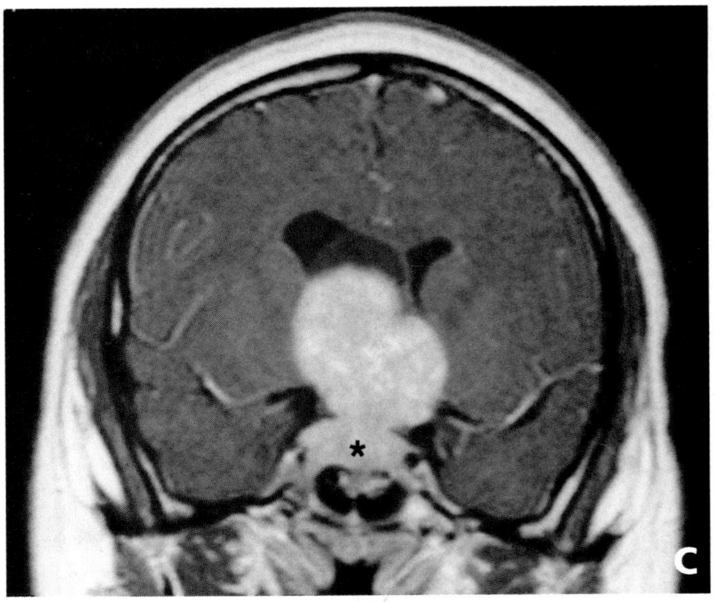

SE 500/17

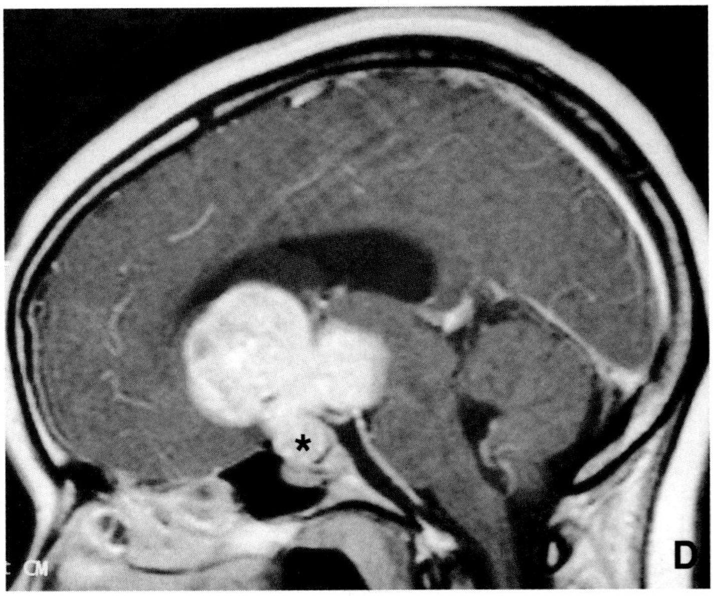

SE 500/17

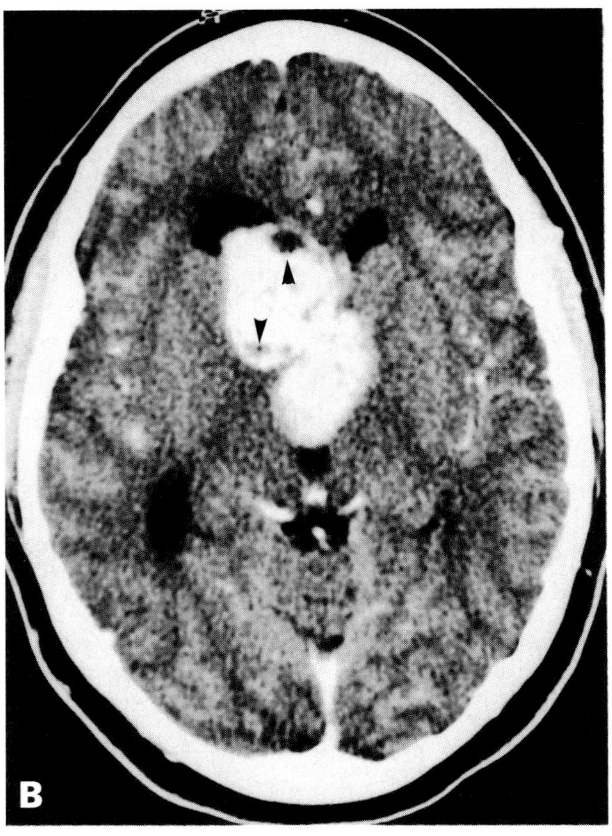

Figure 22-3. Pituitary adenoma in a 15-year-old girl with headache and visual complaints. (A) An axial noncontrast CT scan demonstrates an ill-defined mass, isodense relative to gray matter, causing displacement and compression of the lateral and third ventricles. (B) Following contrast agent administration, homogeneous enhancement of the mass is seen on CT. Small cysts are present within the mass (arrowheads). (C and D) Coronal (C) and sagittal (D) T1-weighted MR images following gadolinium chelate administration demonstrate the intrasellar component (*) of the mass, as well as the lobulated suprasellar extensions. This adenoma was not hormonally active, and the symptoms were related to the mass effect of the tumor on adjacent structures.

Question 108

Concerning intracranial Langerhans cell histiocytosis,

(A) most patients also have extracranial involvement
(B) patients often have precocious puberty
(C) diabetes insipidus is attributable to involvement of the hypothalamic nuclei
(D) an early finding on MRI is thickening of the pituitary stalk
(E) absence of the neurohypophyseal signal on a T1-weighted MR image is a characteristic finding

LCH is one disease in the spectrum of disorders referred to as histiocytoses. Prior to the identification of abnormal Langerhans cell proliferation in 1973, these disorders were referred to as histiocytosis X and were subdivided into eosinophilic granuloma (isolated bone disease), Hand-Schüller-Christian disease (geographic skull lesions, diabetes insipidus, and exophthalmos), and Letterer-Siwe disease (widespread or disseminated disease). It has now been determined that these disorders are unified by the proliferation of cells within the mononuclear phagocytic system and the dendritic cell system. Both of these cell types are derived from the same bone marrow stem cell, the promonocyte. Both are normally responsible for mediating immune and nonimmune inflammatory responses.

When signs or symptoms of LCH are referable to the skull or nervous system, patients typically present with diabetes insipidus attributable to involvement of the hypothalamic-pituitary axis (Figure 22-4). Diabetes insipidus develops when more than 80% of the neurons in the paraventricular and supraoptic nuclei of the hypothalmus are destroyed (**Option (C) is true**). Diabetes insipidus is present in at least 5% of patients with LCH at the time of diagnosis, but in more than 30% of

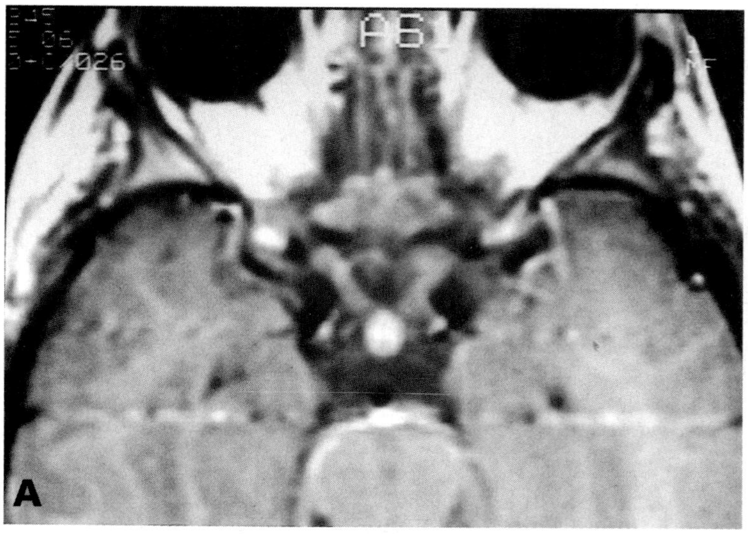

SE 650/30

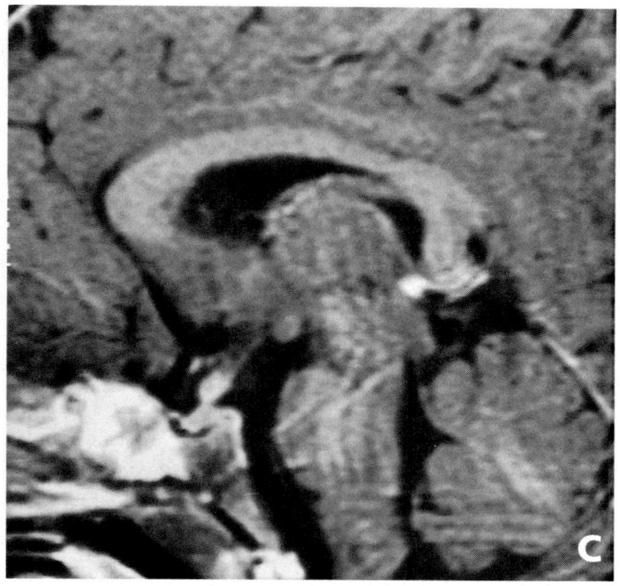

TR 600/11

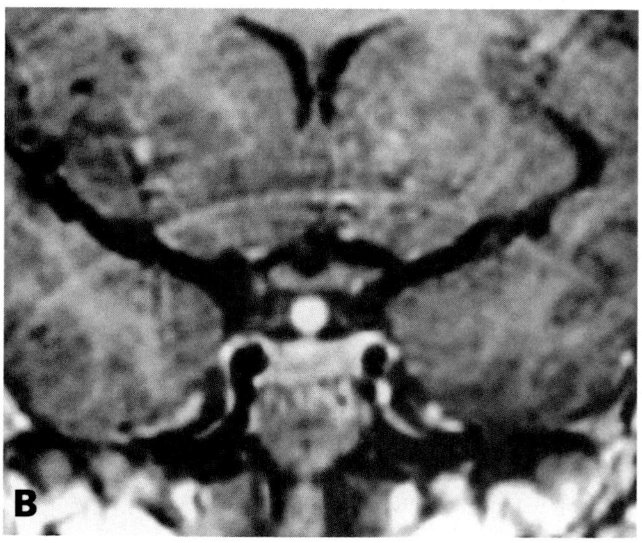

SE 500/23

Figure 22-4. Langerhans cell histiocytosis in a 2-year-old boy with erythematous skin lesions. Axial (A), coronal (B), and sagittal (C) T1-weighted images following gadolinium chelate administration demonstrate thickening and enhancement of the infundibulum. Both of these imaging features are typical of the histiocytic infiltration in LCH. No enlargement or enhancement of the hypothalamus is identified.

patients on follow-up examination. When the pituitary stalk and hypothalamus are involved with LCH, the stalk is thickened (>2.5 mm); this is an early finding of the disease at this site **(Option (D) is true).** The thickening is difficult to see on CT without intravenous contrast agent administration, especially if images are obtained only in the axial plane. When images are obtained in the coronal plane, both the thickening and enhancement of the infundibulum are readily appreciated. MRI is preferred for assessing the hypothalamic region, because the thickening and enhancement can best be appreciated in both the sagittal and coronal planes. The thickened pituitary stalk enhances markedly after intravenous administration of paramagnetic contrast agents.

The normal posterior pituitary exhibits a short T1 relaxation time (appearing as the characteristic pituitary bright spot on T1-weighted images). After the development of diabetes insipidus, the high signal intensity in the posterior pituitary disappears (Figure 22-5) **(Option (E) is true).** The presence of the bright spot is correlated with the concentration of vasopressin in the neurohypophysis. Experimental studies with MRI obtained before and after water deprivation demonstrate a relationship between the brightness of the posterior pituitary and the quantitative vasopressin-neurophysin II content. Also, MRI studies of the posterior pituitary bright spot in normal subjects suggest that it is attributable to an interaction of water with paramagnetic or low-molecular-weight molecules, such as vasopressin and neurophysins.

Infiltration of the hypothalamic nuclei and the pituitary stalk, causing disruption of the hypothalamic-neurohypophyseal axis, results in the clinical syndrome of diabetes insipidus. This syndrome is characterized by polyuria and polydipsia. Diabetes insipidus can be central (vasopressin deficient) or nephrogenic (vasopressin resistant). Diabetes insipidus of central origin can be associated with LCH, trauma, tumor, or infection. MRI is valuable for ascertaining the etiology of diabetes insipidus, first by demonstrating the absence of the normal posterior pituitary bright spot (Figure 22-5) and, second, by allowing examination of the pituitary, suprasellar cistern, and infundibular stalk.

Central precocious puberty is a clinical syndrome defined by the development of secondary sexual characteristics prior to age 8 in girls and age 9 in boys. Activation of the hypothalamic-pituitary-gonadal hormonal axis results in increased secretion of (gonadal) sexual steroids and pituitary gonadotropins. In a 1995 study of patients with central precocious puberty, Kornreich et al. found that the majority (44 of 62) had normal examinations; however, hamartoma of the tuber cinereum and hypothalamic-chiasmatic gliomas were seen in more than 50% of those with demonstrable intracranial pathology. No cases of LCH were documented as a cause for precocious puberty **(Option (B) is false).**

Clinical manifestations of LCH vary with the distribution of the disease. Restricted LCH includes skin rashes and monostotic or polyostotic bone lesions with or without associated diabetes insipidus or lymphadenopathy. More extensive LCH in-

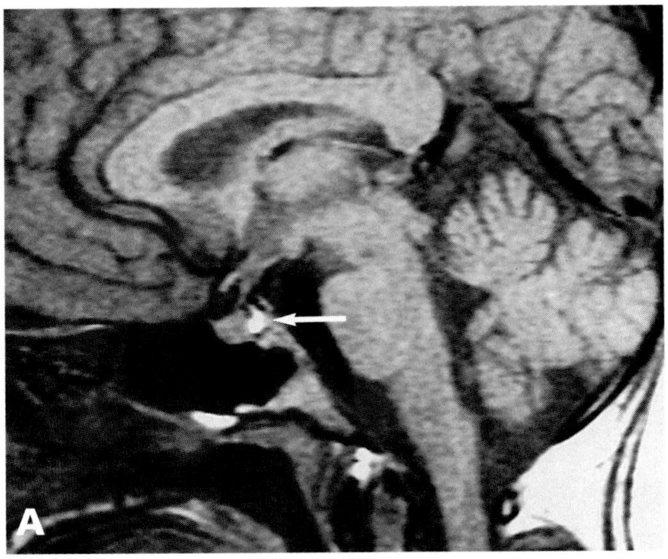

SE 600/20

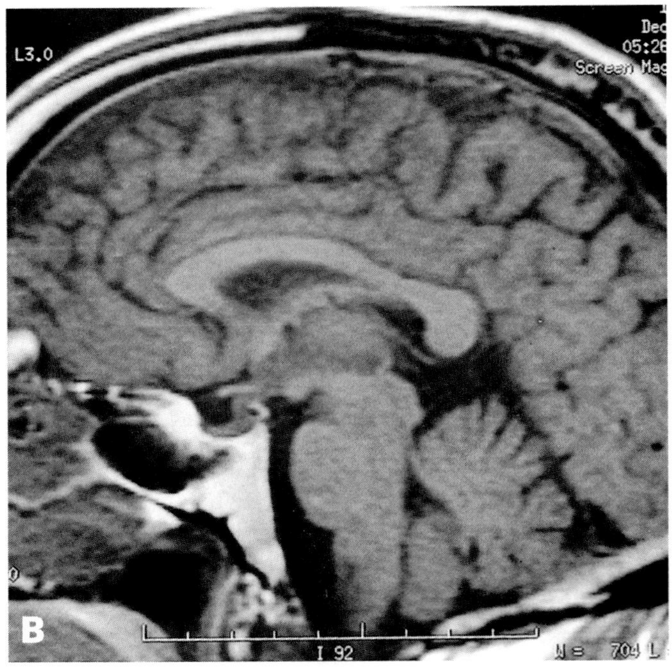

SE 400/8

Figure 22-5. Pituitary bright spot. (A) The posterior pituitary is normally bright on a noncontrast T1-weighted image (arrow). (B) The bright spot is conspicuously absent on an MR image of a patient with diabetes insipidus attributable to histiocytic infiltration in LCH.

cludes visceral organ involvement with or without clinical signs of organ system dysfunction in pulmonary, hepatic, or hemopoietic systems. Bone lesions are found in about 80% of patients with LCH and are associated with painful swelling (Figure 22-6). These lesions are located most commonly in the skull and then in the long and flat bones. Middle ear infiltration can cause destruction of the ossicles, resulting in deafness. "Floating teeth" and vertebra plana also are manifestations of bone infiltration.

Scaly erythematous papules, particularly in intertriginous

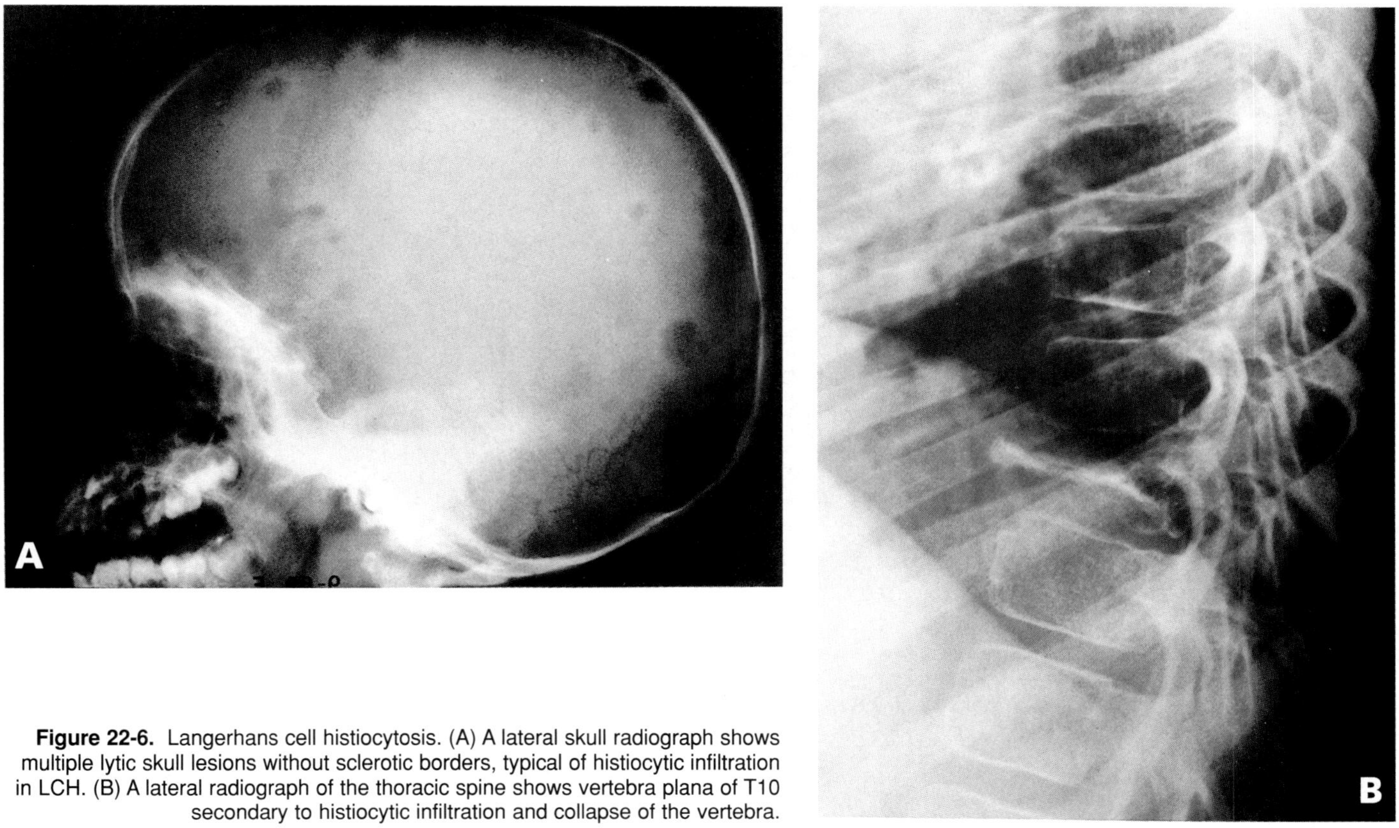

Figure 22-6. Langerhans cell histiocytosis. (A) A lateral skull radiograph shows multiple lytic skull lesions without sclerotic borders, typical of histiocytic infiltration in LCH. (B) A lateral radiograph of the thoracic spine shows vertebra plana of T10 secondary to histiocytic infiltration and collapse of the vertebra.

zones, behind the ear and in the axial and perineal areas, can be present with or without ulceration or lymphadenopathy. Hepatosplenomegaly is caused by histiocytic infiltration, which can lead to cirrhosis and liver failure. Pulmonary involvement can be manifested as tachypnea, with associated fever and weight loss. A micronodular pattern in the lungs is typical. Gastrointestinal involvement can be clinically silent; however, malabsorption syndromes can develop in association with LCH and can contribute to the overall growth retardation seen in affected patients. Growth retardation occurs in less than 1% of LCH patients and may be related more to issues of general nutrition and steroid therapy than to direct pituitary dysfunction.

Although diabetes insipidus can occur before, concurrently, or after the development of bone lesions, patients with widespread or disseminated disease are more likely to develop diabetes insipidus. Skull lesions usually precede the development of diabetes insipidus. The majority of patients with central nervous system involvement in LCH also have involvement of extracranial sites (**Option (A) is true**). Later in the disease course, neurologic deficits can develop because of parenchymal infiltration. This uncommon parenchymal involvement consists of histiocytic infiltration of the cerebellum and periventricular cerebral white matter. These infiltrative lesions develop symmetrically within the cerebellum. Progressive ataxia, dysarthria, and other cerebellar signs are the clinical manifestations of cerebellar infiltration.

Question 109

Concerning hypothalamic hamartoma,

(A) it is a congenital lesion
(B) it involves the tuber cinereum
(C) precocious puberty is the usual presenting symptom
(D) gelastic seizures are characteristic
(E) it usually is 1 to 2 cm in diameter
(F) it usually enhances intensely

Hypothalamic hamartomas are well-defined round or oval congenital lesions projecting from the base of the brain, either the mamillary bodies or tuber cinereum, into the interpeduncular or suprasellar cistern (Figure 22-7) (**Options (A) and (B) are true**). Histologically, the lesions are characterized by neuronal heterotopia with an astrocytic and oligodendrocytic stroma.

These lesions typically are seen in boys less than 2 years old. The majority of these boys present with isosexual precocious puberty (**Option (C) is true**). Gelastic seizures (laughing seizures) are characteristic (**Option (D) is true**). The clinical symptoms of gelastic seizures and precocious puberty are more common when the hamartoma is 1 to 2 cm in diameter, although the usual hamartoma is discovered when it is only 3 to 4 mm in size (**Option (E) is false**).

Obesity and diabetes insipidus have been reported with this tumor. Acromegaly can result secondary to the secretion of growth hormone-releasing factor by a hypothalamic hamartoma.

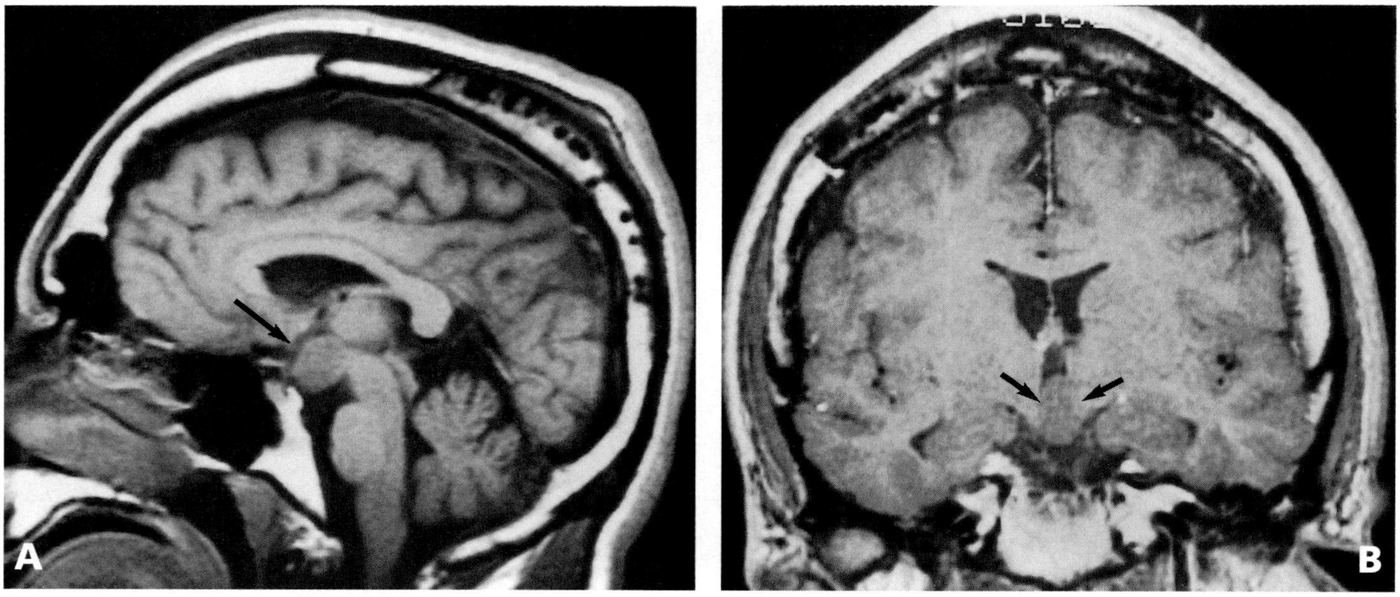

SE 500/11 SE 500/25

Figure 22-7. Hypothalamic hamartoma in a 4-year-old boy with diencephalic syndrome. (A) A noncontrast sagittal T1-weighted image demonstrates a hypointense mass (arrow) arising from the hypothalamus and extending into the suprasellar cistern. (B) A coronal T1-weighted image following gadolinium chelate administration demonstrates no enhancement of the hamartoma (arrows).

This tumor has been seen in conjunction with other congenital abnormalities, including hypoplasia of the olfactory bulb, cardiac and renal malformations, absence of the pituitary gland, and imperforate anus. The etiology of precocious puberty in association with this lesion is not fully understood. The proposed pathophysiologic mechanism includes abnormalities in the inhibitory pathways from the hypothalamus to the posterior pituitary or direct secretory effects from the tumor. Other intracranial tumors can be associated with precocious puberty. These include suprasellar germinomas, third ventricular astrocytoma, and primary intracranial choriocarcinoma.

Hypothalamic hamartomas may be difficult to identify on CT. They sometimes can be recognized as an isodense mass in the suprasellar or interpeduncular cistern. No enhancement is seen following contrast agent infusion **(Option (F) is false).** Occasionally, cystic components can be present and can extend beyond the suprasellar cistern. On MRI, these lesions are typically well defined, and a thin stalk may be identified attaching the hamartoma to the mamillary bodies or tuber cinereum. They are isointense relative to the brain on T1-weighted images and isointense or slightly hyperintense on T2-weighted images. No enhancement is seen on MRI following the injection of a paramagnetic contrast agent (Figure 22-7B).

A variation of the hypothalamic hamartoma is the Pallister-Hall syndrome (Figure 22-8). The syndrome is composed of a hypothalamic hamartoma or hamartoblastoma extending into the suprasellar cistern in association with a variable constellation of extracranial abnormalities. The hamartoma of Pallister-Hall syndrome appears to contain more primitive cells than are seen in the usual or typical small hamartoma of the tuber cinereum. There are frequently associated midline intracranial and facial anomalies. Extracranial manifestations include polydactyly, cleft palate, epiglottic or laryngeal abnormalities, congenital heart defects, imperforate anus, hypopituitarism, and a variety of genitourinary malformations. Affected children frequently do not survive infancy, usually because of the syndrome's extracranial manifestations.

Question 110

Concerning craniopharyngioma,

(A) it is calcified in about 30% of cases
(B) it usually enhances uniformly
(C) intrasellar involvement occurs in about 10% of cases
(D) leptomeningeal spread is common
(E) it is the most common suprasellar mass in childhood

Craniopharyngioma is the most common suprasellar tumor in children, accounting for about 10% of all childhood intracranial neoplasms and 50% of suprasellar lesions **(Option (E) is true).** Craniopharyngiomas are tumors arising from remnants of Rathke's pouch and can arise anywhere from the nasopharynx to the third ventricle. Although histologically benign, craniopharyngiomas are extremely infiltrative, often compromising adjacent structures, such as the pituitary gland, the hypothalamus, and the optic chiasm (Figure 22-9). This invasive characteristic makes complete surgical resection difficult; thus, treatment generally requires adjuvant radiation therapy with or without chemotherapy. Leptomeningeal spread is not a feature of craniopharyngiomas, however **(Option (D) is false).**

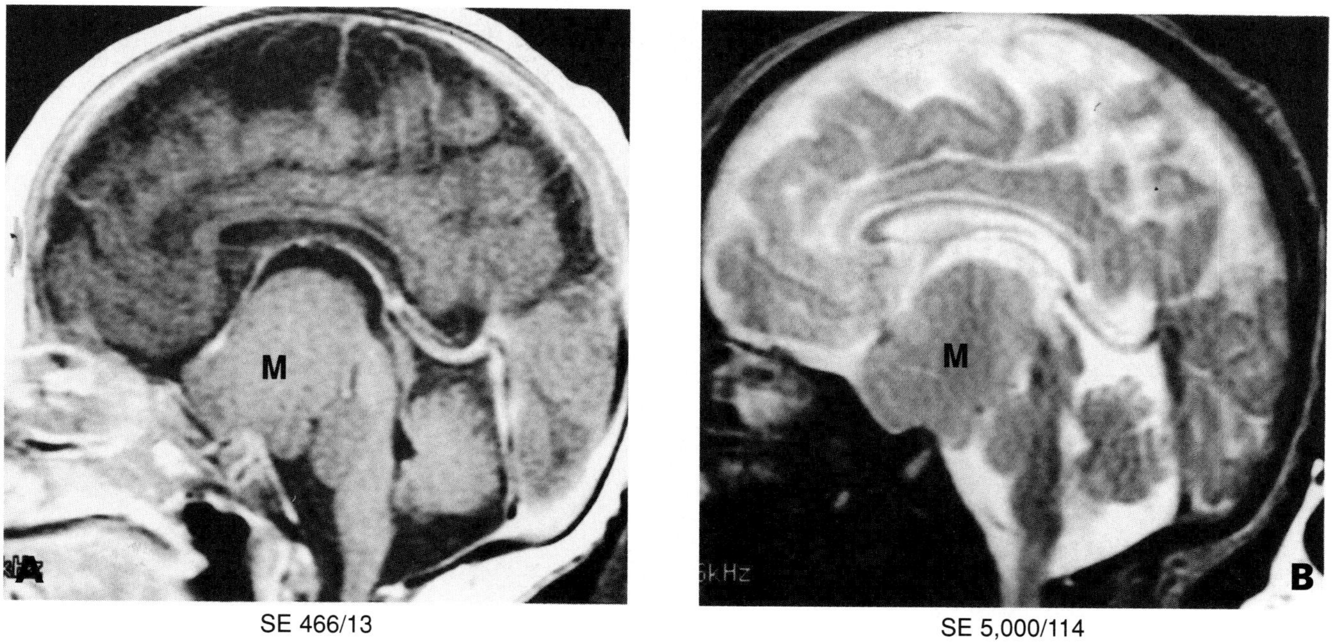

Figure 22-8. Pallister-Hall syndrome with hypothalamic hamartoma in a male newborn with multiple systemic congenital anomalies. A sagittal T1-weighted MR image following gadolinium chelate administration (A) and a sagittal T2-weighted MR image (B) demonstrate a large mass (M) isointense relative to the brain in the hypothalamic region, extending to encroach upon the sella, and displacing the optic chiasm. The absence of enhancement and the lack of increased signal intensity on the T2-weighted image are consistent with the diagnosis of hypothalamic hamartoma. (Case courtesy of A. John Kuta, M.D., Henrico Doctors Hospital, Richmond, VA.)

Craniopharyngiomas have a bimodal age distribution: most occur in children 8 to 12 years old; the second incidence peak occurs in the sixth decade. There is a slight male predominance. Clinical symptoms and signs are related to the location and growth pattern of the tumor. Visual disturbances occur in over 50% of patients and include bitemporal hemianopsia, diplopia, and decreased visual acuity or blindness. Other symptoms and signs include cranial nerve deficits, pituitary dysfunction (30%), and papilledema (because of increased intracranial pressure). The increase in intracranial pressure may result from tumor bulk or from hydrocephalus caused by obstruction of the third ventricle or the foramina of Monro (Figure 22-9). Pituitary dysfunction frequently manifests as growth retardation with delayed or precocious puberty and obesity. Other signs of hypothalamic dysfunction are relatively rare.

Calcifications are present in about 90% of childhood craniopharyngiomas and can be curvilinear, punctate, or clump-like in appearance (**Option (A) is false**). These tumors frequently have a dominant cyst lined by simple stratified squamous epithelium on a collagenous basement membrane. The solid components are composed of columnar basal cells with a vascular connective tissue stroma. The cysts contain cholesterol. Craniopharyngiomas occasionally can be entirely cystic or entirely solid in appearance (Figure 22-10).

On CT, a craniopharyngioma is distinguishable by its suprasellar location, the presence of clumplike or rimlike calcifications, and cystic or solid masses that exhibit intense contrast enhancement in 90% of cases (Figures 22-9 and 22-10). In nearly 80% of cases, the presence of calcifications and the mixed solid and cystic elements contribute to the overall heterogeneous imaging appearance of the craniopharyngioma both before and after contrast agent administration on CT and MRI (**Option (B) is false**). Only 75% of craniopharyngiomas reside in the classic suprasellar location. In 21%, they extend into the sella, and in a minority (4%), they are entirely intrasellar in location (**Option (C) is false**). Large tumors can extend into the posterior fossa.

On MRI, craniopharyngiomas are heterogeneous on all imaging sequences. The cysts can be hypointense, isointense, or hyperintense on T1-weighted images. The signal intensity correlates poorly with the constituents of the cyst fluid, which can contain various combinations of cholesterol, triglycerides, or blood. The solid portion of the tumor usually is hyperintense on T2-weighted images and isointense on T1-weighted images, with enhancement following contrast agent administration (Figures 22-9 and 22-10).

The principal differential diagnostic consideration for the predominantly cystic or intrasellar craniopharyngioma is a Rathke's cleft cyst. Rathke's cleft is located between the pars nervosa and the pars distalis of the pituitary gland. Enlargement of this cleft causes displacement of the infundibulum anteriorly. The cleft is lined with cuboidal epithelium and can contain mucin-producing goblet cells. Within this cleft, a cyst containing mucin, desquamated epithelium, cholesterol, and sometimes blood products can arise. Calcification is rare, and enhancement is unusual (Figure 22-11).

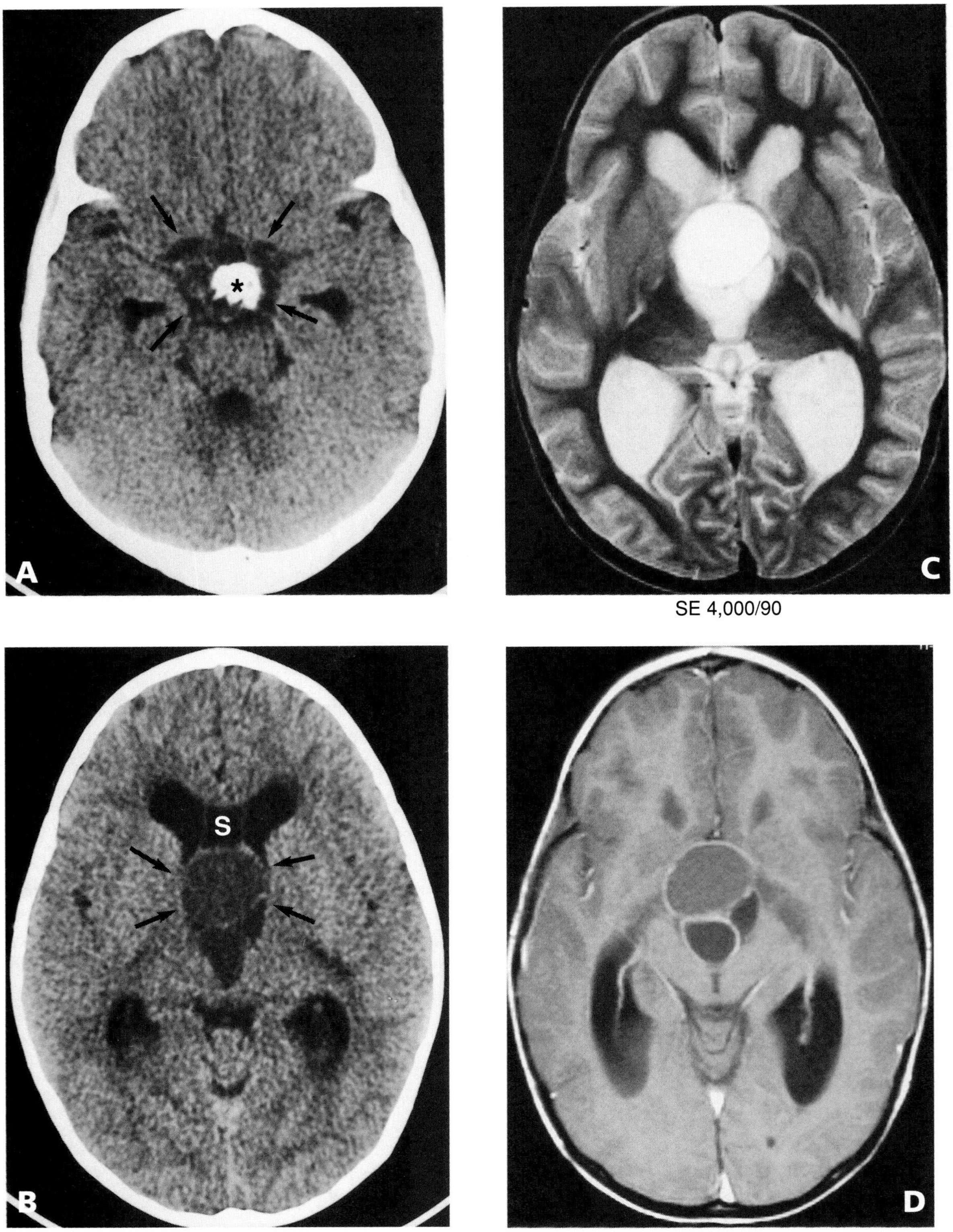

Figure 22-9. Craniopharyngioma in a 4-year-old male with blindness. (A and B) Axial CT scans at the level at the suprasellar cistern (A) and at the level of the foramina of Monro (B) demonstrate a clump of irregular calcification (*) in the midline and to the left of midline and associated hypodense cyst formation (arrows). Note the separation of the leaves of the septum pellucidum (S) and the prominent temporal horns indicating ventricular obstruction at the foramina of Monro. (C) An axial T2-weighted MR image at the level of the foramina of Monro again demonstrates the multicystic mass. The T2 signal characteristics are similar among the multiple cysts. (D) An axial T1-weighted MR image following gadolinium chelate adminstration at a level just below the foramina of Monro demonstrates peripheral enhancement around two of the three cystic lesions, with variations in signal intensity between the cysts indicating slightly different contents. (E) A sagittal T1-weighted MR image following gadolinium chelate administration demonstrates two cysts with an enhancing solid component of the tumor extending into the suprasellar cistern and sella.

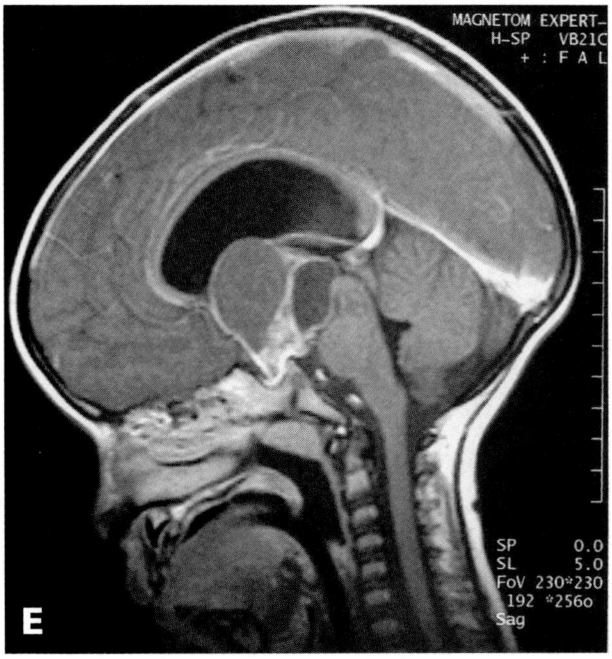

SE 630/17

Figure 22-9 (Continued)

Question 111

Concerning hypothalamic-chiasmatic glioma,

(A) it is associated with diencephalic syndrome
(B) it is associated with neurofibromatosis type 1
(C) cystic components are seen on MRI in most lesions
(D) enhancement occurs in less than 20% of lesions

Hypothalamic-chiasmatic gliomas represent 3.5% to 5% of all pediatric intracranial tumors and 10% to 15% of supratentorial tumors of childhood. Of all tumors arising in the suprasellar region, they are second only to craniopharyngiomas. There is an equal male and female predominance.

The term "hypothalamic-chiasmatic glioma" was derived to describe suprasellar astrocytomas arising from the optic chiasm as well as those arising from the hypothalamus. These tumors are often large when diagnosed; thus, the exact tissue of origin may not be discernible. Hypothalamic tumors can grow inferiorly to involve the chiasm. Likewise, chiasmatic tumors can grow superiorly to involve the hypothalamus, thus resulting in a single mass that invaginates the third ventricle. For this reason, chiasmatic and hypothalamic tumors are generally grouped together as a single entity on the basis of their similar histology, clinical presentation, and therapy.

These lesions frequently are seen in children 2 to 4 years old who present with decreased visual acuity and physical ex-

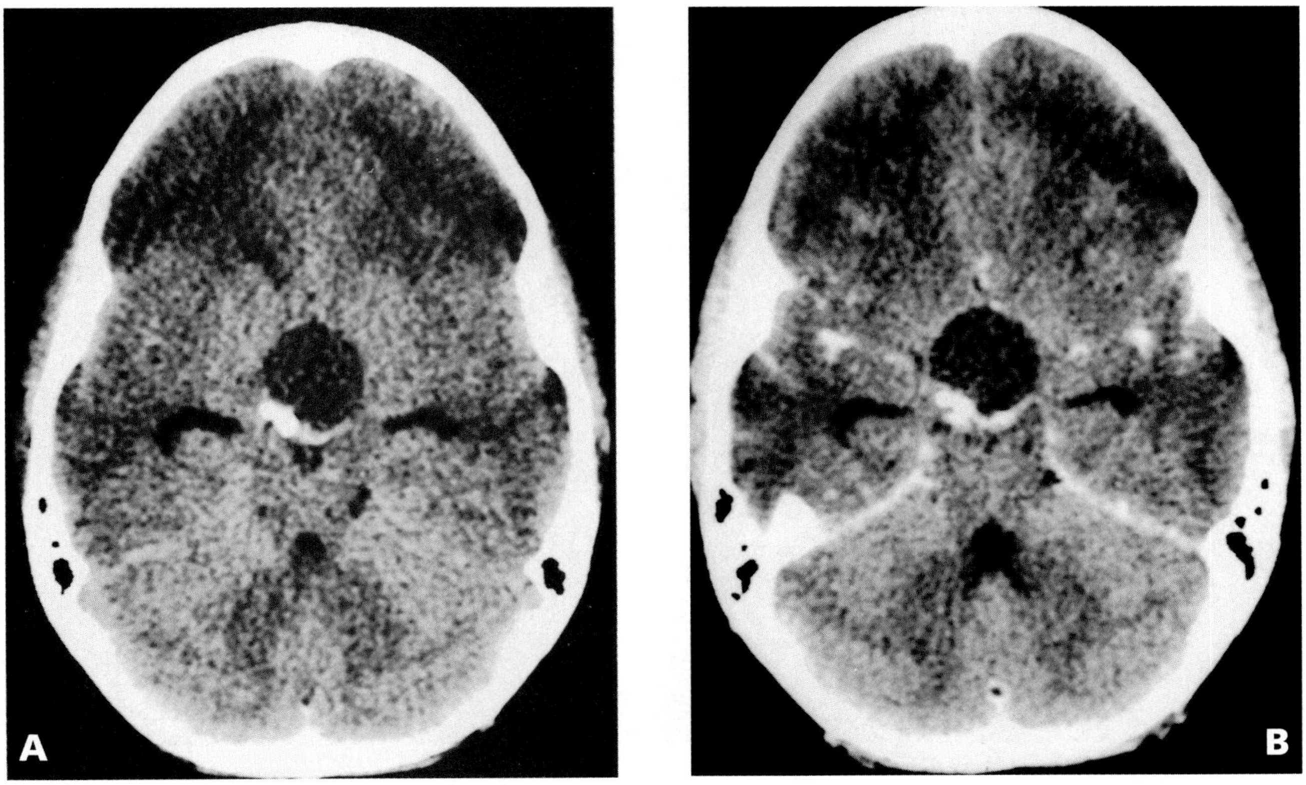

Figure 22-10. Craniopharyngioma in a 12-year-old girl with visual loss. (A) An axial noncontrast CT scan demonstrates a cyst with posterior rim-like calcification in the suprasellar cistern. Note the prominent temporal horns secondary to early ventricular obstruction by the mass. (B) Following contrast agent administration, minimal enhancement of the anterior rim of the cyst was identified.

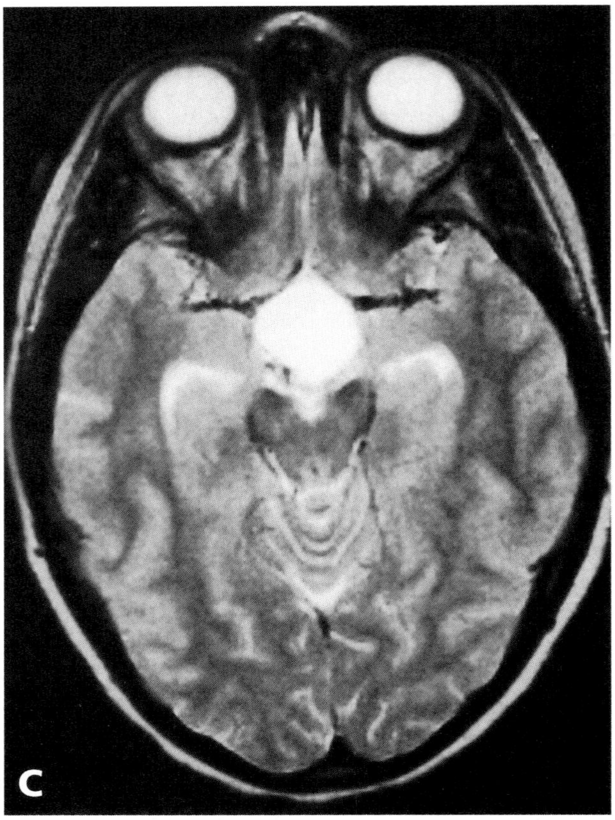

SE 4,000/90

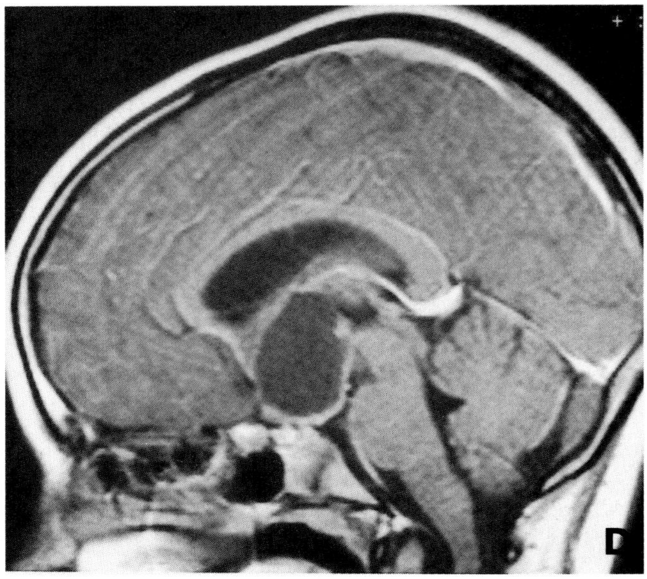

SE 630/17

Figure 22-10 (Continued). Craniopharyngioma in a 12-year-old girl with visual loss. (C) The cyst is homogeneous in signal intensity on an axial T2-weighted MR image, with lower signal intensity corresponding to the calcified portion of the cyst wall. (D) A sagittal T1-weighted image following gadolinium chelate administration demonstrates the well-defined tumor cyst separate from the pituitary gland.

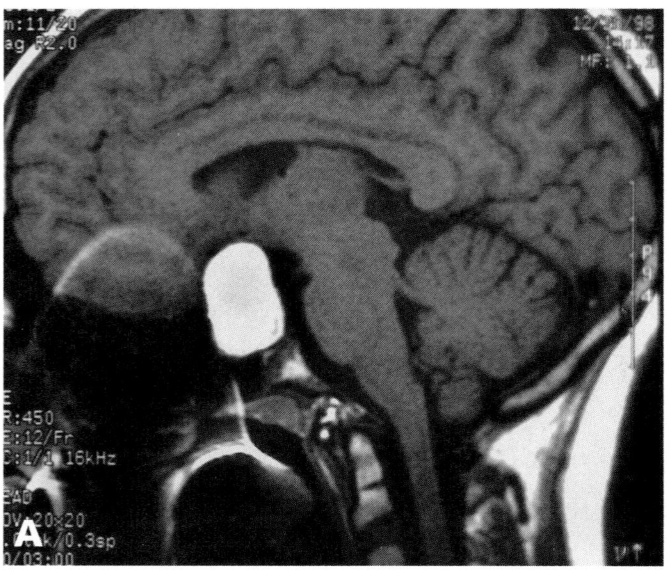

SE 450/12

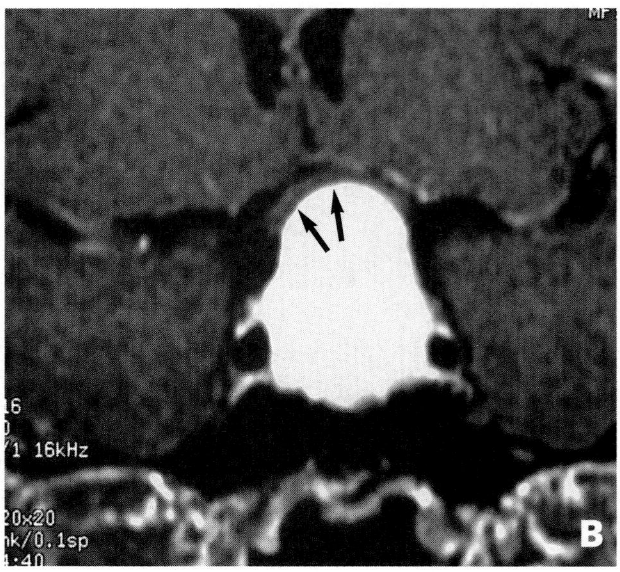

SE 716/20

Figure 22-11. Rathke's cleft cyst in a 14-year-old boy with decreased visual acuity. (A) A sagittal noncontrast T1-weighted MR image demonstrates a hyperintense cystic mass in the sella and suprasellar cistern. (B) A coronal T1-weighted MR image following gadolinium chelate administration demonstrates no enhancement of the cyst. Note the elevation of the optic chiasm (arrows).

amination evidence of optic atrophy. Precocious puberty and hypersomnia are rare. Emaciation, alertness, and hyperactivity are present in 20% of affected patients less than 3 years old and represent the constellation of clinical findings of the diencephalic syndrome (**Option (A) is true**). The emaciation is profound despite a normal dietary intake. Low-grade gliomas of the anterior hypothalamus or optic chiasm generally are associated with this syndrome. Partial resection or chemotherapy and radiation therapy may be useful for restoration of normal endocrine function.

Optic pathway gliomas have a strong association with neurofibromatosis type 1 (NF-1). During the lifetime of patients with NF-1, between 14% and 40% of patients will develop hypothalamic-chiasmatic gliomas (**Option (B) is true**). It should be noted that 50% of children with hypothalamic-chiasmatic gliomas have no evidence of neurofibromatosis. Tumors truly arising from the hypothalamus have no association with NF-1. The typical hypothalamic-chiasmatic glioma is histologically a pilocytic astrocytoma. Such astrocytomas also can arise in the prechiasmatic region or within the optic radiations. They can extend along the entire visual pathway. In patients with NF-1, tumors usually are quiescent and treatment can be conservative. When vision is impaired, aggressive surgical management is indicated.

The 5-year survival rate in patients with hypothalamic-chiasmatic gliomas has been reported to be between 40% and 88%, with a worse prognosis in children less than 5 years old. The principal morbidity of tumors in this location is visual deficit leading to blindness. Medical therapy can be useful for endocrine dysfunction. Increased intracranial pressure causing clinical symptoms is treated aggressively with ventricular shunting and surgical resection.

On CT, a hypothalamic-chiasmatic glioma appears as a low-density lobulated mass in the suprasellar region, inseparable from the optic chiasm. Such tumors may extend anteriorly to enlarge one or both optic nerves. CT shows associated enlargement of the optic foramina to better advantage than does MRI. The majority of these tumors show enhancement (**Option (D) is false**). However, the degree of enhancement is extremely variable, even from one portion of the tumor to another in the same patient. This variable pattern of enhancement includes diffuse tumor enhancement in the region of the chiasm with little or no enhancement in the region of the optic nerves or differential enhancement of the solid component of the chiasmatic tumor. MRI is optimal for showing the relationship of the mass to the chiasm, hypothalamus, and infundibulum (Figure 22-12). These tumors are nearly all solid; hemorrhage, calcification, and cyst formation are very unusual in tumors of the optic nerves prior to therapy (**Option (C) is false**). Fat suppression techniques are usually used for postcontrast MRI when evaluating intraorbital involvement in order to distinguish enhancing tumor from intraorbital fat. The tumor tends to be isodense with white matter on both T1- and T2-weighted images in the prechiasmatic region, with moderate enhancement after gadolinium chelate administration. Chiasmatic and hypothalamic tumors are usually hypodense on T1-weighted images and moderately to markedly hyperintense on T2-weighted images. Whereas tumors in the optic chiasm usually enhance markedly, prechiasmatic and postchiasmatic tumors, as well as intraorbital tumors, enhance much less.

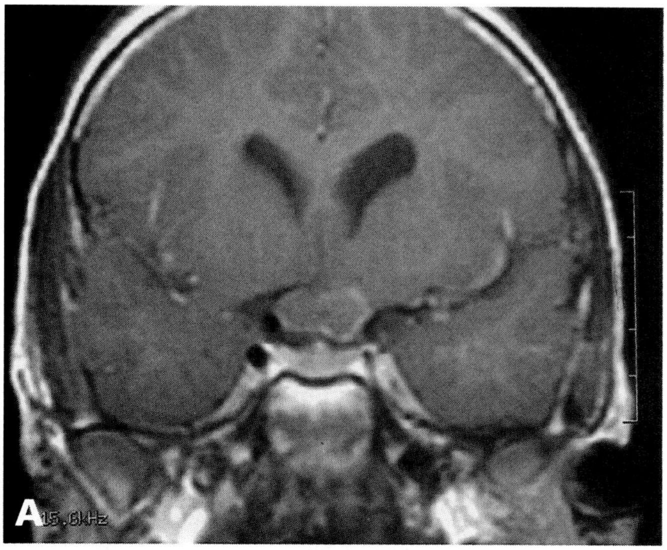

SE 400/20

Figure 22-12. Malignant hypothalamic-chiasmatic glioma in a 6-year-old girl who presented with precocious puberty and bitemporal visual field deficits. (A) A coronal T1-weighted MR image following gadolinium chelate administration demonstrates enlargement of the optic chiasm with peripheral, rim-like enhancement.

SUGGESTED READINGS

HYPOTHALAMIC-CHIASMATIC GLIOMA

1. Alshail E, Rutka JT, Becker LE, Hoffman HJ. Optic chiasmatic-hypothalamic glioma. Brain Pathol 1997; 7:799–806
2. Gropman AL, Packer RJ, Nicholson HS, et al. Treatment of diencephalic syndrome with chemotherapy: growth, tumor response, and long term control. Cancer 1998; 83:166–172
3. Guibaud L, Rode V, Saint-Pierre G, Pracros JP, Foray P, Tran-Minh VA. Giant hypothalamic hamartoma: an unusual neonatal tumor. Pediatr Radiol 1995; 25:17–18
4. Poussaint TY, Barnes PD, Nichols K, et al. Diencephalic syndrome; clinical features and imaging findings. AJNR 1997; 18:1499– 1505
5. Ritter AM, Kubal W, Luo V, Bullock MR. Intrasellar presentation of a cystic optic chiasm fibrillary astrocytoma. Pediatr Neurosurg 1996; 25: 265–268
6. Russell A. A diencephalic syndrome of emaciation in infancy and childhood. Arch Dis Child 1951; 26:274
7. Shuper A, Horev G, Kornreich L, et al. Visual pathway glioma: an erratic tumour with therapeutic dilemmas. Arch Dis Child 1997; 76:259–263
8. Wilson JT, Wald SL, Aitken PA, Mastromateo J, Vieco PT. Primary diffuse chiasmatic germinomas: differentiation from optic chiasm gliomas. Pediatr Neurosurg 1995; 23:1–5

LANGERHANS CELL HISTIOCYTOSIS

9. Angeli SI, Luxford WM, Lo WWM. Magnetic resonance imaging in the evaluation of Langerhans' cell histiocytosis of the temporal bone: case report. Otolaryngol Head Neck Surg 1996; 114:120–124

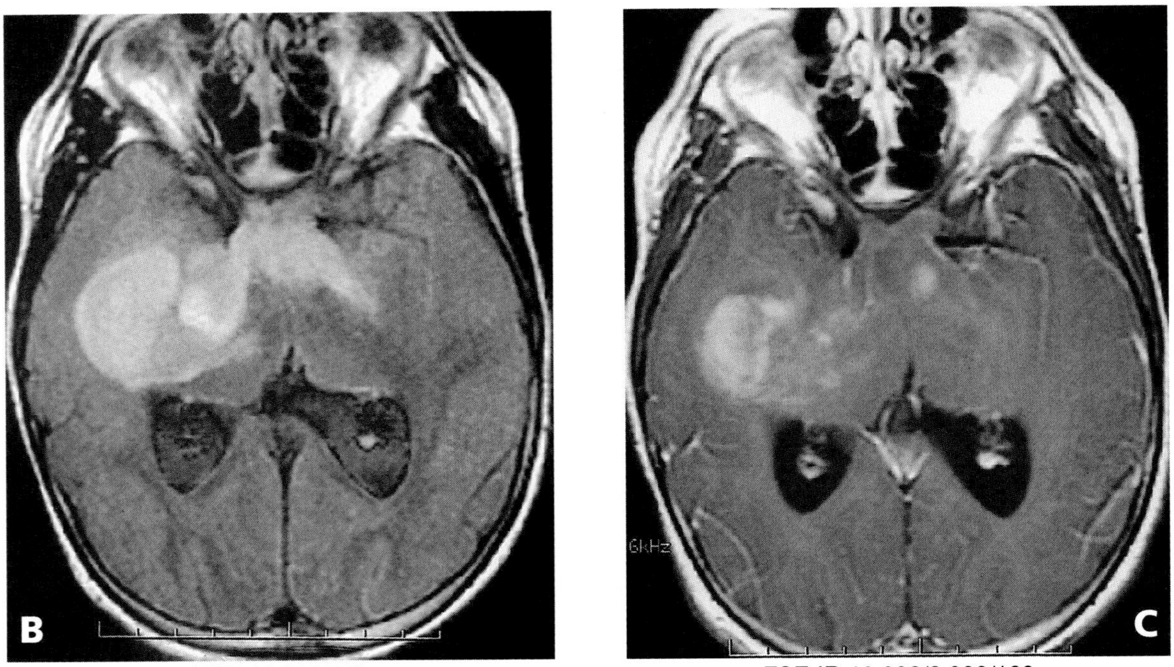

FSE 10,002/160 FSE IR 10,002/2,000/160

Figure 22-12 (Continued). Malignant hypothalamic chiasmatic glioma in a 6-year-old girl who presented with precocious puberty and bitemporal visual field deficits. (B) An axial FLAIR MR image at the level of the chiasm demonstrates a heterogeneous, hyperintense mass extending into the right temporal lobe. (C) The corresponding axial T1-weighted MR image following gadolinium chelate administration demonstrates mild heterogeneous enhancement, which is most marked in the temporal lobe component.

10. Egeler RM, D'Angio GJ. Langerhans cell histiocytosis. J Pediatr 1995; 127:1–11
11. Grois N, Barkovich AJ, Rosenau W, Ablin AR. Central nervous system disease associated with Langerhans' cell histiocytosis. Am J Pediatr Hematol Oncol 1993; 15:245–254
12. Lichtenstein L. Histiocytosis X: integration of eosinophilic granuloma of bone, "Letterer-Siwe disease," and "Schuller-Christian disease" as related manifestations of a single nosologic entity. AMA Arch Pathol 1953; 56: 84–102
13. Meyer JS, Harty MP, Mahboubi S, et al. Langerhans cell histiocytosis: presentation and evolution of radiologic findings with clinical correlation. RadioGraphics 1995; 15:1135–1146
14. Risdall RJ, Dehner LP, Duray P, Kobrinsky N, Robison L, Nesbit ME Jr. Histiocytosis X (Langerhans' cell histiocytosis). Arch Pathol Lab Med 1983; 107:59–63
15. Rosenfield NS, Abrahams J, Komp D. Brain MR in patients with Langerhans cell histiocytosis: findings and enhancement with Gd-DTPA. Pediatr Radiol 1990; 20:433–436

HYPOTHALAMIC HAMARTOMA

16. Arita K, Ikawa F, Kurisu K, et al. The relationship between magnetic resonance imaging findings and clinical manifestations of hypothalamic hamartoma. J Neurosurg 1999; 91:212–220
17. Berkovic SF, Andermann FDM, Melanson D, Ethier RE, Feindel W, Gloor P. Hypothalamic hamartomas and ictal laughter: evolution of a characteristic epileptic syndrome and diagnostic value of magnetic resonance imaging. Ann Neurol 1988; 23:429–439
18. Boyko OB, Curnes JT, Oakes WJ, Burger PC. Hamartomas of the tuber cinereum: CT, MR, and pathologic findings. AJNR 1991; 12:309–314
19. Hall JG, Pallister PD, Clarren SK, et al. Congential hypothalamic hamartoblastoma, hypopituitarism, imperforate anus and postaxial polydactyly—a new syndrome? Part I. Clinical, causal, and pathogenetic considerations. Am J Med Genet 1980; 7:47–74
20. Sisodiya SM, Free SL, Shorvon SD. Surgical treatment of hypothalamic hamartoma. Ann Neurol 1998; 43:273–275
21. Squires LA, Constantini S, Miller DC, Wisoff JH. Hypothalamic hamartoma and the Pallister-Hall syndrome. Pediatr Neurosurg 1995; 22: 303–308

CRANIOPHARYNGIOMA

22. Ahmadi J, Destian S, Apuzzo MLJ, Segall HD, Zee CS. Cystic fluid in craniopharyngiomas: MR imaging and quantitative analysis. Radiology 1992; 182:783–785
23. Carmel PW, Antunes JL, Chang CH. Craniopharyngiomas in children. Neurosurgery 1982; 11:382–389
24. Hald JK, Eldevik OP, Quint DJ, Chandler WF, Kollevold T. Pre- and postoperative MR imaging of craniopharyngiomas. Acta Radiol 1996; 37:806–812
25. Harwood-Nash DC. Neuroimaging of childhood craniopharyngioma. Pediatr Neurosurg 1994; 21 (Suppl 1):2–10
26. Kobayashi T, Kageyama N, Yoshida J, Shibuya N, Yonezawa T. Pathological and clinical basis of the indications for treatment of craniopharyngiomas. Neurol Med Chir 1981; 21:39–47
27. Mark RJ, Lutge WR, Shimizu KT, Tran LM, Selch MT, Parker RG. Craniopharyngioma: treatment in the CT and MR imaging era. Radiology 1995; 197:195–198
28. Pusey E, Kortman KE, Flannigan BD, Tsuruda J, Bradley WG. MR of craniopharyngiomas: tumor delineation and characterization. AJR 1987; 149:383–388

DIABETES INSIPIDUS

29. Holder CA, Elster AD. Magnetization transfer imaging of the pituitary: further insights into the nature of the posterior "bright spot." J Comput Assist Tomogr 1997; 12:171–174
30. Imura H, Nakao K, Shimatsu A, et al. Lymphocytic infundibuloneurohypophysitis as a cause of central diabetes insipidus. N Engl J Med 1993; 329:683–689
31. Maghnie M, Villa A, Arico M, et al. Correlation between magnetic resonance imaging of posterior pituitary and neurohypophyseal function in children with diabetes insipidus. J Clin Endocrinol Metab 1992; 74: 795–800
32. Zucchini S, di Natale B, Ambrosetto P, De Angelis R, Cacciari E, Chiumello G. Role of magnetic resonance imaging in hypothalamic-pituitary disorders. Horm Res 1995; 44(Suppl 3):8–14

PRECOCIOUS PUBERTY

33. Cassio A, Cacciari E, Zucchini S, Balsamo A, Diegoli M, Orsini F. Central precocious puberty: clinical and imaging aspects. J Pediatr Endocrinol Metab 2000; 13 (Suppl 1):703–708
34. De Sanctis V, Corrias A, Rizzo V, et al. Etiology of central precocious puberty in males: the results of the Italian Study Group for Physiopathology of Puberty. J Pediatr Endocrinol Metab 2000; 13 (Suppl 1):687–693
35. Kao SC, Cook JS, Hansen JR, Simonson TM. MR imaging of the pituitary gland in central precocious puberty. Pediatr Radiol 1992; 22:481–484
36. Kornreich L, Horev G, Blaser S, Daneman D, Kauli R, Grunebaum M. Central precocious puberty: evaluation by neuroimaging. Pediatr Radiol 1995; 25:7–11
37. Rieth KG, Comite F, Dwyer AJ, et al. CT of cerebral abnormalities in precocious puberty. AJR 1987; 148:1231–1238

RATHKE'S CLEFT CYST

38. Kucharczyk W, Peck WW, Kelly WM, Norman D, Newton TH. Rathke cleft cysts: CT, MR imaging, and pathologic features. Radiology 1987; 165:491–495
39. Sumida M, Uozumi T, Mukada K, Arita K, Kurisu K, Eguchi K. Rathke cleft cysts: correlation of enhanced MR and surgical findings. AJNR 1994; 15:525–532

SUPRASELLAR TUMORS: GENERAL

40. Donovan JL, Nesbit GM. Distinction of masses involving the sella and suprasellar space: specificity of imaging features. AJR 1996; 167:597–603
41. Kollias SS, Barkovich AJ, Edwards MS. Magnetic resonance analysis of suprasellar tumors of childhood. Pediatr Neurosurg 1992; 17:284–303
42. Lefton DR, Pinto RS, Silvera VM, DeLara FA, Schwartz JB, Haller JO. Radiologic features of pediatric thalamic and hypothalamic tumors. Crit Rev Diagn Imaging 2000; 41:237–278
43. Richmond IL, Wilson CB. Parasellar tumors in children. I. Clinical presentation, preoperative assessment, and differential diagnosis. Child's Brain 1980; 7:73–84
44. Simonetta AB. Imaging of suprasellar and parasellar tumors. Neuroimaging Clin North Am 1999; 9:717–732
45. Zimmerman RA. Imaging of intrasellar, suprasellar, and parasellar tumors. Semin Roentgenol 1990; 25:174–197

CASE 23

Michele H. Johnson, M.D.

Cholesteatoma

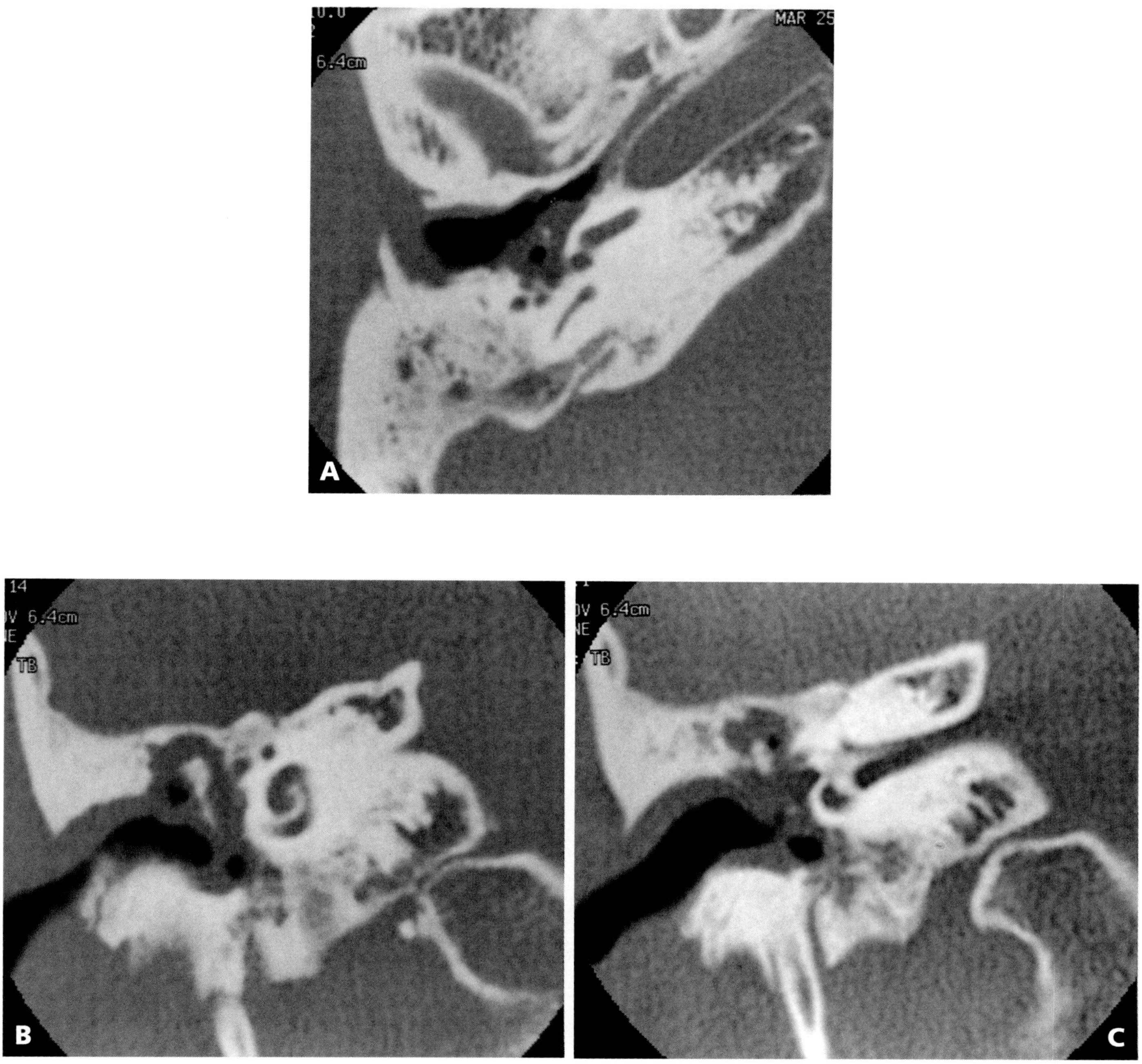

Figure 23-1

Question 112

This 2-year-old boy has impaired hearing. You are shown a 1-mm axial (A) and contiguous 1-mm direct coronal (B and C) CT images of the petrous bone (Figure 23-1).

Which *one* of the following is the MOST likely diagnosis?

(A) Congenital cholesteatoma
(B) Acquired cholesteatoma
(C) Rhabdomyosarcoma
(D) Langerhans cell histiocytosis
(E) Cholesterol granuloma

An axial CT image (Figure 23-1A) at the level of the eustachian tube, filmed at bone-window settings, demonstrates soft tissue thickening within the middle ear cavity (mesotympanum) (Figure 23-2A). A remnant of the ossicular chain embedded within the abnormal soft tissue is identified. There is destruction of the anterior aspect of the mastoid process. The remainder of the mastoid process is sclerotic, with opacification of the mastoid air cells secondary to chronic infection. A coronal CT image at bone-window settings (Figure 23-1B) of the temporal bone at the level of the malleus demonstrates thickened soft tissue within the middle ear cavity, extending inferiorly into the hypotympanum (Figure 23-2B) and superiorly into the epitympanum. There is also soft tissue thickening extending along the external auditory canal (EAC) contiguous with the retracted tympanic membrane (TM). This retracted TM is directly adjacent to the abnormal soft tissue within the middle ear cavity. A second, more anterior coronal CT image

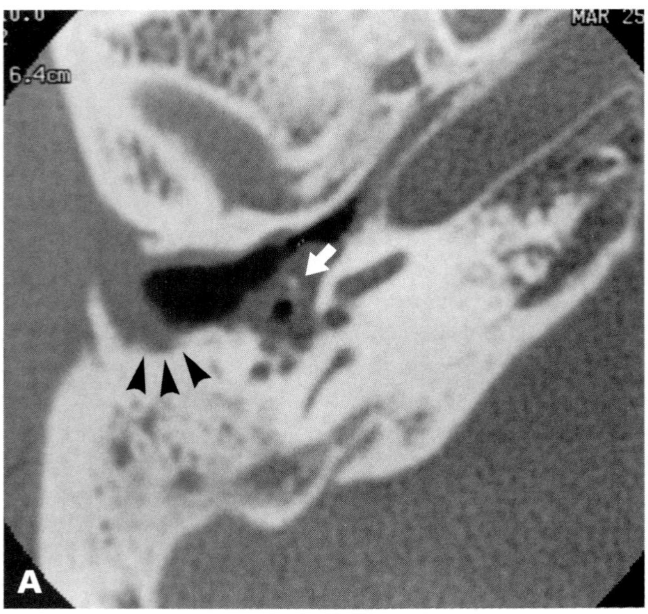

Figure 23-2 (Same as Figure 23-1). Acquired cholesteatoma. (A) A 1-mm axial CT image of the petrous bone shows a remnant of the ossicular chain (arrow) embedded within the abnormal soft tissue. There is also destruction of the anterior aspect of the mastoid process (arrowheads).

(Figure 23-1C) demonstrates erosion of the scutum, a typical feature of acquired cholesteatoma (Figure 23-2C) **(Option (B) is correct)**. Figure 23-3 illustrates the normal appearance of the temporal bone in a coronal section for comparison.

The focal bone destruction within the middle ear cavity and mastoid is caused by the localized accumulation of keratinaceous debris from adjacent squamous epithelium of the EAC. This debris becomes trapped and enveloped in a wall of squamous epithelium with a fibrous stroma. The cholesteatoma increases in size as the debris accumulates, at the expense of adjacent bony structures. Acquired cholesteatoma occurs in the setting of inflammatory disease, most commonly chronic otitis media. The squamous epithelium migrates and becomes trapped adjacent to the edge of the TM. The TM retracts in the presence of inflammatory fluid within the middle ear cavity. Perforation of the TM can occur as a result of inflammation and fluid accumulation, permitting the migration of squamous epithelium from the EAC. Perforation, with the development of an epithelialized scar at the site of perforation, can result in squamous epithelial inclusions and the accumulation of associated keratinized debris.

The CT features of acquired cholesteatoma include a soft tissue mass in the middle ear (Figure 23-2). The middle ear is the most common site for all temporal bone cholesteatomas. Nearly all cholesteatomas are acquired; only about 2% are congenital. Most acquired cholesteatomas arise within Prussak's space from a pars flaccida retraction pocket. The borders of the lesion can be either well or ill defined. There is perforation of the TM posterosuperiorly (Sharpnell membrane). Initially, there is destruction of the lateral wall of the attic, particularly the scutum, with invasion of Prussak's space. There may be extension posteriorly into the mastoid antrum, containing the head of the malleus and the body of the incus. Displacement of the auditory ossicles with erosion of the ossicular chain is not unusual. Erosion frequently affects the long process of the incus first. Also associated with the acquired cholesteatoma is destruction of Körner's septum, which is a small bony projection extending inferiorly from the roof of the mastoid antrum. With large cholesteatomas, there is erosion of the tegmen tympani. Less commonly, the labyrinthine capsule shows erosion involving the lateral semicircular canal first.

Congenital cholesteatoma (Option (A)), also known as epidermoid tumor, arises from rests of squamous epithelium found in the temporal bone. Collections of keratinaceous debris developing from these rests can thus arise in any part of the petrous bone, without prior otitis and with a normal, intact TM. Congenital cholesteatoma can occur in the middle ear, mastoid, EAC, jugular fossa, labyrinth, petrous apex, and cerebellopontine angle. As noted above, the middle ear is the most common site for all cholesteatomas in the temporal bone. Bone destruction results as the collection increases in size, just as with acquired cholesteatoma (Figure 23-4). The smaller congenital cholesteatomas tend to occur near the incudostapedial joint, and the most common sites of erosion are the incus and stapes suprastructure. A congenital cholesteatoma will not erode the tip of the scutum if it is in the attic, but it will extend through

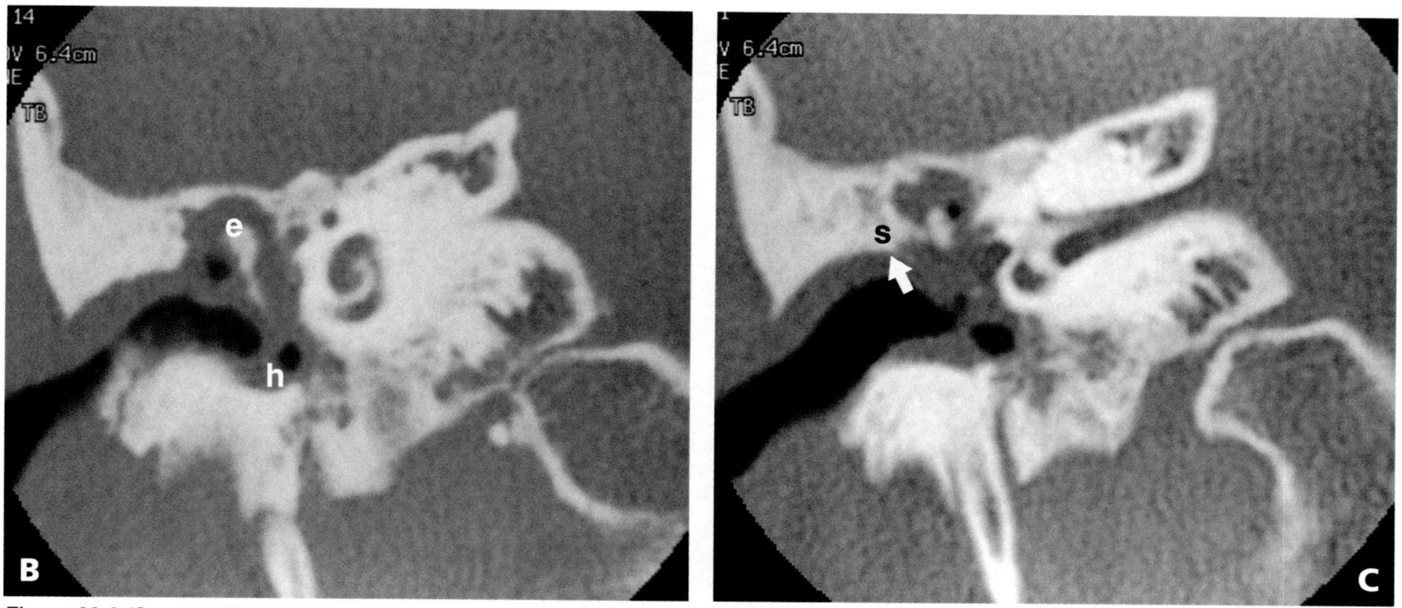

Figure 23-2 (Same as Figure 23-1) (Continued). Acquired cholesteatoma. (B) A 1-mm direct coronal CT image shows thickened soft tissue within the middle ear cavity, extending inferiorly into the hypotympanum (h) and superiorly into the epitympanum (e). (C) A contiguous 1-mm direct coronal CT image further anterior to panel B shows erosion (arrow) of the scutum (s), a typical feature of acquired cholesteatoma.

the lateral epitympanic wall above the spur. Most commonly, however, congenital cholesteatoma appears as an asymptomatic retrotympanic mass. The relative rarity of congenital cholesteatoma and the presence of hearing problems in the test patient make congenital cholesteatoma a less likely diagnosis.

Cholesterol granuloma (Option (E)) also can be considered a cystlike collection of debris within the petrous bone, usually at the petrous apex. It can involve any part of the middle ear. The etiology of cholesterol granuloma is obscure; however, it is believed to occur because of impedance to drainage of the normally aerated temporal bone, resulting in mucosal edema and necrosis, with hemorrhage, inflammation, and granuloma formation. The presence of each of these features, along with the secondary inflammatory process, leads to the pathologic entity of cholesterol granuloma. The granuloma contains cholesterol, lipids, and hemosiderin. Together, these components create a characteristic appearance on MRI (Figure 23-5). A cholesterol granuloma is hyperintense relative to brain on T1-weighted images because of the cholesterol content of the lesion. T2-weighted images detect methemoglobin. On CT, the pattern of bone destruction seen with cholesterol granuloma is smooth and expansile, unlike the irregular destruction typical of acquired cholesteatoma. CT, in addition, will show a cholesterol granuloma as being isodense relative to brain, without enhancement or calcification. For these reasons, cholesterol granuloma is not the most likely diagnosis in the test patient.

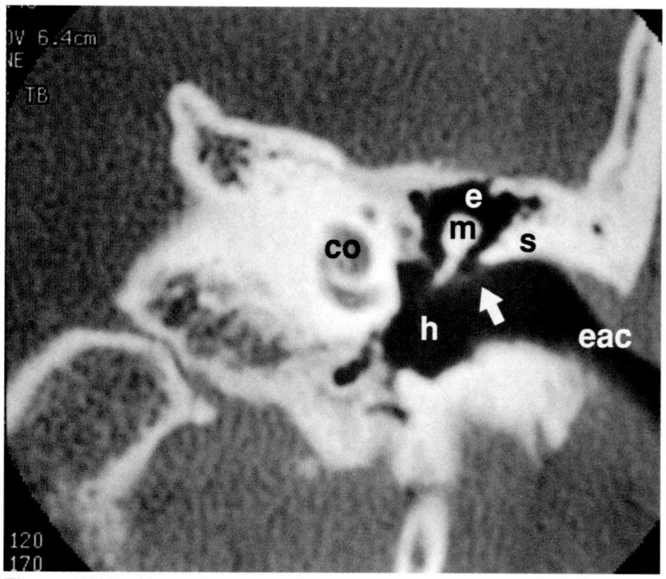

Figure 23-3. Normal coronal CT of the temporal bone. This image through the temporal bone at the level of the cochlea (co) demonstrates the position of the ossicles (m = malleus) within the mesotympanum. Note that there is a slight retraction of the TM (arrow) as it extends from the normal scutum (s). The hypotympanum (h) and the epitympanum (e) are clear, without abnormal soft tissue opacification. The EAC (eac) demonstrates normal soft tissue margins.

Langerhans cell histiocytosis (LCH) (Option (D)) of the temporal bone is a rare disorder consisting of histiocytic infiltration of the bone and resultant bone destruction (Figure 23-6). Most commonly, LCH is manifested as multiple lytic lesions in the calvarium, with or without involvement of the skull base or mastoid. When LCH occurs in the temporal bone, it can be isolated or it can be associated with osseous, endocrine, and other systemic lesions. Involvement of the hypothalamic-pituitary axis is the most common central nervous system manifestation. Between 20% and 40% of patients with multifocal LCH have skull lesions, and 5% to 10% have temporal bone lesions. Bilateral involvement is rare. If the disease is monostotic, the temporal bone may be the only region of involvement. Nearly all instances of temporal bone LCH occur in the mas-

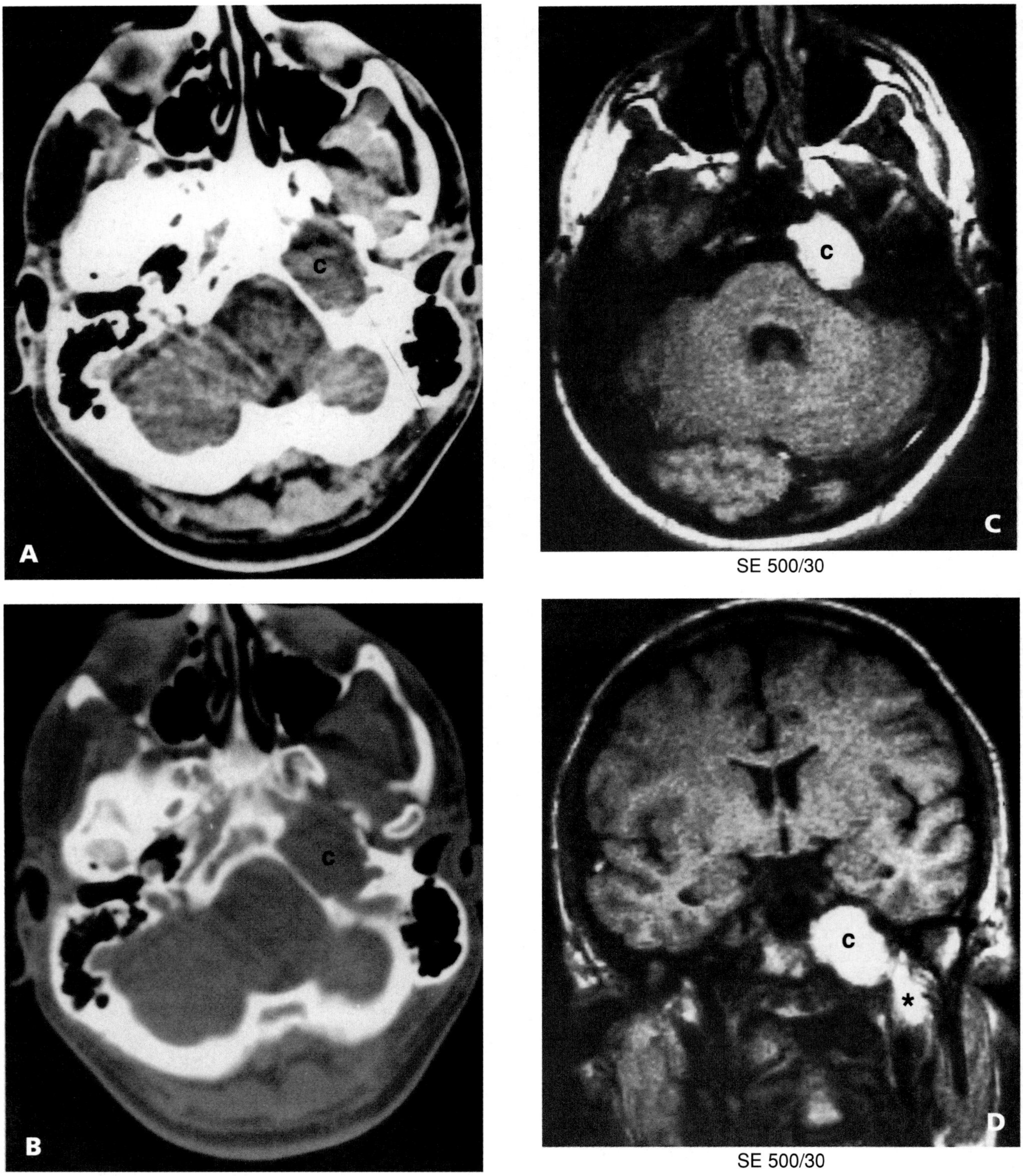

Figure 23-4. Congenital cholesteatoma in a 16-year-old boy with cranial nerve palsies. (A and B) Axial CT images filmed at soft tissue (A) and bone-window (B) settings demonstrate the cholesteatoma (c) as a well-defined expansile mass at the left petrous apex. The mass is isodense relative to brain. Note the absence of inflammatory changes in the mastoid air cells. (C and D) Axial (C) and coronal (D) T1-weighted MR images demonstrate a homogeneous mass (c) that is hyperintense with respect to brain. Note the inferior extension (*) of the cholesteatoma, best seen on the coronal image.

toid; rarely, it can be found in the petrous apex.

CT findings of temporal bone involvement by LCH include nonaeration of the middle ear and mastoid air cell destruction. The bone lesions are irregular and indistinct, without the sclerosis associated with chronic cholesteatoma. The soft tissue mass can expand the mastoid cortex and can erode

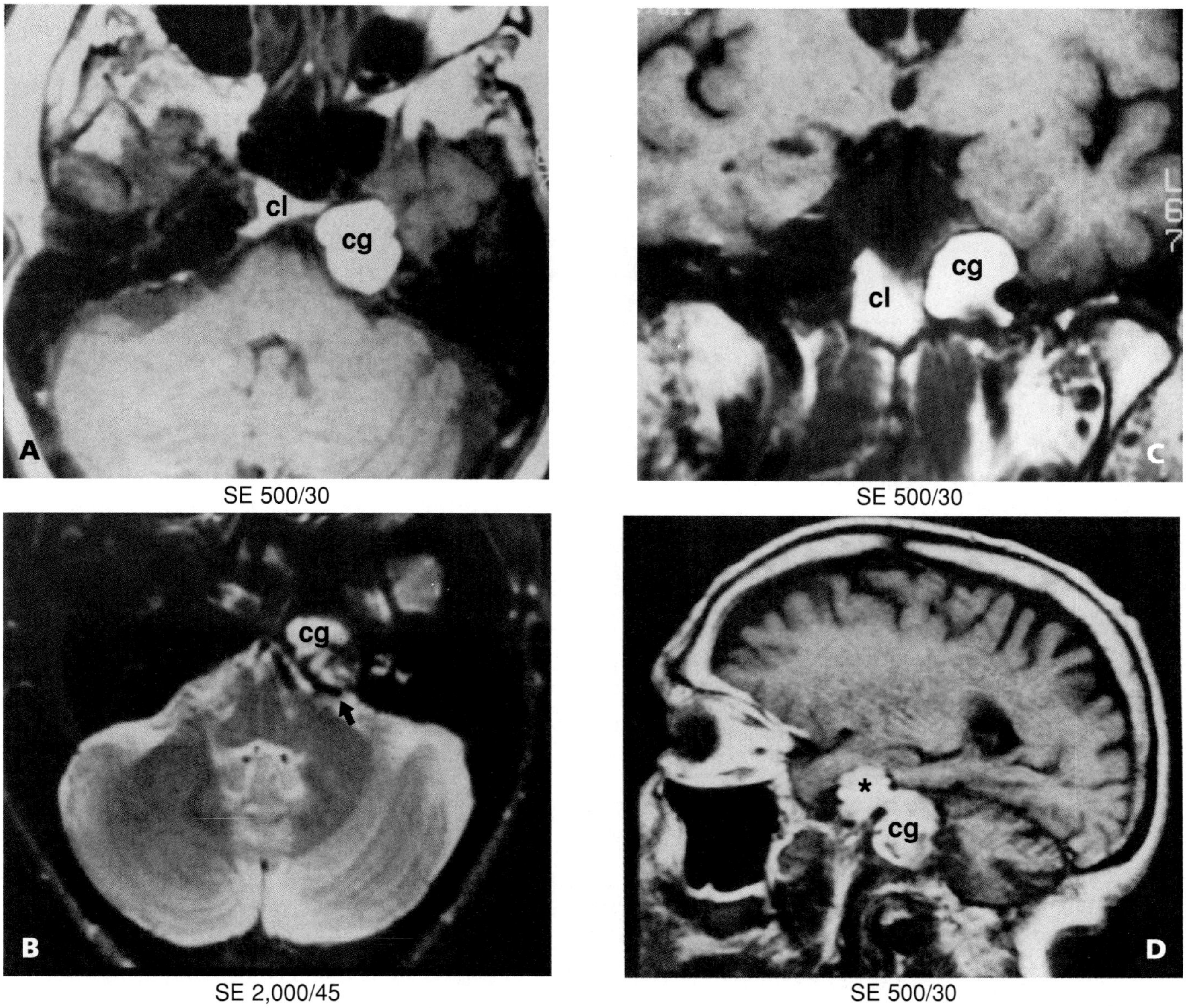

Figure 23-5. Cholesterol granuloma in a 42-year-old woman with headaches. (A) An axial T1-weighted MR image through the petrous bone demonstrates the cholesterol granuloma (cg) as a homogeneous, lobulated mass at the petrous apex, separate from the clivus (cl). (B) The mass is heterogeneous on a T2-weighted image. Note the hypointense hemosiderin ring (arrow) around the posterior aspect of the mass (cg). (C) A coronal T1-weighted image demonstrates the medial extent of the cholesterol granuloma (cg). (D) On a sagittal T1-weighted image, the extension (*) of the cholesterol granuloma (cg) into the middle cranial fossa is defined.

the bone laterally to the EAC. Lesions can be polypoid. When there is posterior extension of LCH, it can destroy the cortex of the sigmoid sulcus and lead to sigmoid sinus compression or thrombosis. In approximately 25% of cases, labyrinthine and ossicular erosion occurs. The predominant involvement of the middle ear, rather than the mastoid air cells, in the test patient makes LCH an unlikely diagnosis.

Rhabdomyosarcoma (Option (C)) accounts for slightly less than 10% of all cases of childhood cancer. It is the most common malignant tumor of the temporal bone. Radiographic findings in temporal bone rhabdomyosarcoma include frank bone destruction with fragmentation, along with an associated soft tissue mass. Although rhabdomyosarcoma usually affects the middle ear and invades the mastoid air spaces, it respects no boundaries and can invade adjacent structures. The tumor readily spreads via the facial nerve canal into the internal auditory canal. The basal cisterns and meninges can be involved at presentation. Very aggressive tumors can extend into the EAC and nasopharynx. CT studies demonstrate an opacified middle ear and mastoid and, in most cases, extensive bone destruction (Figure 23-7). The term "skeletonization" is used to describe the destructive appearance of temporal bone rhabdomyosarcoma on CT. This term refers to incomplete destruction of the petrous bone with sparing of the otic capsule, which can lead to an appearance of the cochlea, vestibule, and semicircular canals seemingly being suspended in soft tissue tumor. The pattern of bone destruction is more extensive than that seen with the typical acquired cholesteatoma. Ear pain and otorrhea

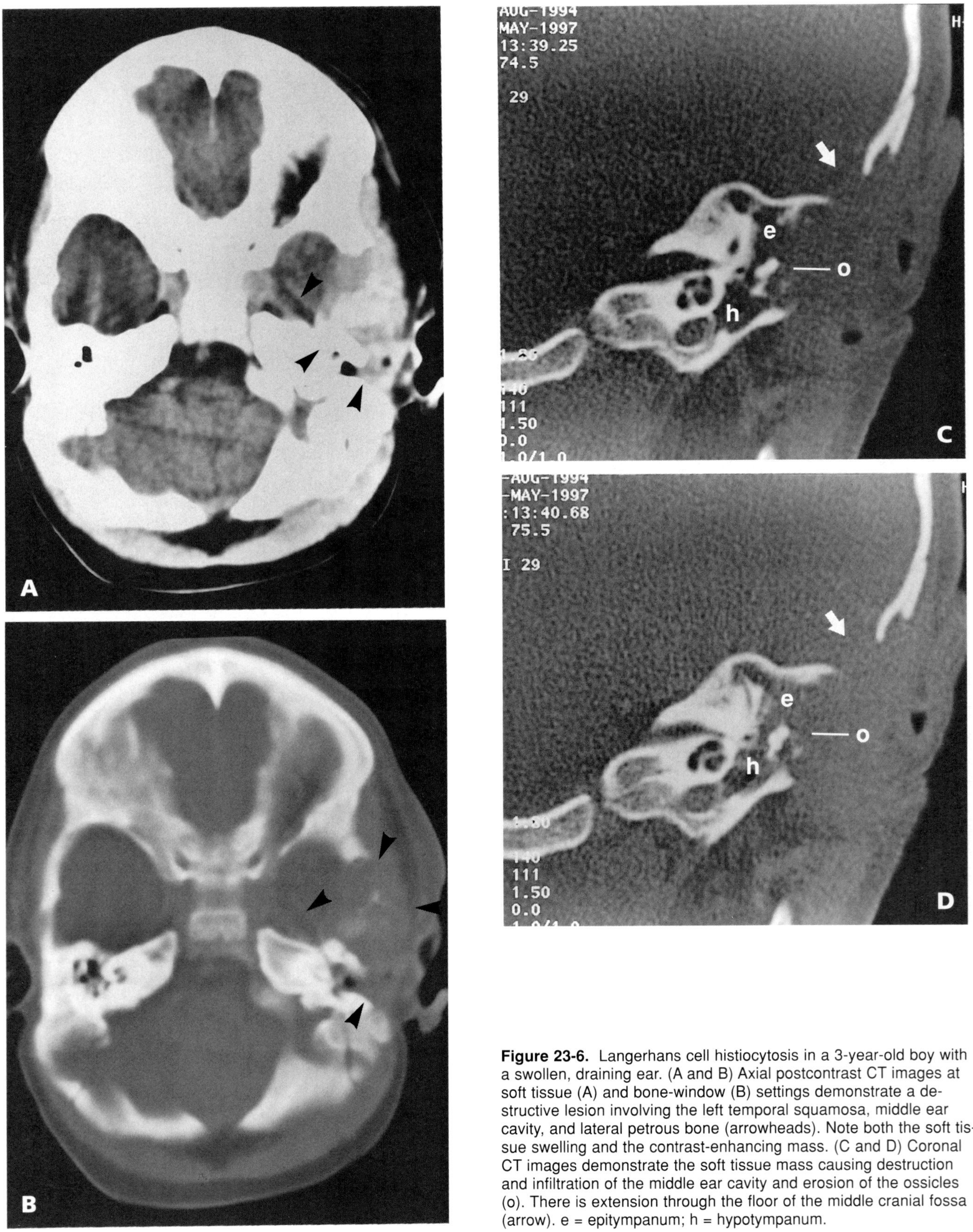

Figure 23-6. Langerhans cell histiocytosis in a 3-year-old boy with a swollen, draining ear. (A and B) Axial postcontrast CT images at soft tissue (A) and bone-window (B) settings demonstrate a destructive lesion involving the left temporal squamosa, middle ear cavity, and lateral petrous bone (arrowheads). Note both the soft tissue swelling and the contrast-enhancing mass. (C and D) Coronal CT images demonstrate the soft tissue mass causing destruction and infiltration of the middle ear cavity and erosion of the ossicles (o). There is extension through the floor of the middle cranial fossa (arrow). e = epitympanum; h = hypotympanum.

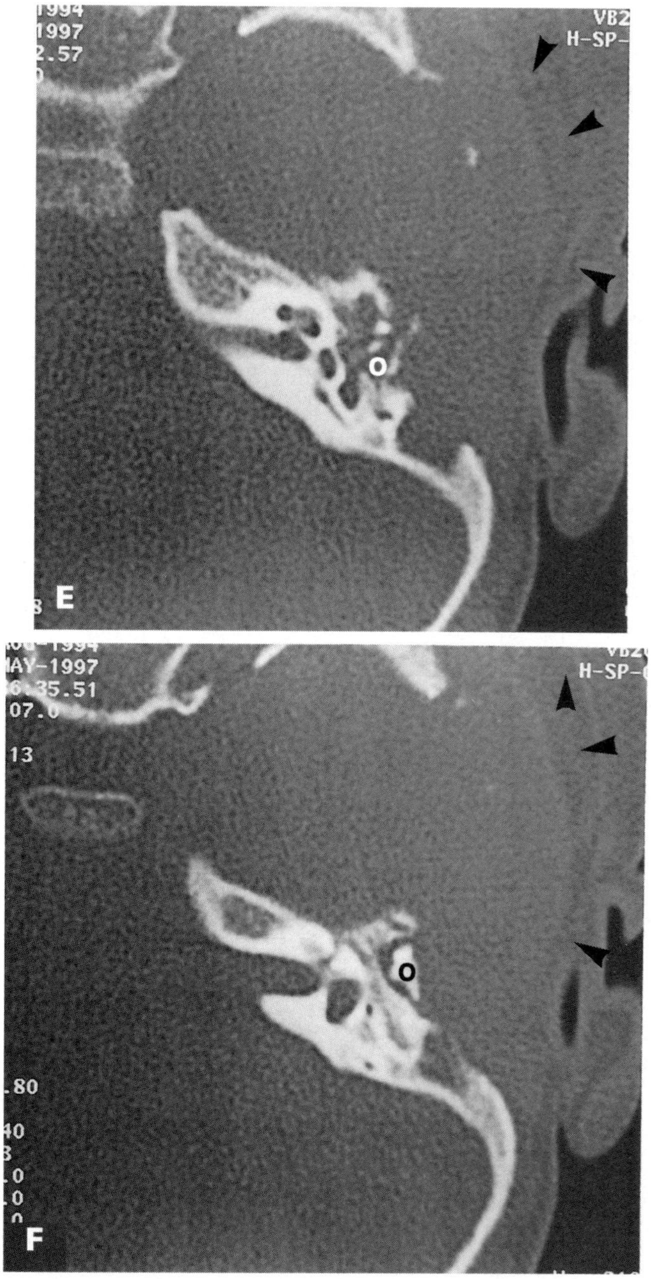

Figure 23-6 (Continued). Langerhans cell histiocytosis in a 3-year-old boy with a swollen, draining ear. (E and F) Axial high-resolution CT images of the temporal bone reveal partial destruction of the ossicles (o) and middle ear cavity. The soft tissue mass as well as the lytic destruction of the temporal squamosa is apparent (arrowheads). These changes are consistent with LCH of the temporal bone, with its typical bone destruction and soft tissue mass.

are common features at presentation. The localized erosion in the test patient would be atypical for rhabdomyosarcoma.

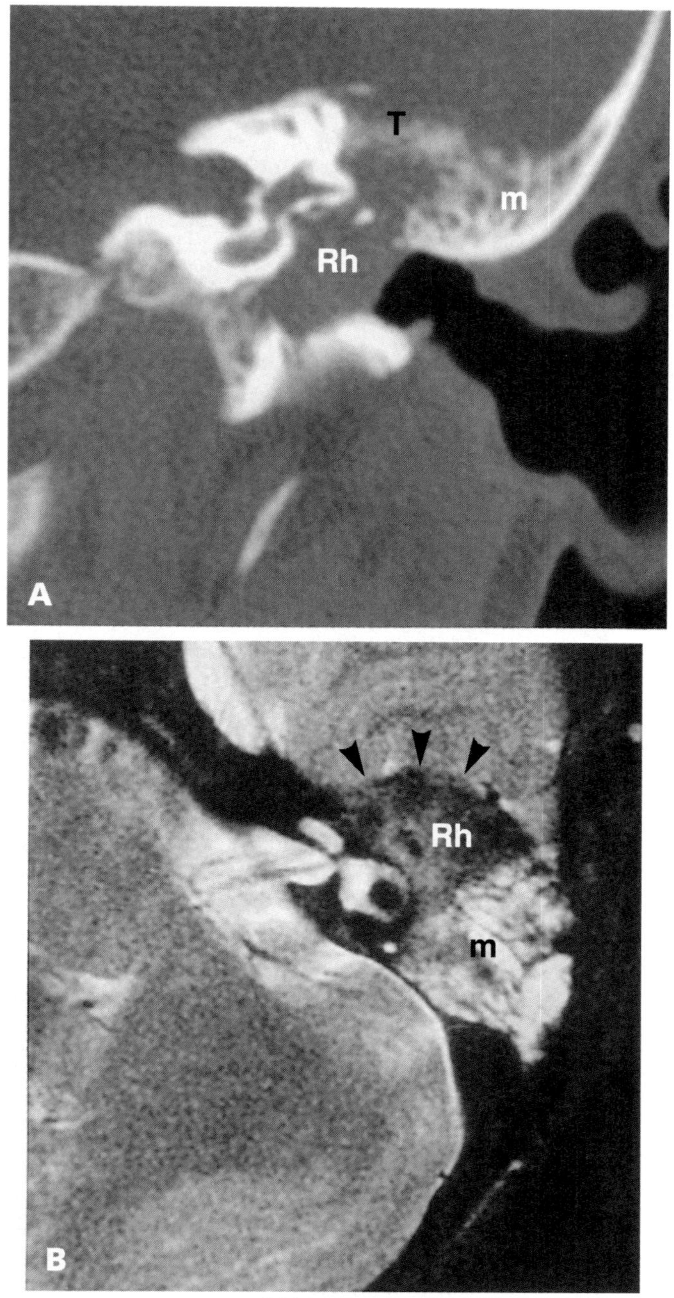

SE 2,000/45

Figure 23-7. Rhabdomyosarcoma in an 11-year-old child with ear pain. (A) A coronal CT image of the temporal bone demonstrates a tumor (Rh) that causes opacification of the middle ear cavity, with extension through the tegmen (T) and destruction of the ossicles. There is extension of the soft tissue mass into the mastoid (m), with opacification of the air cells. Note also the erosion of the wall of the horizontal semicircular canal. (B) An axial T2-weighted MR image demonstrates the soft tissue mass (Rh) centered in the middle ear and extending anteriorly to impress upon the temporal lobe (arrowheads). Note the postobstructive and inflammatory changes in the mastoid air cells (m) laterally and posteriorly. (Case courtesy of Joel D. Swartz, M.D., National Medical Imaging, Philadelphia, PA, and H. Ric Harnsberger, M.D., University of Utah, Salt Lake City, UT.)

Question 113

Concerning congenital cholesteatoma,

(A) it usually appears as an asymptomatic mass behind an intact tympanic membrane
(B) it usually is diagnosed in the neonatal period
(C) it usually originates anterior to the malleus
(D) it is difficult to distinguish from acquired cholesteatoma in most patients

A congenital cholesteatoma commonly appears as an asymptomatic mass behind an intact TM (**Option (A) is true**). Congenital cholesteatomas represent approximately 2% of all cholesteatomas and are seldom bilateral. A cholesteatoma is classified as congenital if the TM is intact and there is no history of prior inflammatory disease or trauma. The lesion can occur in the EAC, TM, mastoid, geniculate ganglion areas, and, rarely, the jugular foramen, petrous apex, or cerebellopontine angle. Congenital cholesteatomas can be referred to as epidermoid tumors of the temporal bone. The average age at diagnosis is approximately 4 years (**Option (B) is false**). In adults, congenital cholesteatoma can be manifested as headache or neck pain because of mass effect on the cerebellum. The pearly, white mass usually is located behind the anterior-superior quadrant of the TM. There can be associated middle ear effusion related to obstruction of the eustachian tube orifice. The presence of ossicular chain erosion or destruction is equally possible with both congenital and acquired cholesteatomas.

Congenital cholesteatoma usually arises anterior to the malleus (**Option (C) is true**). On CT, the lesion has a low density and is expansile, with a smooth border. It can extend to involve the mastoid process, with or without involvement of the middle ear (Figure 23-4). The mass can extend and grow to destroy the adjacent clivus (Figure 23-8). Absence of enhancement on both CT and MRI is typical. Congenital cholesteatomas usually are homogeneous in signal intensity and can be isointense or mildly hyperintense on T1-weighted images and hyperintense on T2-weighted images (Figure 23-4). There is an association of congenital cholesteatoma and congenital ear anomalies, such as external ear atresia. A bony atresia plate typically is identified at the level of the annulus of the TM. The primary distinguishing features of congenital cholesteatoma are the normal TM and the absence of a history of chronic otitis media. The most common sites of erosion are the incus and stapes suprastructure. A congenital cholesteatoma will not erode the tip of the scutum as does the acquired lesion (**Option (D) is false**).

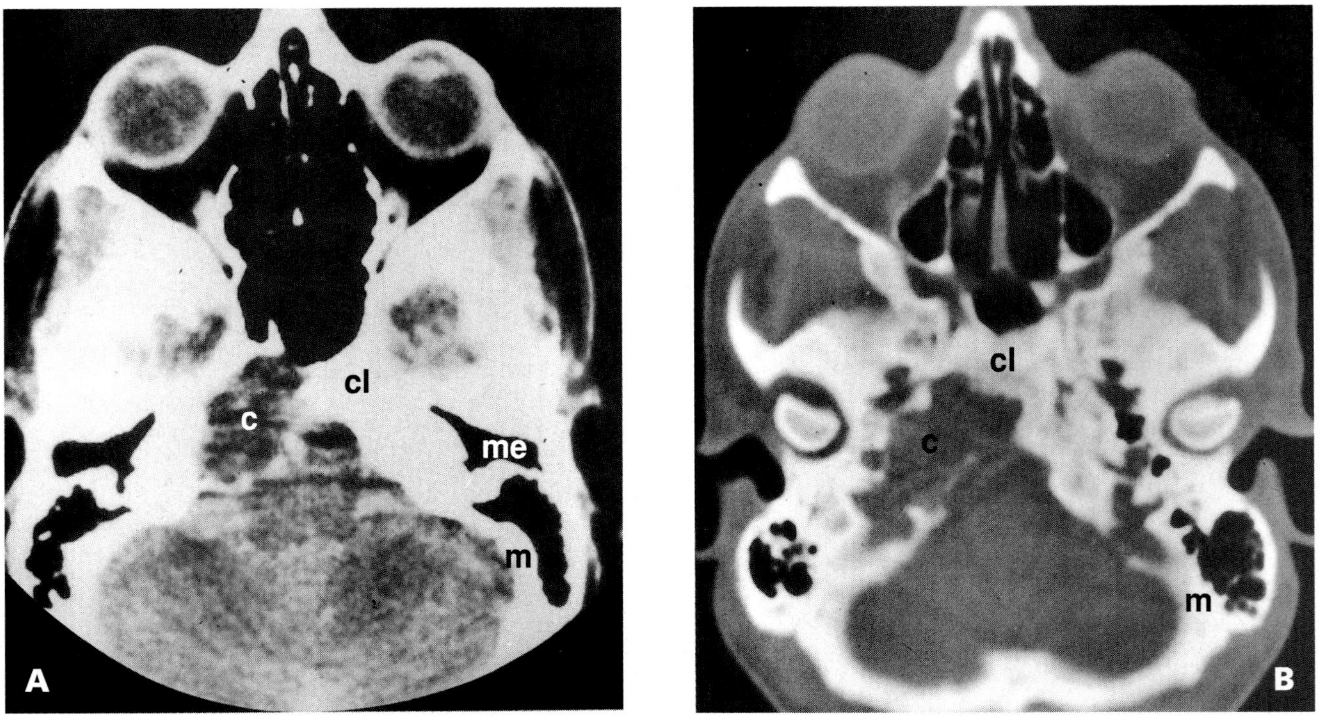

Figure 23-8. Congenital cholesteatoma. Axial postcontrast CT images obtained with soft tissue (A) and bone-window (B) settings demonstrate a nonenhancing destructive lesion (c) involving the right petrous apex and extending into the clivus (cl). There is normal aeration of the middle ear (me) cavity and mastoid (m).

Question 114

Concerning acquired cholesteatoma,

- (A) it is associated with chronic suppurative otitis media in most patients
- (B) it usually can be diagnosed on physical examination
- (C) axial CT images are the most sensitive images for detecting bone destruction
- (D) it usually is treated with antibiotics alone

Children with acquired cholesteatoma usually have a long history of chronic or recurrent otitis media (**Option (A) is true**). Symptomatic children with acquired cholesteatoma can have a chronically draining ear, otorrhea, recurrent otitis, pain, hearing loss, or vertigo. A small percentage of children have an unsuspected retraction pocket on routine physical examination. More commonly, evidence of scarring or retraction of the TM is present in association with a retrotympanic mass (**Option (B) is true**). The acquired variety is more likely to be bilateral (Figure 23-9). A failed school audiogram is a typical reason for a physician referral. Although audiographic abnormalities are common, actual complaints of hearing loss are unusual. The hearing loss associated with cholesteatoma usually is conductive, caused by disruption of sound transduction through the middle ear cavity. If ossicular discontinuity is present, the hearing loss is even greater. Sensory-neural hearing loss in association with cholesteatoma usually reflects destruction of the inner ear structures.

Three mechanisms for the pathogenesis of acquired cholesteatoma have been proposed: (1) implantation and invasion of squamous epithelium into the middle ear secondary to surgery or fracture; (2) extension of squamous epithelium through a perforation or retraction pocket in the TM; and (3) focal metaplasia of the low cuboidal epithelium in the middle ear mucosal surface with secondary squamous epithelial proliferation. Bone destruction by cholesteatoma is caused by a combination of pressure erosion attributable to the expanding mass and enzymatic erosion from enzymes produced by the squamous epithelium.

The development of cholesteatoma is not uncommon given the high incidence and prevalence of otitis media in childhood. Treatment of otitis media includes both antibiotics and tympanostomy tube placement. These treatments speed the resolution of otitis media, but it is unclear whether they change the incidence of cholesteatoma. Surgical removal of the cholesteatoma is necessary in order to prevent the reaccumulation of keratinaceous debris within the middle ear and mastoid (**Option (D) is false**). The treatment goals for patients with acquired cholesteatoma include the elimination of the squamous epithelium from the middle ear cavity and preservation or reconstruction of functional hearing. Surgery can be performed through the middle ear if the lesion is small; mastoidectomy is necessary when the lesion involves the posterior epitympanum or mastoid.

Most acquired cholesteatomas are found adjacent to or within the upper TM (pars flaccida) and adjacent epitympanum (attic) of the middle ear cleft (Figure 23-10). Prussak's space lies between the incus and the lateral wall of the epitympanum. It is best seen in the coronal plane; therefore, coronal CT images are the most useful for defining the extent of disease (Figures 23-1, 23-10, and 23-11) (**Option (C) is false**). The coronal CT projection best demonstrates early and subtle erosion of the scutum, head of the malleus, and incus. These erosive changes are most common with pars flaccida cholesteatoma involving Prussak's space. If erosion is demonstrated on the coronal view, an axial view is obtained to search for erosion in other areas of the ossicles, epitympanum, horizontal semicircular canal, mastoid,

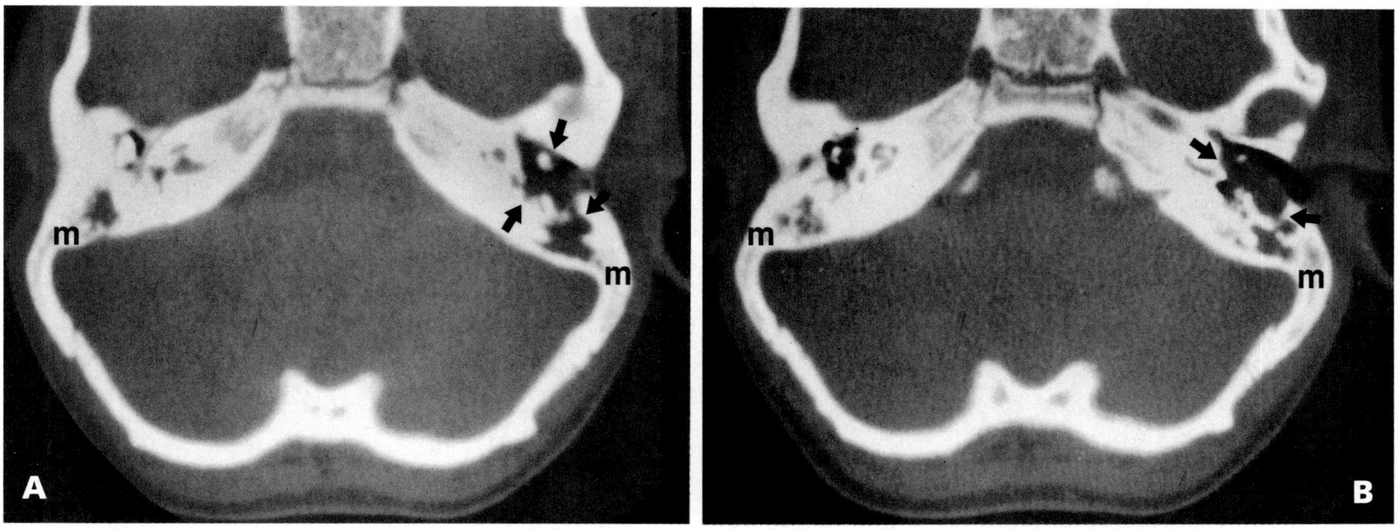

Figure 23-9. Acquired cholesteatoma. (A and B) Axial CT imaging was performed on this 10-year-old boy with chronic otitis media. On the left, a soft tissue mass surrounds the ossicles and extends posteriorly and superiorly into the attic and mastoid process (arrows). Note the mastoid sclerosis. On the right, sclerosis is present with coalescent mastoid air cells, consistent with chronic otitis and chronic mastoiditis. Air is present within the middle ear cavity, surrounding the ossicles on the right, although a small amount of soft tissue mucosal thickening may be identified. m = mastoid.

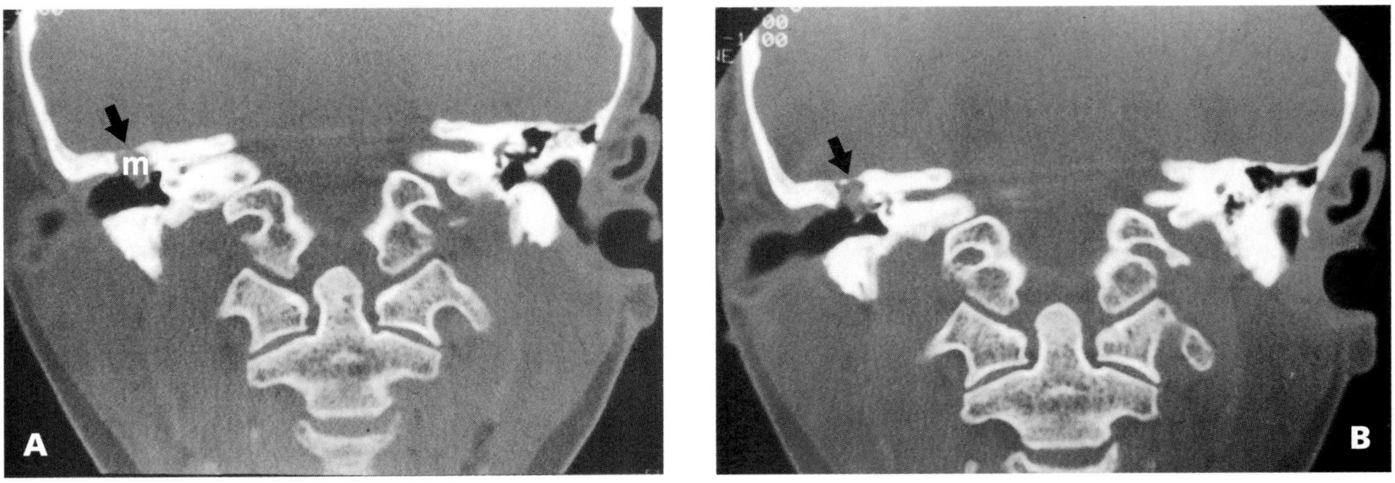

Figure 23-10. Acquired cholesteatoma in an 8-year-old boy with bilateral draining ears. (A and B) Coronal CT images obtained with the bone algorithm demonstrate an epitympanic mass (m) on the right extending up to and eroding the tegmen (arrow). Note also the soft tissue inferiorly within the middle ear cavity on the left, with coalescent air cells, consistent with chronic otitis and mastoiditis.

and bony plate of the sigmoid sinus. Pars tensa cholesteatomas are less common than those arising from the pars flaccida. These spare the scutum, causing erosive changes of the long process of the incus and stapes, and can involve the sinus tympani, the facial recess, and the pyramidal eminence.

CT scanning with the bone algorithm technique has significantly improved the diagnosis and surgical outcome for patients with acquired cholesteatoma (Figures 23-1 and 23-9 through 23-12). Ossicular chain erosion and erosion of the bony labyrinth can be identified preoperatively by CT. This demonstration facilitates surgical removal of the keratinaceous debris. Reconstruction of an ossicular-labyrinthine fistula can be anticipated and dysfunction can be prevented at the time of initial surgery if semicircular canal erosion is documented preoperatively by CT (Figure 23-12).

Complications of cholesteatoma include facial nerve palsy, intracranial extension or infection, fistula of the labyrinth, and vestibular erosion (Figure 23-12). With growth into the mastoid air cells, the cholesteatoma can enter the EAC and then extend into the intracranial or infratemporal spaces. There is a high frequency of postoperative recurrences of cholesteatoma, approximately 3% in children and 3% to 15% in adults. Recurrences can be related to ongoing eustachian tube dysfunction in the setting of recurrent otitis in childhood. Meningitis, brain abscess, and sinus thrombosis are rare complications in all age groups.

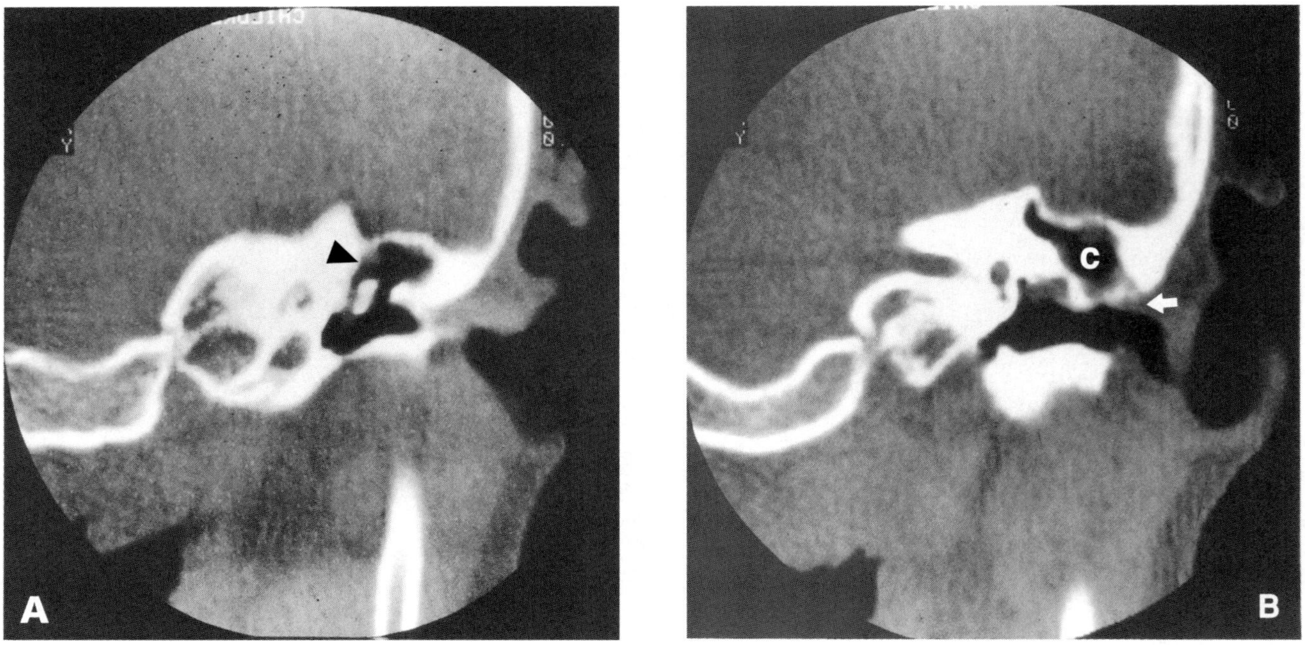

Figure 23-11. Acquired cholesteatoma complications in a 5-year-old boy with new ear drainage. (A and B) Coronal CT bone-window setting images demonstrate minimal soft tissue thickening (arrowhead) within the middle ear cavity, with thinning of the tegmen. Extending posteriorly, note the cavity (c) within the mastoid and the dehiscence of the mastoid floor (arrow). The cavity is lined by soft tissue.

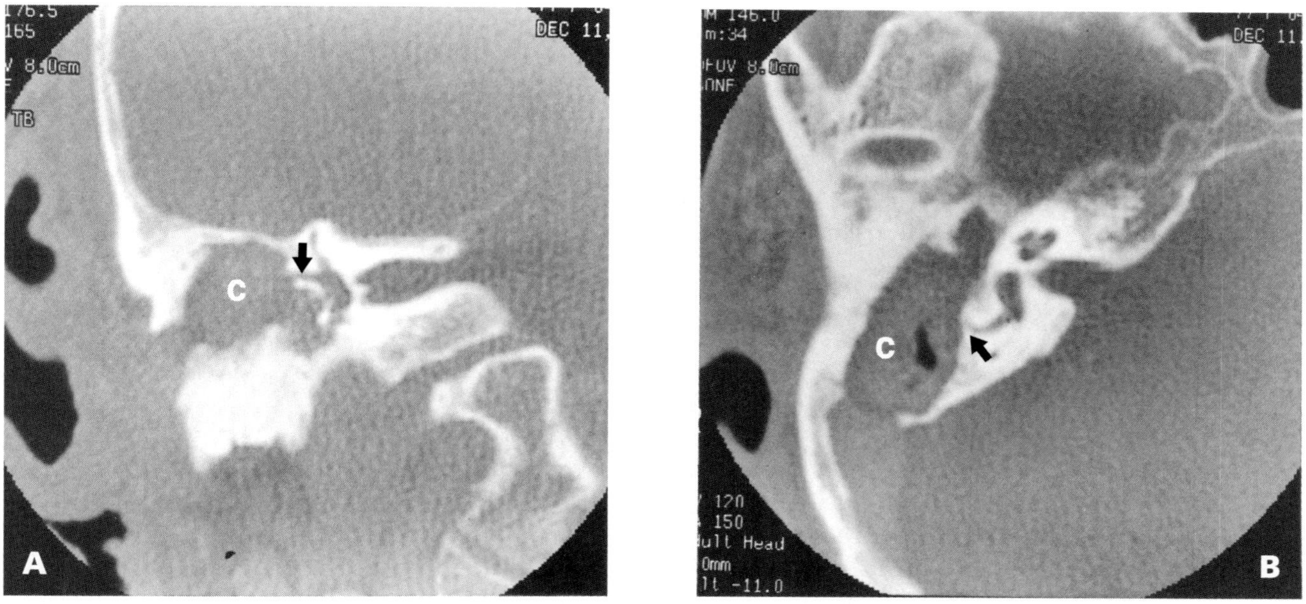

Figure 23-12. Complications of cholesteatoma. Coronal (A) and axial (B) high-resolution temporal bone CT images demonstrate a destructive lesion (c) involving the middle ear cavity and mastoid, consistent with cholesteatoma. Note the bony erosion involving the lateral semicircular canal, consistent with a labyrinthine fistula (arrow). This fistula was surgically corrected. (Case courtesy of James Abrahams, M.D., Yale University School of Medicine, New Haven, CT.)

Question 115

Concerning Langerhans cell histiocytosis of the temporal bone,

(A) it represents the most common site of involvement in the skull
(B) it can present clinically as chronic otitis externa
(C) ossicular sclerosis is characteristic
(D) it usually is a component of the chronic multifocal form of Langerhans cell histiocytosis

The most common site of skull involvement in LCH is the calvarium, in which multiple "punched-out" lesions are identified. Between 25% and 30% of children with LCH have skull lesions, but fewer than 10% have temporal bone involvement (**Option (A) is false**). Bilateral disease is rare.

Lytic destruction of the temporal bone is similar to the typical calvarial lesions of LCH and results from histiocytic infiltration of the normally aerated temporal bone (Figure 23-6). Ossicular sclerosis is not a feature of temporal bone involvement by LCH; 10% to 20% of cases may have ossicular erosion (**Option (C) is false**). The bony labyrinth is more resistant to erosion from the histiocytic infiltration than the aerated mastoid; thus, involvement of inner ear structures is rare. LCH of the temporal bone usually occurs as a component of multifocal histiocytosis. Between 5% and 10% of such patients will have temporal bone involvement (**Option (D) is true**).

Histiocytic infiltration of the skin appears as a scaly erythematous rash. This can precede destruction of the temporal bone. The patient may have chronic otitis externa and otorrhea. Otorrhea is the most common clinical finding, and it may be associated with TM perforation, EAC polyp, otitis externa with histiocytic infiltration of the dermis, ear pain, and postauricular swelling (**Option (B) is true**). Hearing impairment may result from granuloma tissue, ossicular destruction, or labyrinthine erosion. The CT findings include nonaeration of the middle ear and mastoid air cell destruction resembling coalescent mastoiditis. The destructive bone lesions are usually irregular and indistinct. Mastoid granulomas can enlarge the mastoid cortex and erode anteriorly into the EAC with aural polyp development. In approximately 25% of cases, labyrinthine and ossicular erosion occurs. However, cases will present prior to bone destructive changes with only TM perforation, EAC polyp, and thickening of the dermis in the canal. This presentation requires a biopsy for specific diagnosis. The symptoms can mimic those of cholesteatoma, otitis media, chronic eczema, and osteomyelitis.

Question 116

Concerning cholesterol granuloma,

(A) it usually is the result of a viral infection
(B) it usually occurs in children less than 3 years old
(C) physical examination demonstrates a blue tympanic membrane
(D) it is pathologically similar to cholesteatoma
(E) the lesion exhibits high signal intensity on both T1- and T2-weighted images

Cholesterol granuloma of the temporal bone, sometimes called a cholesterol or chocolate cyst, develops in response to the deposition of cholesterol crystals within the air spaces of the temporal bone. The lesion can develop in the setting of granulation tissue and scar from chronic inflammatory disease or secondary to previous middle ear surgery or trauma (**Option (A) is false**). Disturbance in the drainage of normally aerated petrous air cells leads to acute and chronic inflammation, hemorrhage, and granulomatous inflammatory response. The cyst, which develops gradually, can enlarge to occupy the mastoid cavity. The slow expansion causes bony erosion and can impinge upon cranial nerves, dura, brain, or inner ear structures.

Cholesterol granuloma is a disorder usually identified in adulthood (**Option (B) is false**). On physical examination, there is a blue retrotympanic mass (**Option (C) is true**). The blue mass is not specific for cholesterol granuloma; in fact, jugular bulb anomalies and glomus tumors (jugulare or tympanicum) can have a similar appearance. The most frequent locations for cholesterol granuloma of the temporal bone include the petrous apex, the mastoid air cells, and the middle ear cavity. Less commonly, cholesterol granuloma can arise in the frontal and maxillary sinuses or within the frontal bone adjacent to the orbit.

Although both cholesterol granuloma and cholesteatoma arise in response to an accumulation of debris, they are histologically distinct entities (**Option (D) is false**). Histologically, the cholesterol granuloma is made up of a squamous cell lining, keratin debris, cholesterol crystals, and hemorrhage. On CT, cholesterol granuloma is a well-defined, round, low-density mass, similar in density to adjacent soft tissue (Figure 23-13). The soft tissue mass obliterates the normally aerated petrous bone. It can be difficult to differentiate from cholesteatoma on CT. The middle ear cavity may or may not be involved.

Cholesterol granulomas have heterogeneous high signal intensity on both T1- and T2-weighted MR images, attributable to the presence of hemoglobin breakdown products within the cyst (Figures 23-5 and 23-13) (**Option (E) is true**). The heterogeneity, hyperintensity, and characteristic surrounding hemosiderin rim help to distinguish this lesion from cholesteatoma. Cholesteatoma is more likely to be isointense on T1-weighted and hyperintense on T2-weighted images.

Surgical excision and drainage constitute the usual treatment for cholesterol granuloma. The lesion can recur. Follow-up radiographic examination, particularly MRI, is useful for assessment of lesion extirpation.

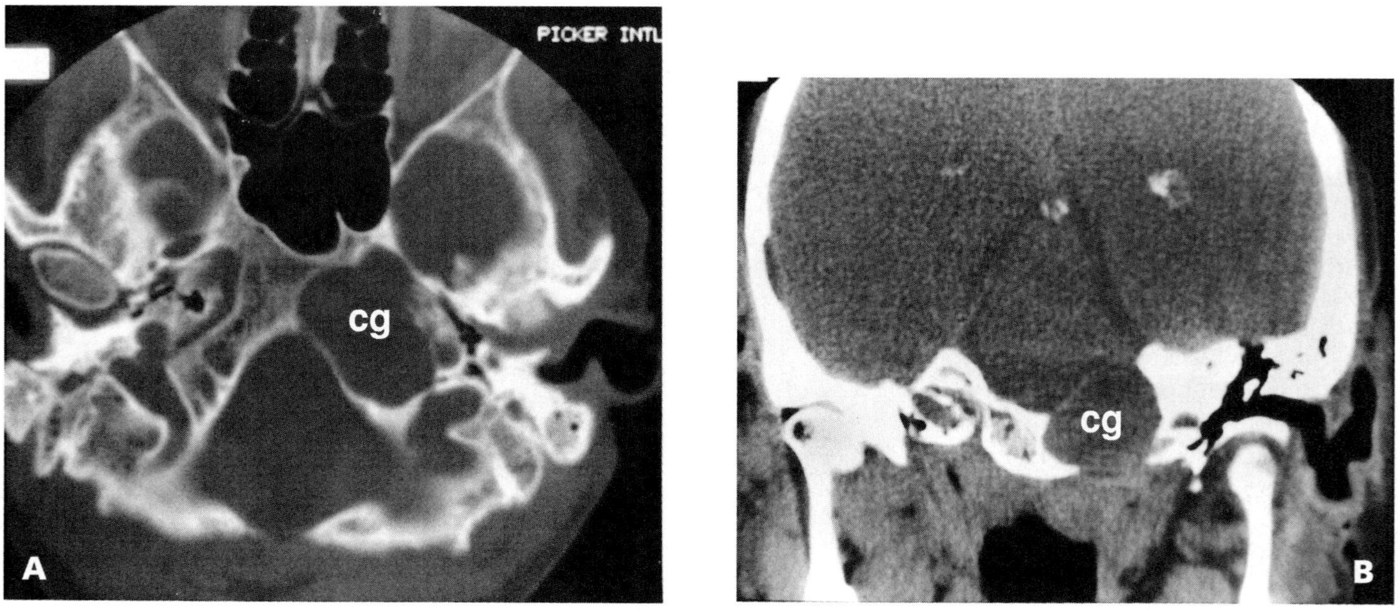

Figure 23-13. Cholesterol granuloma. (A) An axial CT image at bone-window settings demonstrates a well-defined, smoothly marginated, expansile, destructive lesion (cg) involving the inferior aspect of the petrous apex and clivus. (B) A coronal CT image at soft tissue settings confirms the smoothly marginated, expansile, nonenhancing lesion (cg). Note the normal appearance of the middle ear and the external ear.

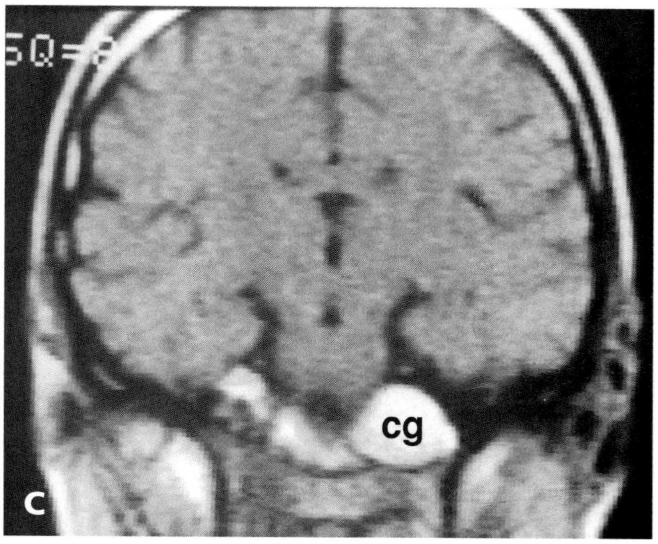

Figure 23-13 (Continued). Cholesterol granuloma. (C) A T1-weighted coronal MR image demonstrates a well-defined, hyperintense lesion (cg), corresponding to the bony defect seen on CT. Surgical exploration confirmed the diagnosis of cholesterol granuloma. (Case courtesy of James Abrahams, M.D.)

SUGGESTED READINGS

ACQUIRED CHOLESTEATOMA

1. Albino AP, Kimmelman CP, Parisier SC. Cholesteatoma: a molecular and cellular puzzle. Am J Otol 1998; 19:7–19
2. Johnson DW, Voorhees RL, Lufkin RB, Hanafee W, Canalis R. Cholesteatomas of the temporal bone: role of computed tomography. Radiology 1983; 148:733–737
3. Sie KCY. Cholesteatoma in children. Pediatr Clin North Am 1996; 43: 1245–1252
4. Swartz JD, Goodman RS, Russell KB, Marlowe FI, Wolfson RJ. High-resolution computed tomography of the middle ear and mastoid. Part II: Tubotympanic disease. Radiology 1983; 148:455–459
5. Watts S, Flood LM, Clifford K. A systematic approach to interpretation of computed tomography scans prior to surgery of middle ear cholesteatoma. J Laryngol Otol 2000; 114:248–253

CONGENITAL CHOLESTEATOMA

6. Latack JT, Kartush JM, Kemink JL, Graham MD, Knake JE. Epidermoidomas of the cerebellopontine angle and temporal bone: CT and MR aspects. Radiology 1985; 157:361–366
7. Luntz M, Telischi F, Bowen B, Ress B, Balkany T. Imaging case study of the month. Congenital cholesteatoma isolated to the mastoid. Ann Otol Rhinol Laryngol 1997; 106:608–610
8. Mafee MF. MRI and CT in the evaluation of acquired and congenital cholesteatomas of the temporal bone. J Otolaryngol 1993; 22:239–248
9. Peron DL, Schuknecht HF. Congenital cholesteatomata with other anomalies. Arch Otolaryngol 1975; 101:498–505
10. Pisaneschi MJ, Langer B. Congenital cholesteatoma and cholesterol granuloma of the temporal bone: role of magnetic resonance imaging. Top Magn Reson Imaging 2000; 11:87–97
11. Rashad U, Hawthorne M, Kumar U, Welsh A. Unusual cases of congenital cholesteatoma of the ear. J Laryngol Otol 1999; 113:52–54

RHABDOMYOSARCOMA

12. Wiatrak BJ, Pensak ML. Rhabdomyosarcoma of the ear and temporal bone. Laryngoscope 1989; 99:1188–1192
13. Yang WT, Kwan WH, Li CK, Metreweli C. Imaging of pediatric head and neck rhabdomyosarcomas with emphasis on magnetic resonance imaging and a review of the literature. Pediatr Hematol Oncol 1997; 14:243–257

LANGERHANS CELL HISTIOCYTOSIS

14. Angeli SI, Luxford WM, Lo WW. Magnetic resonance imaging in the evaluation of Langerhans' cell histiocytosis of the temporal bone: case report. Otolaryngol Head Neck Surg 1996; 114:120–124
15. Devaney KO, Putzi MJ, Ferlito A, Rinaldo A. Head and neck Langerhans cell histiocytosis. Ann Otol Rhinol Laryngol 1997; 106:526–532
16. Goldsmith AJ, Myssiorek D, Valderrama E, Patel M. Unifocal Langerhans' cell histiocytosis (eosinophilic granuloma) of the petrous apex. Arch Otolaryngol Head Neck Surg 1993; 119:113–116
17. Nanduri VR, Pritchard J, Chong WK, Phelps PD, Sirimanna K, Bailey CM. Labyrinthine involvement in Langerhans' cell histiocytosis. Int J Pediatr Otorhinolaryngol 1998; 46:109–115
18. Sellari-Franceschini S, Forli F, Pierini S, Favre C, Berrettini S, Macchia PA. Langerhans' cells histiocytosis. Int J Pediatr Otorhinolaryngol 1999; 48:83–87
19. Shelby JH, Sweet RM. Eosinophilic granuloma of the temporal bone: medical and surgical management in the pediatric patient. South Med J 1983; 76:65–70

CHOLESTEROL GRANULOMA

20. Greenberg JJ, Oot RF, Wismer GL, et al. Cholesterol granuloma of the petrous apex: MR and CT evaluation. AJNR 1988; 9:1205–1214
21. Griffin C, DeLaPaz R, Enzmann D. MR and CT correlation of cholesterol cysts of the petrous bone. AJNR 1987; 8:825–829
22. Latack JT, Graham MD, Kemink JL, Knake JE. Giant cholesterol cysts of the petrous apex: radiologic features. AJNR 1985; 6:409–413
23. Lo W, Solti-Bohman LG, Brackmann DE, Gruskin P. Cholesterol granuloma of the petrous apex: CT diagnosis. Radiology 1984; 153:705–711
24. Martin N, Sterkers O, Mompoint D, Julien N, Nahum H. Cholesterol granulomas of the middle ear cavities: MR imaging. Radiology 1989; 172:521–525
25. Morioka T, Fujii K, Nishio S, et al. Cholesterol granuloma in the middle cranial fossa: report of two cases. Neuroradiology 1995; 37:564–567

TEMPORAL BONE MASSES: GENERAL

26. Bonneville F, Sarrazin JL, Marsot-Dupuch K, et al. Unusual lesions of the cerebellopontine angle: a segmental approach. RadioGraphics 2001; 21:419–438
27. Chang P, Fagan PA, Atlas MD, Roche J. Imaging destructive lesions of the petrous apex. Laryngoscope 1998; 108:599–604
28. Kletzker GR, Smith PG, McIntire LD, Leonetti JP. Presentation and management of uncommon lesions of the middle ear. Am J Otol 1995; 16:634–642
29. Muckle RP, De la Cruz A, Lo WM. Petrous apex lesions. Am J Otol 1998; 19:219–225
30. Swartz JD. High-resolution computed tomography of the middle ear and mastoid. Part I: Normal radioanatomy including normal variations. Radiology 1983; 148:449–454
31. Swartz JD, Harnsberger HR. Imaging of the temporal bone. 3rd ed. New York: Thieme Medical Publishers; 1997

Michele H. Johnson, M.D.

Persistent Hyperplastic Primary Vitreous

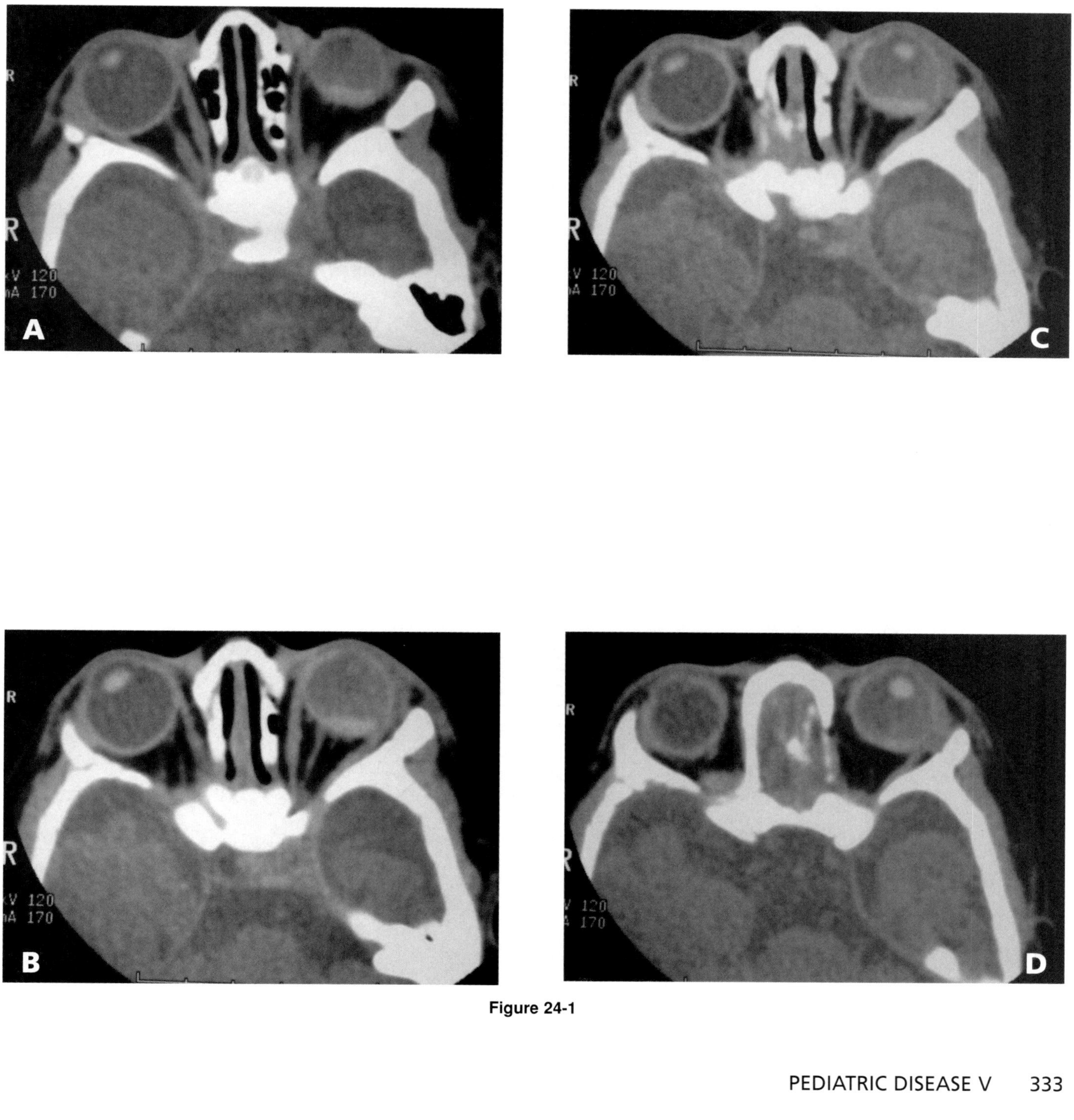

Figure 24-1

Question 117

This 4-week-old girl has an abnormal left-sided light reflex on physical examination. You are shown postcontrast CT scans of the orbits (Figure 24-1).

Which *one* of the following is the MOST likely diagnosis?

(A) Retinoblastoma
(B) Coats' disease
(C) Toxoplasmosis
(D) Coloboma
(E) Persistent hyperplastic primary vitreous

Axial contrast-enhanced CT images of the orbits demonstrate a mildly hyperdense left globe without focal calcifications (Figure 24-1). A dependent fluid-fluid level as well as vague linear opacities within the vitreous can be seen (Figure 24-2). The sclera is not thickened. There is no definite microphthalmia. The optic nerve head is normally shaped and is symmetrical in appearance with that on the right. No retinal mass or detachment is present. These findings are most consistent with persistent hyperplastic primary vitreous (PHPV) **(Option (E) is correct).**

In response to light, the normal retina reflects red light back through the pupil. The reflection of a white or yellow to pinkish white light (an abnormal pupillary light reflex) is defined as leukocoria, or "cat's-eye reflex." This abnormal reflex results when a lesion blocks the normal passage of light through the lens and vitreous to the retina and back. The responsible lesion can involve the lens (e.g., cataracts), the retina (e.g., retinoblastoma, Coats' disease, coloboma, or retinopathy of prematurity), or the vitreous (e.g., PHPV or infectious endophthalmitis).

PHPV occurs in the full-term infant and usually is identified within the neonatal period. It is the second most common cause of leukocoria after retinoblastoma. Usually there is mild unilateral microphthalmia (small hypoplastic globe), although the condition can be seen with a normal-sized globe. The intraorbital segment of the ipsilateral optic nerve is often smaller than normal. The microphthalmia distinguishes PHPV from other causes of leukocoria, such as Coats' disease and retinoblastoma. No calcifications are found within the globe. The vitreous may be increased in attenuation to normal in attenuation on CT. Following contrast agent administration, there is often mild enhancement of the vitreous (Figures 24-2 and 24-3).

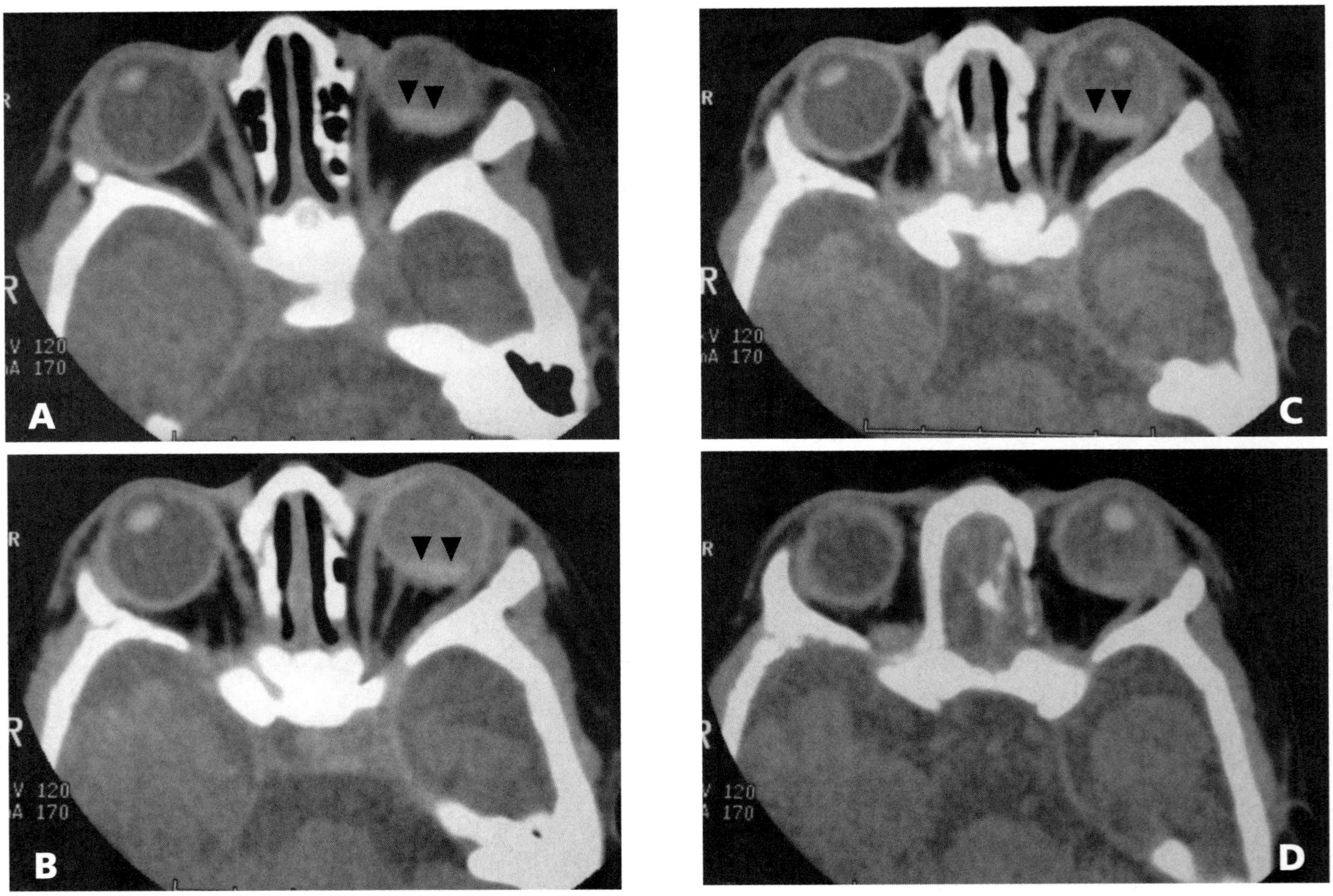

Figure 24-2 (Same as Figure 24-1). Persistent hyperplastic primary vitreous. The CT images show a mildly hyperdense left globe with a dependent fluid-filled level (arrowheads). (Case courtesy of Scott Sullivan, M.D., Yale University School of Medicine, New Haven, CT.)

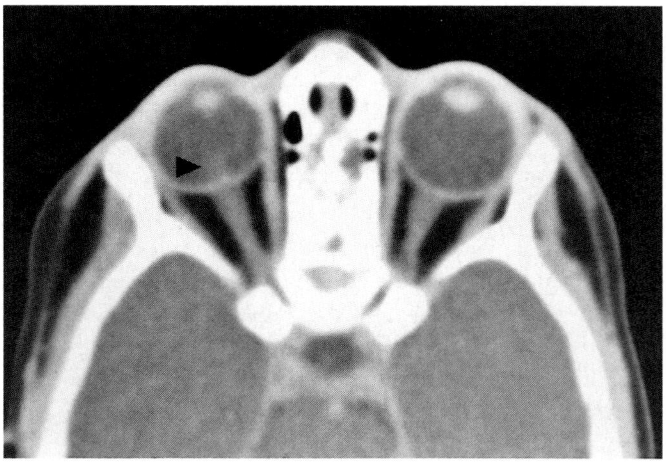

Figure 24-3. Persistent hyperplastic primary vitreous. An axial contrast-enhanced CT image of the orbits demonstrates a mildly hyperdense, mildly microphthalmic right globe in a child with leukocoria secondary to PHPV. Note the cylindrical vitreous body representing the hyaloid remnant within the vitreous.

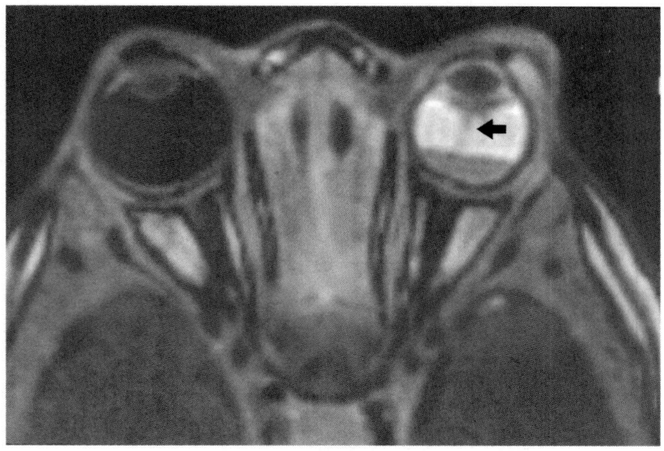

SE 500/20

Figure 24-4. Persistent hyperplastic primary vitreous. An axial T1-weighted MR image of the orbits in a child with leukocoria secondary to PHPV demonstrates a mildly microphthalmic globe on the left with hyperintense vitreous and a dependent fluid-fluid level. There is a linear, hypointense retrolental opacity (arrow) within the vitreous, extending from the lens to the fluid level, consistent with remnants of the primitive hyaloid vascular system. (Case courtesy of Suresh Mukherji, M.D., University of Michigan, Ann Arbor, MI)

Vitreous bodies, tubular, triangular, cylindrical, or irregular in shape, can be found within the globe and behind the lens (retrolental). These represent a remnant of Cloquet's canal. Dependent vitreous fluid-fluid levels can be present, as in the test patient. These result from the breakdown of recurrent hemorrhages in the subhyaloid and subretinal spaces. Bilateral PHPV occurs in about 10% of cases and is most frequently associated with Norrie's disease (congenital progressive oculo-acoustico-cerebral degeneration—a syndome of retinal malformation, deafness, and mental retardation) or Warburg's syndrome (hydrocephalus, agyria, and retinal dysplasia, with or without encephalocele).

The MRI appearance of PHPV can be striking, with increased signal intensity of the vitreous, sometimes associated with fluid-fluid levels on T1-weighted images (Figure 24-4). Postcontrast MRI often demonstrates enhancement of the vitreous bodies not detectable on CT.

Clinically, visual loss with PHPV can be partial or complete. When untreated, the natural course of PHPV includes the development of glaucoma and eventual buphthalmia or end-stage phthisis bulbi.

Pathophysiologically, PHPV is caused by the failure of the primitive hyaloid vascular system to regress, with persistence of the retrolental fibrovascular membrane and the proliferation of reactive connective tissue. In the normal eye, the hyaloid artery arises from the dorsal ophthalmic artery during gestational week 3. It supplies the lens, primary vitreous, retinal tissue, and optic nerve. The primary vitreous is composed of the hyaloid vessels derived from the mesoderm and an ectodermal fibrillar mesh. As growth occurs, between 3 and 8 months of gestation, the primary vitreous regresses and occupies a small area of the anterior chamber, called Cloquet's canal. The latter normally regresses by the time of birth. Sequentially, regression of the vasa hyaloidea propria (horizontal small arteries within the vitreous) occurs first, regression of the tunica vasculosa lentis (small arteries of the posterior lens) occurs second and, finally, regression of the distal portion of the main hyaloid artery occurs. The proximal hyaloid artery persists as the central artery of the retina. The secondary vitreous, consisting of a hyaluronic acid gel and collagen fibers, replaces the primary vitreous as this regression occurs. If the embryonic hyaloid vascular system fails to regress, the primary vitreous, the lens (tunica vasculosa lentis), and the embryonic connective tissue proliferate. This proliferation blocks the normal passage of light through the globe, resulting in loss of the normal papillary reflex, or leukocoria.

Retinoblastoma (Option (A)) is a malignant retinal tumor of childhood that can be diagnosed during the newborn period. The peak age at diagnosis is 13 months, with the majority of cases being diagnosed under the age of 3 years. CT imaging of retinoblastoma shows a solid, smoothly marginated, lobulated, hyperdense, retrolental mass arising within a normal-sized globe. It typically grows subretinally, causing retinal detachment (Figure 24-5). Partial or complete calcification occurs in nearly 90% of cases. The vitreous is often dense. Extraocular extension occurs in 25% of cases and is manifested as optic nerve enlargement, abnormal soft tissue within the orbit, and noncontiguous intracranial enhancing lesions. The lack of a focal mass and the absence of calcifications in the test patient argue against the diagnosis of retinoblastoma. The features of retinoblastoma are considered further in the discussion of Question 118.

Coloboma (Option (D)) is a congenital defect in the posterior retina, usually adjacent to the optic nerve head (Figure 24-6). Microphthalmia is present, and there is often a cyst, referred to as a colobomatous cyst, extending through the retinal defect. The cyst can displace or deform the optic nerve head. The vitreous is of normal density. Thinning and eversion of

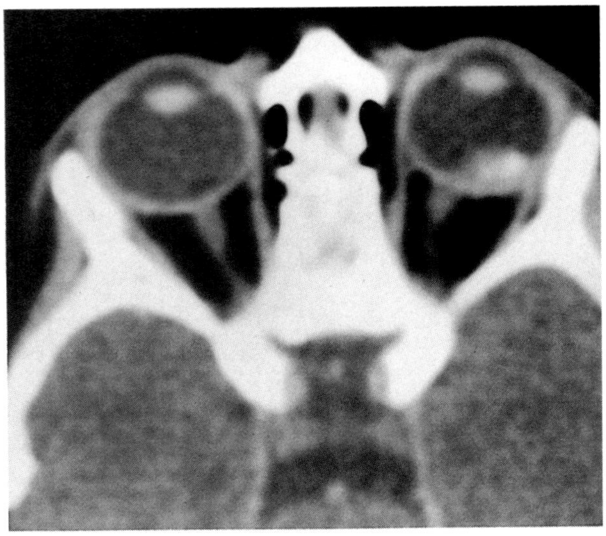

Figure 24-5. Retinoblastoma in a 12-month-old child. An axial contrast-enhanced CT image of the orbits demonstrates a lenticular mass along the posterior aspect of the left globe, emanating from the retina and containing central clumplike calcifications. The optic nerve head appears unremarkable.

the sclera are seen at the margins of the defect. In microphthalmia with cyst formation, the globe is small, and a large cystic intraorbital mass lies adjacent to the globe. The cystic mass is defined by a capsule that represents the thinned sclera. The contents of the cyst are homogeneous and produce CT attenuation values and MRI signal intensities approximately equal to those of normal vitreous. Contrast enhancement does not occur. On sequential thin sections, communication of the cyst with the vitreous cavity of the globe can be demonstrated at some level. This continuity with the globe, along with the presence of microphthalmia and cyst contents with imaging characteristics similar to those of the adjacent vitreous, serves to differentiate this condition from other cystic orbital masses, such as cephalocele, dermoid cyst, and arachnoid cyst. The absence of a focal retinal defect and the presence of hyperdense vitreous on CT in the test patient make coloboma an unlikely diagnosis.

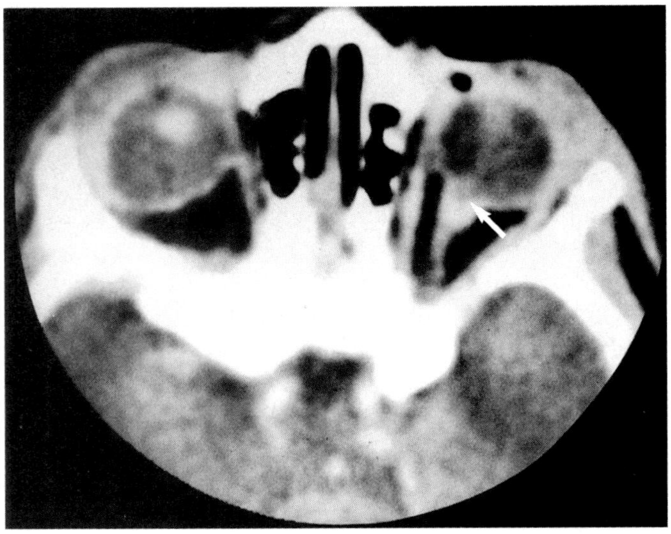

Figure 24-6. Coloboma in a 3-month old child. An axial contrast-enhanced CT image of the orbits demonstrates microphthalmia on the left. There is a congenital defect in the posterior retina (arrow) contiguous with the optic nerve head and consistent with a diagnosis of coloboma. The density of the globe is similar to that on the right.

Coats' disease (Option (B)) (Figure 24-7) and infectious causes of endophthalmitis, such as ocular toxoplasmosis (Option (C)) and toxocariasis (Figure 24-8), each can demonstrate increased attenuation of the vitreous on CT. Congenital ocular toxoplasmosis can be manifested as increased attenuation of the vitreous and bilateral microphthalmia; however, the lack of vitreous bodies and fluid-fluid levels as well as the presence of elevated *Toxoplasma gondii* antibody titers and associated intracranial calcifications distinguish these patients from those with PHPV. Coats' disease, toxocara endophthalmitis, and acquired ocular toxoplasmosis in HIV-infected patients occur within globes of normal size.

Posterior chorioretinitis is the most common manifesta-

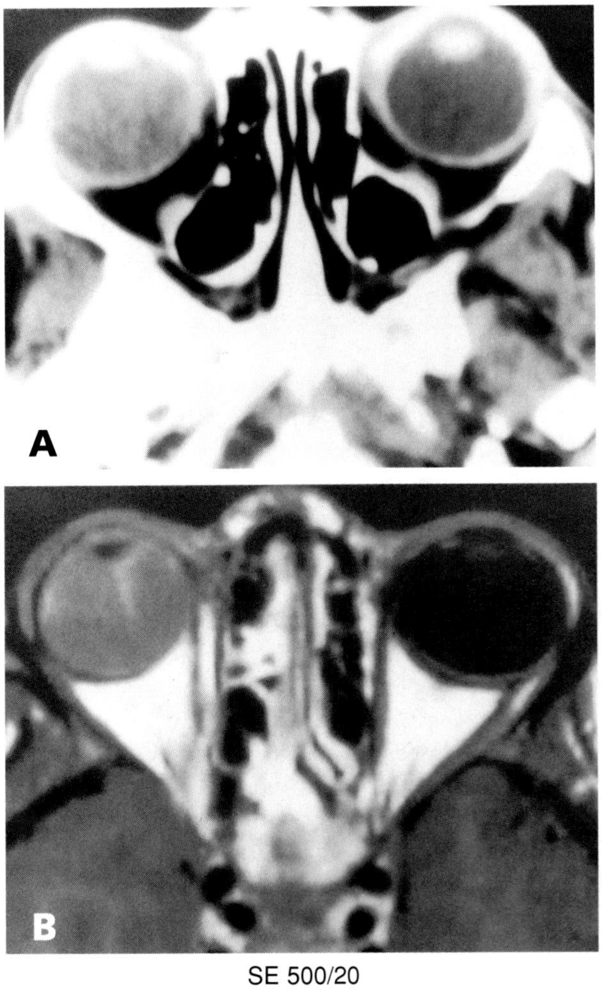

Figure 24-7. Coats' disease. (A) A noncontrast axial CT image shows increased density in the posterior chamber of the right globe. (B) A postcontrast T1-weighted axial MR image shows increased signal intensity in the posterior chamber of the right globe, with a small amount of contrast enhancement. (Reprinted with permission from Kubal [43].)

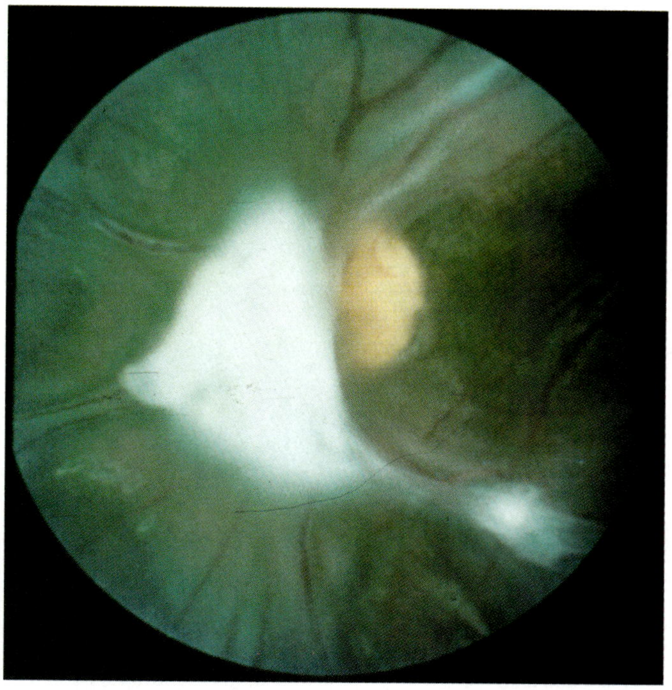

Figure 24-8. Toxocara endophthalmitis. A funduscopic image of a patient with ocular toxocara granuloma demonstrates a typical white mass that blocks the passage of light, leading to the absence of the normal pupillary light reflex. (Case courtesy of Suresh Mukherji, M.D.)

tion of ocular involvement by *T. gondii.* Congenital infection occurs *in utero*, and the active infection usually is over at the time of delivery. Clinical ophthalmologic and neurologic sequelae, including impaired intellectual performance, may not be evident until several years after birth. In the congenital form, the globes are small and show increased attenuation of the vitreous. Mild enhancement of the retina can be identified, particularly in the acquired ocular toxoplasmosis seen in patients with HIV infection.

The incidence of neurologic sequelae in children with subclinical congenital toxoplasmosis is unknown. About 20% of neonates who have congenital infection with *T. gondii* are symptomatic at birth. Evidence of involvement of the central nervous system is almost always present in these patients. The severity and type of clinical manifestations correlate approximately with the gestational age at which fetal infection occurred. Severe forms resulting from early infection can be seen in neonates; the most common neurologic manifestations include microcephaly and signs of meningoencephalitis. The overall mortality of infants with symptomatic congenital toxoplasmosis is approximately 15%. The long-term sequelae include mental retardation in 85%; seizures, spasticity, and other neurologic abnormalities in 75%; severe visual impairment in 50%; and deafness in 10%. CT and MRI may reveal polymicrogyria, hydranencephaly, or multiple large porencephalic cysts. Uncommonly, microphthalmia and ocular calcifications can develop as secondary phenomena.

Toxocara endophthalmitis or sclerosing endophthalmitis is an infection of the globe caused by the ingestion of eggs of the nematode *Toxocara canis.* Pathologically, there is an eosinophilic granuloma or abscess within the globe that contains the secondary-stage toxocara larvae. Cellular infiltration with lymphocytes, eosinophils, plasma cells, and giant cells is typical and is associated with retinal, subretinal, and vitreous hemorrhages. The anterior chamber is generally spared. On CT, there usually is a unilateral process characterized by increased density of the vitreous in association with retinal detachment and thickening of the sclera and episclera. Contrast enhancement of the sclera can be seen with active infection. A noncalcified, focal mass is sometimes present within the globe. MRI demonstrates the changes of hemorrhages and retinal detachment as well as a focal granulomatous mass that usually is isointense relative to the vitreous on T2-weighted images, unlike retinoblastoma, in which the mass is variably hypointense relative to the vitreous on T2-weighted images. An enzyme-linked immunosorbent assay for *T. canis* is available to confirm the diagnosis.

Coats' disease occurs in males, with a peak age at presentation of 4 to 6 years (effectively excluding this diagnosis in the test patient, a 4-week-old girl). It is a unilateral process. Congenital retinal telangiectasia with microaneurysms can leak, with resultant hemorrhage and lipid-laden exudate deposition within the retina. Thus, the normal vitreous is obliterated by the presence of subretinal exudates and hemorrhage, resulting in attenuation values distinctly higher than those of the normal vitreous. Progressive leakage of exudates and hemorrhage result in retinal detachment, which is not present in the test patient. The thin retinal membrane interposed between the vitreous and the exudates forms a distinct linear boundary. Subretinal exudates are homogeneous in density. No contrast enhancement or calcifications are present. These features aid in the distinction between Coats' disease and retinoblastoma on CT. Differentiation from unilateral noncalcifying retinoblastoma is not absolute with CT; however, MRI may provide additional information that is helpful in the diagnosis of Coats' disease. Subretinal exudates have been reported to produce increased signal intensity on both T1- and T2-weighted MR images. The appearance may be related to the presence of lipid in the effusion.

Question 118

Concerning retinoblastoma,

(A) it is inheritable in approximately 40% of cases
(B) the heritable form is associated with an increased incidence of second primary tumors
(C) it spreads chiefly by direct invasion
(D) leukocoria is characteristic
(E) tumor calcification is identified by CT in about 90% of cases
(F) the trilateral form involves the pituitary gland

Retinoblastoma is a malignant neoplasm of childhood that arises from retinal neuroectodermal cells that normally differentiate into photoreceptor cells. At the cellular level, this transformation occurs when both alleles of the Rb gene on chromosome 13, band q14, are inactivated or lost. The incidence of retinoblastoma is one in 15,000 to 18,000 live births.

Over 90% of retinoblastomas are acquired sporadically; 65% of these are manifested as unilateral disease. In the remaining 6% to 10%, the disease follows a familial pattern **(Option (A) is false)**. The transmission is autosomal dominant, with 80% penetrance. About 85% of heritable retinoblastomas are bilateral at the time of initial diagnosis (Figures 24-9 and 10). All patients with bilateral retinoblastomas and about 10% of those with unilateral tumors carry the retinoblastoma gene. The heritable type of retinoblastoma is frequently multicentric, manifesting bilateral tumors or multiple tumor foci in one globe (Figure 24-11). Patients with such retinoblastomas also are at risk of developing pinealomas and suprasellar tumors.

The terms "trilateral retinoblastoma" and "tetralateral retinoblastoma" were coined to describe the coincidence of bilateral retinoblastoma with a pineal tumor (trilateral) **(Option (F) is false)** or with both pineal and suprasellar tumors (tetralateral). These intracranial lesions are not metastatic tumors, but are metachronous, histologically similar tumors of neuroectodermal origin.

For hereditary bilateral tumors, the average age at diagnosis is 12 months; for unilateral tumors (hereditary or sporadic), the average age at diagnosis is 25 months.

Patients with the hereditary form of retinoblastoma have a propensity for the development of nonocular tumors, most commonly sarcomas. Most patients with retinoblastoma are treated with enucleation and irradiation, but not all of the nonocular tumors are related to radiation; 25% to 30% develop outside the radiation field or develop in nonirradiated patients. With hereditary retinoblastoma, the risk of development of secondary neoplasms within the radiation field is 500 to 5,000 times higher than that seen in the normal population; the risk of secondary neoplasms developing outside the radiation field is 200 to 500 times that seen in the normal population **(Option (B) is true)**.

The most common clinical sign associated with retinoblastoma is leukocoria, which is identified on routine examination

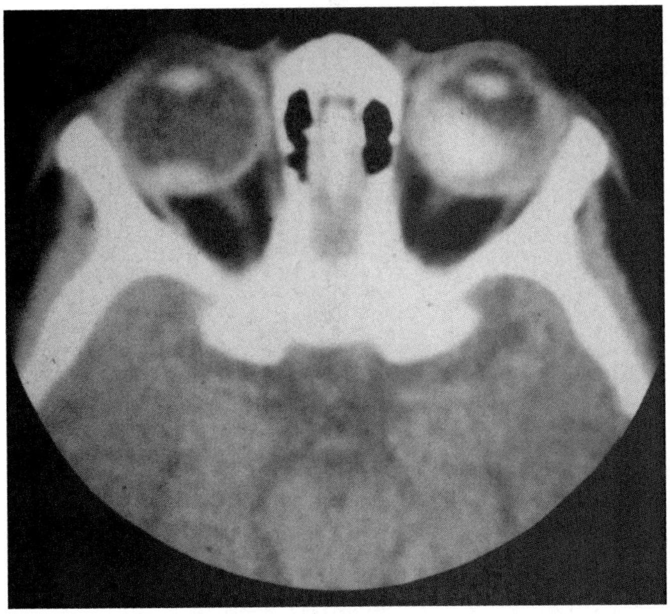

Figure 24-9. Retinoblastoma in an 8-month-old child with bilateral leukocoria. An axial contrast-enhanced CT image demonstrates calcific masses arising from the retinas in both globes. On the right the mass is plaquelike. The mass on the left has both calcific and soft tissue components, consistent with more extensive disease.

(Option (D) is true); ophthalmoscopic and sonographic examinations confirm the presence of an intraocular mass. Other potential clinical findings include strabismus, decreased vision, glaucoma, and nystagmus. Ophthalmoscopic examination demonstrates a pinkish white or gray-white retina-based mass. Three growth patterns of retinoblastoma are recognized. (1) The endophytic pattern describes a tumor based on the retina and projecting into the vitreous. (2) The exophytic growth pattern describes a tumor arising within the retina, with extension

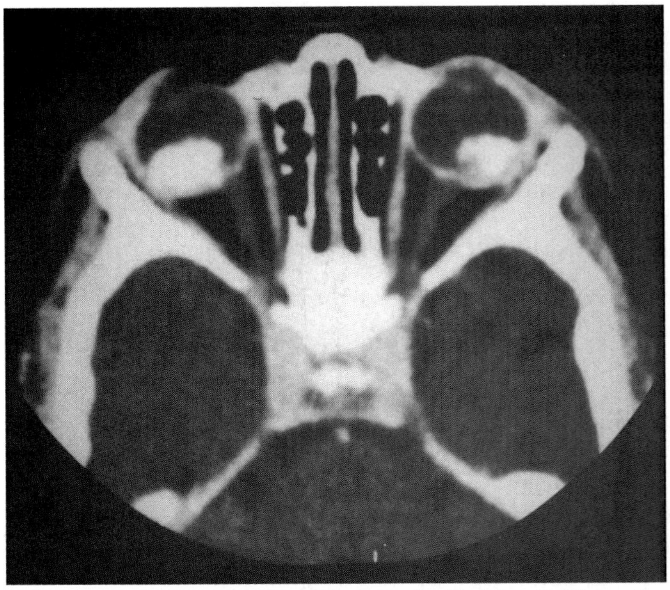

Figure 24-10. Retinoblastoma in a 4-month-old child with bilateral leukocoria. An axial contrast-enhanced CT image demonstrates the symmetric retinal calcifications typical of retinoblastoma.

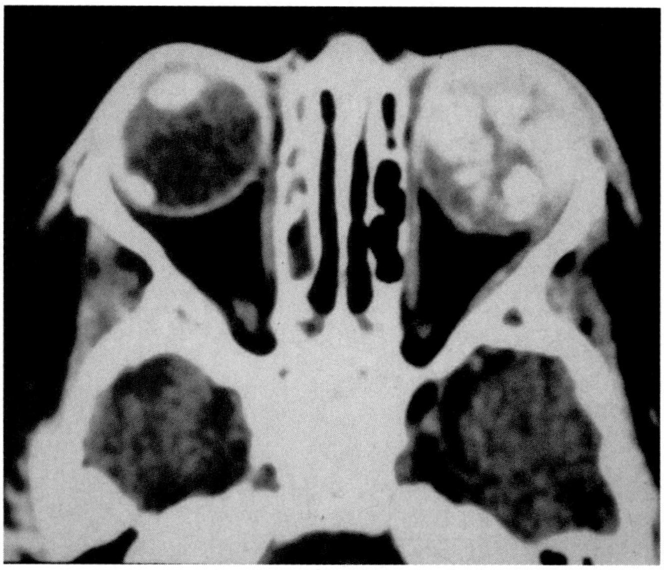

Figure 24-11. Multicentric retinoblastoma. An axial contrast-enhanced CT image demonstrates the typical pattern of a small calcified retinoblastoma on the right. On the left the globe is enlarged, and there are multiple sites of calcification and enhancement representing multicentric foci of a retinoblastoma.

into the subretinal space and with resultant elevation of the retinal vessels by the subretinal mass. (3) The diffusely infiltrating pattern of retinoblastoma describes growth arising as a placode mass on the retina, often associated with retinal detachment. With endophytic retinoblastoma, ophthalmoscopy shows the lobulated mass extending into the vitreous cavity. With exophytic retinoblastoma, ophthalmoscopy demonstrates retinal detachment, but the tumor mass may not be visible. The diffuse type of retinoblastoma can be confused with inflammatory or hemorrhagic conditions ophthalmoscopically and radiographically.

Direct extension of retinoblastoma to the adjacent vitreous or subretinal space, sclera, or optic nerve is the characteristic pattern of spread (**Option (C) is true**). Intracranial extension generally occurs as a result of growth along the optic nerve. Subarachnoid seeding can occur intracranially or along the spinal axis. Hematogenous metastasis probably occurs following invasion of the highly vascular choroid (Figure 24-12). The most common sites for distant metastases include bone, bone marrow, liver, and lymph nodes. Osseous metastasis produces permeative destructive changes that appear radiographically similar to those of metastatic neuroblastoma.

Imaging procedures in patients with retinoblastoma generally are performed for confirmation of diagnosis, characterization of tumor morphology, and detection of local extension or distant metastases. Evaluation with CT usually includes both unenhanced and enhanced images; the axial projection usually is most advantageous. The mass is typically identified along the posterior aspect of the globe, and in most cases the lobulated tumor is visible extending into the vitreous cavity. Tumor calcification is detectable on CT in at least 90% of cases (Figures 24-5 and 9 to 11) (**Option (E) is true**). Calcification can be punctate or clumplike in appearance. Calcification is thought

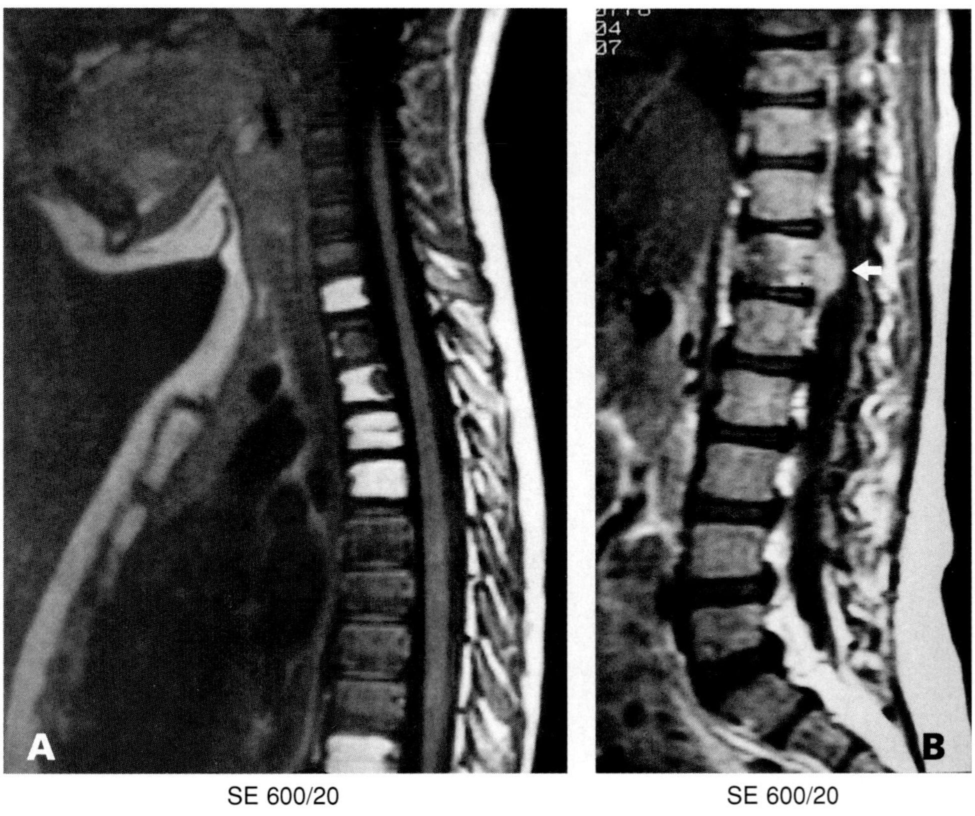

Figure 24-12. Retinoblastoma with hematogenous metastases. (A) A sagittal T1-weighted MR image of the cervicothoracic region demonstrates multiple vertebral bodies with high signal intensity. These represented vertebral body metastases. (B) A T1-weighted MR image of the thoracolumbar region demonstrates an abnormal lower thoracic vertebral body signal with an extradural soft tissue component (arrow) at T12.

to result from the formation of DNA-calcium complexes as DNA is released from the necrotic tumor cells. Detectable calcification can be absent in small tumors (<4 mm) and in the infiltrating type of retinoblastoma. The tumor frequently shows some degree of contrast enhancement. Associated areas of subretinal effusion or hemorrhage are not enhanced. Infiltration of the sclera produces thickening and increased contrast enhancement. Extension of the tumor into the optic nerve is indicated by the enlargement of the nerve. Intracranial extension can be direct or, more commonly, can occur by cerebrospinal fluid dissemination from the subarachnoid space surrounding the optic nerve. Meningeal implants typically demonstrate significant contrast enhancement on CT. The contralateral globe should be closely inspected for evidence of additional primary lesions.

Sonography is slightly less sensitive for the diagnosis of calcifications than CT (80% to 85% sensitive). Retinoblastoma has been reported to appear on T1-weighted MR images as an isointense to slightly hyperintense lesion relative to the signal intensity of the vitreous (Figure 24-13). The lesion is hypointense relative to the vitreous on T2-weighted images, differentiating retinoblastoma from such diseases as Coats' disease, toxocariasis, and PHPV. Although small calcifications are poorly demonstrated on MRI, large calcifications can be recognized as areas of signal void. Differentiation of subretinal effusion or hemorrhage from the primary tumor appears to be somewhat easier with MRI than with CT because the subretinal fluid collection produces high signal intensities on both T1- and T2-weighted images. Enlargement of the optic nerve indicates posterior extension of the neoplasm. Intracranial metastases also are readily identified on MRI.

Retinoblastoma can be confined to the retina, and such small tumors have the best prognosis. Small tumors may be treated with radiation, with preservation of useful vision in 90% of cases.

Question 119

Concerning Coats' disease

(A) it is a vasculitis
(B) it usually is unilateral
(C) CT demonstrates increased attenuation of the posterior chamber of the globe
(D) the subretinal exudate usually is calcified

Coats' disease is a vascular anomaly of the retina characterized by telangiectasia, neovascularity, and an associated lipoproteinaceous exudate that accumulates in the subretinal space, leading to retinal detachment (**Option (A) is false**). First described by George Coats in 1908, this vascular retinopathy is a disorder of young boys 4 to 6 years old (Figure 24-7). Coats' disease is unilateral in 80% to 90% of cases, developing in a globe of normal size (**Option (B) is true**). Affected children have retinal detachment, as noted above, and leukocoria caused by the presence of an exudate that blocks the normal passage of light. Retinal detachment can be recognized on sonography,

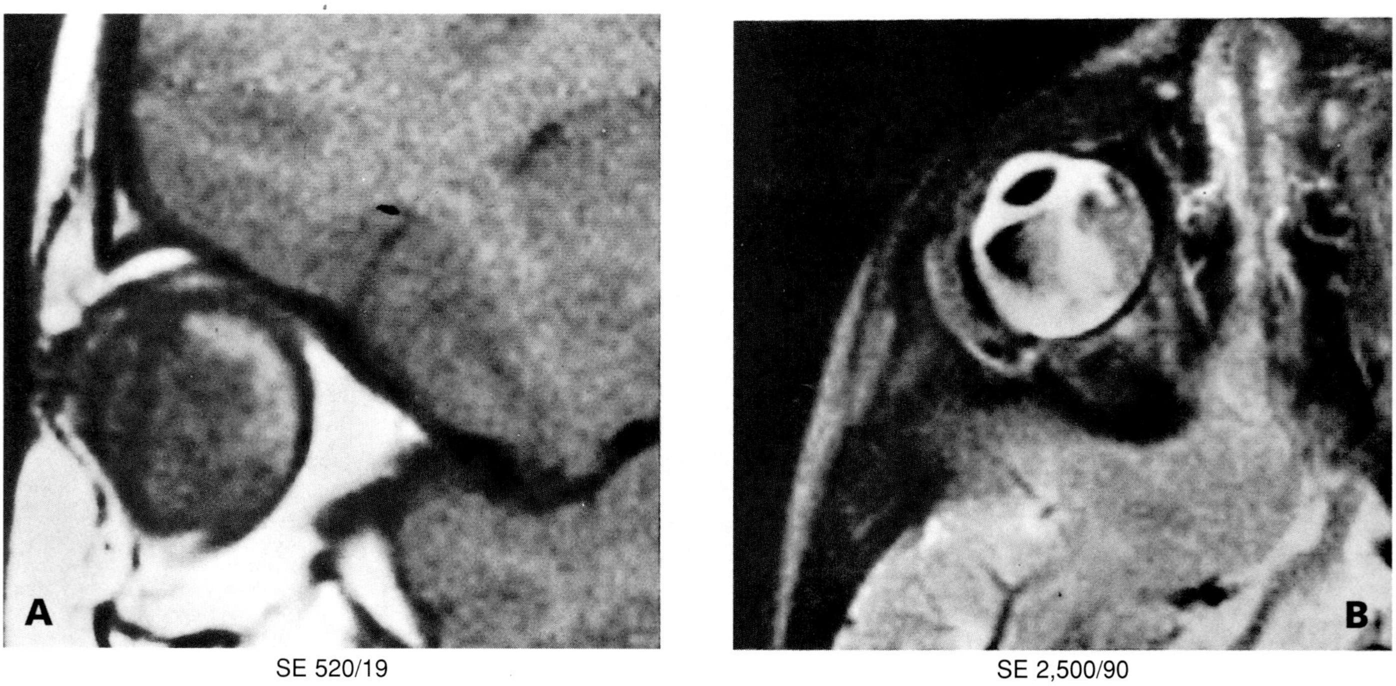

Figure 24-13. Retinoblastoma. (A) A sagittal T1-weighted MR image demonstrates a slightly hyperintense mass along the posterior aspect of the retina, consistent with retinoblastoma. (B) An axial T2-weighted MR image demonstrates heterogeneous signal intensity within the right globe. The globe is normal in size. The heterogeneity is consistent with a mass arising from the retina.

CT, and MRI.

CT in Coats' disease demonstrates a variable degree of obliteration of the vitreous cavity and posterior chamber of the globe by the subretinal exudate. The attenuation value of the exudate is higher than that of the vitreous because of the lipoproteinaceous content (Figure 24-7A) (**Option (C) is true**). Calcification of the subretinal exudate does not occur, however (**Option (D) is false**). Although the retina itself is too thin to be identified, interposition of the exudate between the retina and the vitreous often produces a well-defined boundary. The subretinal exudate is homogeneous and does not demonstrate contrast enhancement.

MRI may provide additional information that is helpful in the diagnosis of Coats' disease. The subretinal exudate invariably produces increased signal intensity on both T1- and T2-weighted MR images. This appearance may be related in part to the presence of lipid in the effusion. Early results of proton MR spectroscopy of the subretinal exudates of Coats' disease have demonstrated a large peak at 1 to 1.6 ppm corresponding to the lipids and phospholipids within the exudates. Spectroscopy may represent a more specific diagnostic tool enabling the differentiation of Coats' disease from retinoblastoma.

As the proliferation of retinal telangiectasia progresses and continual leakage of lipid-laden exudates and hemorrhage occur, exudative retinal detachment occurs, with the development of secondary glaucoma, decreased visual acuity, and pain. Ultimately, blindness ensues. In early stages, phototherapy or cryotherapy may be useful to arrest the growth of the retinal telangiectasis and the subsequent exudation. Unfortunately, many eyes have been enucleated when a diagnosis of retinoblastoma could not be excluded clinically or by imaging assessment.

Question 120

Concerning coloboma,

(A) it results from lack of closure of the choroidal fissure
(B) it involves only the optic nerve
(C) it is associated with midline intracranial anomalies
(D) on CT, there is bulbous enlargement of the optic nerve at its junction with the globe
(E) it is associated with retinal detachment

The embryologic development of the eye begins with paired diverticula that arise from the forebrain and develop into optic vesicles and optic stalks, the precursors of the globes and optic nerves. Invagination of the lateral aspect of the optic vesicle leads to the formation of an optic cup. The sensory retinal epithelium arises from the inner wall of the optic cup, whereas the retinal pigment epithelium arises from the outer wall of the optic cup. Invagination of the optic stalk leads to the formation of the choroidal fissure. The hyaloid artery traverses the choroidal fissure, and mesenchyme migrates along the fissure to form the primary vitreous. The choroidal fissure closes near the time of regression of the primary vitreous, at the site of the developing optic disk.

An abnormality of closure of the choroidal fissure results in a defect, referred to as a coloboma (**Option (A) is true**), that can involve any ocular structure from the optic nerve to the iris (**Option (B) is false**). If only the proximal portion of the fissure fails to close, an isolated optic nerve coloboma is produced. Isolated optic nerve coloboma is uncommon. When the coloboma involves only the optic nerve head, a funduscopic examination reveals the "morning glory anomaly" (described below). Failure of closure of other segments of the choroidal fissure produces iridic, lenticular, ciliary body, or retinochoroidal coloboma. Most often coloboma occurs in the inferomedial quadrant of the globe, corresponding to the line of closure of the fetal choroidal fissure (Figures 24-6 and 24-14). In retinochoroidal coloboma, thinning and outward bulging of the sclera are seen. The term "Fuchs' coloboma" is used when a tilted optic disk is associated with the colobomatous malforma-

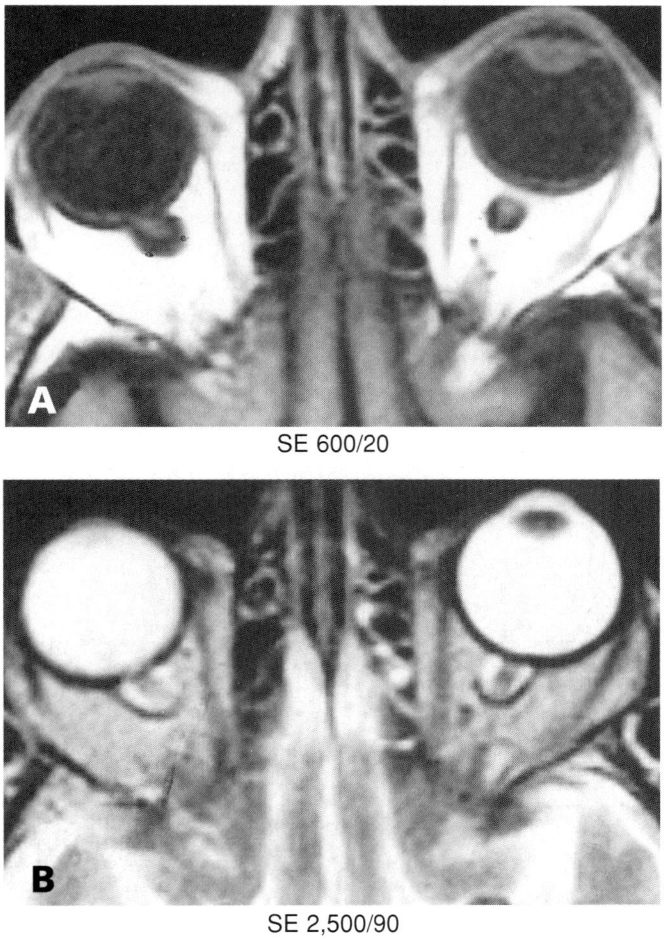

Figure 24-14. Coloboma. Axial T1-weighted (A) and T2-weighted (B) MR images show bilateral defects at the posterior globes. (Reprinted with permission from Kubal [43].)

tion. Colobomas range in size from small defects to large lesions involving the entire length of the choroidal fissure. In some cases, the developing retina prolapses into the residual fissure, creating a colobomatous cyst. This maldevelopment results in hypoplasia of the retina and optic nerve, with associated microphthalmia. Coloboma with microphthalmia and a posterior retinal cyst is often associated with midline intracranial anomalies, including callosal agenesis and encephalocele **(Option (C) is true).**

The morning glory anomaly was first described by Kindler in 1970. This characteristic funduscopic appearance is seen only with coloboma isolated to the optic nerve head. This lesion is characterized by enlargement and excavation of the optic disk. This anatomic derangement leads to a funnel-shaped appearance of the disk on funduscopic examination; a white central zone is surrounded by an annular pattern of lightly pigmented subretinal elevation. The funduscopic appearance is reminiscent of the flower of the same name (Figure 24-15). Ophthalmologic examination reveals a characteristic defect in the posterior retina at the optic nerve head.

Clinically, the eye may be normal in size or microphthalmic, with wide variations in size and appearance depending upon the extent of failure of closure of the embryonic fissure. A colobomatous cyst is sometimes associated with a microphthalmic coloboma. This cyst is created when there is herniation of a portion of ocular neuroectoderm from the globe through an associated scleral defect. On funduscopic examination, typically there is a cleft in the inferior nasal quadrant. Vision varies with the size and extent of the persistent embryonic fissure, the resultant cleft, and the presence of associated scleral or retinal cysts creating mass effect, proptosis, and ocular distortion.

Familial diseases, chromosomal anomalies, and sporadic systemic syndromes varying in severity can have associated coloboma. These include such entities as trisomy 13 and 18, Aicardi syndome, and others. Midline craniofacial anomalies, such as encephalocele, callosal agenesis, and olfactory hypoplasia, also can be associated.

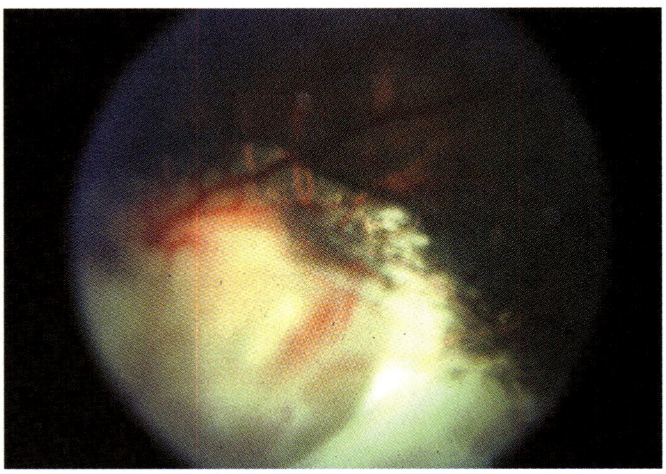

Figure 24-15. Morning glory anomaly. A funduscopic image demonstrates excavation of the optic disk as a result of the failure of closure of the embryonic fissure, mimicking the appearance of the morning glory flower. (Case courtesy of Marcia Carney, M.D., Medical College of Virginia, Virginia Commonwealth University, Richmond, VA.)

On CT or MRI, a coloboma is distinguished by a posterior defect in the retina at the site of the optic nerve head (Figures 24-6 and 24-14). The globe bulges posteriorly through the defect. The optic nerve is not enlarged **(Option (D) is false).** Although the defect is in the retina, there is no association with retinal detachment **(Option (E) is false).** A cyst present in the retrobulbar region can be larger than the microphthalmic globe itself. The cyst contents are homogeneous and produce CT attenuation values and MRI signal intensities approximately equal to those of normal vitreous. Contrast enhancement does not occur. With continuous thin sections, communications of the cyst with the vitreous cavity of the globe can be demonstrated at some level. This continuity with the globe, along with the presence of microphthalmia and imaging characteristics of cyst contents similar to those of vitreous, serves to differentiate this condition from other cystic orbital masses, such as lymphangioma, epithelial implantation cysts, and chocolate cysts, all of which have attenuation values higher than those of normal vitreous.

In morning glory anomaly, CT and MRI demonstrate a funnel-shaped coloboma in the region of the optic nerve head. The retrobulbar portions of the optic nerves are generally normal. Retinal detachment and subretinal exudate occur in approximately one third of cases. Subretinal exudate of sufficient size can be visualized on both CT and MRI as thickening of the subretinal region.

SUGGESTED READINGS

PERSISTENT HYPERPLASTIC PRIMARY VITREOUS

1. Castillo M, Wallace DK, Mukherji SK. Persistent hyperplastic primary vitreous involving the anterior eye. AJNR 1997; 18:1526–1528
2. Goldberg MF, Mafee M. Computed tomography for diagnosis of persistent hyperplastic primary vitreous (PHPV). Ophthalmology 1983; 90: 442–451
3. Kuker W, Ramaekers V. Persistent hyperplastic primary vitreous: MRI. Neuroradiology 1999; 41:520–522
4. Mafee MF, Goldberg MF. Persistent hyperplastic primary vitreous (PHPV): role of computed tomography and magnetic resonance. Radiol Clin North Am 1987; 25:683–692
5. Mafee MF, Goldberg MF, Cohen SB, et al. Magnetic resonance imaging versus computed tomography of leukocoric eyes and use of in vitro proton magnetic resonance spectroscopy of retinoblastoma. Ophthalmology 1989; 96:965–975
6. Mafee MF, Goldberg MF, Valvassori GE, Capek V. Computed tomography in the evaluation of patients with persistent hyperplastic primary vitreous (PHPV). Radiology 1982; 145:713–717
7. Marshman WE, Jan JE, Lyons CJ. Neurologic abnormalities associated with persistent hyperplastic primary vitreous. Can J Ophthalmol 1999; 34:17–22

RETINOBLASTOMA

8. Abramson DH, Ellsworth RM, Kitchin FD, Tung G. Second nonocular tumors in retinoblastoma survivors. Are they radiation-induced? Ophthalmology 1984; 91:1351–1355

9. Bader JL, Miller RW, Meadows AT, Zimmerman LE, Champion LA, Voute PA. Trilateral retinoblastoma. Lancet 1980; 2:582–583
10. Beets-Tan RG, Hendriks MJ, Ramos LM, Tan KE. Retinoblastoma: CT and MRI. Neuroradiology 1994; 36:59–62
11. Haik BG, Saint Louis L, Smith ME, et al. Magnetic resonance imaging in the evaluation of leukocoria. Ophthalmology 1985; 92:1143–1152
12. Hopper KD, Sherman JL, Boel DK, Eggli KD. CT and MR imaging of the pediatric orbit. RadioGraphics 1992; 12:485–503
13. Ibarra MS, O'Brien JM. Is screening for primitive neuroectodermal tumors in patients with unilateral retinoblastoma necessary? J AAPOS 2000; 4:54–56
14. Jaffe MS, Shields JA, Canny CL, Eagle RC, Fry RL. Retinoblastoma simulating Coats' disease: a clinicopathologic report. Ann Ophthalmol 1977; 9:863–868
15. Mafee MF, Goldberg MF, Cohen SB, et al. Magnetic resonance imaging versus computed tomography of leukocoric eyes and use of *in vitro* proton magnetic resonance spectroscopy of retinoblastoma. Ophthalmology 1989; 96:965–976
16. Price HI, Batnitsky S, Danzinger A, et al. The neuroradiology of retinoblastoma. RadioGraphics 1982; 2:7
17. Weber AL, Mafee MF. Evaluation of the globe using computed tomography and magnetic resonance imaging. Isr J Med Sci 1992; 28:145–152
18. Zimmerman RA, Bilaniuk LT. Computed tomography in the evaluation of patients with bilateral retinoblastomas. J Comput Tomogr 1979; 3: 251–257

COATS' DISEASE

19. Chang MM, McLean IW, Merritt JC. Coats' disease: a study of 62 histologically confirmed cases. J Pediatr Ophthalmol Strabismus 1984; 21: 163–168
20. Char DH. Coats' syndrome: long term follow up. Br J Ophthalmol 2000; 84:37–39
21. Coats G. Forms of retinal disease with massive exudation. R Lond Ophthalmol Hosp Rep 1908; 17:440–525
22. Edward DP, Mafee MF, Garcia-Valenzuela E, Weiss RA. Coats' disease and persistent hyperplastic primary vitreous. Role of MR imaging and CT. Radiol Clin North Am 1998; 36:1119–1131
23. Sherman JL, McLean IW, Brallier DR. Coats' disease: CT-pathologic correlation in two cases. Radiology 1983; 146:77–78
24. Steidl SM, Hirose T, Sang D, Hartnett ME. Difficulties in excluding the diagnosis of retinoblastoma in cases of advanced Coats' disease: a clinicopathologic report. Ophthalmologica 1996; 210:336–340

OCULAR TOXOPLASMOSIS AND TOXOCARIASIS

25. Borruat FX, Kapoor R, Sanders MD. Simultaneous retinal and optic nerve lesions in toxoplasmosis: the advantages of magnetic resonance imaging. Br J Ophthalmol 1993; 77:450–452
26. Edwards MG, Pordell GR. Ocular toxocariasis studied by CT scanning. Radiology 1985; 157:685–686
27. Fahnehjelm KT, Malm G, Ygge J, Engman ML, Maly E, Evengard B. Ophthalmological findings in children with congenital toxoplasmosis. Report from a Swedish prospective screening study of congenital toxoplasmosis with two years of follow-up. Acta Ophthalmol Scand 2000; 78:569–575
28. Frezzotti R, Guerra R, Terragna A, Tosi P. A case of congenital toxoplasmosis with active chorioretinitis. Parasitological and histopathological findings. Ophthalmologica 1974; 169:321–325
29. Haik BG, Saint Louis L, Smith ME, Abramson DH, Ellsworth RM. Computed tomography of the nonrhegmatogenous retinal detachment in the pediatric patient. Ophthalmology 1985; 92:1133–1142
30. Hershey BL, Roth TC. Orbital infections. Semin US CT MR 1997; 18: 448–459
31. Holland GN, Engstrom RE Jr, Glasgow BJ, et al. Ocular toxoplasmosis in patients with the acquired immunodeficiency syndrome. Am J Ophthalmol 1988; 106:653–667
32. Lynfield R, Guerina NG. Toxoplasmosis. Pediatr Rev 1997; 18:75–83
33. Margo CE, Katz NN, Wertz, FD, Dorwart RH. Sclerosing endophthalmitis in children: computed tomography with histopathologic correlation. J Pediatr Ophthalmol Strabismus 1983; 20:180–184
34. McAuley J, Boyer KM, Patel D, et al. Early and longitudinal evaluations of treated infants and children and untreated historical patients with congenital toxoplasmosis: the Chicago Collaborative Treatment Trial. Clin Infect Dis 1994; 18:38–72

COLOBOMA

35. Beyer WB, Quencer RM, Osher RH. Morning glory syndrome. A functional analysis including fluorescein angiography, ultrasonography, and computerized tomography. Ophthalmology 1982; 89:1362–1367
36. Corbett JJ, Savino PJ, Schatz NJ, Orr LS. Cavitary developmental defects of the optic disc. Visual loss associated with optic pits and colobomas. Arch Neurol 1980; 37:210–213
37. Gardner TW, Zaparackas ZG, Naidich TP. Congenital optic nerve colobomas: CT demonstration. J Comput Assist Tomogr 1984; 8:95–102
38. Mafee MF, Jampol LM, Langer BG, Tso M. Computed tomography of optic nerve colobomas, morning glory anomaly, and colobomatous cyst. Radiol Clin North Am 1987; 25:693–699
39. Murphy BL, Griffin JF. Optic nerve coloboma (morning glory syndrome): CT findings. Radiology 1994; 191:59–61
40. Polito E, Leccisotti A. Colobomatous ocular cyst excision with globe preservation. Ophthal Plast Reconstr Surg 1995; 11:288–292

GENERAL

41. Hopper KD, Sherman JL, Boal DK, Eggli KD. CT and MR imaging of the pediatric orbit. RadioGraphics 1992; 12:485–503
42. Kaufman LM, Mafee MF, Song CD. Retinoblastoma and simulating lesions. Role of CT, MR imaging and use of Gd-DTPA contrast enhancement. Radiol Clin North Am 1998; 36:1101–1117
43. Kubal WS. The pathological globe: clinical and imaging analysis. Semin US CT MR 1997; 18:423–436
44. O'Brien JM, Char DH, Tucker N, Gordon KB, Norman D. Efficacy of unanesthetized spiral computed tomography scanning in initial evaluation of childhood leukocoria. Ophthalmology 1995; 102:1345–1350
45. Potter PD, Shields CL, Shields JA, Flanders AE. The role of magnetic resonance imaging in children with intraocular tumors and simulating lesions. Ophthalmology 1996; 103:1774–1783
46. Smirniotopoulos JG, Bargallo N, Mafee MF. Differential diagnosis of leukokoria: radiologic-pathologic correlation. RadioGraphics 1994; 14: 1059–1079
47. Smith M, Castillo M. Imaging and differential diagnosis of the large eye. RadioGraphics 1994; 14:721–728

Index

S

T